clinical examination

6th edition

clinical examination

A systematic guide to physical diagnosis

Nicholas J Talley

MD, PhD, Pro Vice Chancellor and Professor, Faculty of Health,
University of Newcastle, Australia; Adjunct Professor of Medicine, Mayo Clinic, USA;
Foreign Guest Professor, Karolinska Institute, Stockholm, Sweden

Simon O'Connor

FRACP, DDU, FCSANZ
Cardiologist, The Canberra Hospital;
Clinical Senior Lecturer, Australian National University Medical School,
Canberra, ACT

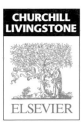

CHURCHILL
LIVINGSTONE

ELSEVIER

Sydney   Edinburgh   London   New York   Philadelphia   St Louis   Toronto

ELSEVIER

Churchill Livingstone
is an imprint of Elsevier

Elsevier Australia. ACN 001 002 357
(a division of Reed International Books Australia Pty Ltd)
Tower 1, 475 Victoria Avenue, Chatswood, NSW 2067

National Library of Australia Cataloguing-in-Publication Data

---

Talley, Nicholas Joseph.

Clinical examination : a systematic guide to physical
   diagnosis / Nicholas J. Talley, Simon O'Connor.

6th ed.

ISBN: 978 0 7295 3905 0

Includes index.
Bibliography.

Physical diagnosis.

O'Connor, Simon.

616.075

Publisher: Sophie Kaliniecki
Developmental Editor: Sabrina Chew
Publishing Services Manager: Helena Klijn
Editorial Coordinator: Lauren Allsop
Edited by Teresa McIntyre
Proofread by Sarah Newton-John
Illustrations by Shelly Communications
Photography, unless otherwise stated, by Glenn McCulloch
Index by Forsyth Publishing Services
Internal design and typesetting by Pindar New Zealand
Cover design by Stan Lamond
Printed in China by China Translation and Printing Services

Foreword

The public face of modern medicine appears to celebrate medical technology and what it can do to diagnose, treat and prevent illness in individuals and communities. While this is understandable in the face of remarkable advances in medical imaging, molecular biology and bio-engineering devices, it does not reflect the very central importance of accurate clinical evaluation in the day-to-day care of people across the world. Without accurate clinical evaluation there is a risk not only to the individual (including incorrect diagnoses and unnecessary tests, procedures and treatments) but also to the financial state of healthcare systems, which in every country of the world operate under increasing cost pressures.

There has never been a more important time than now to have superb clinical skills in history taking, physical examination and synthesis of the data gathered. The increasing age of the population and the expansion of what medicine can do for all illnesses, especially chronic disease, demands more and higher-quality care. Added to this demand is the re-emerging importance of generalist skills across all specialties of medicine, especially in primary care or family practice, emergency medicine, general internal medicine and general surgery. The reality of being able to provide high-quality care to people across metropolitan, rural and remote areas requires the knowledge and skills of the generalist who must, often under great time pressure, take a history and carry out a physical examination that will determine the next stage of investigation or treatment. Depending on the setting, there may not be much assistance from modern technology. These 'old-fashioned' skills of history taking and physical examination have been given new life in recent years by the information gained about their accuracy through clinical epidemiological research: *evidence-based clinical evaluation.*

The challenge for teachers of the art and science of clinical evaluation in the 21st century is to make it attractive and exciting for all clinicians, but especially for medical students and young doctors for whom modern technology may seem to be an alluring shortcut. In the sixth edition of their now classic book, Talley and O'Connor have written an attractive and exciting text that is a joy to read through its clarity of expression, quality of information and engagement with the reader by commentary on historical details and practical hints. The information is made easier to comprehend, assimilate and remember through judicious use of diagrams and pictures. Finally, it has the innovation of the 'Good signs guides' in each chapter giving snapshots of the evidence about how these clinical tests perform.

For over 21 years, *Clinical Examination* by Talley and O'Connor has provided medical students, junior doctors, senior doctors and clinician teachers with the guidance to carry out a rational and thoughtful history and an organised and disciplined physical examination. The information contained in this book is the basis for the hypothetico-deductive process used by most clinicians to reach a provisional diagnosis and a parsimonious list of differential diagnoses. From the first edition in 1988 to today's very different-looking but even better sixth edition, the book has stood not only the test of time but also critical appraisal by thousands of very bright people. This textbook deserves its place on the shelves and in the computers of every medical practitioner.

Michael Hensley
Professor of Medicine and Dean of Medicine,
School of Medicine and Public Health, University
of Newcastle, Australia

Contents

Preface

"And gladly wolde he lerne, and gladly teche."
Chaucer, the prologue to Canterbury Tales.

It is with great pride that we present to you the sixth edition of *Clinical Examination*. The book has been in continuous production for over 20 years and remains one of the most successful textbooks on examination methods in the world today. We have carefully updated and revised the text and illustrations to meet the needs of all medical students, from beginners to advanced practitioners.

Medical education has changed radically in the last decade in many countries. Various medical schools now offer post-graduate medical courses lasting four years; some offer both undergraduate and postgraduate courses, and others only train at the undergraduate level for five to six years. However long the formal training, many new topics have been added to already crowded courses. These changes have meant less emphasis in some programs on the more basic foundations of medicine, regrettably including less anatomy and physiology teaching. A clinical examination textbook cannot teach these subjects in detail, but we have felt the need to introduce basic *examination anatomy* into this book to assist students' understanding of physical examination. We have also added a number of anatomical drawings, X-rays and scans to help explain the structure of key areas being examined.

This edition includes expanded sections on history taking, including a new chapter on *advanced history taking*, and important lists of *differential diagnoses*. Features of the history that may indicate a serious or urgent problem are highlighted.

Unlike most other books teaching examination methods, we have felt it essential to provide references supporting important aspects of examination and history taking. Contemporary medical students are trained to be sceptical and expect evidence for assertions made by their teachers. These references give students the opportunity to follow up areas that interest them in more detail.

The latest evidence-based information on the value of various clinical signs has been included. This area owes much to Professor Steven McGee, and we are very grateful to him for his permission to reproduce some of his published data.

The DVD accompanying the book contains a video guide to the examination of the main systems of the body. For this edition, we have added a selection of examples of *Objective Structured Clinical Examinations* (OSCEs), a library of *electrocardiographs* (ECGs) with notes on ECG interpretation, and a library of important *X-rays and scans*. The ECGs and scans are not a completely comprehensive set, but are an attempt to present the important abnormalities students need to recognise in clinical examinations.

Finally, we are pleased to have brought the list of eponymous signs of aortic regurgitation right up to date with the inclusion of Ashrafian's sign, first described in 2006.

Nicholas J Talley
Simon O'Connor
Jacksonville and Canberra, December 2009

Acknowledgments

We are very grateful for the comments and suggestions from many colleagues over the years who have helped us develop and refine this book. We take responsibility for any errors or omissions.

Dr G Briggs very kindly provided the original chest and abdominal X-ray material. Professor P Boyce provided the original psychiatry chapter, and Dr A Cooper prepared the original chapter on the skin, for which we remain very grateful. Dr A Manoharan and Dr J Isbister provided the original blood film photographs and the accompanying text. A/Professor L Schreiber provided the section on soft-tissue rheumatology, which we have updated. Associate Professor S Posen, Associate Professor IPC Murray, Dr G Bauer, Dr E Wilmshurst, Dr J Stiel and Dr J Webb helped us obtain many of the original photographs.

The dermatology illustrations are reproduced with permission from *Clinical dermatology illustrated: a regional approach,* 3rd edition, by John RT Reeves and Howard Maibach (MacLennan & Petty, Sydney, 2000). Professor John Reeves kindly lent us his transparencies.

The retinal photographs were kindly provided by Dr Chris Kennedy and Professor Ian Constable (and all are copyright Lion's Eye Institute).

A set of photographs come from the Mayo Clinic library and from FS McDonald (editor), *Mayo Clinic images in internal medicine: self-assessment for board exam review* (Mayo Clinic Scientific Press: Rochester MN & CRC Press: Boca Raton FL, 2004). We would like to thank the following from Mayo Clinic College of Medicine for their kind assistance in selecting additional photographic material: Dr Ashok M Patel, Dr Ayalew Tefferi, Dr Mark R Pittelkow and Dr Eric L Matteson.

A number of new X-rays and scans for the 6th edition have been provided by Dr Malcolm Thomson, National Capital Diagnostic Imaging, Canberra. We would also like to thank Professor G Buirski, Director of the Department of Medical Imaging, The Canberra Hospital, for granting permission to use some of the X-rays and scans from The Canberra Hospital X-ray library.

We are particularly indebted to Dr. S. McGee, Associate Professor of Internal Medicine, University of Washington, for permission to use some of his detailed LR figures from his book, *Evidence-based physical diagnosis,* 2nd edn (Saunders, 2007) in the *Good signs guides.* Professor McGee is a pioneer in the field of evidence-based physical examination.

Elsevier Australia and the authors also extend their appreciation to the following reviewers for their comments and insights on the entire manuscript:

Dr Mee Yoke Ling, MBBS (Hons), MPH, FRACGP
Senior Lecturer, Department of General Practice Monash University, Melbourne, Australia.

Dr Craig Mellis, MBBS, MPH, MD, FRACP
Professor of Medicine, Associate Dean & Head, Central Clinical School, Faculty of Medicine, University of Sydney & Royal Prince Alfred Hospital, Sydney, Australia.

Dr John Kolbe, MBBS, FRACP
Head, Dept of Medicine, Faculty of Medical and Health Sciences, University of Auckland Respiratory Physician, Auckland City Hospital, Auckland, New Zealand.

Dr Steve Trumble, MBBS, MD, FRACGP
Associate Professor, Medical Education Unit,

The Melbourne Medical School, University of Melbourne, Victoria, Australia

Dr Andy Wearn, MBChB, MMedSc, MRCGP
Director/Senior Lecturer, Clinical Skills Resource Centre, Faculty of Medical & Health Sciences, The University of Auckland, Auckland, New Zealand.

Dr Neil Scholes, MB ChB FRACS FRCS FRCSE
Senior Lecturer/Academic Coordinator, Rural School of Medicine, University of Queensland

Director of Surgery, Rockhampton Hospital, Central Queensland, Australia

Dr Jonathan Dent, BSc(med), MB, BS
Advanced Trainee in Geriatric Medicine, St Vincent's Hospital, Sydney, Australia

Dr Stephen Allison, MBBS, FRACS
Senior Lecturer, Dept of Surgery, University of Queensland
Director of Surgery, Greenslopes Private Hospital, Brisbane, Australia

Clinical methods: an historical perspective

The best physician is the one who is able to differentiate the possible and the impossible.

Herophilus of Alexandria

From classical Greek times interrogation of the patient has been considered most important because disease was, and still is, viewed in terms of the discomfort it causes. However, the current emphasis on the use of history taking and physical examination for diagnosis developed only in the 19th century. Although the terms 'symptoms and signs' have been part of the medical vocabulary since the revival of classical medicine, until relatively recently they were used synonymously.

During the 19th century, the distinction between *symptoms* (subjective complaints, which the clinician learns from the patient's account of his or her feelings) and *signs* (objective morbid changes detectable by the clinician) evolved.

Until the 19th century, diagnosis was empirical and based on the classical Greek belief that all disease had a single cause, an imbalance of the four humours (yellow bile, black bile, blood and phlegm). Indeed the Royal College of Physicians, founded in London in 1518, believed that clinical experience without classical learning was useless, and physicians who were College members were fined if they ascribed to any other view.

At the time of Hippocrates (460–375 BC) observation (inspection) and feeling (palpation) had a place in the examination of patients. The ancient Greeks, for example, noticed that patients with jaundice often had an enlarged liver that was firm and irregular. Shaking a patient and listening for a fluid splash was also recognised by the Greeks.

Herophilus of Alexandria (335–280 BC) described a method of taking the pulse in the 4th century BC. However, it was Galen of Pergamum (130–200 AD) who established the pulse as one of the major physical signs, and it continued to have this important role up to the 18th century, with minute variations being recorded. These variations were erroneously considered to indicate changes in the body's harmony.

William Harvey's (1578–1657) studies of the human circulation, published in 1628, had little effect on the general understanding of the value of the pulse as a sign. Sanctorius (1561–1636) was the first to time the pulse using a clock, while John Floyer (1649–1734) invented the pulse watch in 1707 and made regular observations of the pulse rate. Abnormalities in heart rate were described in diabetes mellitus in 1776 and in thyrotoxicosis in 1786.

Fever was studied by Hippocrates and was originally regarded as an entity rather than a sign of disease. The thermoscope was devised by Sanctorius in 1625. In association with Gabriel Fahrenheit (1686–1736), Hermann Boerhaave (1668–1738) introduced the thermometer as a research instrument and this was produced commercially in the middle of the 18th century.

In the 13th century Johannes Actuarius (d. 1283) used a graduated glass to examine the urine. In Harvey's time a specimen of urine was sometimes looked at (inspected) and even tasted, and was considered to reveal secrets about the body. Harvey recorded that sugar diabetes (mellitus) and dropsy (oedema) could be diagnosed in this way. The detection of protein in the urine, which Frederik Dekkers (1644–1720) first described in 1673, was ignored until Richard Bright (1789–1858) demonstrated its importance in renal disease. Although Celsus described and valued measurements such as weighing and measuring a patient in the 1st century AD, these methods became widely used only in the 20th century.

A renaissance in clinical methods began with the concept of Battista Morgagni (1682–1771) that disease was not generalised but arose in organs, a conclusion published in 1761. Leopold Auenbrugger invented chest tapping (percussion) to detect disease in the same year. Van Swieten, his teacher, in fact used percussion to detect ascites. The technique was forgotten for nearly half a century until Jean Corvisart (1755–1821) translated Auenbrugger's work in 1808.

The next big step occurred with René Laënnec (1781–1826), a student of Corvisart. He invented the stethoscope in 1816 (at first merely a roll of stiff paper) as an aid to diagnosing heart and lung disease by listening (auscultation). This revolutionised chest examination, partly because it made the chest accessible in patients too modest to allow a direct application of the examiner's ear to the chest wall, as well as allowing accurate clinicopathological correlations. William Stokes (1804–78) published the first treatise in English on the use of the stethoscope in 1825. Josef Skoda's (1805–81) investigations of the value of these clinical methods led to their widespread and enthusiastic adoption after he published his results in 1839.

These advances helped lead to a change in the practice of medicine. Bedside teaching was first introduced in the Renaissance by Montanus (1498–1552) in Padua in 1543. In the 17th century, physicians based their opinion on a history provided by an apothecary (assistant) and rarely saw the patients themselves. Thomas Sydenham (1624–89) began to practise more modern bedside medicine, basing his treatment on experience and not theory, but it was not until a century later that the scientific method brought a systematic approach to clinical diagnosis.

This change began in the hospitals of Paris after the French Revolution, with recognition of the work of Morgagni, Corvisart, Laënnec and others. Influenced by the philosophy of the Enlightenment, which suggested that a rational approach to all problems was possible, the Paris Clinical School combined physical examination with autopsy as the basis of clinical medicine. The methods of this school were first applied abroad in Dublin, where Robert Graves (1796–1853) and William Stokes worked. Later at Guy's Hospital in London the famous trio of Richard Bright, Thomas Addison (1793–1860) and Thomas Hodgkin (1798–1866) made their important contributions. In 1869 Samuel Wilks (1824–1911) wrote on the nail changes in disease and the signs he described remain important. Carl Wunderlich's (1815–77) work changed the concept of temperature from a disease in itself to a symptom of disease.

Spectacular advances in physiology, pathology, pharmacology and the discovery of microbiology in the latter half of the 19th century led to the development of the new 'clinical and laboratory medicine', which is the rapidly advancing medicine of the present day. The modern systematic approach to diagnosis, with which this book deals, is still, however, based on taking the history and examining the patient by looking (inspecting), feeling (palpating), tapping (percussing) and listening (auscultating).

Suggested reading

Reiser SJ. The clinical record in medicine. Part I: Learning from cases. *Ann Intern Med* 1991; 114:902–907.

Bordage G. Where are the history and the physical? *Can Med Assoc J* 1995; 152:1595–1598.

McDonald C. Medical heuristics: the silent adjudicators of clinical practice. *Ann Intern Med* 1996; 124:56–62.

The Hippocratic oath

I swear by Apollo the physician, and Aesculapius, and Hygieia, and Panacea, and all the gods and goddesses that, according to my ability and judgment, I will keep this Oath and this stipulation:

To reckon him who taught me this Art equally dear to me as my parents, to share my substance with him and relieve his necessities if required; to look upon his offspring in the same footing as my own brother, and to teach them this Art, if they shall wish to learn it, without fee or stipulation, and that by precept, lecture, and every other mode of instruction, I will impart a knowledge of the Art to my own sons and those of my teachers, and to disciples bound by a stipulation and oath according to the law of medicine, but to none others.

I will follow that system of regimen which, according to my ability and judgment, I consider for the benefit of my patients, and abstain from whatever is deleterious and mischievous. I will give no deadly medicine to any if asked, nor suggest any such counsel; and in like manner I will not give a woman a pessary to produce abortion.

With purity and with holiness I will pass my life and practise my Art. I will not cut persons labouring under the stone, but will leave this to be done by men who are practitioners of this work. Into whatever houses I enter I will go into them for the benefit of the sick and will abstain from every voluntary act of mischief and corruption; and further from the seduction of females or males, of freemen and slaves.

Whatever, in connection with my professional practice, or not in connection with it, I may see or hear in the lives of men which ought not to be spoken of abroad I will not divulge, as reckoning that all such should be kept secret.

While I continue to keep this Oath unviolated may it be granted to me to enjoy life and the practice of the Art, respected by all men, in all times! But should I trespass and violate this Oath, may the reverse be my lot!

Hippocrates, born on the Island of Cos (460?–357 BC) is agreed by everyone to be the father of medicine. He is said to have lived to the age of 109.

Many of the statements in this ancient oath remain relevant today, while others, such as euthanasia and abortion, remain controversial. The seduction of slaves, however, is less of a problem.

Credits

Every attempt has been made to trace and acknowledge copyright, but in some cases this may not have been possible. The publisher apologises for any accidental infringement and would welcome any information to redress the situation.

Photography new for the 5th edition by Glenn McCulloch, unless stated otherwise.

Illustrations by Shelly Communications Pty Ltd, unless stated otherwise.

Good signs guides based on detailed LR figures from McGee S. *Evidence-based physical diagnosis*, 2nd ed Saunders: Philadelphia, 2007, with permission.

Canberra Hospital X-ray library: Courtesy Professor G Buirsky, Director, Department of Medical Imaging, The Canberra Hospital; reproduced with permission.

Mayo Clinic: From Mayo Clinic Library and FS McDonald, ed. *Mayo Clinic images in internal medicine: self-assessment for board exam review*. © Mayo Clinic Scientific Press: Rochester MN & CRC Press: Boca Raton FL, 2004, with permission.

Macleod: Douglas G, Nicol F, Robertson C. *Macleod's Clinical Examination*, 12th edn. Edinburgh: Churchill Livingstone, 2009.

Mir: From Mir MA. *Atlas of Clinical Diagnosis*, 2nd edn. Edinburgh: Saunders, 2003, with permission.

Reeves & Maibach: From Reeves JT and Maibach H, *Clinical dermatology illustrated: a regional approach*, 3rd edn. McLennan & Petty: Sydney, 2000, with permission.

Thomson: Dr Malcolm Thomson, National Capital Diagnostic Imaging, Canberra.

Page numbers shown in bold face, underlined; figure numbers shown in bold face.

Chapter 3

25 3.2a, 3.2b Mir. **32** 3.3 Adapted from Sackett DL, Richardson WS, Rosenberg W, Haynes RB. *Evidence-based medicine: how to practice and teach EBM*. London: Churchill Livingstone, 1997.

Chapter 4

47 4.5b, 4.5c Adapted from Macleod. **48** 4.6 Adapted from McGee S. *Evidence-based physical diagnosis*, 2nd edn. St Louis: Saunders, 2007. **50** 4.10 From Baker T, Nikoli´c G, O'Connor S. *Practical Cardiology*, 2nd edn. Sydney: Churchill Livingstone, 2008, with permission. **57** 4.19 Mayo Clinic. **64** 4.31 Adapted from Swash M, ed. *Hutchison's clinical methods*, 20th edn. London: Baillière Tindall, 1995. **73** 4.37, **74** 4.38, 4.39 Mayo Clinic. **79** 4.42, **80** 4.43, 4.44 Dr Chris Kennedy & Prof. Ian Constable © Lions Eye Institute, Perth. **101** 4.67 From Baker T, Nikolić G, O'Connor S, *ibid*, with permission.

Chapter 5

121 5.5 Mayo Clinic. **5.6a&b** Mir. **132** 5.14a&b Mayo Clinic.

Chapter 6

153 6.1a&b Thomson. **154** 6.3, 6.4 Mayo Clinic. **156** 6.5a From Jones DV et al, in Feldman M et al, *Sleisenger & Fordtran's gastrointestinal disease*, 6th edn, Chapter 112. Philadelphia: WB Saunders, 1998, with permission. **6.5b** Mayo Clinic. **6.6a&b, 6.7** Mayo Clinic. **159** 6.9 Mayo Clinic. **161** 6.12 Mir. 6.13 Mayo Clinic. **162** 6.14 Mayo Clinic. **164** 6.16 Mayo Clinic. **6.17** Mir. **166** 6.20 Adapted from Swash M, ed. *Hutchison's clinical methods*, 20th edn. London: Baillière Tindall, 1995. **167** 6.21 Mir. 6.22 Based on Swash M, ed, *ibid*. **174** 6.28 Adapted from Clain A, ed. *Hamilton Bailey's Physical signs in clinical surgery*, 17th edn. John Wright & Sons, 1986. **180** 6.33 From Talley NJ, *American Journal of Gastroenterology* 2008; 108:802–803, with permission. **191** 6.36 Mayo Clinic. 6.37 From Misiewisz JJ, Bantrum CI, Cotton PB et al. *Slide atlas of gastroenterology*. London: Gower Medical Publishing, 1985, with permission.

Chapter 7

209 7.5 Mayo Clinic. **216** 7.10 Adapted from Macleod. **217** 7.11 Adapted from Dunphy JE, Botsford TW. *Physical examination of the surgical patient. An introduction to clinical surgery*, 4th edn. Philadelphia: WB Saunders, 1975. **218** 7.13 Adapted from Macleod.

Chapter 8

225 8.1, **230** 8.8 Adapted from Epstein O et al. *Clinical Examination*, 4th edn. Edinburgh: Mosby, 2008. **231** 8.9 Mayo Clinic. **238** 8.23 Mir.

Chapter 9

242 9.1 Adapted from Epstein O et al. *Clinical Examination*, 4th edn. Edinburgh: Mosby, 2008. **242** 9.2, **244** 9.3 Canberra Hospital X-ray library. **249** 9.6 Thomson. **250** 9.7, 9.8, **251** 9.9 Canberra Hospital X-ray library. **258** 9.25b&c, **264** 9.33b Thomson. **265** 9.35 Adapted from Macleod. **266** 9.36a&b, **269** 9.38, **274** 9.45b–d Thomson. **279** 9.52 Canberra Hospital X-ray library. **280** 9.54 Mayo Clinic. **280** 9.55, **281** 9.56, **283** 9.59 Canberra Hospital X-ray library.

Chapter 10

299 10.3 Adapted from McGee S. *Evidence-based physical diagnosis,* 2nd edn. St Louis: Saunders, 2007. **310** 10.12, **314** 10.14a&b Mayo Clinic. **318** 10.18, 10.19 Mayo Clinic. **319** 10.21, 10.22a&b, **320** 10.23 Dr Chris Kennedy & Prof. Ian Constable © Lions Eye Institute, Perth.

Chapter 11

333 11.4, **334** 11.6 Adapted from Snell RS, Westmorland BF. *Clinical neuroanatomy for medical students*, 4th edn. Boston: Little, Brown, 1997. **334** 11.7 Adapted from Bickerstaff ER, Spillane JA. *Neurological examination in clinical practice*, 5th edn. Oxford: Blackwell, 1989. **340** 11.13 Adapted from Lance JW, McLeod JG. *A physiological approach to clinical neurology*, 3ed edn. London: Butterworths, 1981. **344** 11.20 Adapted from Simon RP, Aminoff MJ, Greenberg DA. *Clinical neurology 1989*. Appleton & Lange, 1989. **347** 11.27 Mayo Clinic Image. © Mayo Clinic Scientific Press and CRC Press. **349** 11.31 Adapted from Walton JN. *Brain's diseases of the nervous system*, 10th edn. Oxford: OUP, 1983. **355** 11.38 Adapted from Lance JW, McLeod JG. *A physiological approach to clinical neurology*, 3ed edn. London: Butterworths, 1981. **361** 11.53, **362** 11.55 Adapted from Snell RS, Westmorland BF. *Clinical neuroanatomy for medical students*, 4th edn. Boston: Little, Brown, 1997. **366** 11.61 Adapted from Chusid JG. *Correlative neuroanatomy and functional neurology*, 19th edn. Los Altos: Lange Medical, 1985. **367** 11.62 Mir. **385** 11.94 Adapted from Weiner HL, Levitt LP. *Neurology for the house officer*, 6th edn. Baltimore: Williams & Wilkins. 2000. **388** 11.97 Adapted from Brazis PW. *Localisation in clinical neurology.* Philadelphia: Lippincott, Williams & Wilkins, 2001. **393** 11.103 Mir. **11.104a&b** Mayo Clinic.

Chapter 13

430 13.7, **432** 13.11, 13.12, 13.13, 13.14 Mir.

Chapter 15

443 15.4 Adapted from Schwartz M. *Textbook of physical diagnosis*, 4th edn. Philadelphia: Saunders, 2002. **445** 15.6, 15.7, 15.8, **446** 15.9, 15.10, 15.11, **447** 15.12, 15.13, 15.14, **449** 15.15, **450** 15.16, 15.17, **451** 15.18, 15.19, 15.20, **452** 15.21 Reeves & Maibach.

Chapter 16

458 16.1, 16.2 Reeves & Maibach. **458** 16.3, 16.4 Mayo Clinic. **459** 16.5, 16.6 Dr Chris Kennedy & Prof. Ian Constable © Lions Eye Institute, Perth.

Chapter 1

The general principles of history taking

Medicine is learned by the bedside and not in the classroom.

Sir William Osler (1849–1919)

An extensive knowledge of medical facts is not useful unless a doctor is able to extract accurate and succinct information from a sick person about his or her illness. In all branches of medicine, the development of a rational plan of management depends on a correct diagnosis or sensible, differential diagnosis (list of possible diagnoses). Except for patients who are extremely ill, taking a careful medical history should precede both examination and treatment. A medical history is the first step in making a diagnosis; it will often help direct the physical examination and will usually determine what investigations are appropriate. More often than not, an accurate history suggests the correct diagnosis, whereas the physical examination and subsequent investigations merely serve to confirm this impression.[1,2] The history is also, of course, the least expensive way of making a diagnosis.

Changes in medical education mean that much student teaching is now conducted away from the traditional hospital ward. Students must still learn how to take a thorough medical history, but obviously adjustments to the technique must be made for patients seen in busy surgeries or outpatient departments. Much information about a patient's previous medical history may already be available in hospital or clinic records; the detail needed will vary depending on the complexity of the presenting problem and whether the visit is a follow-up or a new consultation. All students must, however, have a comprehensive understanding of how to take a complete medical history.

Bedside manner and establishing rapport

History taking requires practice and depends very much on the doctor–patient relationship.[3] It is important to try to put the patient at ease immediately, because unless a rapport is established, the history taking is likely to be unrewarding.

There is no doubt that the treatment of a patient begins the moment one reaches the bedside or the patient enters the consulting rooms. The patient's first impressions of a doctor's professional manner will have a lasting effect. One of the axioms of the medical profession is *primum non nocere* (the first thing is to cause no harm).[4] An unkind and thoughtless approach to questioning and examining a patient can cause harm before any treatment has had the opportunity to do so. You should aim to leave the patient feeling better for your visit. This is a difficult technique to teach. Much has been written about the correct way to interview patients, but each doctor has to develop his or her own method, guided by experience gained from clinical teachers and patients.[5–8]

To help establish this good relationship, the student or doctor must make a deliberate point of introducing him- or herself and explaining his or her role. This is especially relevant for students or junior doctors seeing patients in hospital. A student might say: 'Good afternoon, Mrs Evans. My name is Jane Smith; I am Dr Osler's medical student. She has asked me to come and see you.' A patient seen at a clinic should be asked to come and sit down, and be directed to a chair. The door should be shut or, if the patient is in the ward, the curtains drawn to give some privacy. The clinician should sit down beside or near the patient so as to be close to eye level and give the impression that the interview will be an unhurried one.[9,10] It is important here to address the patient respectfully and use his or her name and title. Some general remarks about the weather, hospital food or the crowded waiting room may be appropriate to help put the patient at ease, but these must not be patronising.

Obtaining the history

Allow the patient to tell the whole story, then ask questions to fill in the gaps. Always listen carefully. At the end of the history and examination, a detailed record is made. However, many clinicians find it useful to make rough notes during the interview. With practice this can be done without loss of rapport. In fact, pausing to make a note of a patient's answer to a question suggests that it is being taken seriously.

Many clinics and hospitals use computer records which may be displayed on a computer screen on the desk. Notes are sometimes added to these during the interview via a keyboard. It can be very off-putting for a patient when the interviewing doctor looks entirely at the computer screen rather than at the patient. With practice it is possible to enter data while maintaining eye contact with a patient, but at first it is probably preferable in most cases to make written notes and transcribe them later.

The final record must be a sequential, accurate account of the development and course of the illness or illnesses of the patient (Appendix I, page 461). There are a number of methods of recording this information. Hospitals may have printed forms with spaces for recording specific information. This applies especially to routine admissions (e.g. for minor surgical procedures). Follow-up consultation questions and notes will be briefer than those of the initial consultation; obviously, many questions are only relevant for the initial consultation. When a patient is seen repeatedly at a clinic or in a general practice setting, the current presenting history may be listed as an 'active' problem and the past history as a series of 'inactive' or 'still active' problems.

A sick patient will sometimes emphasise irrelevant facts and forget about very important symptoms. For this reason, a systematic approach to history taking and recording is crucial (Table 1.1).[11]

Introductory questions

In order to obtain a good history the clinician must establish a **good relationship**, interview in a **logical manner**, **listen** carefully, **interrupt** appropriately, note **non-verbal clues**, and **correctly interpret** the information obtained.

TABLE 1.1 History-taking sequence
1 Presenting (principal) symptom (PS)
2 History of presenting illness (HPI) Details of current illnesses Details of previous similar episodes Current treatment and drug history Menstrual and reproductive history for women Extent of functional disability
3 Past history (PH) Past illnesses and surgical operations Past treatments Allergies Blood transfusions
4 Social history (SH) Occupation, education Smoking, alcohol, analgesic use Overseas travel, immunisation Marital status, social support Living conditions
5 Family history (FH)
6 Systems review (SR) See Questions box 1.1, page 9
Also refer to Appendix I.

The next step after introducing oneself should be to find out the patient's major symptoms or medical problems. Asking the patient 'What brought you here today?' can be unwise, as it often promotes the reply 'an ambulance' or 'a car'. This little joke wears thin after some years in clinical practice. It is best to attempt a conversational approach and ask the patient 'What has been the trouble or problem recently?' or 'When were you last quite well?' For a follow-up consultation some reference to the last visit is appropriate, for example: 'How have things been going since I saw you last?' or 'It's about … weeks since I saw you last, isn't it? What's been happening since then?' This lets the patient know the clinician hasn't forgotten him or her. Some writers suggest the clinician begin with questions to the patient about more general aspects of his or her life. There is a danger that this attempt to establish early rapport will seem intrusive to a person who has come for help about a specific problem, albeit one related to other aspects of his or her life. This type of general and personal information may be better approached once the clinician has shown an interest in the presenting problem or as part of the social history. The best approach and timing of this part of the interview must vary, depending on the nature of the presenting problem and the patient's and clinician's attitude. Encourage patients to tell their story in their own words from the onset of the first symptom to the present time.

When a patient stops volunteering information, the question 'What else?' may start things up again.[8] However, some direction may be necessary to keep a garrulous patient on track later during the interview. It is necessary to ask specific questions to test diagnostic hypotheses. For example, the patient may not have noticed an association between the occurrence of chest discomfort and exercise (typical of angina) unless asked specifically. It may also be helpful to give a list of possible answers. A patient with suspected angina who is unable to describe the symptom may be asked if the sensation was sharp, dull, heavy or burning. The reply that it was burning makes angina less likely.

Appropriate (but not exaggerated) reassuring gestures are of value to maintain the flow of conversation. If the patient stops giving the story spontaneously, it can be useful to provide a short summary of what has already been said and encourage him or her to continue.

The clinician must learn to listen with an open mind.[10] The temptation to leap to a diagnostic decision before the patient has had the chance to describe all the symptoms in his or her own words should be resisted. Avoid using pseudo-medical terms; and if the patient uses these, find out exactly what is meant by them, as misinterpretation of medical terms is common.

Patients' descriptions of their symptoms may vary as they are subjected to repeated questioning by increasingly senior medical staff. The patient who has described his chest pain as sharp and left-sided to the medical student may tell the registrar that the pain is dull and in the centre of the chest. These discrepancies come as no surprise to experienced clinicians; they are sometimes the result of the patient's having had time to reflect on his or her symptoms. This does mean, however, that very important aspects of the story should be checked by asking follow-up questions, such as: 'Can you show me exactly where the pain is?' and 'What do you mean by sharp?'

Some patients may have medical problems that make the interview difficult for them; these include deafness and problems with speech and memory. These must be recognised by the clinician if the interview is to be successful. See Chapter 2 for more details.

The presenting (principal) symptom

Not uncommonly, a patient has many symptoms. An attempt must be made to decide which symptom led the patient to present. It must be remembered that the patient's and the doctor's ideas of what constitutes a serious problem may differ. A patient with symptoms of a cold who also, in passing, mentions that he has recently had severe crushing retrosternal chest pain needs more attention to his heart than to his nose. Record each presenting symptom in the patient's own words, avoiding technical terms.

History of the presenting illness

Each of the presenting problems has to be talked about in detail with the patient, but in the first part of the interview the patient should lead the discussion. In the second part the doctor should take more control and ask specific questions. When writing down the history of the presenting illness, the events should be placed in chronological order; this might have to be done later when the whole history has been obtained. If numerous systems are affected, the events should be placed in chronological order for each system.

Current symptoms

Certain information should routinely be sought for each current symptom if this hasn't been volunteered by the patient. The mnemonic SOCRATES summarises the questions that should be asked about most symptoms:

- **Site**
- **Onset**
- **Character**
- **Radiation** (if pain or discomfort)
- **Alleviating factors**
- **Timing**
- **Exacerbating factors**
- **Severity**.

Site

Ask where the symptom is exactly and whether it is localised or diffuse. Ask the patient to point to the actual site on the body.

Some symptoms are not localised. Patients who complain of dizziness do not localise this to any particular site—but vertigo may sometimes involve a feeling of movement within the head and to that extent is localised. Other symptoms that are not localised include cough, shortness of breath (dyspnoea), or change in weight.

Onset (Mode of onset and pattern)

Find out whether the symptom came on rapidly, gradually or instantaneously. Some cardiac arrhythmias are of instantaneous onset and offset. Sudden loss of consciousness (syncope) with immediate recovery occurs with cardiac but not neurological disease. Ask whether the symptom has been present continuously or intermittently. Determine if the symptom is getting worse or better, and, if so, when the change occurred. For example, the exertional breathlessness of chronic obstructive pulmonary disease may come on with less and less activity as it worsens. Find out what the patient was doing at the time the symptom began. For example, severe breathlessness that wakes a patient from sleep is very suggestive of cardiac failure.

Character

Here it is necessary to ask the patient what is meant by the symptom; to describe its character. If the patient complains of dizziness, does this mean the room spins around (vertigo) or is it more a feeling of light-headedness? Does indigestion mean abdominal pain, heartburn, excess wind or a change in bowel habit? If there is pain, is it sharp, dull, stabbing, boring, burning or cramp-like?

Radiation of pain or discomfort

Determine whether the symptom, if localised, radiates; this mainly applies if the symptom is pain. Certain patterns of radiation are typical of a condition or even diagnostic, e.g. the nerve root distribution of pain associated with herpes zoster (shingles).

Alleviating factors

Ask whether anything makes the symptom better. For example, the pain of pericarditis may be relieved when a patient sits up. Have analgesic medications been used to control the pain? Have narcotics been required?

Timing

Find out when the symptom first began and try to date this as accurately as possible. For example, ask the patient what was the first thing he or she noticed that was 'unusual' or 'wrong'. Ask whether the patient has had a similar illness in the past. It is often helpful to ask patients when they last felt entirely well. In a patient with long-standing symptoms, ask why he or she decided to come and see the doctor at this time.

Exacerbating factors

Ask if anything makes the pain or symptom worse. The slightest movement may exacerbate the abdominal pain of peritonitis or the pain in the big toe caused by gout.

Severity

This is subjective. The best way to assess severity is to ask the patient whether the symptom interferes with normal activities or sleep. Severity can be graded from mild to very severe. A mild symptom can be ignored by the patient, while a moderate symptom cannot be ignored but does not interfere with daily activities. A severe symptom interferes with daily activities, while a very severe symptom markedly interferes with most activities. Alternatively, pain or discomfort can be graded on a 10-point scale from 0 (no discomfort) to 10 (unbearable).

The severity of some symptoms can be quantified more precisely; for example, shortness of breath on exertion occurring after walking 10 metres on flat ground is more severe than shortness of breath occurring after walking 90 metres up a hill. Central chest pain from angina occurring at rest is more significant than angina occurring while running 90 metres to catch a bus.

It is crucial to quantify accurately the severity of each symptom—but also to remember that symptoms a patient considers mild may be very significant.

Associated symptoms

Here an attempt is made to uncover in a systematic way symptoms that might be expected to be associated with disease of a particular area. Initial and most thorough attention must be given to the system that includes the presenting complaint (see *Questions box 1.1*, page 9). Remember that while a single symptom may provide the clue that leads to the correct diagnosis, usually it is the combination of characteristic symptoms that most reliably suggests the diagnosis.

Current treatment and drug allergies

Ask the patient whether he or she is currently taking any tablets or medicines (the use of the word 'drug' may cause alarm); the patient will often describe these by colour or size rather than by name and dose. Then ask the patient to show you all his or her medications, if possible, and list them. Note the dose, length of use, and the indication for each drug. This list may provide a useful clue to chronic or past illnesses, otherwise forgotten. Remember that some drugs are prescribed as transdermal patches or subcutaneous implants (e.g. contraceptives and hormonal treatment of carcinoma of the prostate). Ask whether the drugs were taken as prescribed. Always ask specifically whether a woman is taking the contraceptive pill, because this is not considered a medicine or tablet by many who take it. The same is true of inhalers, or what many patients call their 'puffers'.

To remind the patient, it is often useful to ask about the use of classes of drugs. A basic list should include questions about treatment for blood pressure, high cholesterol, diabetes, arthritis, anxiety or depression, impotence, contraception, hormone replacement, epilepsy, anticoagulation and the use of antibiotics. Also ask the patient if he or she is taking any over-the-counter preparations (e.g. aspirin, antihistamines, vitamins). Aspirin and standard non-steroidal anti-inflammatory drugs (NSAIDs), but not paracetamol, can cause gastrointestinal bleeding. Patients with chronic pain may consume large amounts of analgesics, including drugs containing opioids such as codeine or morphine. A careful history of the period of use of opioids and the quantities used is important because they are drugs of dependence.

Approximately 50% of people now use 'natural remedies' of various types. They may not feel these are a relevant part of their medical history, but these chemicals, like any drug, may have adverse effects. Indeed, some of these have been found to be adulterated with drugs such as steroids and NSAIDs. More information about these substances and their effects is becoming available and there is an increasing responsibility for clinicians to be aware of them.

There may be some medications or treatments the patient has had in the past which remain relevant. These include corticosteroids, chemotherapeutic agents (anti-cancer drugs) and radiotherapy. Often patients, especially those with a chronic disease, are very well informed about their condition and their treatment. However, some allowance must be made for patients' non-medical interpretation of what happened.[10]

Note any **adverse reactions** in the past. Also ask specifically about any **allergy to drugs** (often a skin reaction or episode of bronchospasm) and what the allergic reaction actually involved, to help judge if it was really an allergic reaction.[12] The patient often confuses an allergy with a side-effect of a drug.

Ask about 'recreational' drug use. The use of intravenous drugs has many implications for the patient's health. Ask whether any attempt has been made to avoid sharing needles. This may protect against the injection of viruses, but not against bacterial infection from the use of impure substances.

Not all medical problems are treated with drugs. Ask about courses of physiotherapy or rehabilitation for musculoskeletal problems or injuries, or to help recovery following surgery or a severe illness. Certain gastrointestinal conditions are treated with dietary supplements (e.g. pancreatic enzymes for chronic pancreatitis) or restrictions (e.g. of gluten for coeliac disease).

Menstrual history

For women, a menstrual history should be obtained; it is particularly relevant for a patient with abdominal pain, a suspected endocrine disease or genitourinary symptoms. Write down the date of the last menstrual period. Ask about the age at which menstruation began, if the periods are regular, or whether menopause has occurred. Ask if the symptoms are related to the periods. Do not forget to ask a woman of childbearing age if there is a possibility of pregnancy; this, for example, may preclude the use of certain investigations or drugs.[13] Observing the well-known axiom that 'every woman of childbearing years is pregnant until proven otherwise' can prevent unnecessary danger to the unborn child and avoid embarrassment for the unwary clinician. Ask about any miscarriages. Record *gravida* (the number of pregnancies) and *para* (the number of births of babies over 20 weeks' gestation).

The effect of the illness

A serious illness can change a person's life—for example, a chronic illness may prevent work or further education. The psychological and physical effects of a serious health problem may be devastating and, of course, people respond differently to similar problems. Even after full recovery from a life-threatening illness, some people may be permanently affected by loss of confidence or self-esteem. There may be continuing anxieties about the capability of supporting a family. Try to find out how the patient and his or her family have been affected. How has he or she coped so far, and what are the patient's expectations and hopes for the future with regard to health? What explanations of the condition has the patient been given or obtained (e.g. from the internet)?

Helping a patient manage ill-health is a large part of the clinician's duty. This depends on sympathetic and realistic explanations of the probable future course of the disease and the effects of treatment.

The past history

Ask the patient whether he or she has had any serious illnesses, operations or admissions to hospital in the past. Don't forget to inquire about childhood illnesses and any obstetric or gynaecological problems. Previous illnesses or operations may have a direct bearing on the current health of the patient. It is worth asking specifically about certain operations that have a continuing effect on the patient's health; for example, operations for malignancy, bowel surgery or cardiac surgery—especially valve surgery. Implanted prostheses are common in surgical, orthopaedic and cardiac procedures. These may involve a risk of infection of the foreign body, while magnetic metals—especially cardiac pacemakers—are a contraindication to magnetic resonance imaging (MRI). Chronic kidney disease may be a contraindication to X-rays using iodine contrast materials and MRI scanning using gadolinium contrast. Pregnancy is usually a contraindication to radiation exposure (X-rays and nuclear scans—remember that CT scans cause hundreds of times the radiation exposure of simple X-rays).

The patient may believe that he or she has had a particular diagnosis made in the past, but careful questioning may reveal this as unlikely. For example, the patient may mention a previous duodenal ulcer, but not have had any investigations or treatment for it, which makes the diagnosis less certain. Therefore it is important to obtain the particulars of each relevant past illness, including the symptoms experienced, tests performed and treatments prescribed.

Patients with chronic illnesses such as diabetes mellitus will probably have had their condition managed with the help of various doctors and at specialised clinics where diabetic educators, nurses and dieticians will have had a primary role in management of the illness. Find out what supervision and treatment these have provided. For example, who does the patient contact if there is a problem with the insulin dose, and does the patient know what to do (an action plan) if there is an urgent or dangerous complication? Patients with chronic diseases are often very much involved in their own care and are very well informed about aspects of their treatment. For example, diabetics should keep records of their home-measured blood sugar levels; heart failure patients should monitor their weight daily, and so on. These patients will often make their own adjustments to their medication doses. Assessing a patient's understanding of and confidence in making these changes should be part of the history taking.

The social and personal history

This is the time to find out more about the patient as a person. The questions should be asked in an interested and conversational way and should not sound like a routine learned by rote. This history includes the whole economic, social, domestic and industrial situation of the patient. Ask first about the places of birth and residence, and the level of education obtained. Recent migrants may have been exposed to infectious diseases like tuberculosis; ethnic background is important in some diseases, such as thalassaemia and sickle cell anaemia.

Smoking

The patient may claim to be a non-smoker if he or she stopped smoking that morning. Therefore, ask whether the patient has ever smoked and, if so, how many cigarettes (or cigars or pipes) were smoked a day and for how many years. Find out if the patient has stopped smoking, and if so when that was. Calculate the number of packet-years of smoking (20 cigarettes a day for 1 year = a packet-year).

Cigarette smoking is a risk factor for vascular disease, chronic lung disease, several cancers and peptic ulceration, and may damage the fetus (Table 1.2). Cigar and pipe smokers typically inhale less smoke than cigarette smokers, and overall mortality rates are correspondingly lower in this group, except from carcinoma of the oral cavity, larynx and oesophagus.

TABLE 1.2 Smoking and clinical associations*
1 Cardiovascular disease
Premature coronary artery disease
Peripheral vascular disease
Cerebrovascular disease
2 Respiratory disease
Lung cancer
Chronic obstructive pulmonary disease (chronic airflow limitation)
Increased incidence of respiratory infection
Increased incidence of postoperative respiratory complications
3 Other cancers
Larynx, oral cavity, oesophagus, nasopharynx, bladder, kidney, pancreas, stomach, uterine cervix
4 Gastrointestinal disease
Peptic ulceration
5 Pregnancy
Increased risk of spontaneous abortion, fetal death, neonatal death, sudden infant death syndrome
6 Drug interactions
Induces hepatic microsomal enzyme systems, e.g. increased metabolism of propranolol, theophylline
* Individual risk is influenced by the duration, intensity and type of smoke exposure, as well as by genetic and other environmental factors. Passive smoking is also associated with respiratory disease.

Alcohol

Ask whether the patient drinks alcohol.[14] If so, ask what type, how much and how often. If the patient claims to be a social drinker, find out exactly what this means. In a glass of wine, a nip (or shot) of spirits, a glass of port or sherry, or a 200 mL (7 oz) glass of beer, there are approximately 8–10 g of alcohol (1 unit = 8 g). In the UK, the current recommended safe limits are 21 units (168 g of ethanol) a week for men and 14 units (112 g of ethanol) for women; weekly consumption of more than 50 units for men and 35 units for women defines a high-risk group. Alcohol becomes a major risk factor for liver disease in men if more than 80 g and in women if more than 40 g are taken daily for 5 years or longer. The National Health & Medical Research Council (NHMRC) in Australia recommends a maximum alcohol intake of no more than 40 g per day for males on average (and 20 g per day for females) with two alcohol-free days a week. Alcoholics are notoriously unreliable about describing their alcohol intake, so it may be important to suspend belief and sometimes (with the patient's permission) talk to the relatives.

Certain questions can be helpful in making a diagnosis of alcoholism; these are referred to as the CAGE questions:[15]

1 Have you ever felt you ought to *Cut* down on your drinking?
2 Have people *Annoyed* you by criticizing your drinking?
3 Have you ever felt bad or *Guilty* about your drinking?
4 Have you ever had a drink first thing in the morning to steady your nerves or get rid of a hangover? (*Eye opener*)

If the patient answers 'yes' to any of these questions, this suggests there may be a serious alcohol

---

TABLE 1.3 Alcohol (ethanol) abuse: complications

Gastrointestinal system
- Acute gastric erosions
- Gastrointestinal bleeding from varices, erosions, Mallory-Weiss tear, peptic ulceration
- Pancreatitis (acute, recurrent or chronic)
- Diarrhoea (watery, due to alcohol itself, or steatorrhoea from chronic alcoholic pancreatitis or, rarely, liver disease)
- Hepatomegaly (fatty liver, chronic liver disease)
- Chronic liver disease (alcoholic hepatitis, cirrhosis) and associated complications
- Cancer (oesophagus, cardia of stomach, liver, pancreas)

Cardiovascular system
- Cardiomyopathy
- Arrhythmias
- Hypertension

Nervous system
- 'Blackouts'
- Nutrition-related conditions, e.g. Wernicke's encephalopathy, Korsakoff's psychosis, peripheral neuropathy (thiamine deficiency), pellagra (dementia, dermatitis and diarrhoea from niacin deficiency)
- Withdrawal syndromes, e.g. tremor, hallucinations, 'rum fits', delirium tremens
- Cerebellar degeneration
- Alcoholic dementia
- Alcoholic myopathy
- Autonomic neuropathy

Haematopoietic system
- Anaemia (dietary folate deficiency, iron deficiency from blood loss, direct toxic suppression of the bone marrow, rarely B_{12} deficiency with chronic pancreatitis, or sideroblastic anaemia)
- Thrombocytopenia (from bone marrow suppression or hypersplenism)

Genitourinary system
- Erectile dysfunction (impotence), testicular atrophy in men
- Amenorrhoea, infertility, spontaneous abortion, fetal alcohol syndrome in women

Other effects
- Increased risk of fractures and osteonecrosis of the femoral head

dependence problem. The complications of alcohol abuse are summarised in Table 1.3.

Occupation and education

Ask the patient about present occupation;[16] the WHACS mnemonic is useful here:[17]

1 **What** do you do?
2 **How** do you do it?
3 **Are** you concerned about any of your exposures or experiences?
4 **Co-workers** or others exposed?
5 **Satisfied** with your job?

Finding out exactly what the patient does at work can be helpful (page 113). Note particularly any work exposure to dusts, chemicals or disease; for example, mine and industrial workers may have the disease asbestosis. Find out if any similar complaints have affected fellow workers.

Ask about the education level attained; this can influence the way things are explained. Checking on hobbies can also be informative (e.g. bird fanciers and lung disease).

Overseas travel and immunisation

If an infectious disease is a possibility, ask about recent overseas travel, destinations reached, and how the patient lived when away (e.g. did he or she drink unbottled water and eat local foods, or dine at expensive international hotels). Ask about immunisation status and whether any prophylactic drugs (e.g. for malaria) were taken during the travel period. Find out whether the patient has had recent immunisations (e.g. for hepatitis B, pneumococcal disease, *Haemophilus influenzae* or influenza).

Marital status, social support and living conditions

To determine the patient's marital status, ask who is living at home with the patient. Find out about the health of the spouse and of any children. Check if there are any other household members. Establish who is the patient's main 'caregiver'. Discreet questions about sexual activity may be very relevant. For example, erectile dysfunction may occur in neurological conditions, debilitating illness or psychiatric disease. Questions about living arrangements are particularly important for chronic or disabling illnesses, where it is necessary to know what social support is available and whether the patient is able to manage at home (for example, the number of steps required for access to the house, or the location of the toilet).

Ask if the patient considers him- or herself to be a spiritual person. Spirituality is an important factor, especially in the care of dying patients, in the creation of living wills and in understanding the support network available for the patient.

Ask about the adequacy of the patient's diet, who does the cooking, availability of 'meals on wheels' and other services such as house cleaning. Also ask about the amount of physical activity undertaken. The presence of pets in the home may be important if infections or allergies are suspected.

The family history

Many diseases run in families. For example, ischaemic heart disease that has developed at a young age in parents or siblings is a major risk factor for ischaemic heart disease in the offspring. Various malignancies, such as breast and large-bowel carcinoma, are more common in certain families. Both genetic and common environmental exposures may explain these familial associations. Some diseases (e.g. haemophilia) are directly inherited.[18]

Ask about any history of a similar illness in the family. Inquire about the health and, if relevant, the causes of death and ages of death of the parents and siblings. If there is any suggestion of a hereditary disease, a complete family tree should be compiled showing all members affected (Figure 1.1). Patients can be reluctant to mention that they have relatives with mental illnesses, epilepsy or cancer, so ask tactfully about these diseases. Consanguinity (usually first cousins marrying) increases the probability of autosomal recessive abnormalities in the children; ask about this if the pedigree is suggestive.

Systems review

As well as detailed questioning about the system likely to be diseased, it is essential to ask about important symptoms and disorders in other systems (*Questions box 1.1*), otherwise important diseases may be missed.[19,20] An experienced clinician will perform a targeted systems review, based on information already obtained from the patient; clearly it is not realistic to put all of the listed questions to a patient.

When recording the systems review, list important negative answers ('relevant negatives'). Remember: if other recent symptoms are unmasked, more details must be sought; relevant information is then added to the history of the presenting illness. Before completing the history, it is often valuable to ask what the patient thinks is wrong, and what he or she is most concerned about. General and sympathetic questions about the effect of a chronic or severe illness on the patient's life are important for establishing rapport and for finding out what

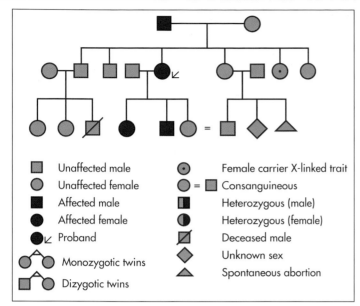

Figure 1.1 Preparing a family tree: note the symbols used for the documentation

Legend for Figure 1.1:
- Unaffected male
- Unaffected female
- Affected male
- Affected female
- Proband
- Monozygotic twins
- Dizygotic twins
- Female carrier X-linked trait
- Consanguineous
- Heterozygous (male)
- Heterozygous (female)
- Deceased male
- Unknown sex
- Spontaneous abortion

else might be needed (both medical and non-medical) to help the patient.

Major presenting symptoms for each system are described in the following chapters. Examples of supplementary important questions to ask about past history, social history and family history are also given there for each system.

Questions box 1.1

The systems review

Enquire about common symptoms and three or four of the common disorders in each major system listed below. Not all these questions should be asked of every patient. Adjust the detail of questions based on the presenting problem, the patient's age and the answers to the preliminary questions.

! denotes symptoms for the possible diagnosis of an urgent or dangerous (alarm) problem.

Cardiovascular system

! 1 Have you had any pain or pressure in your chest, neck or arm?—Myocardial ischaemia

2 Are you short of breath on exertion? How much exertion is necessary?

! 3 Have you ever woken up at night short of breath?—Cardiac failure

4 Can you lie flat without feeling breathless?

5 Have you had swelling of your ankles?

6 Have you noticed your heart racing or beating irregularly?

! 7 Have you had blackouts without warning?—Stokes-Adams attacks

! 8 Have you felt dizzy or blacked out when exercising?—Severe aortic stenosis or hypertrophic cardiomyopathy

9 Do you have pain in your legs on exercise?

10 Do you have cold or blue hands or feet?

11 Have you ever had rheumatic fever, a heart attack, or high blood pressure?

Respiratory system

! 1 Are you ever short of breath? **Has this come on suddenly?**—Pulmonary embolism

2 Have you had any cough?

! 3 Is your cough associated with shivers and shakes (rigors) and breathlessness and chest pain?—Pneumonia

4 Do you cough up anything?

! 5 Have you coughed up blood?—Bronchial carcinoma

6 What type of work have you done?—Occupational lung disease

7 Do you snore loudly? Do you fall asleep easily during the day? When? Have you fallen asleep while driving? (Sleep history)

8 Do you ever have wheezing when you are short of breath?

9 Have you had fevers?

10 Do you have night sweats?

(Continues over page)

Respiratory system continued

11 Have you ever had pneumonia or tuberculosis?

12 Have you had a recent chest X-ray?

! 13 Have you had any bleeding or discharge from your breasts or felt any lumps there?—Carcinoma of the breast

Gastrointestinal system

1 Are you troubled by indigestion?

2 Do you have heartburn?

! 3 Have you had any difficulty swallowing?—Oesophageal cancer

! 4 Have you had nausea or vomiting, or vomited blood?—Gastrointestinal bleeding

5 Have you had pain or discomfort in your abdomen?

6 Have you had any abdominal bloating or distension?

! 7 Has your bowel habit changed recently?—Carcinoma of the colon

8 How many bowel motions a week do you usually pass?

9 Have you lost control of your bowels or had accidents (faecal incontinence)?

! 10 Have you seen blood in your motions or vomited blood?—Gastrointestinal bleeding

! 11 Have your bowel motions been black?—Gastrointestinal bleeding

! 12 Have you lost weight recently without dieting?—Carcinoma of the colon

13 Have your eyes or skin ever been yellow?

14 Have you ever had hepatitis, peptic ulceration, colitis, or bowel cancer?

15 Tell me about your diet recently.

Genitourinary system

1 Do you have difficulty or pain on passing urine?

2 Is your urine stream as good as it used to be?

3 Is there a delay before you start to pass urine? (Applies mostly to men)

4 Is there dribbling at the end?

5 Do you have to get up at night to pass urine?

6 Are you passing larger or smaller amounts of urine?

7 Has the urine colour changed?

! 8 Have you seen blood in your urine?—Urinary tract malignancy

9 Have you any problems with your sex life? Difficulty obtaining or maintaining an erection?

10 Have you noticed any rashes or lumps on your genitals?

11 Have you ever had a sexually transmitted disease?

12 Have you ever had a urinary tract infection or kidney stone?

13 Are your periods regular?

14 Do you have excessive pain or bleeding with your periods?

Haematological system

1 Do you bruise easily?

2 Have you had fevers, or shivers and shakes (rigors)?

! 3 Do you have difficulty stopping a small cut from bleeding?—Bleeding disorder

! 4 Have you noticed any lumps under your arms, or in your neck or groin?—Haematological malignancy

5 Have you ever had blood clots in your legs or in the lungs?

Musculoskeletal system

1 Do you have painful or stiff joints?

! 2 Are any of your joints red, swollen and painful?—Septic arthritis

3 Have you had a skin rash recently?

4 Do you have any back or neck pain?

5 Have your eyes been dry or red?

6 Have you ever had a dry mouth or mouth ulcers?

7 Have you been diagnosed as having rheumatoid arthritis or gout?

8 Do your fingers ever become painful and become white and blue in the cold?

Endocrine system

1 Have you noticed any swelling in your neck?

2 Do your hands tremble?

3 Do you prefer hot or cold weather?

4 Have you had a thyroid problem or diabetes?

5 Have you noticed increased sweating?

6 Have you been troubled by fatigue?

7 Have you noticed any change in your appearance, hair, skin or voice?

! 8 Have you been unusually thirsty lately?—New onset of diabetes

Reproductive history (women)

1 How many pregnancies have you had?

2 Have you had any miscarriages?

3 Have you had high blood pressure or diabetes in pregnancy?

4 Were there any other complications during your pregnancies or deliveries?

5 Have you had a Caesarean section?

Neurological system and mental state

1 Do you get headaches?

! 2 Is your headache very severe and did it begin very suddenly?—Sub-arachnoid haemorrhage

3 Have you had memory problems or trouble concentrating?

4 Have you had fainting episodes, fits or blackouts?

5 Do you have trouble seeing or hearing?

6 Are you dizzy?

7 Have you had weakness, numbness or clumsiness in your arms or legs?

8 Have you ever had a stroke or head injury?

9 Have you had difficulty sleeping?

10 Do you feel sad or depressed, or have problems with your 'nerves'?

11 Have you ever been sexually or physically abused?

The elderly patient

! 1 Have you had problems with falls or loss of balance?—High fracture risk

2 Do you walk with a frame or stick?

3 Do you take sleeping tablets or sedatives? —Falls risk

4 Do you take blood pressure tablets?— Postural hypotension and falls risk

5 Have you been tested for osteoporosis?

6 Can you manage at home without help?

7 Are you affected by arthritis?

8 Have you had problems with your memory or with managing things like paying bills?— Cognitive decline

9 How do you manage your various tablets?— Risk of polypharmacy and confusion of doses

Concluding the interview

Is there *anything else* you would like to talk about?

Skills in history taking

In summary, several skills are important in obtaining a useful and accurate history.[21] First, establish rapport and understanding. Second, ask questions in a logical sequence. Start with open-ended questions. Listen to the answers and adjust your interview accordingly. Third, observe and provide non-verbal clues carefully. Encouraging, sympathetic gestures and concentration on the patient that makes it clear he or she has your undivided attention are most important and helpful, but are really a form of normal politeness. Fourth, proper interpretation of the history is crucial.

Your aim should be to obtain information that will help establish the likely anatomical and physiological disturbances present, the aetiology of the presenting symptoms and the impact of the symptoms on the patient's ability to function. (In Chapter 2, some advice on how to take the history in more challenging circumstances is considered.) This type of information will help you plan the diagnostic investigations and treatment, and to discuss the findings with, or present them to, a colleague if necessary (see page 462). First, however, a comprehensive and systematic physical examination is required.

These skills can be obtained and maintained only by practice.

References

1. Longson D. The clinical consultation. *J R Coll Physicians Lond* 1983; 17:192–195. Outlines the principles of hypothesis generation and testing during the clinical evaluation.

2. Nardone DA, Johnson GK, Faryna A et al. A model for the diagnostic medical interview: nonverbal, verbal and cognitive assessments. *J Gen Intern Med* 1992; 7:437–442. Verbal and non-verbal questions and diagnostic reasoning are reviewed in this useful article.

3. Bellet PS, Maloney MJ. The importance of empathy as an interviewing skill in medicine. *JAMA* 1991; 266:1831–1832. Distinguishes between empathy, reassurance and patient education.

4. Brewin T. Primum non nocere? *Lancet* 1994; 344:1487–1488. Review of a key principle in clinical management.

5. Platt FW, McMath JC. Clinical hypocompetence: the interview. *Ann Intern Med* 1979; 91:898–902. A valuable review of potential flaws in interviewing, condensed into five syndromes: inadequate content, database flaws, defects in hypothesis generation, failure to obtain primary data and a controlling style.

6. Coulehan JL et al. 'Tell me about yourself': the patient-centred interview. *Ann Intern Med* 2001; 134:1079–1084.

7. Fogarty L et al. Can 40 seconds of compassion reduce patient anxiety? *J Clin Oncol* 1999; 17:371–379.

8. Barrier P et al. Two words to improve physician–patient communication: What else? *Mayo Clin Proc* 2003; 78:211–214.

9. Blau JN. Time to let the patient speak. *BMJ* 1999; 298:39. The average doctor's uninterrupted narrative with a patient lasts less than 2 minutes (and often much less!), which is too brief. Open interviewing is vital for accurate history taking.

10. Smith RC, Hoppe RB. The patient's story: integrating the patient- and physician-centered approaches to interviewing. *Ann Intern Med* 1991; 115:470 477. Patients tell stories of their illness, integrating both the medical and psychosocial aspects. Both need to be obtained, and this article reviews ways to do this and to interpret the information.

11. Beckman H, Markakis K, Suchman A, Frankel R. Getting the most from a 20-minute visit. *Am J Gastroenterol* 1994; 89:662–664. A lot of information can be obtained from a patient even when time is limited, if the history is taken logically.

12. Salkind AR, Cuddy PG, Foxworth JW. The rational clinical examination. Is this patient allergic to penicillin? An evidence-based analysis of the likelihood of penicillin allergy. *JAMA* 2001; 285(19):2498–2505.

13. Ramosaka EA, Sacchetti AD, Nepp M. Reliability of patient history in determining the possibility of pregnancy. *Ann Emerg Med* 1989; 18:48–50. One in ten women who denied the possibility of pregnancy, in this study, had a positive pregnancy test.

14. Kitchens JM. Does this patient have an alcohol problem? *JAMA* 1994; 272:1782–1787. A useful guide to making this assessment.

15. Beresford TP, Blow FC, Hill E, Singer K, Lucey MR. Comparison of CAGE questionnaire and computer-assisted laboratory profiles in screening for covert alcoholism. *Lancet* 1990; 336:482–485.

16. Newman LS. Occupational illness. *N Engl J Med* 1995; 333:1128–1134. The importance of knowing the occupation for the diagnosis of an illness cannot be overemphasised.

17. Blue AV, Chessman AW, Gilbert GE, Schuman SH, Mainous AG. Medical students' abilities to take an occupational history: use of the WHACS mnemonic. *J Occup Environ Med* 2000; 42(11):1050–1053.

18. Rich EC, Burke W, Heaton CJ, Haga S, Pinsky L, Short MP, Acheson L. Reconsidering the family history in primary care. *J Gen Intern Med* 2004; 19(3):273–280.

19. Hoffbrand BI. Away with the system review: a plea for parsimony. *BMJ* 1989; 198:817–819. Presents the case that the systems review approach is not valuable. A focused review still seems to be useful in practice (see below).

20. Boland BJ, Wollan PC, Silverstein MD. Review of systems, physical examination, and routine test for case-finding in ambulatory patients. *Am J Med Sci* 1995; 309:194–200. A systems review can identify unsuspected clinically important conditions.

21. Simpson M, Buchman R. Stewart M et al. Doctor–patient communication: the Toronto consensus statement. *BMJ* 1991; 303:1385–1387. Most complaints about doctors relate to failure of adequate communication. Encouraging patients to discuss their major concerns without interruption or premature closure enhances satisfaction and yet takes little time (average 90 seconds). Factors that improve communication include use of appropriate open-ended questions, giving frequent summaries, and the use of clarification and negotiation. Giving premature advice or reasurance, or inappropriate use of closed questions, badly affects the interview. These skills can be learned but require practice.

Chapter 2

Advanced history taking

'First the doctor told me the good news: I was going to have a disease named after me.'

Steve Martin

Most complaints about doctors relate to the failure of adequate communication.[1,2] Encouraging patients to discuss their major concerns without interruption enhances satisfaction and yet takes little time (on average 90 seconds).[3,4] Giving premature advice or reassurance, or inappropriate use of closed questions, badly affects the interview.

Taking a good history

Communication and history taking skills can be learnt but require constant practice. Factors that improve communication include use of appropriate open-ended questions, giving frequent summaries, and the use of clarification and negotiation.[3,4] See Table 2.1.

The differential diagnosis

As the interview proceeds, the clinician will need to begin to consider the possible diagnosis or diagnoses – the **differential diagnosis**. This usually starts as a long and ill-defined mental list in the mind of the doctor. As more detail of the symptoms emerges, the list becomes more defined. This mental list must be used as a guide to further questioning in the later part of the interview. Specific questions should then be used to help confirm or eliminate various possibilities. The physical examination and investigations may then be directed to help further narrow the differential. At the end of the history and examination, a likely diagnosis and list of differential diagnoses should be drawn up. This will often be modified as results of tests emerge.

This method of history taking is called, rather grandly, the *hyopthetico-deductive approach*. It

TABLE 2.1 Taking a better history
1 Ask open questions to start with (and resist the urge to interrupt), but finish with specific questions to narrow the differential diagnosis.
2 Do not hurry (or at least do not appear to be in a hurry, even if you have only limited time).
3 Ask the patient 'What else?' after he or she has finished speaking, to ensure that all problems have been identified. Repeat the 'What else?' question as often as required.
4 Maintain comfortable eye contact and an open posture.
5 Use the head nod appropriately, and use silences to encourage the patient to express him- or herself.
6 When there are breaks in the narrative, provide a summary for the patient by briefly re-stating the facts or feelings identified, to maximise accuracy and demonstrate active listening.
7 Clarify the list of chief or presenting complaints with the patient, rather than assuming that you know them.
8 If you are confused about the chronology of events or other issues, admit it and ask the patient to clarify.
9 Make sure the patient's story is internally consistent and, if not, ask more questions to verify the facts.
10 If emotions are uncovered, name the patient's emotion and indicate that you understand (e.g. 'You seem sad'). Show respect and express your support (e.g. 'It's understandable that you would feel upset').
11 Ask about any other concerns the patient may have, and address specific fears.
12 Express your support and willingness to cooperate with the patient to help solve the problems together.

is in fact used by most experienced clinicians. History taking does not mean asking a series of set questions of every patient, but rather knowing what questions to ask as the differential diagnosis begins to become clearer.

Fundamental considerations when taking the history

As any medical interview proceeds, the clinician should keep in mind four underlying principles:

1 What is the probable diagnosis so far?

   This is a basic differential diagnosis. As you complete the history of the presenting illness, ask yourself: 'For *this* patient based on *these* symptoms and what I know so far, what are the most likely diagnoses?' Then direct additional questions accordingly.

2 Could any of these symptoms represent an urgent or dangerous diagnosis – **red-flag** (alarm) symptoms?

   Such diagnoses may have to be considered and acted upon even though they are not the most likely diagnosis for this patient. For example, the sudden occurrence of breathlessness in an asthmatic who has had surgery this week is more likely to be due to a worsening of asthma than to a pulmonary embolism, but an embolism must be considered because of its urgent seriousness. Ask yourself: 'What diagnoses must not be missed?'

3 Could these symptoms be due to one of the mimicking diseases which can present with a great variety of symptoms in different parts of the body?

   Tuberculosis used to be the great example of this, but HIV infection, syphilis and sarcoidosis are also important disease 'mimickers'. Anxiety and depression commonly present with many somatic symptoms.

4 Is the patient trying to tell me about something more than these symptoms alone?

   Apparently trivial symptoms may be worrying to the patient because of an underlying anxiety about something else. Asking 'What is it that has made you concerned about these problems now?' or 'Is there anything else you want to talk about?' may help to clarify this aspect. Ask the patient 'What else?' as natural breaks occur in the conversation.

Personal history taking

Certain aspects of history taking go beyond routine questioning about symptoms. This part of the art needs to be learnt by taking lots of histories; practice is absolutely essential. With time you will gain confidence in dealing with patients whose medical, psychiatric or cultural situation makes standard questioning difficult or impossible.[5,6]

Most illnesses are upsetting, and can induce feelings of anxiety or depression. On the other hand, patients with primary psychiatric illnesses often present with physical rather than psychological symptoms. This brain–body interaction is bi-directional, and this must be understood as you obtain the story.

Discussion of **sensitive issues** may actually be therapeutic in some cases. '*Sympathetic confrontation*' can be helpful in some situations. For example, if the patient appears sad, angry or frightened, referring to this in a tactful way may lead to the volunteering of appropriate information.

If an emotional response is obtained, use **emotion-handling skills** (**NURS**) to deal with this during the interview (see Table 2.2). *Name* the emotion, show *Understanding*, deal with the issue with great *Respect*, and show *Support* (e.g. 'It makes sense you were angry after you husband left you. This must have been very difficult to deal with. Can I be of any help to you now?').

TABLE 2.2 Emotion-handling skills—NURS
• **N**ame the emotion
• Show **U**nderstanding
• Deal with the issue with **R**espect
• Show **S**upport

There may be reluctance or initial inability on the part of the patient to discuss sensitive problems with a stranger. Here, gaining the patient's confidence is critical. Although this type of history taking can be difficult, it can also be the most satisfying of all interviews, since interviewing can be directly therapeutic for the patient.

Any medical illness may affect the psychological status of a patient. Moreover, pre-existing psychological factors may influence the way a medical problem presents. Psychiatric disease can also present with medical symptoms. Therefore, an essential part of the history-taking process is to obtain information about psychological distress and the mental state. A **sympathetic**, unhurried approach using **open-ended questions** will provide much information that can then be systematically recorded after the interview.

It is important for the history taker to maintain an objective demeanour, particularly when asking about delicate subjects such as sexual problems, grief reactions or abuse. It is not the clinician's role to appear judgmental about patients or their lives.

Questions box 2.1

Personal questions to consider asking a patient

1. Where do you live (e.g. a house, flat or hostel)?
2. What work do you do now, and what have you done in the past?
3. Do you get on well with people at home?
4. Do you get on well with people at work?
5. Do you have any money problems?
6. Are you married or have you been married?
7. Could you tell me about your close relationships?
8. Would you describe your marriage (or living arrangements) as happy?
9. Have you been hit, kicked or physically hurt by someone (physical abuse)?
10. Have you been forced to have sex (sexual abuse)?
11. Would you say you have a large number of friends?
12. Are you religious?
13. Do you feel you are too fat or too thin?
14. Has anyone in the family had problems with psychiatric illness?
15. Have you ever had a nervous breakdown?
16. Have you ever had any psychiatric problem?

Questions box 2.2

Questions to ask the patient who may have depression

1. Have you been feeling sad, down or blue?
2. Have you felt depressed or lost interest in things daily for 2 or more weeks in the past?
3. Have you ever felt like taking your own life?—Risk of self-harm
4. Do you find you wake very early in the morning?
5. Has your appetite been poor recently?
6. Have you lost weight recently?
7. How do you feel about the future?
8. Have you had trouble concentrating on things?
9. Have you had guilty thoughts?
10. Have you lost interest in things you usually enjoy?

Questions box 2.3

Questions to ask the patient who may have anxiety

1. Do you worry excessively about things?
2. Do you have trouble relaxing?
3. Do you have problems getting to sleep at night?
4. Do you feel uncomfortable in crowded places?
5. Do you worry excessively about minor things?
6. Do you feel suddenly frightened, or anxious or panicky, for no reason in situations in which most people would not be afraid?
7. Do you find you have to do things repetitively, such as washing your hands multiple times?
8. Do you have any rituals (such as checking things) that you feel you have to do, even though you know it may be silly?
9. Do you have recurrent thoughts that you have trouble controlling?

The formal psychological or psychiatric interview differs from general medical history taking. It takes considerable time for patients to develop rapport with, and confidence in, the interviewer. There are certain standard questions that may give valuable insights into the patient's state of mind (see *Questions boxes 2.1–2.3*). It may be important to obtain much more detailed information about each of these problems, depending on the clinical circumstances (see Chapter 12).

The sexual history

The sexual history is important, but these questions are not appropriate for all patients, at least not at the first visit when the patient has not yet had time to develop confidence and trust. The patient's permission should be sought before questions of this sort are asked. This request should include some explanation as to why the questions are necessary.[7]

A sexual history is most relevant if there is presentation with a urethral discharge, painful urination (dysuria), vaginal discharge, a genital ulcer or rash, abdominal pain, pain on intercourse (dyspareunia), or anorectal symptoms, or if human immunodeficiency virus (HIV) or hepatitis are suspected.[8]

Ask about the last date of intercourse, number of contacts, homosexual or bisexual partners, and contacts with sex workers. The type of sexual practice may also be important: for example, oro-anal contact may predispose to colonic infection, and rectal contact to hepatitis B or C, or HIV.

It is also often relevant to ask diplomatic and 'matter of fact' questions about a history of sexual abuse. One way to start is: 'You may have heard that some people have been sexually or physically victimised, and this can affect their illness. Has this ever happened to you?' Such events may have important and long-lasting physical and psychological effects.[9]

Accurate answers to some of these questions may not be obtained until the patient has had a number of consultations and has developed trust in the treating doctor. If an answer seems unconvincing, it may be reasonable to ask the question again at a later stage.

Cross-cultural history taking

If the patient's first language is not the same as yours, he or she may find the medical interview very difficult. Maintain eye contact (unless this is considered rude in the cultural context) and be attentive as you ask questions.[10]

If language is an issue, an **interpreter** who is *not* a relative should be used to assist these patients. Some patients may be embarrassed to discuss medical problems in front of a relative, and relatives are often tempted to explain (or change) the patient's answers instead of just translating them. Professional translators are trained to avoid this and can often provide simultaneous and accurate translation, but not all patients feel comfortable with a third person present. It is important to continue to make eye contact with the patient while asking questions, even though it will be the interpreter who responds; otherwise the patient may feel left out of the discussion. Questions should be directed as if going straight to the patient: 'Have you had any problems with shortness of breath?' rather than 'Has he had any breathlessness?' It always takes longer to interview a patient using an interpreter, and more time should be allowed for the consultation.

It is alarmingly common for relatives who accompany patients to interrupt and contradict the patient's version of events even when they are not acting as translators. The interposition of a relative between the clinician and the patient always makes the history taking less direct and the patient's symptoms more subject to 'filtering' or interpretation before the information reaches the clinician. Try tactfully to direct relatives to let the patient answer in his or her own words.

Attitudes to illness and disease vary in different cultures. Problems considered shameful by the patient may be very difficult for him or her to discuss. In some cultures (and increasingly in Australia), women may object to being questioned or examined by male doctors or students. Male students may need to be accompanied by a female chaperone for even the interview with sensitive female patients, and certainly should have one during the physical examination of the patient. It is most important that cultural sensitivities on either side are not allowed to prevent a thorough medical assessment.

Aboriginal patients may have a large extended family. These relatives may be able to provide invaluable support to the patient, but their own medical or social problems may interfere with the patient's ability to manage his or her own health. Commitments to family members may make it difficult for the patient to come to medical appointments or to travel for specialist treatment. Detailed questioning about family contacts and responsibilities may help with the planning of the patient's treatment.

Recent concepts in indigenous health care include the notions of *cultural awareness, cultural sensitivity* and *cultural safety*.[11,12] Cultural awareness can be thought of as the first step towards understanding the rituals, beliefs, customs and practices of a culture. Cultural sensitivity means accepting the importance and roles of these differences. Cultural safety means using this knowledge to protect patients and communities from danger, and making sure that there is a genuine partnership between the health workers and their indigenous patients. These skills have general application for all cultural groups but vary in detail from one to another.

All of these problems require an especially sensitive approach. You as a clinician need to be impartial and objective. Students may need to discuss specific problems with members of the medical faculty and find out what the university and hospital policies are on these matters.

The 'uncooperative' or 'difficult' patient and the history

Most clinical encounters are a cooperative effort on the part of the patient and clinician. The patient wants help to find out what is wrong and to get better. This should make the meeting satisfying and friendly for both parties. However, interviews do not always run smoothly.[13] Resentment may occur on both sides if the patient seems not to be taking the doctor's advice seriously, or will not cooperate with attempts at history taking or examination. Unless there is a serious psychiatric or neurological problem that impairs the patient's judgment, taking or not taking advice remains his or her prerogative. The clinician's role is to give advice and explanation, not to dictate. Indeed, it must be realised that the advice may not always be correct. Keeping this in mind will help prevent that most unsatisfactory and unprofessional of outcomes—becoming angry with the patient.

This approach, however, must not be an excuse for not providing a proper, sympathetic and thorough explanation of the problem and the consequences of ignoring medical advice, to the extent that the patient will allow. A clinician whose advice is rarely accepted should begin to wonder about his or her clinical acumen.

Patients who are **aggressive and uncooperative** may have a medical reason for their behaviour. The possibilities to be considered include alcohol or drug withdrawal, an intracranial lesion such as a tumour or subdural haematoma, or a psychiatric disease such as paranoid schizophrenia. In other cases, resentment at the occurrence of illness may be the problem.

Some patients may seem difficult because they are **too cooperative**. The patient concerned about his blood pressure may have brought printouts of his own blood pressure measurements at half-hour intervals for several weeks. It is important to show restrained interest in these recordings, without encouraging excessive enthusiasm in the patient. Other patients may bring with them information about their symptoms or a diagnosis obtained from the internet. It is important to remember, and perhaps point out, that information obtained in this way may not have been subjected to any form of peer review. People with chronic illnesses, on the other hand, may know more about their conditions than their medical attendants.

Sometimes the interests of the patient and the doctor are not the same. This is especially so in cases where there is the possibility of compensation for an illness or injury. These patients may, consciously or unconsciously, attempt to manipulate the encounter. This is a very difficult situation and can be approached only by rigorous application of clinical methods.

Occasionally, attempted manipulation takes the form of flattery or inappropriate personal interest directed at the clinician. This should be dealt with by carefully maintaining professional detachment. The clinician and the patient must be conscious that their meeting is a professional and not a social one.

History taking for the maintenance of good health

There has never been more public awareness of the influence the way people live has on their health. Most people have some understanding of the dangers of smoking, excessive alcohol consumption and obesity. People have more varied views on what constitutes a healthy diet and exercise regime, and many are ignorant of what constitutes risky sexual activity.

Part of the thorough assessment of patients includes obtaining and conveying some idea of what measures may help them maintain good health (*Questions box 2.4*). This includes a comprehensive approach to the combination of risk factors for various diseases, which is much more important than each individual risk factor. For example, advising a patient about the risk of premature cardiovascular disease will involve knowing about the family history, smoking history, previous and current blood pressure, current and historical cholesterol levels, dietary history, assessment for diabetes mellitus and how much exercise the patient undertakes.

Ask about screening tests being done for any serious illnesses, such as mammograms for breast cancer, Pap smears for cervical cancer or colonoscopy for colon cancer.

The first interview with a patient is an opportunity to make an assessment of the known risk factors for a number of important medical conditions. Even when the patient has come about an unconnected problem, there is often the opportunity for a quick review. Constant matter-of-fact reminding about these can make a great difference to the way people protect themselves from ill-health.

The patient's awareness and understanding of these basic measures for maintaining good health can be assessed throughout the interview. Even when they are unrelated to the presenting problem, serious examples of risky behaviour should be pointed out. This should not be done in an aggressive way. For example, you might say: 'This might be a good time to make a big effort to give up smoking, because it's especially unwise for someone like you with a family history of heart disease.'

Certain questions can be helpful in making a diagnosis of alcoholism; these are referred to as the CAGE questions (see Chapter 1). Another approach is to ask, 'Have you ever had a drinking problem?' and 'Did you have your last drink within the last 24 hours?' The patient who answers 'yes' to both questions is likely to be a high-risk drinker.

Questions box 2.4

Questions related to the maintenance of good health

1 Are you a smoker? When did you stop?
2 Do you know what your cholesterol level is?
3 Do you think you have a healthy diet?
4 Has your blood pressure been high?
5 Have you had diabetes or a raised sugar level?
6 Do you drink alcohol? Every day? How many drinks?
7 Do you do any sort of regular exercise?
8 How much do you weigh? Has your weight changed recently?
9 Do you think you have engaged in any risky sexual activity? What was that?
10 What vaccinations have you had? Include questions about tetanus, influenza, pneumococcal and meningococcal vaccination and *Haemophilus influenzae* (these last three are essential for patients who have had a splenectomy as they are especially vulnerable to infection with these encapsulated organisms), hepatitis A & B, papilloma virus, travel vaccinations
11 Have you had any regular screening for breast cancer or ovarian cancer? (Family history or age over 50 years)
12 Have you had screening for colon cancer screening? What was it? (Age 50+ years or family history of colon cancer or inflammatory bowel disease)
13 Is there a history of inherited diseases, e.g. a family history of sudden death?

The patient's vaccination record should be reviewed regularly and brought up to date when indicated. The dead virus vaccines include influenza and polio (injectable); hepatitis A and B vaccines are recombinant vaccines. Dead bacteria vaccines include the pneumococcal, meningococcal and *H. influenzae* vaccines; tetanus, diphtheria and pertussis are bacterial toxins modified to be non-toxic. The attenuated live-virus vaccines include measles-mumps-rubella (MMR), herpes zoster and influenza (nasal); an attenuated live-bacteria vaccine is bacille Calmette-Guérin (BCG—for tuberculosis). Pregnant women and immunosuppressed people should ***not*** be given attenuated live vaccines. Travel to rural Asia and other exotic places may be an indication for additional vaccinations (e.g. Japanese encephalitis, typhoid).

The elderly patient

Patients who are in their seventies or older present with similar illnesses to younger patients but certain problems are more likely in older patients. History taking should address these potential problems as part of the 'maintenance of good health' aspect of history taking.

Activities of daily living (ADL)

For elderly patients and those with a chronic illness, ask some basic screening questions about **functional activity**.

Ask specific questions about the patient's ability to bathe, walk, use the toilet, eat and dress (ADL). Find out whether the patient needs help to perform these tasks and who provides it. It may be necessary to ask, 'How do you manage?' or 'What do you do about that problem?' Help may come from relatives, neighbours, friends, the health service or charitable organisations. The proximity and availability of these services vary, and more details should be sought. Try to find out whether the patient is happy to accept help or not.

You should also ask questions about the **instrumental activities** of daily living (IADL), such as shopping, cooking and cleaning, the use of transport, and managing money and medications.

Establish whether the patient has ever been assessed by an occupational therapist or whether there has been a 'home visit'. Ask whether alterations been made to the house (e.g. installation of ramps, railings in the bathroom, emergency call buttons, etc.).

Find out who else lives with the patient and how those people seem to be coping with the patient's illness. Obviously, the amount of detail required depends on the severity and chronicity of the patient's illness.

The risk of complications of infections is increased, and most elderly people should have routine influenza vaccinations—ask if vaccinations are up to date.

Mental state

Ask questions that may help to assess cognitive function. Is there a family history of dementia? Has the patient noticed problems with memory or with aspects of life such as paying bills?

Delirium refers to confusion and altered consciousness. Don't confuse this with *dementia*, where consciousness is not altered but there is progressive loss of long-term memory and other cognitive functions. Perform a mini-mental examination (refer to Chapter 12) and record the score.

Specific problems in the elderly

Falls and loss of balance are common and dangerous for these patients. Hip fractures and head injuries are life-threatening events. Ask about falls and near-falls. Does the patient use a stick or a frame? Are there hazards in the house that increase the risk (e.g. steep and narrow stairs)? The use of sedatives like sleeping tablets or anti-anxiety (anxiolytic) drugs and of some anti-hypertensive drugs increases falls risk and must be assessed.

Screening for osteoporosis is recommended for all women over 65 years and all men 70 and older. Risk factors for osteoporosis include being underweight, heavy alcohol use, use of corticosteroids or early menopause, or a history of previous fractures.

General questions about mobility should also include asking about reasons for immobility. These may include arthritis, obesity, general muscle weakness and proximal muscle weakness (sometimes due to corticosteroid use).

Elderly patients may have strong feelings about the extent of treatment they want if their condition deteriorates. These should be recorded before a deteriorating medical illness makes the patient incapable of expressing his or her wishes. This is a difficult area. If a patient expresses a wish not to have certain treatments, the clinician must make very sure that the nature and likely success of these is understood by the patient. For example, a patient who expresses a wish not to be revived if his or her heart stops after a myocardial infarct may not understand that early ventricular fibrillation is almost always successfully treated by cardioversion without long-term sequelae. Patients' decisions must be *informed* decisions.

Polypharmacy (use of four or more regular medications) is a particular problem for old people. Take a detailed drug history and attempt to find out the indications for each of the drugs, and consider possible drug interactions. Find out how the patient manages the medications and whether they seem to be taken accurately. Does the patient use a prepared weekly drug box (a 'Webster pack')?

Evidence-based history taking and differential diagnosis

The principles of evidence-based clinical examination are discussed in the next chapter in more detail, but they also have an application to history taking. The starting point of the differential diagnosis of a certain symptom is the likelihood (or probability) that a certain condition will occur in this person. Most clinicians still rely on their own experience when making this assessment, although some information of disease prevalence in different populations is becoming available. Unfortunately, one person's experience is a relatively small sample, and past experience may bias the clinician in favour of or against a certain diagnosis.

Some diagnoses may largely be excluded from the differential diagnosis list at once. This may be based, for example, on the patient's age, sex or race or the extreme rarity of the disease in a particular country. For example, chronic obstructive pulmonary disease would be very unlikely in a 20-year-old non-smoker who presents with breathlessness.

The differential diagnosis is gradually narrowed as more information about the patient's symptoms comes from the patient directly, and as a result of specific questioning about features of the symptoms that will help to refine the list.

A symptom typical of a certain condition will increase the likelihood of the diagnosis by a certain percentage. If the prevalence of the condition is already high, a high likelihood ratio (LR) should bring that condition towards the top of the differential list. For example, a patient's description of 'typical angina' has a strong LR of 5.8 for the diagnosis of significant coronary artery disease. This would make the diagnosis highly likely in a patient from a population with a high prevalence of coronary disease (e.g. a man over the age of 50 with typical anginal chest pain) but still very unlikely in someone from a very low risk population (e.g. a 19-year-old woman). Likelihood ratios are discussed in more detail in Chapter 3.

The clinical assessment

After the physical examination, the interview with the patient concludes with an assessment by the clinician of what the diagnosis or possible diagnoses are, in order of probability.[14] This will, not unreasonably, be the most important part of the whole process from the patient's point of view.

The explanation must relate to the patient's symptoms or perception of the problem. The clinician should explain how the symptoms and any examination findings relate to the diagnosis. For example, if a patient presents with dyspnoea, the clinician should begin by saying, 'I believe your shortness of breath is probably the result of pneumonia, but there are a few other possibilities'. The complexity of the explanation will depend on the clinician's understanding of the patient's ability to follow any technical aspects of the diagnosis. The patient's desire for a detailed explanation is also variable, and this must be taken into account.

If the diagnosis is fairly definite, then the prognosis and the implications of this must be outlined. A serious diagnosis must be discussed frankly but always in the context of the variability of outcome for most medical conditions and the benefits of correct treatment. When a patient seems unwilling to accept a serious diagnosis and seems likely to decline treatment, the clinician must attempt to find out the reason for the patient's decision. Have there been previous bad experiences with medical treatment, or has a friend or relative had a similar diagnosis and a difficult time with treatment or complications?

Sometimes blunt language may be justified. For example, 'It is important for you to realise that this is a life-threatening illness which needs urgent treatment.' Patients who seem unable to accept advice of this sort should be offered a chance to discuss the matter with another doctor or with their family. This must be done sympathetically: 'This is obviously a difficult time for you. Would you like me to arrange for you to see someone for another opinion about it? Or would you like to come back with some of your family to talk about it again?' The patient's response should be carefully documented in the notes.

Patients may need to be cautioned about certain activities until the condition is treated. For example, a patient with a possible first epileptic seizure must be told that he or she may not legally drive a motor vehicle.

Concluding the interview

After talking to the patient about the assessment and prognosis, the need for investigations and any urgency involved should be discussed. Admission to hospital may be recommended if the problem is a serious one. This may involve major inconvenience to a patient; the clinician must be ready to justify the recommendation and attempt to predict the likely length of stay. If the investigations are onerous or involve risk, this must also be explained and alternatives discussed, if they are available.

If drug treatment is being prescribed, the patient is entitled to know why this is necessary, what it is likely to achieve and what possible important adverse effects might occur. This is a complex topic. On the clinician's part, it requires a comprehensive understanding of drug interactions and adverse effects, as well as an assessment of what it is reasonable to tell a patient without causing alarm or symptoms by suggestion. Patients must at least know what dangerous symptoms should lead to immediate cessation of the drug. Pharmacies often provide patients with long and unedited lists of possible adverse effects when they dispense drugs. Patients may be too frightened to take the prescription unless these are explained at the time of the consultation. Dealing with this difficult area takes time and experience.

There is no shame in telling a patient you will look up possible side-effects and interactions of a drug before you prescribe it or if a patient expresses concern about it. You could say 'I haven't heard of that problem with this drug but let me look it up and check.'

Finally, the patient must be given the opportunity to ask questions. Few people, given a complicated diagnosis, can absorb everything that has been said to them. The patient should be reminded that there will be an opportunity to ask further questions at the next consultation, when the results of tests or the effects of treatment can be assessed.

References

1. Nardone DA, Johnson GK, Faryna A, Coulehan JL, Parrino TA. A model for the diagnostic medical interview: nonverbal, verbal, and cognitive assessments. *J Gen Intern Med* 1992; 7:437–442.
2. Balint J. Brief encounters: speaking with patients. *Ann Intern Med.* 1999; 131:231–234.
3. Simpson M, Buchman R, Stewart M et al. Doctor–patient communication: the Toronto consensus statement. *BMJ* 1991; 303:1385–1387.
4. Stewart MA. Effective physician–patient communication and health outcomes in review. *Can Med Assoc J* 1995; 152:1423–1433. The outcome of an illness can be affected by the first part of the medical intervention, the doctor's history taking.
5. Smith RC, Hoppe RB. The patient's story: integrating the patient- and physician-centered approaches to interviewing. *Ann Intern Med* 1991; 115:470–477. Patients tell stories of their illness, integrating both the medical and psychosocial aspects. Both need to be obtained, and this article reviews ways to do this and to interpret the information.
6. Ness DE, Ende J. Denial in the medical interview: recognition and management. *JAMA* 1994; 272:1777–1781. Denial is not always maladaptive, but can be addressed using appropriate techniques. This is a good guide to the problem and process.
7. Ende J, Rockwell S, Glasgow M. The sexual history in general medicine practice. *Arch Intern Med* 1984; 144:558–561. This study emphasises the importance of obtaining the sexual history as a routine.
8. Furner V, Ross M. Lifestyle clues in the recognition of HIV infection. How to take a sexual history. *Med J Aust* 1993; 158:40–41. This review guides the shy medical student through this difficult task.

9. Drossman DA, Talley NJ, Leserman J et al. Sexual and physical abuse and gastrointestinal illness. *Ann Intern Med* 1995; 123:782–794. Abuse is common, has occurred more often in women, causes a poorer adjustment to illness and usually remains a fact not discussed with the doctor.

10. Qureshi B. How to avoid pitfalls in ethnic medical history, examination, and diagnosis. *J R Soc Med* 1992; 85:65–66. Provides information on transcultural issues, including taboos on anogenital examinations.

11. Ngyuen T. Patient centered care. Cultural safety in indigenous health. *Aust Fam Physician* 2008; 37(12):900–904.

12. Ramsden I. Cultural safety. *N Z Nurs J* 1990; 83:18–19.

13. Groves JE. Taking care of the hateful patient. *N Engl J Med* 1978; 298:833–837. Describes groups of patients that induce negative feelings, and provides important management insights.

14. Hampton JR, Harrison MJG, Mitchell JAR, Pritchard JS, Seymour C. Relative contributions of history-taking, physical examination, and the laboratory to the diagnosis and management of medical outpatients. *BMJ* 1975; 2:486–489. In 66 out of 80 new patients the diagnosis based on the history was correct; physical examination was useful in only 7 patients and laboratory tests in another 7. Take a good history: it's the key to success!

Suggested reading

Billings JA. *The clinical encounter: a guide to the medical interview and case presentation*, 2nd edn. St Louis: Mosby Year Book Medical Publishers, 1999.

Cohen-Cole SA. *The medical interview: the three function approach*, 2nd edn. St Louis: Mosby, 2000.

Coulehan JL, Block MR. *The medical interview: a primer for students of the art*, 4th edn. Philadelphia: FA Davis Company, 2001.

Mysercough PR. *Talking with patients—a basic clinical skill*, 3rd edn. Oxford: Oxford University Press, 1996.

Chapter 3

The general principles of physical examination

More mistakes are made from want of a proper examination than for any other reason.

Russell John Howard (1875–1942)

Students beginning their training in physical examination will be surprised at the formal way this examination is taught and performed.[1,2] There are, however, a number of reasons for this formal approach. The first is that it ensures the examination is thorough and that important signs are not overlooked because of a haphazard method.[3] The second is that the most convenient methods of examining patients in bed, and for particular conditions in various other postures, have evolved with time. By convention, patients are usually examined from the right side of the bed, even though this may be more convenient only for right-handed people. When students learn this, they often feel safer standing on the left side of the bed with their colleagues in tutorial groups, but many tutors are aware of this device, particularly when they notice all students standing as far away from the right side of the bed as possible.

It should be pointed out here that there is only limited evidence-based information concerning the validity of clinical signs. Many parts of the physical examination are performed as a matter of tradition. As students develop their examination skills, experience and new evidence-based data will help them refine their use of examination techniques. We have included information about the established usefulness of signs where it is available, but have also included signs that students will be expected to know about despite their unproven value.

For clinical *viva voce* (with live voice) examinations and objective structured clinical examinations (OSCEs), the examiners expect all candidates to have a polished and thorough examination method.

This formal approach to the physical examination leads to the examination of the parts of the body by **body system**. For example, examination of the cardiovascular system, which includes the heart and all the major accessible blood vessels, begins with positioning the patient correctly. This is followed by a quick general inspection and then, rather surprisingly for the uninitiated, seemingly prolonged study of the patient's fingernails. From there, a set series of manoeuvres brings the doctor to the heart. This type of approach applies to all major systems, and is designed to discover peripheral signs of disease in the system under scrutiny. The attention of the examining doctor is directed particularly towards those systems identified in the history as possibly being diseased, but of course proper physical examination requires that all the systems be examined.

The danger of a systematic approach is that time is not taken to stand back and look at the patient's *general appearance*, which may give many clues to the diagnosis. Doctors must be observant, like a detective (Conan Doyle based his character Sherlock Holmes on an outstanding Scottish surgeon).[4] Taking the time to make an appraisal of the patient's **general appearance**, including the face, hands and body, conveys the impression to the patient (and to the examiners) that the doctor or student is interested in the person as much as the disease. This general appraisal usually occurs at the bedside when patients are in hospital, but for patients seen in the consulting room it should begin as the patient walks into the room and during the history taking, and continue at the start of the physical examination.

Diagnosis has been defined as 'the crucial process

that labels patients and classifies their illnesses, that identifies (and sometimes seals) their likely fates or prognoses and that propels us towards specific treatments in the confidence (often unfounded) that they will do more good than harm'.[5]

In normal clinical practice, the detail of the physical examination performed will be 'targeted' and will depend on clues from the history and whether the consultation is a follow-up or new consultation. Students however must know how to perform a complete examination of the body systems even though they will not often perform this in practice (except perhaps during examinations).

First impressions

First impressions of a patient's condition must be deliberately sought; they cannot be passively acquired. Make a conscious point of assessing the patient's general condition right at the start. The specific changes that occur in particular illnesses (e.g. myxoedema) will be discussed in detail in the appropriate chapters. However, certain abnormalities should be obvious to the trained or training doctor.

First, decide how sick the patient seems to be: that is, does he or she look generally ill or well? The cheerful person sitting up in bed reading Proust (Figure 3.1) is unlikely to require urgent attention to save his life. At the other extreme, the patient on the verge of death may be described as *in extremis* or moribund. The patient in this case may be lying still in bed and seem unaware of the surroundings. The face may be sunken and expressionless, respiration may be shallow and laboured; at the end of life, respiration often becomes slow and intermittent, with longer and longer pauses between rattling breaths.

When a patient walks into the consulting room or undresses for the examination, there is an opportunity to look for problems with mobility and breathlessness.

Apart from gaining a general impression of a patient's state of health, certain general physical signs must be sought.

Vital signs

Certain important measurements must be made during the assessment of the patient. These relate primarily to cardiac and respiratory function, and include pulse, blood pressure, temperature and respiratory rate. For example, an increasing respiratory rate has been shown to be an accurate predictor of respiratory failure.[6] Patients in hospital may have continuous ECG and pulse oximetry monitoring on display on a monitor; these

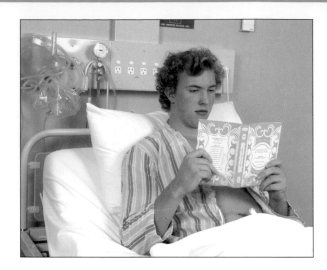

Figure 3.1 'For a long time I used to go to bed early.'

measurements may be considered an extension of the physical examination.

The vital signs must be assessed at once if a patient appears unwell. Patients in hospital have these measurements taken regularly and charted. They provide important basic physiological information.

TABLE 3.1 Some important diagnostic facies
Amiodarone (anti-arrhythmic drug)—deep blue discoloration around malar area and nose
Acromegalic (page 307)
Cushingoid (page 309)
Down syndrome (page 314)
Hippocratic (advanced peritonitis)—eyes are sunken, temples collapsed, nose is pinched with crusts on the lips and the forehead is clammy (page 27)
Marfanoid (page 50)
Mitral (page 57)
Myopathic (page 391)
Myotonic (page 392)
Myxoedematous (prolonged hypothyroidism) (page 305)
Pagetic (page 320)
Parkinsonian (page 396)
Ricketic (page 314)
Thyrotoxic (page 302)
Turner's syndrome (page 314)
Uraemic (page 207)
Virile facies (page 315)

Facies

A specific diagnosis can sometimes be made by inspecting the face, its appearance giving a clue to the likely diagnosis. Other physical signs must usually be sought to confirm the diagnosis. Some facial characteristics are so typical of certain diseases that they immediately suggest the diagnosis, and are called the **diagnostic facies** (Table 3.1 and Figure 3.2). Apart from these, there are several other important abnormalities that must be looked for in the face.

Jaundice

When the serum bilirubin level rises to about twice the upper limit of normal, bilirubin is deposited in the tissues of the body. It then causes yellow discoloration of the skin (*jaundice*) and, more dramatically, the apparent discoloration of the sclerae. The usual term *scleral icterus* is misleading, since the bilirubin is actually deposited in the vascular conjunctiva rather than the avascular sclerae. The sclerae (conjunctivae) are rarely affected by other pigment changes. In fact, jaundice is the only condition causing yellow sclerae. Other causes of yellow discoloration of the skin, but where the sclerae remain normal, are carotenaemia (usually due to excess consumption of carotene, often from intemperate eating of carrots or mangoes), acriflavine, fluorescein and picric acid ingestion.

Jaundice may be the result of excess production of bilirubin, usually from excessive destruction of red blood cells (termed haemolytic anaemia), when it can produce a pale lemon-yellow scleral discoloration. Alternatively, jaundice may be due to obstruction to bile flow from the liver, which, if severe, produces a dark yellow or orange tint. Scratch marks may be prominent due to associated itching (pruritus). The other main cause of jaundice is hepatocellular failure. Gilbert's disease is also a common cause of jaundice. It causes a mild elevation of unconjugated bilirubin and is due to an inherited enzyme deficiency that limits bilirubin conjugation; it has a benign prognosis.

Jaundice is discussed in detail in Chapter 6.

Cyanosis

This refers to a blue discoloration of the skin and mucous membranes; it is due to the presence of deoxygenated haemoglobin in superficial blood vessels. The haemoglobin molecule changes colour from blue to red when oxygen is added to it in the lungs. If more than about 50 g/L of deoxygenated haemoglobin is present in the capillary blood, the skin will have a bluish tinge.[7] Cyanosis does *not* occur in anaemic hypoxia because the total

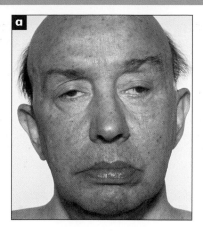

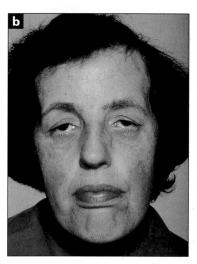

Figure 3.2 Some important diagnostic facies: (a) myopathic; (b) myotonic

(From Mir MA, *Atlas of Clinical Diagnosis*, 2nd edn. Edinburgh: Saunders, 2003, with permission.)

haemoglobin content is low. Cyanosis is more easily detected in fluorescent light than in daylight.

Central cyanosis means that there is an abnormal amount of deoxygenated haemoglobin in the arteries and that a blue discoloration is present in parts of the body with a good circulation, such as the tongue. This must be distinguished from *peripheral cyanosis*, which occurs when the blood supply to a certain part of the body is reduced and the tissues extract more oxygen than normal from the circulating blood: for example, the lips in cold weather are often blue, but the tongue is spared. The presence of central cyanosis should lead one to a careful examination of the cardiovascular (Chapter 4) and respiratory (Chapter 5) systems (see also Table 3.2).

TABLE 3.2 Causes of cyanosis

Central cyanosis

1 Decreased arterial oxygen saturation
   - Decreased concentration of inspired oxygen: high altitude
   - Hypoventilation: coma, airway obstruction
   - Lung disease: chronic obstructive pulmonary disease with cor pulmonale, massive pulmonary embolism
   - Right-to-left cardiac shunt (cyanotic congenital heart disease)
2 Polycythaemia
3 Haemoglobin abnormalities (rare)
   - Methaemoglobinaemia
   - Sulfhaemoglobinaemia

Peripheral cyanosis

1 All causes of central cyanosis cause peripheral cyanosis
2 Exposure to cold
3 Reduced cardiac output: left ventricular failure or shock
4 Arterial or venous obstruction

GOOD SIGNS GUIDE 3.1 Anaemia

Sign	Positive LR*	Negative LR†
Pallor at multiple sites	4.5	0.7
Facial pallor	3.8	0.6
Palm crease pallor	7.9	NS
Conjunctival pallor	16.7	–

* Positive likelihood ratio: when the finding is *present*, describes the probability change. The higher the LR is above 1, the more likely there is disease.
† Negative likelihood ratio: when the finding is *absent*, describes the probability change. The closer the LR is to 0, the more likely there is *not* disease.

NS = not significant.

From McGee S, *Evidence-based physical diagnosis*, 2nd edn. St Louis: Saunders, 2007.

TABLE 3.3 Causes of shock

1 Hypovolaemia
   - External fluid loss, e.g. blood, vomitus, diarrhoea, urine, burns, excess sweating
   - Sequestration of body fluids in the abdomen (e.g. ascites), chest (e.g. haemothorax) or limbs (e.g. fracture)
2 Cardiac
   - Pump failure, e.g. myocardial infarction, acute mitral regurgitation
   - Cardiac tamponade
   - Dissecting aortic aneurysm
   - Arrhythmia
3 Massive pulmonary embolus
4 Sepsis, e.g. gram-negative bacteria (endotoxin)
5 Anaphylaxis
6 Endocrine failure, e.g. adrenal failure, hypothyroidism
7 Neuropathic—from drugs (e.g. antihypertensives, anaesthesia), spinal cord injury of autonomic neuropathy

Pallor

A deficiency of haemoglobin (*anaemia*) can produce pallor of the skin and should be noticeable, especially in the mucous membranes of the sclerae if the anaemia is severe (less than 70 g/L of haemoglobin). Pull the lower eyelid down and compare the colour of the anterior part of the palpebral conjunctiva (attached to the inner surface of the eyelid) with the posterior part where it reflects off the sclera. There is usually a marked difference between the red anterior and creamy posterior parts (see Figure 13.3a, page 425). This difference is absent when significant anaemia is present. Although this is at best a crude way of screening for anaemia, it can be specific (though not sensitive) when anaemia is suspected for other reasons as well (*Good signs guide 3.1*). It should be emphasised that pallor is a sign, while anaemia is a diagnosis based on laboratory results.

Facial pallor may also be found in *shock*, which is usually defined as a reduction of cardiac output such that the oxygen demands of the tissues are not being met (Table 3.3). These patients usually appear clammy and cold and are significantly hypotensive (have low blood pressure) (page 27). Pallor may also be a normal variant due to a deep-lying venous system and opaque skin.

Hair

Bearded or bald women and hairless men not uncommonly present to doctors. These conditions may be a result of more than the rich normal variations of life, and occasionally are due to endocrine disease (Chapter 10).

Weight, body habitus and posture

Look specifically for obesity. This is most objectively assessed by calculation of the body mass index (BMI), where the weight in kilograms is divided by the height in metres squared. Normal is less than 25 kg/m². A BMI of ≥30 indicates frank obesity. *Morbid* obesity is a BMI ≥40. Medical risks are increasingly recognised in association with obesity (Table 3.4).

There are racial differences in BMIs associated with medical risk. Australian Aboriginals and Asians may have increased medical risk once the BMI exceeds 20.

The waist–hip ratio (WHR) is also predictive of health risk. This measurement is of the circumference of the waist (at the midpoint between the costal margin and the iliac crest) divided by that at the hips (at the widest part around the buttocks). Increased risk occurs when this exceeds 1.0 for men and 0.85 for women. Simple waist measurement correlates with the risks of obesity. A female waist circumference of more than 88 cm or male circumference of more than 102 cm indicates increased risk. These measurements can usefully be made repeatedly and recorded.

Severe underweight (BMI <18.5) is called cachexia.[8] Look for wasting of the muscles, which

may be due to neurological or debilitating disease, such as malignancy.

Note excessively short or tall stature, which may be rather difficult to judge when the patient is lying in bed (page 313). Inspect for limb deformity or missing limbs (rather embarrassing if missed in viva voce examinations) and observe if the physique is consistent with the patient's stated chronological age. A number of body shapes are almost diagnostic of different conditions (Table 3.5). If the patient walks into the examining room, the opportunity to examine gait should not be lost: the full testing of gait is described in Chapter 11.

TABLE 3.4 Medical conditions associated with obesity (BMI ≥30)

Endocrine
Type 2 diabetes
Amenorrhoea
Dyslipidaemia
Infertility
Polycystic ovary syndrome
Hypogonadism

Respiratory
Sleep apnoea
Dyspnoea

Cardiovascular
Hypertension
Cardiac failure
Ischaemic heart disease
Cor pulmonale (right heart failure secondary to lung disease)
Pulmonary embolism

Musculoskeletal
Arthritis
Immobility

Skin
Skin abscesses
Cellulitis
Venous stasis
Fungal infections

Gut
Gastro-oesophageal reflux disease
Non-alcoholic steatohepatitis
Hernias

TABLE 3.5 Some body habitus syndromes

Endocrine
Acromegaly (Figure 10.9)
Cushing's syndrome (Figure 10.12)
Hypopituitarism (page 306)
Pseudohypoparathyroidism (Figure 10.14)
Rickets
Paget's disease (Figure 10.24)

Musculoskeletal
Marfan's syndrome (Figure 4.8)
Turner's syndrome
Klinefelter's syndrome (page 316)
Achondroplasia (page 314)

Hydration

Although this is not easy to assess, all doctors must be able to estimate the approximate state of *hydration* of a patient.[9–11] For example, a severely dehydrated patient is at risk of death from developing acute renal failure, while an overhydrated patient may develop pulmonary oedema.

For a traditional assessment of dehydration (Table 3.6), inspect for sunken orbits, dry mucous membranes and the moribund appearance of severe dehydration. Reduced skin turgor (pinch the skin: normal skin returns immediately on being released) occurs in moderate and severe dehydration (this traditional test is not of proven value, especially in the elderly, whose skin may always be like that). The presence of dry axillae increases the likelihood of dehydration and a moist tongue reduces the likelihood, but the other signs are in fact of little proven value (*Good signs guide 3.2*).

Take the blood pressure (page 54) and look for a fall in blood pressure when the patient sits or stands up after lying down. The patient should stand, if he or she can, for at least 1 minute before the blood pressure is taken again (the inability of the patient to stand because of postural dizziness is probably

TABLE 3.6 Classical physical signs of dehydration (of variable reliability—see *Good signs guide 3.2*)

Mild (<5%): = 2.5 L deficit
Mild thirst
Dry mucous membranes
Concentrated urine

Moderate (5%–8%): = 4 L deficit
As above
Moderate thirst
Reduced skin turgor (elasticity), especially arms, forehead, chest, abdomen
Tachycardia

Severe (9%–12%): = 6 L deficit
As above
Great thirst
Reduced skin turgor and decreased eyeball pressure
Collapsed veins, sunken eyes, 'gaunt' face
Postural hypotension
Oliguria (<400 mL urine/24 hours)

Very severe (>12%): >6 L deficit
As above
Comatose
Moribund
Signs of shock

Note: Total body water in a man of 70 kg is about 40 L.

GOOD SIGNS GUIDE 3.2 Hypovolaemia

Sign	Positive LR	Negative LR
Dry axillae	2.8	NS
Dry mucous membranes; nose and mouth	NS	0.3
Sunken eyes	NS	0.5
Confusion	NS	NS
Speech not clear	NS	0.5

NS = not significant.
From McGee S, *Evidence-based physical diagnosis*, 2nd edn. St Louis: Saunders, 2007.

a more important sign than the blood pressure difference). This is called *postural hypotension*. An increase in the pulse rate of 30 or more, when the patient stands, is also a sign of *hypovolaemia*.

Weigh the patient. Following the body weight daily is the best way to determine changes in hydration over time. For example, a 5% decrease in body weight over 24 hours indicates that about 5% of body water has been lost (use the same set of scales).

Assessment of the patient's jugular venous pressure is one of the most sensitive ways of judging intravascular volume overload, or overhydration (see Chapter 4).

The hands and nails

Changes occur in the hands in many different diseases. It is useful as an introduction to shake a patient's hand when meeting him or her. Apart from being polite, this may help make the diagnosis of dystrophia myotonica, a rare muscle disease in which the patient may be unable to let go. Shaking hands is also an acceptable and gentle way of introducing the physical examination. Physical examination is an intrusive event that is tolerated only because of the doctor's (and even the medical student's) professional and cultural standing.

There is probably no subspecialty of internal medicine in which examination of the hands is not rewarding. The shape of the nails may change in some cardiac and respiratory diseases, the whole size of the hand may increase in acromegaly (page 307), gross distortion of the hands' architecture occurs in some forms of arthritis (page 250), tremor or muscle wasting may represent neurological disease (page 354), and pallor of the palmar creases may indicate anaemia (Table 3.7). These and other changes in the hands await you later in the book.

Temperature

The temperature should always be recorded as part of the initial clinical examination of the patient. The normal temperature (in the mouth) ranges from 36.6°C to 37.2°C (98°F to 99°F) (Table 3.8). The rectal temperature is normally higher and the axillary and tympanic temperature lower than the oral temperature (Table 3.8). In very hot weather the temperature may rise by up to 0.5°C. Patients who report they have a fever are usually correct, as is a mother who reports that her child's forehead is warm and that fever is present (*Good signs guide 3.3*).

There is a diurnal variation; body temperature is lowest in the morning and reaches a peak between 6.00 and 10.00 p.m. The febrile pattern of most diseases follows this diurnal variation. The pattern of the fever (pyrexia) may be helpful in diagnosis (Table 3.9).

Very high temperatures (*hyperpyrexia*, defined as above 41.6°C) are a serious problem and may result in death. The causes include heat stroke from exposure or excessive exertion (e.g. in marathon runners), malignant hyperthermia (a group of genetically determined disorders in which hyperpyrexia occurs in response to various anaes-

TABLE 3.7 Nail signs in systemic disease

Nail sign	Some causes	Page no.
Blue nails	Cyanosis, Wilson's disease, ochronosis	25
Red nails	Polycythaemia (reddish-blue), carbon monoxide poisoning (cherry-red)	236
Yellow nails	Yellow nail syndrome	132
Clubbing	Lung cancer, chronic pulmonary suppuration, infective endocarditis, cyanotic heart disease, congenital, HIV infection, chronic inflammatory bowel disease, etc.	50
Splinter haemorrhages	Infective endocarditis, vasculitis	50
Koilonychia (spoon-shaped nails)	Iron deficiency, fungal infection, Raynaud's disease	224
Pale nail bed	Anaemia	224
Onycholysis	Thyrotoxicosis, psoriasis	301
Non-pigmented transverse bands in the nail bed (Beau's lines)	Fever, cachexia, malnutrition	208
Leuconychia (white nails)	Hypoalbuminaemia	159
Transverse opaque white bands (Muehrcke's lines)	Trauma, acute illness, hypoalbuminaemia (also caused by chemotherapy)	208
Single transverse white band (Mees' lines)	Arsenic poisoning, renal failure (also caused by chemotherapy or severe illness)	208
Nailfold erythema and telangiectasia	Systemic lupus erythematosus	282
'Half and half nails' (proximal portion white to pink and distal portion red or brown: Terry's nails)	Chronic renal failure, cirrhosis	208

thetic agents [e.g. halothane] or muscle relaxants [e.g. suxamethonium]), the neuroleptic malignant syndrome, and hypothalamic disease.

Hypothermia is defined as a temperature of less than 35°C. Normal thermometers do not record below 35°C and therefore special low-reading thermometers must be used if hypothermia is suspected. Causes of hypothermia include hypothyroidism and prolonged exposure to cold (page 304).

Smell

Certain medical conditions are associated with a characteristic odour.[12] These include the sickly sweet acetone smell of the breath of patients with ketoacidosis, the sweet smell of the breath in patients with liver failure, the ammoniacal fish breath ('uraemic fetor') of kidney failure and, of course, the stale cigarette smell of the patient who smokes. This smell will be on his or her clothes and even on the referral letter kept in a bag or pocket next to a packet of cigarettes. The recent consumption of alcoholic drinks may be obvious and 'bad breath', although often of uncertain cause, may be related to poor dental hygiene, gingivitis (infection of the gums) or nasopharyngeal tumours. Chronic suppurative infections of the lung can make the breath and saliva foul-smelling. Skin abscesses may be very offensive, especially if caused by anaerobic organisms or *Pseudomonas* spp. Urinary

TABLE 3.8 Average temperature values

	Normal	Fever
Mouth	36.8°C	>37.3°C
Axilla*	36.4°C	>36.9°C
Rectum	37.3°C	>37.7°C

* Tympanic temperatures are similar to axillary ones.

GOOD SIGNS GUIDE 3.3 Fever

Sign	Positive LR	Negative LR
Patient says has fever	4.9	0.2
Warm forehead	2.5	0.4

From McGee S, *Evidence-based physical diagnosis,* 2nd edn. St Louis: Saunders, 2007.

TABLE 3.9 Types of fever

Type	Character	Examples
Continued	Does not remit	Typhoid fever, typhus, drug fever, malignant hyperthermia
Intermittent	Temperature falls to normal each day	Pyogenic infections, lymphomas, miliary tuberculosis
Remittent	Daily fluctuations >2°C, temperature does not return to normal	Not characteristic of any particular disease
Relapsing	Temperature returns to normal for days before rising again	Malaria: Tertian—3-day pattern, fever peaks every other day (*Plasmodium vivax, P. ovale*); Quartan—4-day pattern, fever peaks every 3rd day (*P. malariae*) Lymphoma: Pel-Ebstein* fever of Hodgkin's disease (very rare) Pyogenic infection

* Pieter Pel (1859–1919), Professor of Medicine, Amsterdam; Wilhelm Ebstein (1836–1912), German physician
Note: The use of antipyretic and antibiotic drugs has made these patterns unusual today.

incontinence is associated with the characteristic smell of stale urine, which is often more offensive if the patient has a urinary tract infection. The smell of bacterial vaginosis is usually just described as offensive. Severe bowel obstruction and the rare gastrocolic fistula can cause faecal contamination of the breath when the patient belches. The black faeces (*melaena*) caused by gastric bleeding and the breakdown of blood in the gut has a strong smell, familiar to anyone who has worked in a ward for patients with gastrointestinal illnesses. The metallic smell of fresh blood, sometimes detectable during invasive cardiological procedures, is very mild by comparison.

Preparing the patient for examination

An accurate physical examination is best performed when the examining conditions are ideal. This means that, if possible, the patient should be in a well-lit room (preferably daylight) from which distracting noises and interruptions have been excluded (rarely possible in busy hospital wards). Screens must be drawn around patients before they are examined. Consulting rooms and outpatient clinics should be set up to ensure privacy and comfort for patients.

Patients have a right to expect that students and doctors will have washed their hands or rubbed them with anti-microbial hand sanitisers before they perform an examination. This is as important in clinics and surgeries as in hospital wards. Many hospitals now have notices telling patients that they may ask their doctors if their hands have been washed.

The examination should not begin until permission has been asked of the patient and the nature of the examination has been explained.

The patient must be undressed so that the parts to be examined are accessible. Modesty requires that a woman's breasts be covered temporarily with a towel or sheet while other parts of the body are being examined. Male doctors and students should be accompanied by a female *chaperone* when they examine a woman's pelvis, rectum or breasts. Both men and women should have the groin covered— for example, during the examination of the legs. Outpatients should be provided with a gown to wear. However, important physical signs will be missed in some patients if excessive attention is paid to modesty.

The position of the patient in bed or elsewhere should depend on what system is to be examined. For example, a patient's abdomen is best examined if he or she lies flat with one pillow placed so that the abdominal muscles are relaxed. This is discussed in detail in subsequent chapters.

Within each of the examining systems, four elements comprise the main parts of the physical examination: looking—*inspection*; feeling— *palpation*; tapping—*percussion*; and listening— *auscultation*. For many systems a fifth element, *assessment of function*, is added. *Measuring* is also relevant in some systems. Each of these will be discussed in detail in the following chapters.

Evidence-based clinical examination

History taking and physical examination are latecomers to evidence-based medicine. There are big efforts in all areas of medicine to base practice on evidence of benefit.

By their nature, physical signs tend to be subjective and one examiner will not always agree with another. For example, the loudness of a murmur or the presence or absence of fingernail changes may be controversial. There are often different accepted methods of assessing the presence or absence of a sign, and experienced clinicians will often disagree about whether, for example, the apex beat is in the normal position or not. Even apparently objective measurements such as the blood pressure can vary depending on whether Korotkov sound IV or V (page 55) is used, and from minute to minute for the same patient. Some physical signs are present only intermittently; the pericardial rub may disappear before students can be found in the games room to come and listen to it.

A way of looking at the usefulness of a sign or a test is to measure or estimate its *specificity* and *sensitivity*.

- The specificity of a sign is the proportion of people *without* the disease who do *not* have the sign ('negative in health').[5] For example, an 80% specificity means that 8 out of 10 people *without* that sign *do not have* the condition.
- The sensitivity of a sign is the proportion of people *with* the disease who *have* the sign— that is, those who are correctly identified by the test ('positive in disease').[5] A sensitivity of 80% means that assessment of the presence of that sign will pick up 80% of people with the condition (but will not pick up 20%).

You may find it helpful to use the following mnemonics to help you remember this: **SpIn** = *Specific* tests when *positive* help to rule *In* disease and **SnOut** = *Sensitive* tests when *negative* help rule *Out* disease.

The perfect test or sign (if there were such a thing) is 100% sensitive and specific. A sign or test that is present or 'positive' in a person who does not have the condition is called a *false positive*. The absence of a sign, or a negative test, in a patient who has the condition is called a *false negative*. Another way of looking at this is the positive or negative predictive value of a test—that is, the probability that a positive result means the condition is present or that a negative result means it is absent.

The likelihood that a test or sign result will be a true positive or negative depends on the pre-test probability of the presence of the condition. For example, if splinter haemorrhages (page 50) are found in the nails of a well manual labourer they are likely to represent a false positive sign of infective endocarditis. This sign is not very sensitive or specific and in this case the pre-test probability

of the condition is low. If splinters are found in a sick patient with known valvular heart disease and a new murmur, the sign is likely to be a true positive in this patient with a high pre-test probability of endocarditis. This pre-test probability analysis of the false and true positive rate is based on Bayes' theorem.

A useful way to look at sensitivity and specificity is the **likelihood ratio** (LR). A positive LR,

$$\text{Positive LR} = \frac{\text{sensitivity}}{1 - \text{specificity}}$$

indicates that the presence of a sign is likely to occur that much more often in an individual with the disease than in one without it. The higher the positive LR, the more useful is a positive sign. A negative likelihood ratio increases the likelihood that the disease is absent if the sign is not present.

$$\text{Negative LR} = \frac{1 - \text{sensitivity}}{\text{specificity}}$$

Remember that if the LR is greater than 1 there is an increased probability of disease; if the LR is less than 1 there is a decreased probability of disease.

For example, the presence of a third heart sound in a patient who might have heart failure (e.g. breathlessness on exertion) has a positive likelihood ratio of 3.8 and a negative LR around 1. This means that a third heart sound is specific for heart failure (increases likelihood of the condition nearly four times) but not sensitive (the absence of a third heart sound does not reduce the likelihood).

All these figures are calculated on a population suspected of disease; it would be quite incorrect to apply them to an asymptomatic group of people. Fagan's nomogram (Figure 3.3) can be used to apply LRs to clinical problems if the pre-test probability of the condition is known or can be estimated. Remember, positive LRs of 2, 5 and 10 increase the probability of disease by 15%, 30% and 45%, respectively. Similarly, negative LRs of 0.5, 0.2 and 0.1 decrease the probability of disease by 15%, 30% and 45% respectively.

When the pre-test probability is very low, even a high positive LR does not make the disease very likely. A line is drawn from the pre-test probability number through the known LR and ends up on the post-test probability number. For example, if the pre-test probability of the condition is low, say 10 (10%) and a sign is present which has an LR of 2, the post-test probability of the condition being present is only about 20%. We have included the LRs in tables of *Good signs guides* in most chapters of this book.

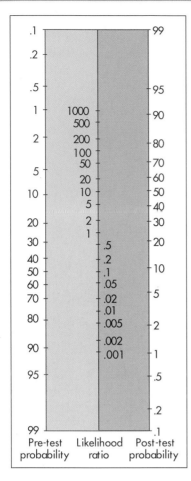

Figure 3.3 Fagan's nomogram for interpreting a diagnostic test result
(Adapted from Sackett DL, Richardson WS, Rosenberg W, Haynes RB. *Evidence-based medicine: how to practice and teach EBM*. Churchill-Livingstone: London, 1997.)

TABLE 3.10 Important reasons for inter-observer disagreement

1 The sign comes and goes; e.g. basal crackles in heart failure, a fourth heart sound

2 Some of the observers' technique may be imperfect; e.g. not asking the patient to cough before declaring the presence of lung crackles consistent with heart failure

3 Some signs are intrinsically subjective; e.g. the grading of the loudness of a murmur

4 Preconceptions about the patient based on other observations or the history may influence the observer; e.g. goitre may seem readily palpable when a patient is known to have thyroid disease

5 The examination conditions may not be ideal; e.g. attempting to listen to the heart in a noisy clinic when the patient is sitting in a chair and not properly undressed

Inter-observer agreement (reliability) and the κ-statistic

The LR of a sign assumes that the sign is present but there is considerable variability in the agreement between observers about the presence of many signs. There are a number of reasons for this low reliability (Table 3.10).

The κ (kappa) statistic is a way of expressing the inter-observer variation for a sign or test. Values are between 0 and 1, where 0 means the agreement about the sign is the same as it would be by chance and 1 means complete (100%) agreement. Occasionally values of less than 0 are obtained when inter-observer agreement is worse than should occur by chance. By convention a κ-value of 0.8 to 1 means almost or perfect agreement, 0.6 to 0.8 substantial agreement, 0.2 to 0.4 fair agreement, and 0 to 0.2 slight agreement. A selection of signs and their κ-values is listed in Table 3.11. Remember that a high κ-value means agreement about the presence of a sign, *not* that the sign necessarily has a high LR. A low κ-value may be an indication that the sign is a difficult one to elicit accurately, especially for beginners, but it does not always mean that the sign is not useful.

Although some of these values appear low, κ-values for the reporting of a number of diagnostic tests have also been calculated and are not much more impressive—e.g. the reporting of cardiomegaly on a chest X-ray is 0.48, while cholestasis reported on a liver biopsy is 0.40.

In medical practice, multiple factors are taken into account when diagnostic decisions are made. Only very rarely is one symptom or sign or test diagnostic of a condition. The evidence supporting the usefulness of most signs is based on looking at the sign in isolation. It is much more difficult to study the combined importance of the range of historical and physical findings that are present. However, the skilled and experienced clinician uses many pieces of information and is sceptical when an unexpected or illogical finding or test result is obtained.

References

1. Sacket DL. The science of the art of clinical examination. *JAMA* 1992; 267:2650–2652. Examines the limitations of current research in the field of clinical examination.
2. Sackett DL. A primer on the precision and accuracy of the clinical examination (the rational clinical examination). *JAMA* 1992; 267:2638–2644. An important article examining the relevance of understanding both precision (reproducibility among various examiners) and accuracy

TABLE 3.11 Selected signs and their kappa (κ) values

	κ-value		κ-value
Skin		**Heart**	
Jaundice	0.65	Third heart sound	−0.17−+0.75
Cyanosis	0.36−0.70	Systolic murmur present or absent; >2/6	0.19; 0.59
Palmar erythema	0.37−0.49	Abdominojugular test	0.92
Hydration		Neck veins elevated or normal	0.38−0.69
Axillary dryness	0.50	**Abdomen**	
Patient appears dehydrated	0.44−0.53	Abdominal distension	0.35−0.42
Vital signs		Ascites	0.63−0.75
Tachycardia (>100/min)	0.85	Guarding	0.36−0.49
Bradycardia (<60/min)	0.87	Palpable spleen	0.33−0.75
Tachypnoea	0.25−0.60	Palpable liver edge	0.44−0.53
Goitre	0.38−0.77	Liver span by percussion > 9cm	0.11
Lungs		**Extremities**	
Clubbing	0.33−0.45	Peripheral pulse present or absent	0.52−0.92
Displaced trachea	0.01	Peripheral pulse normal or reduced	0.01−0.15
Decreased tactile fremitus	0.24	Oedema	0.39
Increased tactile fremitus	0.01	Shoulder: painful arc	0.64
Hyper-resonant percussion note	0.26−0.50	**Knee**	
Dull percussion note	0.16−0.52	Effusion	0.28−0.59
Reduced breath sounds	0.16−0.51	McMurray's sign	0.16−0.35
Bronchial breathing	0.19−0.32	**Neurological**	
Crackles	0.21−0.63	Pharyngeal sensation present or absent	1.0
Wheezes	0.43−0.93	Facial weakness present or absent	0.47
Pleural rub	0.51	Dysarthria present or absent	0.61−0.77
Forced expiratory time	0.27−0.70	Muscle strength (MRC scale)	0.69−0.93
Hoover's sign	0.74	Light touch sensation normal, increased or reduced	0.63
		Vibration sense normal, increased or diminished	0.45−0.54

Adapted with permission from McGee S, *Evidence-based physical diagnosis*, 2nd edn. St Louis: Saunders, 2007.

(determining the truth) in clinical examination.

3. Wiener S, Nathanson M. Physical examination: frequently observed errors. *JAMA* 1976; 236:852–855. This article categorises errors, including poor skills, under-reporting and over-reporting of signs, use of inadequate equipment and inadequate recording.

4. Fitzgerald FT, Tierney LM Jr. The bedside Sherlock Holmes. *West J Med* 1982; 137:169–175. Here deductive reasoning is discussed as a tool in clinical diagnosis.

5. Sackett DL, Haynes RB, Tugwell P. *Clinical epidemiology. A basic science for clinical medicine.* Boston: Little, Brown & Co, 1985. The perceived commonness of diseases affects our approach to their diagnosis.

6. Cretikos MA, Bellomo R, Hillman K, Chen J, Finfer S, Flabouris A. Respiratory rate: the neglected vital sign. *Med J Aust* 2008;188(11):657-659.

7. Martin L, Khalil H. How much reduced hemoglobin is necessary to generate central cyanosis? *Chest* 1990; 97:182–185. This useful article explains the chemistry of haemoglobin and its colour change.

8. Detsky AS, Smalley PS, Chang J. Is this patient malnourished? *JAMA* 1994; 271:54–58. Assessment

of nutrition is an important part of the examination but needs a scientific approach.

9. Gross CR, Lindquist RD, Woolley AC, et al. Clinical indicators of dehydration severity in elderly patients. *J Emerg Med* 1992; 10:267–274. This important and urgent assessment is more difficult in elderly sick patients.

10. Koziol-McLain J, Lowenstein SR, Fuller B. Orthostatic vital signs in emergency medicine department patients. *Ann Emerg Med* 1991; 20:606–610. These signs help in the assessment of the severity of illness in emergency patients but there is a wide range of normal.

11. McGee S, Abernethy WB III, Simel DL. Is this patient hypovolemic? *JAMA* 1999, 281.1022–1029. The most sensitive clinical features for large-volume blood loss are severe postural dizziness and a postural rise in pulse rate of >30 beats a minute, not tachycardia or supine hypotension. A dry axilla supports dehydration. Moist mucous membranes and a tongue without furrows make hypovolaemia unlikely; assessing skin turgor, surprisingly, is not of proven value.

12. Hayden GF. Olfactory diagnosis in medicine. *Postgrad Med* 1980; 67:110–115, 118. Describes characteristic patient odours and their connections with disease, although the diagnostic accuracy is uncertain.

Suggested reading

Beaven DW. *Color atlas of the nail in clinical diagnosis*, 3rd edn. Chicago: Mosley Year Book 1996.

Browse NL. *An introduction to the symptoms and signs of surgical disease*, 4th edn. London: Edward Arnold, 2005.

Joshua AM, Celermajer DS, Stockler MR. Beauty is in the eye of the examiner: reaching agreement about physical signs and their value. *Intern Med J* 2005; 35:178–187.

Lumley JJP, ed. *Hamilton Bailey's demonstrations of physical signs in clinical surgery*, 18th edn. Oxford: Butterworth-Heinemann, 1997.

McGee S. *Evidence-based physical diagnosis*, 2nd edn. St Louis: Saunders, 2007.

McHardy KC et al. *Illustrated signs in clinical medicine*. Edinburgh: Churchill-Livingstone, 1997.

Orient JM. *Sapira's art and science of bedside diagnosis*, 3rd edn. Baltimore: Lippincott, Williams & Wilkins, 2005.

Schneiderman H, Peixoto AJ. *Bedside diagnosis. An annotated bibliography of literature on physical examination and interviewing*, 3rd edn. Philadelphia: American College of Physicians, 1997. A superb summary of the evidence base for clinical examination.

Zatouroff M. *Color atlas of physical signs in general medicine*, 2nd edn. Chicago: Mosby Year Book, 1996.

Chapter 4
The cardiovascular system

The heart ... moves of itself and does not stop unless for ever.

Leonardo da Vinci (1452–1519)

This chapter deals with the history and the examination of the heart and blood vessels, as well as other parts of the body where symptoms and signs of heart disease may appear. Not only is this fundamental to the assessment of any patient, but it is also an extremely common system tested in viva voce examinations. It is believed by cardiologists to be the most important system in the body.

The cardiovascular history
Presenting symptoms (Table 4.1)
Chest pain

The mention of chest pain by a patient tends to provoke more urgent attention than other symptoms. The surprised patient may find himself whisked into an emergency ward with the rapid appearance of worried-looking doctors. This is because ischaemic heart disease, which may be a life-threatening condition, often presents in this manner (Table 4.2). The pain of *angina* and *myocardial infarction* tends to be similar in character; it may be due to the accumulation of metabolites from ischaemic muscle following complete or partial obstruction of a coronary artery, leading to stimulation of the cardiac sympathetic nerves.[1,2] Patients with cardiac transplants who develop coronary disease in the transplanted heart may not feel angina, presumably because the heart is denervated. Similarly, patients with diabetes are more likely to be diagnosed with 'silent infarcts'.

To help determine the cause of chest pain, it is important to ascertain the duration, location, quality, and precipitating and aggravating factors (the **four cardinal features**), as well as means

---

TABLE 4.1 Cardiovascular history

Major symptoms
Chest pain or heaviness
Dyspnoea: exertional (note degree of exercise necessary), orthopnoea, paroxysmal nocturnal dyspnoea
Ankle swelling
Palpitations
Syncope
Intermittent claudication
Fatigue

Past history
History of ischaemic heart disease: myocardial infarction, coronary artery bypass grafting
Rheumatic fever, chorea, sexually transmitted disease, recent dental work, thyroid disease
Prior medical examination revealing heart disease (e.g. military, school, insurance)
Drugs

Social history
Tobacco and alcohol use
Occupation

Family history
Myocardial infarcts, cardiomyopathy, congenital heart disease, mitral valve prolapse, Marfan's syndrome

Coronary artery disease risk factors
Previous coronary disease
Smoking
Hypertension
Hyperlipidaemia
Family history of coronary artery disease
Diabetes mellitus
Obesity and physical inactivity
Male sex and advanced age
Raised homocysteine levels

Functional status in established heart disease
Class I—disease present but no symptoms, or angina* or dyspnoea† during unusually intense activity
Class II—angina or dyspnoea during ordinary activity
Class III—angina or dyspnoea during less than ordinary activity
Class IV—angina or dyspnoea at rest

* Canadian Cardiovascular Society (CCVS) classification
† New York Heart Association (NYHA) classification

TABLE 4.2 Causes (differential diagnosis) of chest pain and typical features

Pain	Causes	Typical features
Cardiac pain	Myocardial ischaemia or infarction	Central, tight or heavy; may radiate to the jaw or left arm
Vascular pain	Aortic dissection	Very sudden onset, radiates to the back
	Aortic aneurysm	
Pleuropericardial pain	Pericarditis +/– myocarditis	Pleuritic pain, worse when patient lies down
	Infective pleurisy	Pleuritic pain
	Pneumothorax	Sudden onset, sharp, associated with dyspnoea
	Pneumonia	Often pleuritic, associated with fever and dyspnoea
	Autoimmune disease	Pleuritic pain
	Mesothelioma	Severe and constant
	Metastatic tumour	Severe and constant, localised
Chest wall pain	Persistent cough	Worse with movement, chest wall tender
	Muscular strains	Worse with movement, chest wall tender
	Intercostal myositis	Sharp, localised, worse with movement
	Thoracic zoster	Severe, follows nerve root distribution, precedes rash
	Coxsackie B virus infection	Pleuritic pain
	Thoracic nerve compression or infiltration	Follows nerve root distribution
	Rib fracture	History of trauma, localised tenderness
	Rib tumour, primary or metastatic	Constant, severe, localised
	Tietze's syndrome	Costal cartilage tender
Gastrointestinal pain	Gastro-oesophageal reflux	Not related to exertion, may be worse when patient lies down—common
	Diffuse oesophageal spasm	Associated with dysphagia
Airway pain	Tracheitis	Pain in throat, breathing painful
	Central bronchial carcinoma	
	Inhaled foreign body	
Other causes	Panic attacks	Often preceded by anxiety, associated with breathlessness and hyperventilation
Mediastinal pain	Mediastinitis	
	Sarcoid adenopathy, lymphoma	

of relief and accompanying symptoms (the SOCRATES questions; see Chapter 1).[3]

The term **angina**[a] was coined by Heberden from the Greek and Latin words meaning 'choking' or strangling; and the patient may complain of crushing pain, heaviness, discomfort or a choking sensation in the retrosternal area or in the throat. It is best to ask if the patient experiences chest 'discomfort' rather than 'pain', because angina is often dull and aching in character and may not be perceived as pain.

The pain or discomfort is usually central rather

---

a   William Heberden's (1710–1801) description of angina (1768) is difficult to improve upon: 'They who are afflicted with it, are seized while they are walking (more especially if it be up hill and soon after eating) with a painful and most disagreeable sensation in the breast, which seems as if it would extinguish life, if it were to increase or continue; but the moment they stand still, all this uneasiness vanishes.'

Questions box 4.1

Questions to ask the patient with suspected angina

! denotes symptoms for the possible diagnosis of an urgent or dangerous problem.

1 Can you tell me what the pain or discomfort is like? Is it sharp or dull, heavy or tight?

2 When do you get the pain? Does it come out of the blue, or come on when you do physical things? Is it worse if you exercise after eating?

3 How long does it last?

4 Where do you feel it?

5 Does it make you stop or slow down?

6 Does it go away quickly when you stop exercising?

! 7 Is it coming on with less effort or at rest?—Unstable symptoms

8 Have you had angina before, and is this the same?

TABLE 4.3 Clinical classification of angina from the European Society of Cardiology

Typical angina	Meets all 3 of the following characteristics:
	1 Characteristic retrosternal chest discomfort—typical quality and duration
	2 Provoked by exertion or emotion
	3 Relieved by rest or GTN (glyceryl trinitrate) or both
Atypical angina	Meets 2 of the above characteristics
Non-cardiac chest pain	Meets 1 or none of the above characteristics

continuously for many days is unlikely to be either. Associated symptoms of myocardial infarction include dyspnoea, sweating, anxiety, nausea and faintness.

Other causes of retrosternal pain are listed in Table 4.2. Chest pain made worse by inspiration is called *pleuritic pain*. This may be due to pleurisy (page 110) or pericarditis (page 78). Pleurisy may occur because of inflammation of the pleura as a primary problem (usually due to viral infection), or secondary to pneumonia or pulmonary embolism. Pleuritic pain is not usually brought on by exertion and is often relieved by sitting up and leaning forwards. It is caused by the movement of inflamed pleural or pericardial surfaces on one another.

Chest wall pain is usually localised to a small area of the chest wall, is sharp and is associated with respiration or movement of the shoulders rather than with exertion. It may last only a few seconds or be present for prolonged periods. Disease of the *cervical or upper thoracic spine* may also cause pain associated with movement. This pain tends to radiate around from the back towards the front of the chest.

Pain due to a *dissecting aneurysm* of the aorta is usually very severe and may be described as tearing. This pain is usually greatest at the moment of onset and radiates to the back. These three features—quality, rapid onset and radiation—are very specific for aortic dissection. A proximal dissection causes anterior chest pain and involvement of the descending aorta causes interscapular pain. A history of hypertension or of a connective tissue disorder such as Marfan's syndrome or Ehlers-Danlos syndrome puts the patient at increased risk of this condition.

Massive pulmonary embolism causes pain of very sudden onset which may be retrosternal and associated with collapse, dyspnoea and cyanosis

than left-sided. The patient may dismiss his or her pain as non-cardiac because it is not felt over the heart on the left side. It may radiate to the jaw or to the arms, but very rarely travels below the umbilicus. The severity of the pain varies.

Angina characteristically occurs with exertion, with rapid relief once the patient rests or slows down. The amount of exertion necessary to produce the pain may be predictable to the patient. A change in the pattern of onset of previously stable angina must be taken very seriously.

These features constitute *typical angina* (Table 4.3).[4] Although angina typically occurs on exertion, it may also occur at rest or wake a patient from sleep. Ischaemic chest pain is usually unaffected by respiration. The use of sublingual nitrates characteristically brings relief within a couple of minutes, but this is not specific as nitrates may also relieve oesophageal spasm and also have a pronounced placebo effect.

The pain associated with an acute coronary syndrome (myocardial infarction or unstable angina) often comes on at rest, is usually more severe and lasts much longer. Acute coronary syndromes are usually caused by the rupture of a coronary artery plaque which leads to the formation of thrombus in the arterial lumen. Stable exertional angina is a result of a fixed coronary narrowing. Pain present for more than half an hour is more likely to be due to an acute coronary syndrome than to stable angina, but pain present

TABLE 4.4A Differential diagnosis of chest pain		
Favours angina	**Favours pericarditis or pleurisy**	**Favours oesophageal pain**
Tight or heavy	Sharp or stabbing	Burning
Onset predictable with exertion	Not exertional	Not exertional
Relieved by rest	Present at rest	Present at rest
Relieved rapidly by nitrates	Unaffected	Unaffected unless spasm
Not positional	Worse supine (pericarditis)	Onset may be when supine
Not affected by respiration	Worse with respiration Pericardial or pleural rub	Unaffected by respiration

TABLE 4.4B Differential diagnosis of chest pain	
Favours myocardial infarction (acute coronary syndrome)	**Favours angina**
Onset at rest	Onset with exertion
May be severe	Less severe
Sweating	No sweating
Anxiety (angor)	Mild or no anxiety
No relief with nitrates	Rapid relief with nitrates
Associated symptoms (nausea and vomiting)	Associated symptoms absent
Favours myocardial infarction	**Favours aortic dissection**
Central chest pain	Radiates to back
Subacute onset (minutes)	Instantaneous onset
May be severe	Very severe
Favours myocardial ischaemia	**Favours chest wall pain**
Exertional	Positional
Occurs with exertion	Often worse at rest
Brief episodes	Prolonged
Diffuse	Localised
No chest wall tenderness (only discriminates between infarction and chest wall pain)	Chest wall tenderness

(page 136). It is often pleuritic, but can be identical to anginal pain, especially if associated with right ventricular ischaemia.

Spontaneous pneumothorax may result in pain and severe dyspnoea (page 132). The pain is sharp and localised to one part of the chest.

Gastro-oesophageal reflux can quite commonly cause angina-like pain without heartburn. It is important to remember that these two relatively common conditions may co-exist. *Oesophageal spasm* may cause retrosternal chest pain or discomfort and can be quite difficult to distinguish from angina, but is rare. The pain may come on after eating or drinking hot or cold fluids, may be associated with dysphagia (difficulty swallowing) and may be relieved by nitrates.

Cholecystitis can cause chest pain and be confused with myocardial infarction. Right upper quadrant abdominal tenderness is usually present (page 170).

The cause of severe, usually unilateral, chest pain may not be apparent until the typical vesicular rash of *herpes zoster* appears in a thoracic nerve root distribution.

Dyspnoea

Shortness of breath may be due to cardiac disease. Dyspnoea (Greek *dys* 'bad', *pnoia* 'breathing') is often defined as an unexpected awareness of breathing. It occurs whenever the work of breathing is excessive, but the mechanism is uncertain. It is probably due to a sensation of increased force required of the respiratory muscles to produce a volume change in the lungs, because of a reduction in compliance of the lungs or increased resistance to air flow. Cardiac dyspnoea is typically chronic and occurs with exertion because of failure of the left ventricular output to rise with exercise; this in turn leads to an acute rise in left ventricular end-diastolic pressure, raised pulmonary venous pressure, interstitial fluid leakage and thus reduced lung compliance. However, the dyspnoea of chronic cardiac failure does not correlate well with measurements of pulmonary artery pressures, and clearly the origin of the symptom of cardiac dyspnoea is complicated.[5] Left ventricular function may be impaired because of ischaemia (temporary or permanent reduction in myocardial blood supply), previous infarction (damage) or hypertrophy (often related to hypertension). As it becomes more severe, cardiac dyspnoea occurs at rest.

Orthopnoea (from the Greek *ortho* 'straight'; see Table 4.5), or dyspnoea that develops when a patient is supine, occurs because in an upright position the patient's interstitial oedema is redistributed; the lower zones of the lungs become worse and the upper zones better. This allows improved overall blood oxygenation. Patients with severe orthopnoea spend the night sitting up in a chair or propped up on numerous pillows in bed. The absence of orthopnoea suggests that left ventricular failure is unlikely to be the cause of a patient's dyspnoea (negative likelihood ratio [LR] = 0.04[6]).

TABLE 4.5 Causes of orthopnoea
Cardiac failure
Uncommon causes
Massive ascites
Pregnancy
Bilateral diaphragmatic paralysis
Large pleural effusion
Severe pneumonia

Paroxysmal[b] *nocturnal dyspnoea* (PND) is severe dyspnoea that wakes the patient from sleep so that he or she is forced to get up gasping for breath. This occurs because of a sudden failure of left ventricular output with an acute rise in pulmonary venous and capillary pressures; this leads to transudation of fluid into the interstitial tissues, which increases the work of breathing. The sequence may be precipitated by resorption of peripheral oedema at night while supine. Acute cardiac dyspnoea may also occur with acute pulmonary oedema or a pulmonary embolus.

Cardiac dyspnoea can be difficult to distinguish from that due to lung disease or other causes (page 109)[7]. One should inquire particularly about a history of any cardiac disease that could be responsible for the onset of cardiac failure. For example, a patient with a number of known previous myocardial infarctions who develops dyspnoea is more likely to have decreased left ventricular contractility. A patient with a history of hypertension or a very heavy alcohol intake may have hypertensive heart disease or an alcoholic cardiomyopathy. The presence of orthopnoea or paroxysmal nocturnal dyspnoea is more suggestive of cardiac failure than of lung disease.

Dyspnoea is also a common symptom of anxiety. These patients often describe an inability to take a big enough breath to fill the lungs in a satisfying way. Their breathing may be deep and punctuated with sighs.

Ankle swelling

Some patients present with bilateral ankle swelling due to *oedema* from cardiac failure. Patients with the recent onset of oedema and who take a serious interest in their weight may have noticed a gain in weight of 3 kg or more. Ankle oedema of cardiac origin is usually symmetrical and worst in the evenings, with improvement during the night. It may be a symptom of biventricular failure or right ventricular failure secondary to a number of possible underlying aetiologies. As failure progresses, oedema ascends to involve the legs, thighs, genitalia and abdomen. There are usually other symptoms or signs of heart disease.

It is important to find out whether the patient is taking a vasodilating drug (e.g. a calcium channel blocker), which can cause peripheral oedema. There are other (more) common causes of ankle oedema than heart failure that also need to be considered (page 71). Oedema that affects the face is more likely to be related to nephrotic syndrome (page 213).

Palpitations

This is not a very precise term. It is usually taken to mean an unexpected awareness of the heartbeat.[8] Ask the patient to describe exactly what he or she notices and whether the palpitations are slow or fast, regular or irregular, and how long they last (*Questions box 4.2*).

There may be the sensation of a missed beat followed by a particularly heavy beat; this can be due to an *atrial* or *ventricular ectopic beat* (which produces little cardiac output) followed by a compensating pause and then a normally conducted beat (which is more forceful than usual because there has been a longer diastolic filling period for the ventricle).

If the patient complains of a rapid heartbeat, it is important to find out whether the palpitations are of sudden or gradual onset and offset. Cardiac arrhythmias are usually instantaneous in onset and offset, whereas the onset and offset of *sinus tachycardia* is more gradual. A completely irregular rhythm is suggestive of *atrial fibrillation*, particularly if it is rapid.

It may be helpful to ask the patient to tap the rate and rhythm of the palpitations with his or her finger. Associated features including pain, dyspnoea or faintness must be inquired about. The awareness of rapid palpitations followed by syncope suggests *ventricular tachycardia*. These patients usually have a past history of significant heart disease. Any rapid rhythm may precipitate angina in a patient with ischaemic heart disease.

---

b   Paroxysmal symptoms or signs occur suddenly and intermittently.

TABLE 4.6 Causes (differential diagnosis) of dyspnoea, palpitations and oedema

Favours heart failure	Favours lung disease
History of myocardial infarction	History of smoking
	Onset after some exertion (asthma)
No wheeze	Wheezing
PND	PND absent
Orthopnoea	Orthopnoea absent
Abnormal apex beat	
Third heart sound (S3)	
Mitral regurgitant murmur	
	Overexpanded chest
	Pursed-lips breathing
Early and mid-inspiratory crackles	Fine end-inspiratory crackles
Cough only on lying down	Productive cough

Palpitations differential diagnosis		Ankle oedema differential diagnosis
Feature	**Suggests**	**Favours heart failure**
Heart misses and thumps	Ectopic beats	History of cardiac failure
Worse at rest	Ectopic beats	Other symptoms of heart failure
Very fast, regular	SVT (VT)	Jugular venous pressure elevated (+ve LR 9.0*)
Instantaneous onset	SVT (VT)	**Favours hypoproteinaemia**
Offset with vagal manoeuvres	SVT	Jugular venous pressure normal
Fast and irregular	AF	Oedema pits and refills rapidly, 2–3s†
Forceful and regular—not fast	Awareness of sinus rhythm (anxiety)	**Favours deep venous thrombosis or cellulitis**
		Unilateral
Severe dizziness or syncope	VT	Skin erythema
Pre-existing heart failure	VT	Calf tenderness
		Favours drug-induced oedema
		Patient takes calcium channel blocker
		Favours lymphoedema
		Not worse at end of day
		Not pitting when chronic
		Favours lipoedema
		Not pitting
		Spares foot
		Obese woman

PND = paroxysmal nocturnal dyspnoea.
SVT = supraventricular tachycardia.
VT = ventricular tachycardia.
AF = atrial fibrillation.
* McGee S, *Evidence-based clinical diagnosis*, 2nd edn. St Louis: Saunders, 2007.
† Khan NA, Rahim SA, Avand SS et al. Does the clinical examination predict lower extremity peripheral arterial disease? *JAMA* 2006 Feb 1; 295(5):536–546.

TABLE 4.7 Differential diagnosis of syncope and dizziness

Favours vasovagal syncope (most common cause)

Onset in teens or 20s

Occurs in response to emotional distress, e.g. sight of blood

Associated with nausea and clamminess

Injury uncommon

Unconsciousness brief, no neurological signs on waking

Favours orthostatic hypotension

Onset when getting up quickly

Brief duration

Injury uncommon

More common when fasted or dehydrated

Known low systolic blood pressure

Use of antihypertensive medications

Favours 'situational syncope'

Occurs during micturition

Occurs with prolonged coughing

Favours syncope due to left ventricular outflow obstruction (AS, HCM)

Occurs during exertion

Favours cardiac arrhythmia

Family history of sudden death (Brugada or long QT syndrome)

Anti-arrhythmic medication (prolonged QT)

History of cardiac disease (ventricular arrhythmias)

History of rapid palpitations

No warning (heart block—Stokes-Adams attack)

Favours vertigo

No loss of consciousness

Worse when turning head

Head or room seems to spin

Favours seizure

Prodrome—aura

Tongue bitten

Jerking movements during episode

Sleepiness afterwards

Head turns during episode

Follows emotional stress

Cyanosis

Muscle pain afterwards

Favours metabolic cause of syncope (coma)

Hypoglycaemic agents, low blood sugar

AS = aortic stenosis.
HCM = hypertrophic cardiomyopathy.

Questions box 4.2

Questions to ask the patient with palpitations

! denotes symptoms for the possible diagnosis of an urgent or dangerous problem.

1 Is the sensation one of the heart beating abnormally, or something else?

2 Does the heart seem fast or slow? Have you counted how fast? Is it faster than it ever goes at any other time, e.g. with exercise?

3 Does the heart seem regular or irregular—stopping and starting? If it is irregular, is this the feeling of normal heart beats interrupted by missed or strong beats—ectopic beats; or is it completely irregular?—Atrial fibrillation

4 How long do the episodes last?

5 Do the episodes start and stop very suddenly?—Supraventricular tachycardia (SVT)

6 Can you terminate the episodes by deep breathing or holding your breath?—SVT

7 Is there a sensation of pounding in the neck?—some types of SVT[9]

8 Has an episode ever been recorded on an ECG?

! 9 Have you lost consciousness during an episode?—Ventricular arrhythmias

! 10 Have you had other heart problems such as heart failure or a heart attack in the past?—Ventricular arrhythmias?

11 Is there heart trouble of this sort in the family?

Patients may have learned manoeuvres that will return the rhythm to normal. Attacks of *supraventricular tachycardia* (SVT) may be suddenly terminated by increasing vagal tone with the Valsalva manoeuvre (page 70), carotid massage, by coughing, or by swallowing cold water or ice cubes.

Syncope, presyncope and dizziness

Syncope is a transient loss of consciousness resulting from cerebral anoxia, usually due to inadequate blood flow. Presyncope is a transient sensation of weakness without loss of consciousness. (See *Questions box 11.4*, page 326.)

Syncope may represent a simple faint or be a symptom of cardiac or neurological disease. One must establish whether the patient actually loses consciousness and under what circumstances the syncope occurs—e.g. on standing for prolonged

TABLE 4.8 Drugs and syncope

Associated with QT interval prolongation and ventricular arrhythmias

Anti-arrhythmics; flecainide, quinidine, sotalol, procainamide, amiodarone

Gastric motility promoter; cisapride

Antibiotics; clarithromycin, erythromycin

Antipsychotics; chlorpromazine, haloperidol

Associated with bradycardia

Beta-blockers

Some calcium channel blockers (verapamil, diltiazem)

Digoxin

Associated with postural hypotension

Most antihypertensive drugs, but especially prazosin and calcium channel blockers

Anti-Parkinsonian drugs

Questions box 4.3

Questions to ask the patient with suspected peripheral vascular disease

! denotes symptoms for the possible diagnosis of an urgent or dangerous problem.

1. Have you had problems with walking because of pains in the legs?
2. Where do you feel the pain?
3. How far can you walk before it occurs?
4. Does it make you stop?
5. Does it go away when you stop walking?
! 6. Does the pain ever occur at rest?—Severe ischaemia may threaten the limb
7. Have there been changes in the colour of the skin over your feet or ankles?
8. Have you had any sores or ulcers on your feet or legs that have not healed?
9. Have you needed treatment of the arteries of your legs in the past?
10. Have you had diabetes, high blood pressure, or problems with strokes or heart attacks in the past?
11. Have you been a smoker?

periods or standing up suddenly (*postural syncope*), while passing urine (*micturition syncope*), on coughing (*tussive syncope*), or with sudden emotional stress (*vasovagal syncope*). Find out whether there is any warning, such as dizziness or palpitations, and how long the episodes last. Recovery may be spontaneous or the patient may require attention from bystanders.

If the patient's symptoms appear to be postural, inquire about the use of anti-hypertensive or anti-anginal drugs and other medications that may induce postural hypotension. If the episode is vasovagal, it may be precipitated by something unpleasant like the sight of blood, or occur in a crowded, hot room; patients often sigh and yawn and feel nauseated and sweaty before fainting and may have previously had similar episodes, especially during adolescence and young adulthood.

If syncope is due to an *arrhythmia*, there is a sudden loss of consciousness regardless of the patient's posture; chest pain may also occur if the patient has ischaemic heart disease or aortic stenosis.[10] Recovery is equally quick. Exertional syncope may occur with obstruction to left ventricular outflow by *aortic stenosis* or *hypertrophic cardiomyopathy*. Profound and sudden bradycardia, usually a result of complete heart block, causes sudden and recurrent syncope (Stokes-Adams[c] attacks[d]). These patients may have a history of atrial fibrillation. Typically they have periods of tachycardia (fast heart rate) as well as periods of bradycardia (slow heart rate). This condition is called the *sick sinus syndrome*. The patient must be asked about drug treatment that could cause bradycardia, e.g. beta-blockers, digoxin, calcium channel blockers.

It is important to ask about a family history of sudden death. An increasing number of *ion channelopathies* are being identified as a cause of syncope and sudden death. These inherited conditions include the long QT syndrome and the Brugada syndrome. They are often diagnosed from typical ECG changes. In addition, certain drugs can cause the acquired long QT syndrome (Table 4.8).

Neurological causes of syncope are associated with a slow recovery and often residual neurological symptoms or signs. Bystanders may also have noticed abnormal movements if the patient has epilepsy. Dizziness that occurs even when the patient is lying down or which is made worse by movements of the head is more likely to be of neurological origin, although recurrent tachyarrhythmias may occasionally cause dizziness in any position. One

c   William Stokes (1804–1878) succeeded his father as Regius professor of physic in 1840. He was a member of the 'Dublin School' of medicine along with famous physicians like Graves, Cheyne, Adams and Corrigan. He was an art lover, and insisted his students have an arts degree before studying medicine.
    Robert Adams (1791–1875) was Regius professor of surgery in Dublin, and became Queen Victoria's surgeon. He was affected by gout, and wrote a famous paper on it.
d   Stokes-Adams attacks were probably described first by Gerbezius in 1691 and then by Morgagni in 1761; the latter was a pupil of Valsalva and also described Turner's syndrome 170 years before Turner.

should attempt to decide whether the dizziness is really *vertiginous* (where the world seems to be turning around), or whether it is a presyncopal feeling.

Intermittent claudication and peripheral vascular disease

The word claudication[e] comes from the Latin meaning to limp. Patients with claudication notice pain in one or both calves, thighs or buttocks when they walk more than a certain distance. This distance is called the 'claudication distance'. The claudication distance may be shorter when patients walk up hills. A history of claudication suggests peripheral vascular disease with a poor blood supply to the affected muscles. The most important risk factors are smoking, diabetes, hypertension and a history of vascular disease elsewhere in the body, including cerebrovascular disease and ischaemic heart disease. More severe disease causes the feet or legs to feel cold, numb and finally painful at rest. Rest pain is a symptom of severely compromised arterial supply. Remember the six P's of peripheral vascular disease:

Pain
Pallor
Pulselessness
Paraesthesiae
Perishingly cold
Paralysed.

Popliteal artery entrapment can occur, especially in young men with intermittent claudication on walking but *not* running. Also, *lumbar spinal stenosis* causes pseudo-claudication: unlike vascular claudication, the pain in the calves is not relieved by standing still, but is relieved by sitting (flexing the spine) and may be exacerbated by extending the spine (e.g. walking downhill).

Fatigue

Fatigue is a common symptom of cardiac failure. It may be associated with a reduced cardiac output and poor blood supply to the skeletal muscles. There are many other causes of fatigue, including lack of sleep, anaemia and depression.

Risk factors for coronary artery disease

An essential part of the cardiac history involves obtaining detailed information about a patient's

---

> **Questions box 4.4**
>
> **Questions to ask about possible cardiovascular risk factors**
>
> 1 Have you had angina or a heart attack in the past?
> 2 Do you know what your cholesterol level is? Before or after treatment?
> 3 Are you a diabetic?
> 4 Have you had high blood pressure and has it been treated?
> 5 Are you now or have you been a smoker? How long since you stopped?
> 6 Has anyone in the family had angina or heart attacks? Who? How old were they?
> 7 Have you had kidney problems?

risk factors—the patient's **cardiovascular risk factor profile** (*Questions box 4.4*).

Previous ischaemic heart disease is the most important risk factor for further ischaemia. The patient may know of previous infarcts or have had a diagnosis of angina in the past.

Hypercholesterolaemia is the next most important risk factor for ischaemic heart disease. Many patients now know their serum cholesterol levels because widespread testing has become fashionable. The total serum cholesterol is a useful screening test, and levels above 5.2 mmol/L are considered undesirable. Cholesterol measurements (unlike triglyceride measurements) are accurate even when a patient has not been fasting. Patients with established coronary artery disease benefit from lowering of total cholesterol to below 4 mmol/L. An elevated total cholesterol level is even more significant if the high-density lipoprotein (HDL) level is low (less than 1.0 mmol/L). Significant elevation of the triglyceride level is a coronary risk factor in its own right and also adds further to the risk if the total cholesterol is high. If a patient already has coronary disease, *hyperlipidaemia* is even more important. Control of risk factors for these patients is called 'secondary prevention'. Patients who have multiple risk factors for ischaemic heart disease (e.g. diabetes and hypertension) should have their cholesterol controlled aggressively. If the patient's cholesterol is known to be high, it is worth obtaining a dietary history. This can be very trying. It is important to remember that not only foods containing cholesterol but those containing saturated fats contribute to the serum cholesterol level. High alcohol consumption and obesity are associated with hypertriglyceridaemia.

---

e   The Roman Emperor Tiberius Claudius Drusus Nero Germanicus (10 BC–54 AD) limped owing to some form of paralysis. 'Claudication' and 'Claudius', however, are etymologically unrelated, which seems rather a cruel coincidence for Claudius. 'Claudicant' first appeared in English in 1624.

Smoking is probably the next most important risk factor for cardiovascular disease and peripheral vascular disease. Some patients describe themselves as non-smokers even though they stopped smoking only a few hours before. The number of years the patient has smoked and the number of cigarettes smoked per day are both very important (and are recorded as packet-years, page 6). The significance of a history of smoking for a patient who has not smoked for many years is controversial. The risk of symptomatic ischaemic heart disease falls gradually over the years after smoking has been stopped. After about 2 years the risk of myocardial infarction falls to the same level as for those who have never smoked. After 10 years the risk of developing angina falls close to that of non-smokers.

Hypertension is another important risk factor for coronary artery disease. Find out when hypertension was first diagnosed and what treatment, if any, has been instituted. The treatment of hypertension probably does reduce the risk of ischaemic heart disease, and certainly reduces the risk of hypertensive heart disease, cardiac failure and cerebrovascular disease. Treatment of hypertension has also been shown to reverse left ventricular hypertrophy.

A family history of coronary artery disease increases a patient's risk, particularly if it has been present in first-degree relatives (parents or siblings) and if it has affected these people below the age of 60. Not all heart disease, however, is ischaemic; a patient whose relatives suffered from rheumatic heart disease is at no greater risk of ischaemic heart disease than anybody else.

A history of *diabetes mellitus* increases the risk of ischaemic heart disease very substantially. A diabetic without a history of ischaemic heart disease has the same risk of myocardial infarction as a non-diabetic who has had an infarct. It is important to find out how long a patient has been diabetic and whether insulin treatment has been required. Good control of the blood sugar level of diabetics reduces this risk. An attempt should therefore be made to find out how well a patient's diabetes has been controlled.

Chronic kidney disease is associated with a very high risk of vascular disease. This is possibly related to high calcium-times-phosphate product and may be reduced by dietary intervention, 'phosphate binders', efficient dialysis, in renal transplant. Ischaemic heart disease is the most common cause of death in renal failure patients on dialysis.

The presence of multiple risk factors makes control of each one more important. Aggressive control of risk factors is often indicated in these patients.

It is interesting to note that in the diagnosis of angina the patient's description of typical symptoms is more discriminating than is the presence of risk factors which only marginally increase the likelihood that chest pain is ischaemic. Previous ischaemic heart disease is an exception. Certainly a patient who has had angina before and says he or she has it again, is usually right.

Teeth

A history of dental decay or infection is important for patients with valvular heart disease, since it puts them at risk of infective endocarditis. Dental caries may also be associated with an increased risk of ischaemic heart disease. Ask about the regularity of visits to the dentist and the patient's awareness of the need for antibiotic prophylaxis before dental (and some surgical) procedures.

Treatment

The medications a patient is taking often give a good clue to the diagnosis. Find out about any ill-effects from current or previous medications. The surgical history must also be elicited. The patient may have had a previous angioplasty or coronary artery bypass grafting, and may know how many arteries were dilated or bypassed. If the patient is unable to provide a history, a midline sternotomy scar and scars consistent with previous saphenous vein harvesting support this diagnosis.

Past history

Patients with a history of definite previous angina or myocardial infarction remain at high risk for further ischaemic events. It is very useful at this stage to find out how a diagnosis of ischaemic heart disease was made and in particular what investigations were undertaken. The patient may well remember exercise testing or a coronary angiogram, and some patients can even remember how many coronary arteries were narrowed, how many coronary bypasses were performed (having more than three grafts often leads to a certain amount of boasting). The angioplasty patient may know how many arteries were dilated and whether *stents* (often called coronary stunts by patients and cardiac surgeons) were inserted. Acute coronary syndromes are now usually treated with early coronary angioplasty.

Patients may recall a diagnosis of rheumatic fever in their childhood, but many were labelled as having 'growing pains'.[11] A patient who was put to bed for a long period as a child may well have had rheumatic fever. A history of rheumatic fever places patients at risk of rheumatic valvular disease.

Hypertension may be caused or exacerbated by aspects of the patient's activities and diet (*Questions box 4.5*). A high salt intake, moderate or greater alcohol use, lack of exercise, obesity and kidney disease may all be factors contributing to high blood pressure. Non-steroidal anti-inflammatory drugs cause salt and fluid retention and may also worsen blood pressure. Ask about these, about previous advice to modify these factors, and about any drug treatment of hypertension when interviewing any patient with high blood pressure.

Social history

Both ischaemic heart disease and rheumatic heart disease are chronic conditions that may affect a patient's ability to function normally. It is therefore important to find out whether the patient's condition has prevented him or her from working and over what period. Patients with severe cardiac failure, for example, may need to make adjustments to their living arrangements so that they are not required to walk up and down stairs at home.

Most hospitals run cardiac rehabilitation programmes for patients with ischaemic heart disease or chronic heart failure. They provide exercise classes that help patients regain their confidence and physical fitness, along with information classes about diet and drug treatment, and can help with psychological problems. Find out if the patient has been enrolled in one of these and whether it has been helpful. Is this service used as a point of contact for the patient if he or she has concerns about new symptoms or the management of medications?

The return of confidence and self-esteem are very important issues for patients and for their families after a life-threatening illness.

Examination anatomy

The contraction of the heart results in a wringing or twisting movement that is often palpable (the *apex beat*) and sometimes visible on the part of the chest that lies in front of it—the *praecordium* (from the Latin *prae* 'in front of', and *cor* 'heart'). The passage of blood through the heart and its valves and on into the great vessels of the body produces many interesting sounds, and causes pulsation in arteries and movement in veins in remote parts of the body. Signs of cardiac disease may be found by examining the praecordium and the many accessible arteries and veins of the body.

The surface anatomy of the heart and of the cardiac valves (Figure 4.1) and the positions of the palpable arteries (Figure 4.2) must be kept in mind during the examination of the cardiovascular system. In addition the physiology of blood flow through the systemic and pulmonary circuits need to be understood if the cardiac cycle and causes of cardiac murmurs are to be understood (Figure 4.3).

The cardiac valves separate the atria from the ventricles (the atrioventricular or mitral and tricuspid valves) and the ventricles from their corresponding great vessels. Figure 4.4 shows the fibrous skeleton that supports the four valves and their appearance during systole (cardiac contraction) and diastole (cardiac relaxation).

The filling of the right side of the heart from the systemic veins can be assessed by inspection of the jugular veins in the neck (Figure 4.5) and by palpation of the liver. These veins empty into the right atrium.

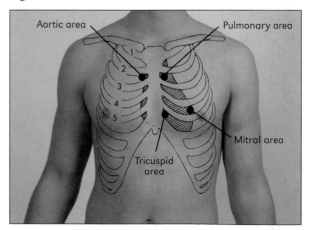

Figure 4.1 The areas best for auscultation do not exactly correlate with the anatomical location of the valves

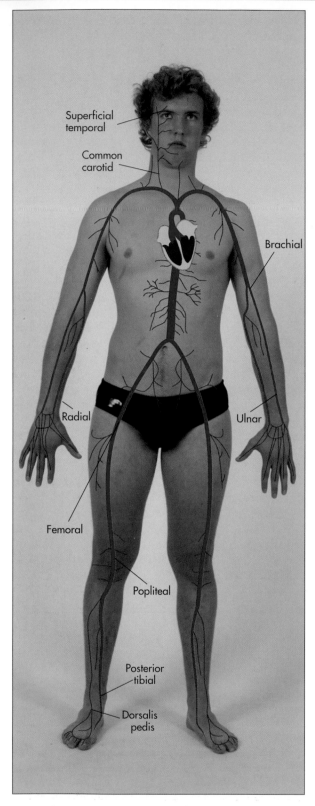

Figure 4.2 Palpable arteries

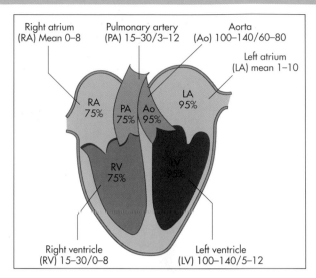

Figure 4.3 Normal pressures (mmHg) and saturations (%) in the heart

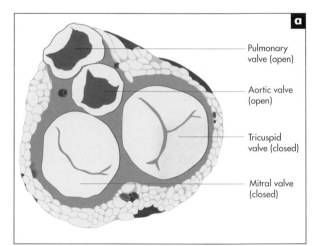

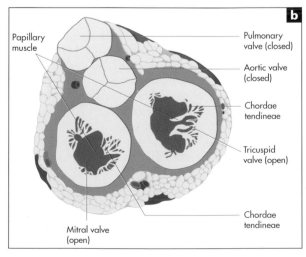

Figure 4.4 The cardiac valves in systole (a) and diastole (b)

The internal jugular vein is deep in the sterno-mastoid muscle, while the external jugular vein is lateral to it. Traditionally, use of the external jugular vein to estimate venous pressure is discouraged,

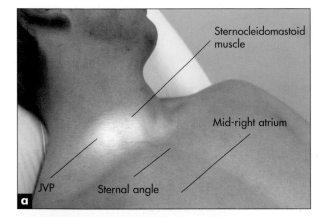

Sternocleidomastoid muscle

Mid-right atrium

JVP Sternal angle

a

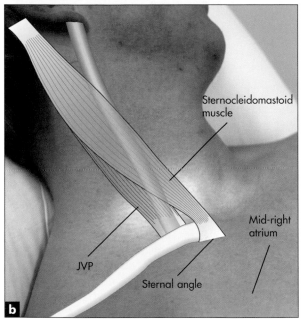

Sternocleidomastoid muscle

Mid-right atrium

JVP

Sternal angle

b

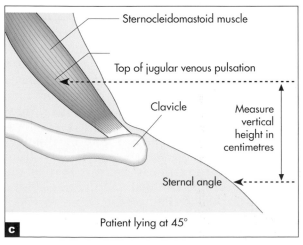

Sternocleidomastoid muscle

Top of jugular venous pulsation

Clavicle

Measure vertical height in centimetres

Sternal angle

Patient lying at 45°

c

but the right internal and external jugular veins usually give consistent readings. The left-sided veins are less accurate because they cross from the left side of the chest before entering the right atrium. Pulsations that occur in the right-sided veins reflect movements of the top of a column of blood that extends directly into the right atrium. This column of blood may be used as a manometer and enables us to observe pressure changes in the right atrium. By convention, the sternal angle is taken as the zero point and the maximum height of pulsations in the internal jugular vein, which are visible above this level when the patient is at 45 degrees, is measured in centimetres. In the average person the centre of the right atrium lies 5 cm below this zero point (Figures 4.5a and 4.6).

The cardiovascular examination

The cardiovascular system lends itself particularly well to the formal examination approach. There are a number of equally satisfactory methods, but the precise approach used is not as important as having a method which is comprehensive, gives the impression of being (and is) proficient, and ensures that no important part of the examination is omitted.

First, one should appropriately expose and position the patient properly and pause to get an impression of the general appearance. Then detailed examination begins with the hands and pulses and progresses smoothly to the neck, face, and then on to the praecordium. A summary of a suggested method of examination is found at the end of this chapter.

Positioning the patient

It is important to have the patient lying in bed with enough pillows to support him or her at 45 degrees (Figure 4.7). This is the usual position in which the jugular venous pressure (JVP) is assessed. Even a 'targeted' cardiovascular examination in an outpatients' clinic or surgery can only be performed adequately if the patient is lying down and an examination couch should be available. During

Figure 4.5 (left) The jugular venous pressure (JVP) (a) Assessment of the JVP. The patient should lie at 45 degrees. The relationships between the sternomastoid muscle, the JVP, the sternal angle and the mid-right atrium are shown. (b, c) The anatomy of the neck showing the relative positions of the main vascular structures, clavicle and sternocleidomastoid muscle. See also Figure 4.6. (Figures (b) and (c) adapted from Douglas G, Nicol F, Robertson C, *Macleod's Clinical Examination*, 11th edn. Edinburgh: Churchill Livingstone, 2005.)

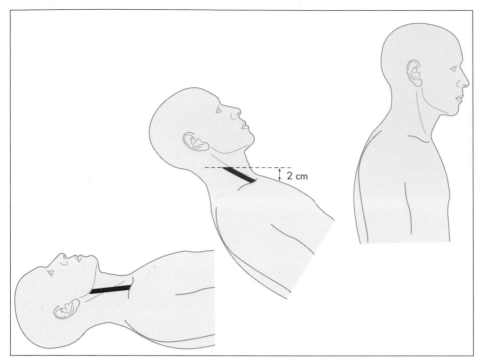

Figure 4.6 Changes in the height of the JVP as the patient sits up (Adapted from McGee S, *Evidence-based physical diagnosis*, 2nd edn. St Louis: Saunders, 2007.)

auscultation, optimal examination requires further positioning of the patient, as discussed later.

General appearance

Look at the general state of health. Does the patient appear to be ill? If he or she looks ill, try to decide why you have formed that impression. Note whether the patient at rest has rapid and laboured respiration, suggesting dyspnoea (see Table 5.6, page 110).

The patient may look *cachectic*: that is, there may be severe loss of weight and muscle wasting. This is commonly caused by malignant disease, but severe cardiac failure may also have this effect (*cardiac cachexia*). It probably results from a combination of anorexia (due to congestive enlargement of the liver), impaired intestinal absorption (due to congested intestinal veins) and increased levels of inflammatory cytokines such as TNF-α.

There are also some syndromes that are associated with specific cardiac disease. Marfan's syndrome[f] (Figure 4.8, page 50), Down syndrome[g] (page 314) and Turner's syndrome[h] (page 314) are important examples.

---

[f] Bernard-Jean Antonin Marfan (1858–1942), French physician and first professor of hygiene in Paris.
[g] John Langdon Down (1828–96), Assistant Physician to the London Hospital and founder of the Normansfield Mental Hospital. He described the clinical picture of mongolism in 1866.
[h] Henry Hubert Turner (1892–1970), Clinical Professor of Medicine, Oklahoma University. He described the syndrome in 1938.

The hands

Pick up the right hand. Look first at the nails. Now is the time for a decision as to the presence or absence of *clubbing*. Clubbing is an increase in the soft tissue of the distal part of the fingers or toes. The causes of clubbing are surprisingly varied (Table 4.9). The mechanism is unknown but there are, of course, several theories. One current theory is that platelet-derived growth factor (PDGF), released from megakaryocyte and platelet emboli in the nail beds, causes fibrovascular proliferation. Megakaryocytes and clumps of platelets do not normally reach the arterial circulation. Their large size (up to 50 μm) prevents their passing through the pulmonary capillaries when they are released from the bone marrow. In conditions where platelets may clump in the arterial circulation (infected cardiac valve) or bypass the pulmonary capillaries (right to left shunt associated with congenital heart disease), they can reach the systemic circulation and become trapped in the terminal capillaries of the fingers and toes. Damage to pulmonary capillaries from various lung disorders can have the same effect.

Proper examination for clubbing involves inspecting the fingernails (and toenails) from the side to determine if there is loss of the angle between the nail bed and the finger—the *hyponychial angle* (Figure 4.9). One accepted measurement is the *interphalangeal depth ratio*. The anteroposterior (AP) dimension of the finger

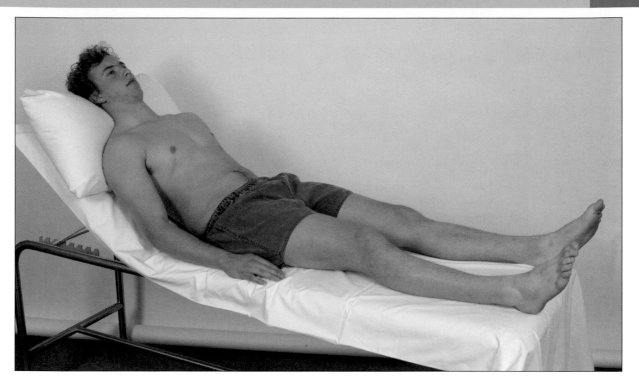

Figure 4.7 Cardiovascular examination: positioning the patient

is measured at the distal interphalangeal joint and compared with the AP diameter at the level of the point where the skin joins the nail. A ratio of more than 1 means clubbing.[12,i] Eventually, the distal phalanx becomes enlarged, due to soft-tissue swelling. This angle can be measured with a *shadowgraph*, which projects the silhouette of the finger so that it can be measured with a protractor. It is not in common use. If the angle is greater than 190°, clubbing is generally agreed to be present. Patients hardly ever notice that they have clubbing, even when it is severe. They often express surprise at their doctor's interest in such an unlikely part of their anatomy.

Before leaving the nails, look for *splinter haemorrhages* in the nail beds (Figure 4.10). These are linear haemorrhages lying parallel to the long axis of the nail. They are most often due to trauma, particularly in manual workers. However, an important cause is infective endocarditis (page 79), which is a bacterial or other infection of the heart valves or part of the endocardium. In this disease splinter haemorrhages are probably the result of a vasculitis in the nail bed, but this is controversial.

Other rare causes of splinter haemorrhages include vasculitis, as in rheumatoid arthritis, polyarteritis nodosa or the antiphospholipid syndrome, sepsis elsewhere in the body, haematological malignancy or profound anaemia.

Osler's nodes[j] are a rare manifestation of infective endocarditis. These are red, raised, tender palpable nodules on the pulps of the fingers (or toes), or on the thenar or hypothenar eminences. They are reported to have occurred in 50% of patients before antibiotic treatment of endocarditis became available. Currently they are seen in fewer than 5% of patients. *Janeway lesions*[k] (Figure 4.11) are non-tender erythematous maculopapular lesions containing bacteria, which occur very rarely on the palms or pulps of the fingers in patients with infective endocarditis.[l]

Tendon xanthomata are yellow or orange deposits of lipid in the tendons that occur in type II hyperlipidaemia. These can be seen over the

i   The eminent South African cardiologist Leo Schamroth developed clubbing as a result of endocarditis in 1976. As the condition advanced, he observed in his own fingers that the diamond-shaped space formed when the nails of two similar fingers were held facing each other disappeared, only to reappear as he improved.

j   Sir William Osler (1849–1919), Canadian physician, Professor of Medicine at McGill University at 25, and later famous Regius professor of medicine at Oxford and renowned medical historian. He was made a baronet. His only son was killed at Ypres.
k   Edward Janeway (1841–1911), American physician.
l   These signs are now mostly of historical interest. They date from the period when endocarditis could be diagnosed but not treated. Physicians were able to describe and name interesting signs but were unable to provide treatment (cf the eponymous signs of aortic regurgitation, page 87).

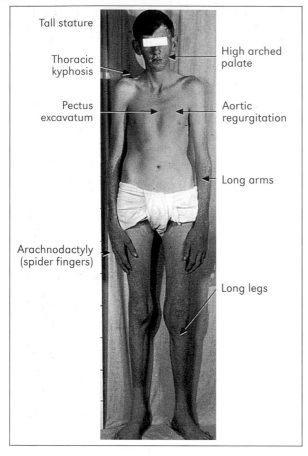

Figure 4.8 Marfan's syndrome
Tall stature, thoracic kyphosis, pectus excavatum, arachnodactyly (spider fingers), long limbs, aortic regurgitation and a high, arched palate

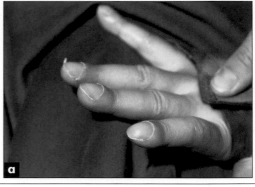

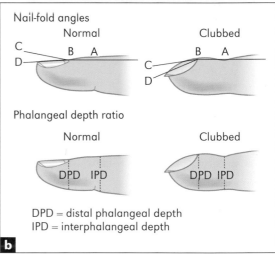

Figure 4.9 Finger clubbing: (a) appearance; (b) phalangeal depth ratio

tendons of the hand and arm. *Palmar xanthomata*, and *tuboeruptive xanthomata* over the elbows and knees, are characteristic of type III hyperlipidaemia (Figure 4.12).

The arterial pulse

The accomplished clinician is able, while inspecting the hands, to palpate the radial artery at the wrist. Patients expect to have the pulse taken as part of a proper medical examination. The clinician can feel the pulse while talking to the patient and while looking for other signs. When this traditional part of the examination is performed with some ceremony, it may help to establish rapport between patient and doctor.

Although the radial pulse is distant from the central arteries, certain useful information may be gained from examining it. The pulse is usually felt just medial to the radius, using the forefinger and middle finger pulps of the examining hand (Figure 4.13). The following observations should be made:

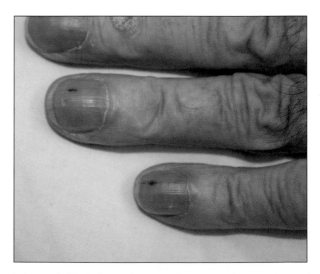

Figure 4.10 Splinter haemorrhages in the fingernails of a patient with staphylococcal aortic valve endocarditis
(From Baker T, Nikolić G, O'Connor S, *Practical Cardiology*, 2nd edn. Sydney: Churchill Livingstone, 2008, with permission.)

TABLE 4.9 Causes of clubbing

Common

Cardiovascular

Cyanotic congenital heart disease

Infective endocarditis

Respiratory

Lung carcinoma (usually *not* small cell carcinoma)

Chronic pulmonary suppuration:
- Bronchiectasis
- Lung abscess
- Empyema

Idiopathic pulmonary fibrosis

Uncommon

Respiratory

Cystic fibrosis

Asbestosis

Pleural mesothelioma (benign fibrous type) or pleural fibroma

Gastrointestinal

Cirrhosis (especially biliary cirrhosis)

Inflammatory bowel disease

Coeliac disease

Thyrotoxicosis

Familial (usually before puberty) or idiopathic

Rare

Neurogenic diaphragmatic tumours

Pregnancy

Secondary hyperparathyroidism

Unilateral clubbing

Bronchial arteriovenous aneurysm

Axillary artery aneurysm

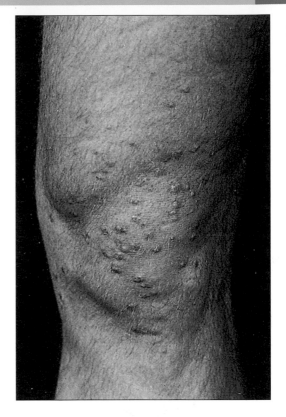

Figure 4.12 Tuboeruptive xanthomata of the knee

(i) rate of pulse, (ii) rhythm and (iii) presence or absence of delay of the femoral pulse compared with the radial pulse (*radiofemoral delay*). The character and volume of the pulse are better assessed from palpation of the brachial or carotid arteries.

Rate of pulse

Practised observers can estimate the rate quickly. Formal counting over 30 seconds is accurate and

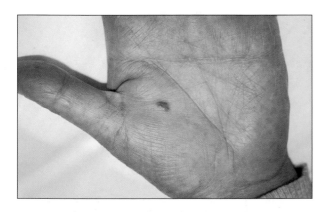

Figure 4.11 Janeway lesion

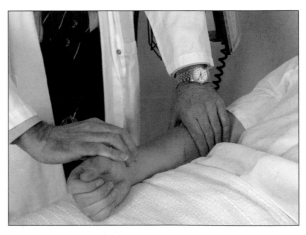

Figure 4.13 Taking the radial pulse

requires only simple mathematics to obtain the rate per minute. The normal resting heart rate in adults is usually said to be between 60 and 100 beats per minute but a more sensible range is probably 55 to 95 (95% of normal people). *Bradycardia* (Greek *bradys* 'slow', *kardia* 'heart') is defined as a heart rate of less than 60 beats per minute. *Tachycardia* (Greek *tachys* 'swift', *kardia* 'heart') is defined as a heart rate over 100 beats per minute. The causes of bradycardia and tachycardia are listed in Table 4.10.

TABLE 4.10 Causes of bradycardia and tachycardia

Bradycardia

Regular rhythm	Irregular rhythm
Physiological (athletes, during sleep: due to increased vagal tone)	*Irregularly irregular*
Drugs (e.g. beta-blockers, digoxin, amiodarone)	Atrial fibrillation (in combination with conduction system disease or AV nodal blocking drugs) due to:
Hypothyroidism (decreased sympathetic activity secondary to thyroid hormone deficiency)	• alcohol, post-thoracotomy, idiopathic
Hypothermia	• mitral valve disease or any cause of left atrial enlargement
Raised intracranial pressure (due to an effect on central sympathetic outflow)—a late sign	Frequent ectopic beats
Third degree atrioventricular (AV) block, or second degree (type 2) AV block	*Regularly irregular rhythm*
Myocardial infarction	Sinus arrhythmia (normal slowing of the pulse with expiration)
Paroxysmal bradycardia: vasovagal syncope	Second degree AV block (type 1)
Jaundice (in severe cases only, due to deposition of bilirubin in the conducting system)	Apparent
	Pulse deficit* (atrial fibrillation, ventricular bigeminy)

Tachycardia

Regular rhythm	Irregular rhythm
Hyperdynamic circulation, due to:	Atrial fibrillation, due to:
• exercise or emotion (e.g. anxiety)	• myocardial ischaemia
• fever (allow 15–20 beats per minute per °C above normal)	• mitral valve disease or any cause of left atrial enlargement
• pregnancy	• thyrotoxicosis
• thyrotoxicosis	• hypertensive heart disease
• anaemia	• sick sinus syndrome
• arteriovenous fistula (e.g. Paget's disease or hepatic failure)	• pulmonary embolism
• beri-beri (thiamine deficiency)	• myocarditis
Congestive cardiac failure	• fever, acute hypoxia or hypercapnia (paroxysmal)
Constrictive pericarditis	• other: alcohol, post-thoracotomy, idiopathic
Drugs (e.g. salbutamol and other sympathomimetics, atropine)	Multifocal atrial tachycardia
Normal variant	Atrial flutter with variable block
Denervated heart e.g. diabetes (resting rate of 106–120 beats per minute)	
Hypovolaemic shock	
Supraventricular tachycardia (usually >150)	
Atrial flutter with regular 2:1 AV block (usually 150)	
Ventricular tachycardia (often >150)	
Sinus tachycardia, due to:	
• thyrotoxicosis	
• pulmonary embolism	
• myocarditis	
• myocardial ischaemia	
• fever, acute hypoxia or hypercapnia (paroxysmal)	
Multifocal atrial tachycardia	
Atrial flutter with variable block	

* This is the difference between the heart rate counted over the praecordium and that observed at the periphery. In beats where diastole is too short for adequate filling of the heart, too small a volume of blood is ejected during systole for a pulse to be appreciated at the wrist.

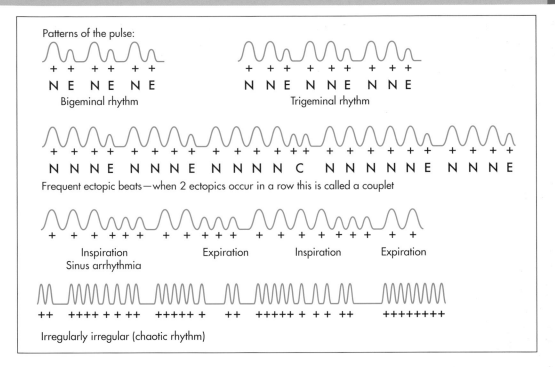

Figure 4.14 Common pulse patterns
N = normal; E = ectopic; C = couplet.

Rhythm

The rhythm of the pulse can be regular or irregular. An irregular rhythm can be completely irregular with no pattern (*irregularly irregular* or *chaotic* rhythm); this is usually due to atrial fibrillation (Table 4.10). In atrial fibrillation coordinated atrial contraction is lost, and chaotic electrical activity occurs with bombardment of the atrioventricular (AV) node with impulses at a rate of over 600 per minute. Only a variable proportion of these is conducted to the ventricles because (fortunately) the AV node is unable to conduct at such high rates. In this way, the ventricles are protected from very rapid rates, but beat irregularly, usually at rates between 150 and 180 per minute (unless the patient is being treated with drugs to slow the heart rate). The pulse also varies in amplitude from beat to beat in atrial fibrillation because of differing diastolic filling times. This type of pulse can occasionally be simulated by frequent irregularly occurring supraventricular or ventricular ectopic beats.

Patients with atrial fibrillation or frequent ectopic beats may have a detectable *pulse deficit*. This means the heart rate when counted by listening to the heart with the stethoscope is higher than that obtained when the radial pulse is counted at the wrist. In these patients the heart sounds will be audible with every systole, but some early contractions preceded by short diastolic filling periods will not produce enough cardiac output for a pulse to be palpable at the wrist.

An irregular rhythm can also be *regularly irregular*. For example, in patients with *sinus arrhythmia* the pulse rate increases with each inspiration and decreases with each expiration; this is a normal finding. It is associated with changes in venous return to the heart.

Patterns of irregularity (Figure 4.14) can also occur when patients have frequent ectopic beats. These may arise in the atrium (atrial ectopic beats—AEBs) or in the ventricle (ventricular ectopic beats—VEBs). Ectopic beats quite commonly occur in a fixed ratio to normal beats. When every second beat is an ectopic one, the rhythm is called *bigeminy*. A bigeminal rhythm caused by ectopic beats has a characteristic pattern: normal pulse, weak pulse, delay, normal pulse, ... Similarly, every third beat may be ectopic—*trigeminy*. A pattern of irregularity is also detectable in the *Wenckebach phenomenon*.[m] Here the AV nodal conduction time increases progressively until a non-conducted atrial systole occurs. Following this, the AV conduction time shortens and the cycle begins again.

---

m   Marel Frederik Wenckebach (1864–1940), Dutch physician who practised in Vienna.

Radiofemoral and radial–radial delay

This is an important sign and often neglected. While palpating the radial pulse, the clinician places the fingers of the other hand over the femoral pulse, which is situated below the inguinal ligament, one-third of the way up from the pubic tubercle (Figure 4.15). A noticeable delay in the arrival of the femoral pulse wave suggests the diagnosis of *coarctation of the aorta*, where a congenital narrowing in the aortic isthmus occurs at the level where the ductus arteriosus joins the descending aorta. This is just distal to the origin of the subclavian artery. This lesion can cause upper limb hypertension.

It can also be useful to palpate both radial pulses together to detect radial–radial inequality in timing or volume, usually due to a large arterial occlusion by an atherosclerotic plaque or aneurysm, or to subclavian artery stenosis on one side. It can also be a sign of dissection of the thoracic aorta.

Character and volume

These are poorly assessed by palpating the radial pulse; the carotid or brachial arteries should be used to determine the character and volume of the pulse, as these more accurately reflect the form of the aortic pressure wave. However, the collapsing (bounding) pulse of *aortic regurgitation*, and *pulsus alternans* (alternating strong and weak pulse) of advanced left ventricular failure, may be readily apparent in the radial pulse.

Condition of the vessel wall

Only changes in the medial layer of the radial artery can be assessed by palpation. Thickening or tortuosity will be detected commonly in the arteries of elderly people. These changes, however, do not indicate the presence of luminal narrowing

due to atherosclerosis. Therefore, this sign is of little clinical value.

The blood pressure

Measurement of the arterial blood pressure[n] is an essential part of the examination of almost any patient. Usually, indirect measurements of the systolic and diastolic pressures are obtained with a *sphygmomanometer* (Greek *sphygmos* 'pulsing', *manos* 'thin').[13] The systolic blood pressure is the peak pressure that occurs in the artery following ventricular systole, and the diastolic blood pressure is the level to which the arterial blood pressure falls during ventricular diastole. Normal blood pressure is defined as a systolic reading of less than 140 mmHg *and* a diastolic reading of less than 90 mmHg. In some circumstances, lower pressures may be considered normal (e.g. in pregnancy) or desirable (e.g. for diabetics).

Measuring the blood pressure with the sphygmomanometer

The usual blood pressure cuff width is 12.5 cm. This is suitable for a normal-sized adult forearm. However, in obese patients with large arms (up to 30% of the adult population) the normal-sized cuff will overestimate the blood pressure and therefore a large cuff must be used. A range of smaller sizes are available for children. Use of a cuff that is too large results in only a small underestimate of blood pressure.

The cuff is wrapped around the upper arm with the bladder centred over the brachial artery (Figure 4.16). This is found in the antecubital fossa, one-third of the way over from the medial epicondyle. For an approximate estimation of the systolic blood pressure, the cuff is fully inflated and then deflated slowly (3–4 mmHg per second) until the radial pulse returns. Then, for a more accurate estimation of the blood pressure, this manoeuvre is repeated with the diaphragm of the stethoscope placed over the brachial artery, slipped underneath the distal end of the cuff's bladder.

The patient's brachial artery should be at about the level of the heart which is at the level of the fourth intercostal space at the sternum. If the arm is too high, e.g. at the level of the supraclavicular notch, the blood pressure reading will be about 5 mmHg lower; and if the arm is too low the reading will be higher than is accurate.

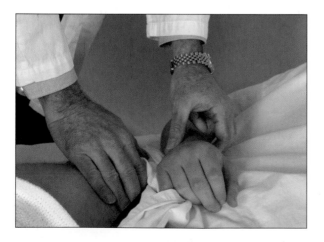

Figure 4.15 Feeling for the radiofemoral delay

n   Blood pressure was first measured in a horse in 1708 by Stephen Hales, an English clergyman. Measurement of the blood pressure was the last of the traditional vital signs measurements to come into regular use. It wasn't until early in the 20th century that work by Korotkoff and Janeway led to its routine use.

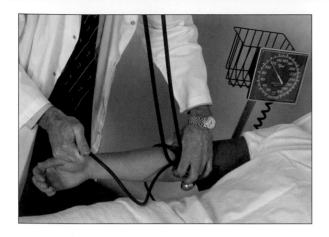

Figure 4.16 Measuring the blood pressure, with the patient lying at 45 degrees

Five different sounds will be heard as the cuff is slowly released (Figure 4.17). These are called the Korotkoff° sounds. The pressure at which a sound is first heard over the artery is the systolic blood pressure (Korotkoff I). As deflation of the cuff continues, the sound increases in intensity (KII), then decreases (KIII), becomes muffled (KIV) and then disappears (KV). Different observers have used KIV and KV to indicate the level of the

diastolic pressure. KV is probably the best measure. However, this provides a slight underestimate of the arterial diastolic blood pressure. Although diastolic pressure usually corresponds most closely to KV, in severe aortic regurgitation KIV is a more accurate indication. KV is absent in some normal people and KIV must then be used.

Occasionally, there will be an auscultatory gap (the sounds disappear just below the systolic pressure and reappear before the diastolic pressure) in healthy people. This can lead to an underestimate of the systolic blood pressure if the cuff is not pumped up high enough.

The systolic blood pressure may normally vary between the arms by up to 10 mmHg; in the legs the blood pressure is normally up to 20 mmHg higher than in the arms, unless the patient has coarctation of the aorta. Measurement of the blood pressure in the legs is more difficult than in the arms. It requires a large cuff that is placed over the mid-thigh. The patient lies prone and the stethoscope is placed in the popliteal fossa, behind the knee.

During inspiration, the systolic and diastolic blood pressures normally decrease (because intrathoracic pressure becomes more negative, blood pools in the pulmonary vessels, so left-heart filling is reduced). When this normal reduction in blood pressure with inspiration is *exaggerated*, it is termed *pulsus paradoxus*. Kussmaul meant by this that there was a fall in blood pressure and a paradoxical rise in pulse rate. A fall in arterial pulse

---

°   Nikolai Korotkoff (1874–1920), a St Petersburg surgeon, described the auscultatory method of determining blood pressure in 1905, although his findings were scoffed at.

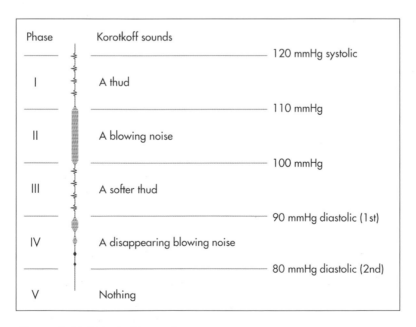

Figure 4.17 Korotkoff sounds
Systolic pressure is determined by the appearance of the first audible sound, and diastolic pressure is determined by its disappearance.

pressure on inspiration of more than 10 mmHg is abnormal and may occur with *constrictive pericarditis, pericardial effusion*, or severe asthma. To detect this: lower the cuff pressure slowly until KI sounds are heard intermittently (expiration) and then until KI is audible with every beat. The difference between the two readings represents the level of the pulsus paradoxus.

Variations in blood pressure

When blood pressure is measured with an intra-arterial catheter it becomes clear that blood pressure varies from minute to minute in normal people. Short-term changes of 4 mmHg in the systolic and 3 mmHg in the diastolic readings are common. Hour-to-hour and day-to-day variations are even greater. The standard deviation between visits is up to 12 mmHg for systolic pressure and 8 mmHg for diastolic. This means that when there is concern about an abnormal reading, repeat measurements are necessary.

When the heart is very irregular (most often because of atrial fibrillation), the cuff should be deflated slowly, and the point at which most of the cardiac contractions are audible (KI) taken as the systolic pressure and the point at which most have disappeared (KV) taken as diastole.

High blood pressure

This is difficult to define.[13] The most helpful definitions of hypertension are based on an estimation of the level associated with an increased risk of vascular disease. There have been many classifications of blood pressure, as what is considered normal or abnormal changes as more information comes to hand. Table 4.11 gives a useful guide to current definitions. If recordings above 140/90 mmHg are considered abnormal, high blood pressure may occur in up to 20% of the adult population.[p] Blood pressure measured by the patient at home, or by a 24-hour monitor, should be up to 10/5 mmHg less than that measured in the surgery.

Postural blood pressure

The blood pressure should routinely be taken with the patient both lying down and standing (Figure 4.18).[15] A fall of more than 15 mmHg in systolic blood pressure or 10 mmHg in diastolic blood

TABLE 4.11 A classification of blood pressure readings*		
Category	**Systolic (mmHg)**	**Diastolic (mmHg)**
Optimal	< 120	< 80
Normal	120–129	80–84
High normal	130–139	85–89
Mild hypertension (grade 1)	140–159	90–99
Moderate hypertension (grade 2)	160–179	100–109
Severe hypertension (grade 3)	> 180	> 110

* Khan NA, Rahim SA, Avand SS et al. Does the clinical examination predict lower extremity peripheral arterial disease? *JAMA* 2006 Feb 1; 295(5):536–546.

pressure on standing is abnormal and is called *postural hypotension* (Table 4.12). It may cause dizziness or not be associated with symptoms. The most common cause is the use of antihypertensive drugs, α-adrenergic antagonists in particular.

TABLE 4.12 Causes of postural hypotension (HANDI)
Hypovolaemia (e.g. dehydration, bleeding); **H**ypopituitarism
Addison's* disease
Neuropathy—autonomic (e.g. diabetes mellitus), amyloidosis, Shy-Drager syndrome)
Drugs (e.g. vasodilators and other antihypertensives, tricyclic antidepressants, diuretics, antipsychotics)
Idiopathic orthostatic hypotension (rare progressive degeneration of the autonomic nervous system, usually in elderly men)

* Thomas Addison (1793–1860), London physician.

The face

Inspect the sclerae for *jaundice* (page 25). This can occur with severe congestive cardiac failure and hepatic congestion. Prosthetic heart valve induced haemolysis of red blood cells, due to excessive turbulence, is an uncommon but cardiac cause of jaundice. *Xanthelasmata* (Figure 4.19) are intracutaneous yellow cholesterol deposits around the eyes and are relatively common. These may be a normal variant or may indicate type II or III hyperlipidaemia, though they are not always associated with hyperlipidaemia.

Look at the pupils for an *arcus senilis* (Figure 4.20). This half or complete grey circle is seen around

---

p   In pseudohypertension the blood pressure, as measured by the sphygmomanometer, is artificially high because of arterial wall calcification. Osler's manoeuvre traditionally detects this condition: inflate the cuff above systolic pressure and palpate the radial artery, which in pseudohypertension may be palpable despite being pulseless. However, the value of Osler's manoeuvre has been questioned.[14]

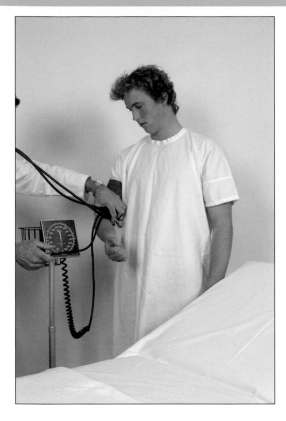

Figure 4.18 Measuring the blood pressure, with patient standing

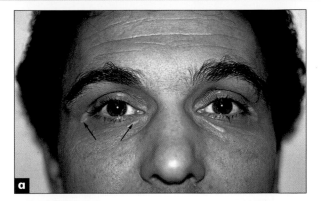

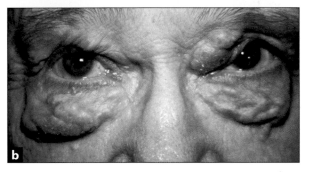

Figure 4.19 Xanthelasmata
(Figure b from McDonald FS, ed., *Mayo Clinic images in internal medicine*, with permission. © Mayo Clinic Scientific Press and CRC Press.)

the outer perimeter of the pupil and is probably associated with some increase in cardiovascular risk.[q]

Next look for the presence of a *mitral facies*, which refers to rosy cheeks with a bluish tinge due to dilatation of the malar capillaries. This is associated with pulmonary hypertension and a low cardiac output such as occurs in severe mitral stenosis, and is now rare.

Now look in the mouth using a torch to see if there is a *high arched palate*. This occurs in Marfan's syndrome, a condition that is associated with congenital heart disease, including aortic regurgitation secondary to aortic root dilatation, and also mitral regurgitation due to mitral valve prolapse. Notice whether the teeth look diseased, as they can be a source of organisms responsible for infective endocarditis. Look at the tongue and lips for central cyanosis. Inspect the mucosa for petechiae that may indicate infective endocarditis.

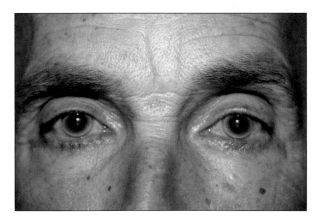

Figure 4.20 Arcus senilis

The neck
Oddly enough, this small area of the body is packed with cardiovascular signs which must be elicited with great care and skill.

Carotid arteries
The carotids are not only easily accessible, medial to the sternomastoid muscles (Figure 4.21), but provide a great deal of information about the wave

---

q   The connection of arcus senilis with old age and cardiovascular disease has been made from early in the 19th century. The pathologist Virchow was convinced it was an indicator of vascular disease.

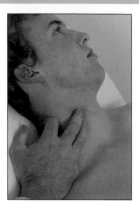

Figure 4.21 Palpating the carotid pulse

TABLE 4.13 Arterial pulse character	
Type of pulse	**Cause(s)**
Anacrotic	Aortic stenosis
	Small volume, slow uptake, notched wave on upstroke
Plateau	Aortic stenosis
	Slow upstroke
Bisferiens	Aortic stenosis *and* regurgitation
	Anacrotic and collapsing
Collapsing	Aortic regurgitation
	Hyperdynamic circulation
	Patent ductus arteriosus
	Peripheral arteriovenous fistula
	Arteriosclerotic aorta (elderly patients in particular)
Small volume	Aortic stenosis
	Pericardial effusion
Alternans	Left ventricular failure
	Alternating strong and weak beats

form of the aortic pulse, which is affected by many cardiac abnormalities. Never palpate both carotid arteries simultaneously as they provide much of the blood supply to the *brain* (a vital organ).

Evaluation of the pulse wave form (the amplitude, shape and volume) is important in the diagnosis of various underlying cardiac diseases and in assessing their severity. It takes considerable practice to distinguish the different important types of carotid wave forms (Table 4.13). Auscultation of the carotids may be performed now or in association with auscultation of the praecordium.

Jugular venous pressure (JVP)—pulsation

Just as the carotid pulse tells us about the aorta and left ventricular function, the *jugular venous pressure* (JVP) (Figure 4.5, page 47) tells us about right atrial and right ventricular function.[16] The positioning of the patient and lighting are important for this examination to be done properly. The patient must be lying down at 45 degrees to the horizontal with his or her head on pillows and in good lighting conditions. This is a difficult examination and there is considerable inter- (and intra-)observer variation in the findings.

When the patient is lying at 45 degrees, the sternal angle is also roughly in line with the base of the neck (Figure 4.5c). This provides a convenient zero point from which to measure the vertical height of the column of blood in the jugular vein. The jugular venous pulsation (movement) can be distinguished from the arterial pulse because: (i) it is visible but not palpable and has a more prominent *inward* movement than the artery; (ii) it has a complex wave form, usually seen to flicker twice with each cardiac cycle (if the patient is in sinus rhythm); (iii) it moves on respiration—normally the JVP decreases on inspiration; and (iv) it is at first obliterated and then filled from above when light

pressure is applied at the base of the neck.

The JVP must be assessed for *height* and *character*. When the JVP is more than 3 cm above the zero point, the right-heart filling pressure is raised (a normal reading is less than 8 cm of water: 5 cm + 3 cm). This is a sign of right ventricular failure, volume overload or of some types of pericardial disease.

The assessment of the *character* of JVP is difficult even for experienced clinicians. There are two positive waves in the normal JVP.[r] The first is called the *a wave* and coincides with right atrial systole.[s] It is due to atrial contraction. The *a* wave also coincides with the first heart sound and precedes the carotid pulsation. The second impulse is called the *v wave* and is due to atrial filling, in the period when the tricuspid valve remains closed during ventricular systole. Between the *a* and *v* waves there is a trough caused by atrial relaxation. This is called the *x descent*. It is interrupted by the *c point,* which is due to transmitted carotid pulsation and coincides with tricuspid valve closure; it is not usually visible. Following the *v* wave, the tricuspid

---

[r] The waves visible in the JVP were named by Sir James Mackenzie (1853–1925), British physician and one of the founders of the specialty of cardiology.

[s] Sir James Mackenzie first applied these labels to the jugular waveforms in the late 19th century.

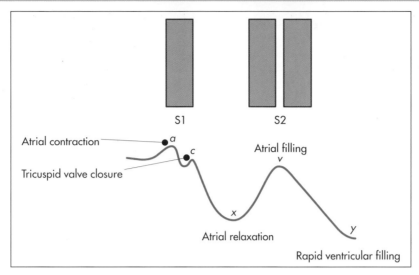

Figure 4.22 The jugular venous pressure, and its relationship to the first (S1) and second (S2) heart sounds

valve opens and rapid ventricular filling occurs; this results in the *y descent* (Figure 4.22).

In Table 4.14, characteristic changes in the JVP are described. Any condition in which right ventricular filling is limited (e.g. *constrictive pericarditis, cardiac tamponade* or *right ventricular infarction*) can cause elevation of the venous pressure, which is more marked on inspiration when venous return to the heart increases. This rise in the JVP on inspiration, called *Kussmaul's*[t] sign, is the opposite of what normally happens. This sign is best elicited with the patient sitting up at 90 degrees and breathing quietly through the mouth.

The abdominojugular reflux test *(hepatojugular reflux)* is a way of testing for right or left ventricular failure or reduced right ventricular compliance.[17] Pressure exerted over the middle of the abdomen for 10 seconds will increase venous return to the right atrium. The JVP normally rises transiently following this manoeuvre.[u] If there is right ventricular failure or left atrial pressures are elevated (left ventricular failure), it may remain elevated (>4cm) for the duration of the compression—a positive hepatojugular reflux. The sudden fall in the JVP (>4 cm) as the pressure is released may be easier to see than the initial rise. It is not necessary to compress the liver and so the older name, *hepatojugular reflux*, is not so appropriate. It is important that the patient be relaxed, breathe through the mouth and not perform a Valsalva

manoeuvre. The examiner should press firmly with the palm over the middle of the abdomen. It is

TABLE 4.14 Jugular venous pressure (pulse)
Causes of an elevated central venous pressure
Right ventricular failure
Tricuspid stenosis or regurgitation
Pericardial effusion or constrictive pericarditis
Superior vena caval obstruction
Fluid overload
Hyperdynamic circulation
Wave form
Causes of a dominant *a* wave
Tricuspid stenosis (also causing a slow *y* descent)
Pulmonary stenosis
Pulmonary hypertension
Causes of cannon *a* waves
Complete heart block
Paroxysmal nodal tachycardia with retrograde atrial conduction
Ventricular tachycardia with retrograde atrial conduction or atrioventricular dissociation
Cause of a dominant *v* wave
Tricuspid regurgitation
***x* descent**
Absent: atrial fibrillation
Exaggerated: acute cardiac tamponade, constrictive pericarditis
***y* descent**
Sharp: severe tricuspid regurgitation, constrictive pericarditis
Slow: tricuspid stenosis, right atrial myxoma

---

t   Adolf Kussmaul (1822–1909), German physician who also described laboured breathing ('air hunger') in diabetic coma (1874) and was the first to use an oesophagoscope. He coined the word 'hemiballismus'.
u   First described by Louis Pasteur in 1885.

not necessary to apply pressure for more than 10 seconds.

Cannon a waves occur when the right atrium contracts against the closed tricuspid valve. This occurs intermittently in complete heart block where the two chambers beat independently.

Giant a waves are large but not explosive *a* waves with each beat. They occur when right atrial pressures are raised because of elevated pressures in the pulmonary circulation or obstruction to outflow (tricuspid stenosis).

The *large v waves* of tricuspid regurgitation should never be missed. They are a reliable sign of tricuspid regurgitation and are visible welling up into the neck during each ventricular systole.

The praecordium

Now at last the examiner has reached the praecordium.

Inspection

Inspect first for scars. Previous cardiac operations will have left scars on the chest wall. The position of the scar can be a clue to the valve lesion that has been operated on. Most valve surgery requires cardiopulmonary bypass and for this a *median sternotomy* (a cut down the middle of the sternum) is very commonly used. This type of scar is occasionally hidden under a forest of chest hair. It is not specifically helpful, as it may also be a result of previous coronary artery bypass grafting. Alternatively, left- or even right-sided lateral thoracotomy scars, which may be hidden under a pendulous breast, may indicate a previous closed mitral valvotomy. In this operation a stenosed mitral valve is opened through an incision made in the left atrial appendage; cardiopulmonary bypass is not required. Coronary artery bypass grafting and even valve surgery are now sometimes performed using small lateral 'port' incisions for video-assisted instruments.

Skeletal abnormalities such as *pectus excavatum* (funnel chest, page 121) or *kyphoscoliosis* (Greek *kyphos* 'hunchbacked', *skolios* 'curved'), a curvature of the vertebral column (page 121), may be present. Skeletal abnormalities such as these, which may be part of Marfan's syndrome, can cause distortion of the position of the heart and great vessels in the chest and thus alter the position of the apex beat. Severe deformity can interfere with pulmonary function and cause pulmonary hypertension (page 81).

Another surgical 'abnormality' that must not be missed, if only to avoid embarrassment, is a pacemaker or cardioverter-defibrillator box. These are usually under the right or left pectoral muscle just below the clavicle, are usually easily palpable and obviously metallic. The pacemaker leads may be palpable under the skin, leading from the top of the box. The box is normally mobile under the skin. Fixation of the skin to the box or stretching of the skin over the box may be an indication for repositioning. Erosion of the box through the skin is a serious complication because of the inevitable infection that will occur around this foreign body. Rarely, a loose lead connection will lead to twitching of the muscles of the chest wall around the box. Penetration of the right ventricular lead into or through the right ventricular wall may lead to disconcerting paced diaphragmatic contractions (hiccups) at whatever rate the pacemaker is set. Defibrillator boxes are larger than pacemakers. They are currently about 10×5 cm and a little less than 1 cm thick.

Look for the apex beat. Its normal position is in the fifth left intercostal space, 1 cm medial to the midclavicular line (Figure 4.23). It is due primarily to recoil of the heart as blood is expelled in systole. There may be other visible pulsations—for example, over the pulmonary artery in cases of severe pulmonary hypertension.

Palpation

The *apex beat* must be palpated (Figures 4.23 and 4.24).[18] It is important to count down the number of interspaces. The first palpable interspace is the second. It lies just below the manubriosternal angle. The position of the apex beat is defined as the most lateral and inferior point at which the palpating

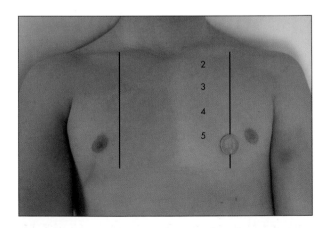

Figure 4.23 The apex beat
Coin is over the apex. Intercostal spaces are numbered. Vertical lines show right and left midclavicular and left anterior axillary lines. Care must be taken in identifying the midclavicular line; the inter-observer variability can be as much as 10 cm!

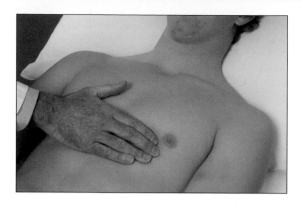

Figure 4.24 Feeling for the apex beat

fingers are raised with each systole. The normal apex is felt over an area the size of a 20 cent (50 p) coin (Figure 4.23). Use firm pressure with the tips of the fingers into the rib interspaces. The heel of the examiner's hand is lifted off the patient's sternum. Note that the apex beat is palpable in only about 50% of adults.

It is worth noting that the palpable apex beat is not the anatomical apex of the heart but a point above it. At the time the apex beat is palpable,[v] the heart is assuming a more spherical shape and the apex is twisting away from the chest wall. The area above the apex, however, is moving closer to the chest and is palpable. If the apex beat is displaced laterally or inferiorly, or both, this usually indicates enlargement,[18] but may sometimes be due to chest wall deformity, or pleural or pulmonary disease (page 121).

The character of the apex beat may provide the examiner with vital diagnostic clues. The normal apex beat gently lifts the palpating fingers. There are a number of types of abnormal apex beats. The *pressure loaded* (heaving, hyperdynamic or systolic overloaded) apex beat is a forceful and sustained impulse. This occurs with aortic stenosis or hypertension. The *volume loaded* (thrusting) apex beat is a displaced, diffuse, non-sustained impulse. This occurs most commonly in advanced mitral regurgitation or dilated cardiomyopathy. The *dyskinetic* apex beat is an uncoordinated impulse felt over a larger area than normal in the praecordium and is usually due to left ventricular dysfunction (e.g. in anterior myocardial infarction). The *double impulse* apex beat, where two distinct

impulses are felt with each systole, is characteristic of hypertrophic cardiomyopathy (page 91). The *tapping* apex beat will be felt when the first heart sound is actually palpable (heart sounds are not palpable in health) and indicates mitral or very rarely tricuspid stenosis. The character, but not the position, of the apex beat may be more easily assessed when the patient lies on the left side.

In many patients the apex beat may not be palpable. This is most often due to a thick chest wall, emphysema, pericardial effusion, shock (or death) and rarely to dextrocardia (where there is inversion of the heart and great vessels). The apex beat will be palpable to the right of the sternum in many cases of dextrocardia.

Other praecordial impulses may be palpable in patients with heart disease. A *parasternal impulse* may be felt when the heel of the hand is rested just to the left of the sternum with the fingers lifted slightly off the chest (Figure 4.25). Normally no impulse or a slight inward impulse is felt. In cases of right ventricular enlargement or severe left atrial enlargement, where the right ventricle is pushed anteriorly, the heel of the hand is lifted off the chest wall with each systole. Palpation with the fingers over the pulmonary area may reveal the palpable tap of pulmonary valve closure (*palpable P2*) in cases of pulmonary hypertension (Figure 4.26).

Turbulent blood flow, which causes cardiac murmurs on auscultation, may sometimes be palpable. These palpable murmurs are called *thrills*. The praecordium should be systematically palpated for thrills with the flat of the hand, first over the apex and left sternal edge, and then over the *base of the heart* (this is the upper part of the chest and includes the aortic and pulmonary areas) (Figure 4.26).

Apical thrills can be more easily felt with the patient rolled over to the left side (the left lateral position) as this brings the apex closer to the chest

---

v   James Hope was the first to demonstrate (in 1830) that the apex beat was caused by ventricular contraction. Jean-Nicholas Corvisant (Napoleon's personal doctor) was the first to associate abnormal palpation of the heart with cardiac chamber enlargements.

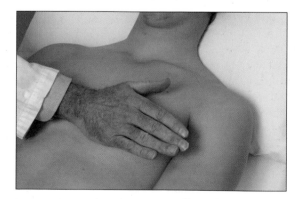

Figure 4.25 Feeling for the parasternal impulse

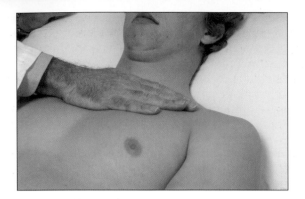

Figure 4.26 Palpating the base of the heart

wall. Thrills may also be palpable over the base of the heart. These may be maximal over the pulmonary or aortic areas, depending on the underlying cause, and are best felt with the patient sitting up, leaning forwards and in full expiration. In this position the base of the heart is moved closer to the chest wall. A thrill that coincides in time with the apex beat is called a *systolic thrill*; one that does not coincide with the apex beat is called a *diastolic thrill*.

The presence of a thrill usually indicates an organic lesion. Careful palpation for thrills is a useful, but often neglected, part of the cardiovascular examination.

Percussion

It is possible to define the cardiac outline by means of percussion[w] but this is not routine (page 124).[19] Percussion is most accurate when performed in the fifth intercostal space. The patient should lie supine and the examiner percusses from the anterior axillary line towards the sternum. The point at which the percussion note becomes dull represents the left heart border. A distance of more than 10.5 cm between the border of the heart and the middle of the sternum indicates cardiomegaly. The sign is not useful in the presence of lung disease.

Auscultation

Now at last the stethoscope is required.[20] However, in some cases the diagnosis should already be fairly clear. In the viva voce examination, the examiners will occasionally stop a candidate before auscultation and ask for an opinion.

Auscultation of the heart begins in the mitral area with the bell of the stethoscope (Figures 4.1, page 45, and 4.27). The bell is designed as a resonating chamber and is particularly efficient in amplifying low-pitched sounds, such as the diastolic murmur of mitral stenosis or a third heart sound. It must be applied to the chest wall lightly, because forceful application will stretch the skin under the bell so that it forms a diaphragm. Some modern stethoscopes do not have a separate bell; the effect of a bell is produced when the diaphragm is placed lightly on the chest, and of a diaphragm when it is pushed more firmly.

Next, listen in the mitral area with the diaphragm of the stethoscope (Figure 4.28), which best reproduces higher-pitched sounds, such as the systolic murmur of mitral regurgitation or a fourth heart sound. Then place the stethoscope in the tricuspid area (fifth left intercostal space) and listen. Next inch up the left sternal edge to the pulmonary (second left intercostal space) and aortic (second

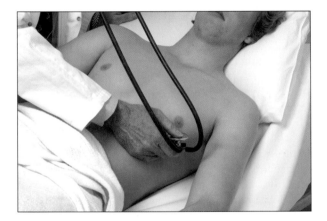

Figure 4.27 Auscultation in the mitral area with the bell of the stethoscope
Listening for mitral stenosis in the left lateral position.

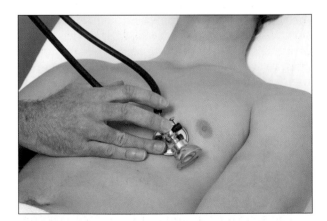

Figure 4.28 Auscultation at the apex with the diaphragm of the stethoscope

---

w   Percussion of the heart and other organs was enthusiastically promoted by Pierre Poiry, a student of Laënnec, in the early 19th century. He performed indirect percussion using an ivory plate instead of his left middle finger.

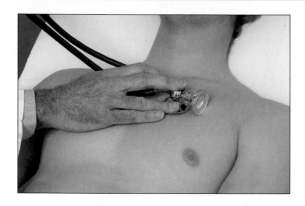

Figure 4.29 Auscultation at the base of the heart (pulmonary area)

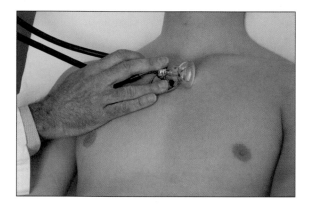

Figure 4.30 Auscultation at the base of the heart (aortic area)

right intercostal space) areas (Figures 4.29 and 4.30), listening carefully in each position with the diaphragm.

For accurate auscultation, experience with what is normal is important. This can be obtained only through constant practice. Auscultation of the normal heart reveals two sounds called, not surprisingly, the first and second heart sounds. The explanation for the origin of these noises changes from year to year; the sounds are probably related to vibrations caused by the closing of the heart valves in combination with rapid changes in blood flow and tensing within cardiac structures that occur as the valves close.

The *first heart sound* (S1) has two components: mitral and tricuspid valve closure. Mitral closure occurs slightly before tricuspid, but usually only one sound is audible. The first heart sound indicates the beginning of ventricular systole.

The *second heart sound* (S2), which is softer, shorter and at a slightly higher pitch than the first and marks the end of systole, is made up of sounds arising from aortic and pulmonary valve closures. In normal cases, although left and right ventricular systole end at the same time, the lower pressure in the pulmonary circulation compared with the aorta means that flow continues into the pulmonary artery after the end of right ventricular systole. As a result, closure of the pulmonary valve occurs later than that of the aortic valve. These components are usually (in 70% of normal adults) sufficiently separated in time so that splitting of the second heart sound is audible. Because the pulmonary component of the second heart sound (P2) may not be audible throughout the praecordium, splitting of the second heart sound may best be appreciated in the pulmonary area and along the left sternal edge. Pulmonary valve closure is further delayed (by 20 or 30 milliseconds) with inspiration because of increased venous return to the right ventricle; thus, splitting of the second heart sound is wider on inspiration. The second heart sound marks the beginning of diastole, which is usually longer than systole.

It can be difficult to decide which heart sound is which. Palpation of the carotid pulse will indicate the timing of systole and enable the heart sounds to be more easily distinguished. It is obviously crucial to define systole and diastole during auscultation so that cardiac murmurs and abnormal sounds can be placed in the correct part of the cardiac cycle. Students are often asked to time a cardiac murmur; this is not a request to measure its length, but rather to say in which part of the cardiac cycle it occurs. Even the experts can mistake a murmur if they do not time it. It is important, during auscultation, to concentrate separately on the components of the cardiac cycle. The clinician should attempt to identify each and listen for abnormalities. There can be more than 12 components to identify in patients with heart disease. An understanding of the cardiac cycle is helpful when interpreting the auscultatory findings (Figure 4.31).

Abnormalities of the heart sounds

Alterations in intensity. The **first heart sound** (S1) is *loud* when the mitral or tricuspid valve cusps remain wide open at the end of diastole and shut forcefully with the onset of ventricular systole. This occurs in mitral stenosis because the narrowed valve orifice limits ventricular filling so that there is no diminution in flow towards the end of diastole. The normal mitral valve cusps drift back towards the closed position at the end of diastole as ventricular filling slows down. Other causes of a loud S1 are related to reduced diastolic filling time (e.g. tachycardia or any cause of a short atrioventricular conduction time).

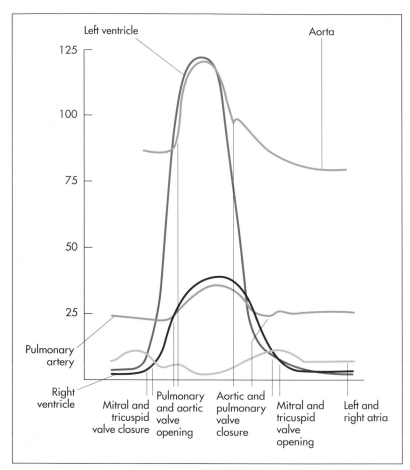

125

100

75

50

25

Left ventricle

Aorta

Pulmonary artery

Right ventricle

Mitral and tricuspid valve closure

Pulmonary and aortic valve opening

Aortic and pulmonary valve closure

Mitral and tricuspid valve opening

Left and right atria

Figure 4.31 The cardiac cycle
Normally the onset of left ventricular systole precedes the onset of pressure rise in the right ventricle. The mitral valve, therefore, closes before the tricuspid valve. Because the pulmonary artery diastolic pressure is lower than aortic diastolic pressure, the pulmonary valve opens before the aortic valve. Therefore, pulmonary ejection sounds occur closer to the first heart sound than do aortic ejection sounds. During systole the pressure in the ventricles slightly exceeds the pressure in the corresponding great arteries. Towards the end of systole, the ventricular pressure falls below the pressure in the great arteries, and when diastolic pressure is reached the semilunar valves close. Normally, aortic valve closure precedes pulmonary valve closure. The mitral and tricuspid valves begin to open at the point at which the ventricular pressures fall below the corresponding atrial pressures.
(Adapted from Swash M, ed. *Hutchison's clinical methods*, 20th edn. Philadelphia: Baillière Tindall, 1995, with permission.)

Soft first heart sounds can be due to a prolonged diastolic filling time (as with first-degree heart block) or a delayed onset of left ventricular systole (as with left bundle branch block), or to failure of the leaflets to coapt normally (as in mitral regurgitation).

The **second heart sound** (S2) will have a *loud* aortic component (A2) in patients with systemic hypertension. This results in forceful aortic valve closure secondary to high aortic pressures. Congenital aortic stenosis is another cause, because the valve is mobile but narrowed, and closes suddenly at the end of systole. The pulmonary component of the second heart sound (P2) is traditionally said to be *loud* in pulmonary hypertension, where the valve closure is forceful because of the high pulmonary pressure. In fact, a palpable P2 correlates better with raised pulmonary pressures than a loud P2.[21]

A *soft* A2 will be found when the aortic valve is calcified and leaflet movement is reduced, and in aortic regurgitation when the leaflets cannot coapt.

Splitting. Splitting of the heart sound is usually most obvious during auscultation in the pulmonary area. Splitting of the **first heart sound** is usually not detectable clinically; however, when it occurs it is most often due to the cardiac conduction abnormality known as complete right bundle branch block.

Increased normal splitting (wider on inspiration) of the **second heart sound** occurs when there is any delay in right ventricular emptying, as in right bundle branch block (delayed right ventricular depolarisation), pulmonary stenosis (delayed right ventricular ejection), ventricular septal defect (increased right ventricular volume load), and mitral regurgitation (because of earlier aortic valve closure, due to more rapid left ventricular emptying).

In the case of *fixed splitting* of the second heart sound, there is no respiratory variation (as is normal) and splitting tends to be wide. This is caused by an atrial septal defect where equalisation of volume loads between the two atria occurs through the defect. This results in the atria acting as a common chamber.

In the case of *reversed splitting*, P2 occurs first and splitting occurs in expiration. This can be due to delayed left ventricular depolarisation (left bundle branch block), delayed left ventricular emptying (severe aortic stenosis, coarctation of the aorta) or increased left ventricular volume load (large patent ductus arteriosus). However, in the last-mentioned, the loud machinery murmur means that the second heart sound is usually not heard.

Extra heart sounds. The **third heart sound** (S3) is a low-pitched (20–70 Hz) mid-diastolic sound that is best appreciated by listening for a triple rhythm.[22] Its low pitch makes it more easily heard with the bell of the stethoscope. It has been likened (rather accurately) to the galloping of a horse and is often called a *gallop rhythm*. Its cadence is similar to that of the word 'Kentucky'. It is more likely to be appreciated if the clinician listens not to the individual heart sounds but to the rhythm of the heart. It is probably caused by tautening of the mitral or tricuspid papillary muscles at the end of rapid diastolic filling, when blood flow temporarily stops. A physiological left ventricular S3 sometimes occurs in children and young people and is due to very rapid diastolic filling. A pathological S3 is due to reduced ventricular compliance, so that a filling sound is produced even when diastolic filling is not especially rapid. It is strongly associated with increased atrial pressure.

A *left ventricular* S3 is louder at the apex than at the left sternal edge, and is louder on expiration. It can be associated with an increased cardiac output, as occurs in pregnancy and thyrotoxicosis. Otherwise, it is an important sign of left ventricular failure and dilatation, but may also occur in aortic regurgitation, mitral regurgitation, ventricular septal defect and patent ductus arteriosus.[23]

A *right ventricular* S3 is louder at the left sternal edge and with inspiration. It occurs in right ventricular failure or constrictive pericarditis.

The **fourth heart sound** (S4) is a late diastolic sound pitched slightly higher than the S3.[24] The cadence of an S4 is similar to that of the word 'Tennessee'. Again, this is responsible for the impression of a triple (gallop) rhythm. It is due to a high-pressure atrial wave reflected back from a poorly compliant ventricle. It does not occur if the patient is in atrial fibrillation, because the sound depends on effective atrial contraction, which is lost when the atria fibrillate. Its low pitch means that unlike a split first heart sound it disappears if the bell of the stethoscope is pressed firmly onto the chest.

A *left ventricular* S4 occurs whenever left ventricular compliance is reduced due to aortic stenosis, acute mitral regurgitation, systemic hypertension, ischaemic heart disease or advanced age. It is often present during an episode of angina or with a myocardial infarction, and may be the only physical sign of that condition.

A *right ventricular* S4 occurs when right ventricular compliance is reduced in pulmonary hypertension or pulmonary stenosis.

If the heart rate is greater than 120 per minute, S3 and S4 may be superimposed, resulting in a **summation gallop**. In this case, two inaudible sounds may combine to produce an audible one. This does not necessarily imply ventricular stress, unless one or both of the extra heart sounds persists when the heart rate slows or is slowed by carotid sinus massage. When both S3 and S4 are present, the rhythm is described as a quadruple rhythm. It usually implies severe ventricular dysfunction.

Additional sounds. An **opening snap** is a high-pitched sound that occurs in mitral stenosis at a variable distance after S2. It is due to the sudden opening of the mitral valve and is followed by the diastolic murmur of mitral stenosis. It can be difficult to distinguish from a widely split S2, but normally occurs rather later in diastole than the pulmonary component of the second heart sound. It is pitched higher than a third heart sound and so is not usually confused with this. It is best heard at the lower left sternal edge with the diaphragm of the stethoscope. Use of the term 'opening snap' implies the diagnosis of mitral or rarely of tricuspid stenosis.

A **systolic ejection click** is an early systolic high-pitched sound that is heard over the aortic or pulmonary and left sternal edge areas, and which may occur in cases of congenital aortic or pulmonary stenosis where the valve remains mobile; it is followed by the systolic ejection murmur of aortic or pulmonary stenosis. It is due to the abrupt doming of the abnormal valve early in systole.

A **non-ejection systolic click** is a high-pitched sound heard during systole and is best appreciated at the mitral area. It is a common finding. It may be followed by a systolic murmur. The click may be due to prolapse of one or more redundant mitral valve leaflets during systole. Non-ejection clicks may also be heard in patients with *atrial septal defects* or *Ebstein's anomaly* (page 89).

An *atrial myxoma* is a very rare tumour which may occur in either atrium. During atrial systole a loosely pedunculated tumour may be propelled into the mitral or tricuspid valve orifice causing an early diastolic plopping sound, a **tumour plop**. This sound is only rarely heard even in patients with a myxoma (about 10%).

A **diastolic pericardial knock** may occur when there is sudden cessation of ventricular filling because of constrictive pericardial disease.[25]

Prosthetic heart valves produce characteristic sounds (page 90). Rarely, a right ventricular pacemaker produces a late diastolic high-pitched click due to contraction of the chest wall muscles (the **pacemaker sound**).[26]

Murmurs of the heart

In deciding the origin of a cardiac murmur, a number of different features must be considered. These are: timing, the area of greatest intensity, the loudness and pitch, associated features (peripheral signs), and the effect of dynamic manoeuvres, including respiration and the Valsalva manoeuvre (Figure 4.32). The presence of a characteristic murmur is very reliable for the diagnosis of certain valvular abnormalities, but for others less so.

Associated features. As already mentioned, the cause of a cardiac murmur can sometimes be elicited by careful analysis of the peripheral signs.

Timing (Table 4.15). **Systolic murmurs** (which occur during ventricular systole) may be pansystolic, ejection systolic or late systolic.

The *pansystolic murmur* extends throughout systole, beginning with the first heart sound, then going right up to the second heart sound. Its loudness and pitch vary during systole. Pansystolic murmurs occur when a ventricle leaks to a lower pressure chamber or vessel. As there is a pressure difference from the moment the ventricle begins to contract (S1), blood flow and the murmur both begin at the first heart sound and continue until the pressures equalise (S2). Causes of pansystolic murmurs include mitral regurgitation,[x] tricuspid regurgitation and ventricular septal defect.

With an *ejection (mid)systolic* murmur, the murmur does not begin right at the first heart sound; its intensity is greatest in midsystole or later,

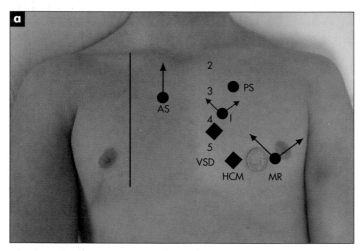

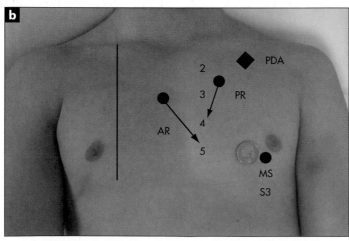

Figure 4.32 Sites of maximum intensity and radiation of murmurs and heart sounds
(a) Systolic murmurs:
   AS = aortic stenosis;
   MR = mitral regurgitation;
   HCM = hypertrophic cardiomyopathy;
   PS = pulmonary stenosis;
   VSD = ventricular septal defect;
   I = innocent.
(b) Diastolic murmurs and sounds:
   AR = aortic regurgitation;
   MS = mitral stenosis;
   S3 = third heart sound;
   PR = pulmonary regurgitation;
   PDA = patent ductus arteriosus
      (continuous murmur).

GOOD SIGNS GUIDE 4.1 Characteristic murmurs and valvular heart disease

Sign	Positive LR	Negative LR
Characteristic systolic murmur		
Aortic stenosis	3.3	0.1
Mild mitral regurgitation or worse (moderate or severe)	5.4	0.4
Mild tricuspid regurgitation or worse	14.6	0.8
Moderate to severe tricuspid regurgitation	10.1	0.4
Characteristic diastolic murmur		
Mild aortic regurgitation or worse	9.9	0.3
Pulmonary regurgitation	17.4	NS

NS = not significant.
From McGee S, *Evidence-based physical diagnosis*, 2nd edn. St Louis: Saunders, 2007.

and wanes again late in systole. This is described as a *crescendo-decrescendo* murmur. These murmurs are usually caused by turbulent flow through the aortic or pulmonary valve orifices or by greatly increased flow through a normal-sized orifice or outflow tract.

With a *late systolic* murmur it is possible to distinguish an appreciable gap between the first heart sound and the murmur, which then continues right up to the second heart sound. This is typical of mitral valve prolapse or papillary muscle dysfunction where mitral regurgitation begins in midsystole.

Diastolic murmurs occur during ventricular diastole. They are more difficult for students to hear than systolic murmurs and are usually softer. A loud murmur is unlikely to be diastolic.

The *early diastolic* murmur begins immediately with the second heart sound and has a decrescendo quality (it is loudest at the beginning and extends for a variable distance into diastole). These early diastolic murmurs are typically high pitched and are due to regurgitation through leaking aortic or pulmonary valves. The murmur is loudest at the beginning because this is when aortic and pulmonary artery pressures are highest.

Mid-diastolic murmurs begin later in diastole and may be short or extend right up to the first heart sound. They have a much lower-pitched quality than early diastolic murmurs. They are due to impaired flow during ventricular filling and can be caused by mitral stenosis and tricuspid stenosis, where the valve is narrowed, or rarely by an atrial myxoma, where the tumour mass obstructs the valve orifice.

In severe aortic regurgitation, the regurgitant jet from the aortic valve may cause the anterior leaflet of the mitral valve to shudder, producing a diastolic murmur. Occasionally, normal mitral or tricuspid valves can produce flow murmurs, which are short and mid-diastolic, and occur when there is torrential flow across the valve. Causes include a high cardiac output or intracardiac shunting (atrial or ventricular septal defects).

Presystolic murmurs may be heard when atrial systole increases blood flow across the valve just before the first heart sound. They are extensions of the mid-diastolic murmurs of mitral stenosis and tricuspid stenosis, and usually do not occur when atrial systole is lost in atrial fibrillation.

As the name implies, **continuous murmurs** extend throughout systole and diastole. They are produced when a communication exists between two parts of the circulation with a permanent pressure gradient so that blood flow occurs continuously. They can usually be distinguished from combined systolic and diastolic murmurs (due, for example, to aortic stenosis and aortic regurgitation), but this may sometimes be difficult. The causes are presented in Table 4.15.

A **pericardial friction rub** is a superficial scratching sound; there may be up to three distinct components occurring at any time during the cardiac cycle. They are not confined to systole or diastole. A rub is caused by movement of inflamed pericardial surfaces; it is a result of pericarditis. The sound can vary with respiration and posture; it is often louder when the patient is sitting up and breathing out. It tends to come and go, and is often absent by the time students can be found to come and listen for it. It has been likened to the crunching sound made when *walking on snow*.

---

x The term incompetence is synonymous with regurgitation, but the latter better describes the pathophysiology.

TABLE 4.15 Cardiac murmurs

Timing	Lesion
Pansystolic	Mitral regurgitation
	Tricuspid regurgitation
	Ventricular septal defect
	Aortopulmonary shunts
Midsystolic	Aortic stenosis
	Pulmonary stenosis
	Hypertrophic cardiomyopathy
	Pulmonary flow murmur of an atrial septal defect
Late systolic	Mitral valve prolapse
	Papillary muscle dysfunction (due usually to ischaemia or hypertrophic cardiomyopathy)
Early diastolic	Aortic regurgitation
	Pulmonary regurgitation
Mid-diastolic	Mitral stenosis
	Tricuspid stenosis
	Atrial myxoma
	Austin Flint* murmur of aortic regurgitation
	Carey Coombs[†] murmur of acute rheumatic fever
Presystolic	Mitral stenosis
	Tricuspid stenosis
	Atrial myxoma
Continuous	Patent ductus arteriosus
	Arteriovenous fistula (coronary artery, pulmonary, systemic)
	Aortopulmonary connection (e.g. congenital, Blalock[‡] shunt)
	Venous hum (usually best heard over right supraclavicular fossa and abolished by ipsilateral internal jugular vein compression)
	Rupture of sinus of Valsalva into right ventricle or atrium
	'Mammary souffle' (in late pregnancy or early postpartum period)

Note: The combined murmurs of aortic stenosis and aortic regurgitation, or mitral stenosis and mitral regurgitation, may sound as if they fill the entire cardiac cycle, but are not continuous murmurs by definition.
* See footnote mm, page 87.
[†] Carey F Coombs (b. 1879), Bristol physician.
[‡] Alfred Blalock (1899–1965), Baltimore physician.

A **mediastinal crunch** (Hamman's sign[y]) is a crunching sound heard in time with the heartbeat but with systolic and diastolic components. It is caused by the presence of air in the mediastinum, and once heard it is not forgotten. It is very often present after cardiac surgery and may occur associated with a pneumothorax or after aspiration of a pericardial effusion.

Area of greatest intensity. Although the place on the praecordium where a murmur is heard most easily is a guide to its origin, this is not a particularly reliable physical sign. For example, mitral regurgitation murmurs (*Good signs guide 4.1*) are usually loudest at the apex, over the mitral area, and tend to radiate towards the axillae, but they may be heard widely over the praecordium and even right up into the aortic area or over the back. Conduction of an ejection murmur up into

[y]   Louis Hamman (1877–1946), physician, Johns Hopkins Hospital, Baltimore.

GOOD SIGNS GUIDE 4.2   Dynamic auscultation

Sign	Positive LR	Negative LR
Louder on inspiration—right-sided murmur	7.8	0.2
Louder with Valsalva strain—hypertrophic cardiomyopathy	14.0	0.3
Louder squatting to standing—hypertrophic cardiomyopathy	6.0	0.1
Softer with isometric handgrip—hypertrophic cardiomyopathy	3.6	0.1
Louder with isometric handgrip—mitral regurgitation	5.8	0.3

From McGee S, *Evidence-based physical diagnosis*, 2nd edn. St Louis: Saunders, 2007.

TABLE 4.16   Dynamic manoeuvres and systolic cardiac murmurs

Manoeuvre	Lesion			
	Hypertrophic cardiomyopathy	Mitral valve prolapse	Aortic stenosis	Mitral regurgitation
Valsalva strain phase (decreases preload)	Louder	Longer	Softer	Softer
Squatting or leg raise (increases preload)	Softer	Shorter	Louder	Louder
Hand grip (increases afterload)	Softer	Shorter	Softer	Louder

the carotid arteries strongly suggests that this arises from the aortic valve.

Loudness and pitch. Unfortunately, the *loudness* of the murmur is not always helpful in deciding the severity of the valve lesion. For example, in the severest forms of valve stenosis, murmurs may be soft. However, murmurs are usually graded according to loudness. Cardiologists most often use a classification with six grades (Levine's grading system):[27]

Grade 1/6: very soft and not heard at first (often audible only to consultants and to those students who have been told the murmur is present)
Grade 2/6: soft, but can be detected almost immediately by an experienced auscultator
Grade 3/6: moderate; there is no thrill
Grade 4/6: loud; thrill just palpable
Grade 5/6: very loud; thrill easily palpable
Grade 6/6: very, very loud; can be heard even without placing the stethoscope right on the chest.

This grading is useful, particularly because a change in the intensity of a murmur may be of great significance—for example, after a myocardial infarction.

It requires practice to appreciate the *pitch* of the murmur, but this may be of use in identifying its type. In general, low-pitched murmurs indicate turbulent flow under low pressure, as in mitral stenosis, and high-pitched murmurs indicate a high velocity of flow, as in mitral regurgitation.

Dynamic manoeuvres (*Good signs guide 4.2*). All patients with a newly diagnosed murmur should undergo dynamic manoeuvre testing (Table 4.16).[28]

• **Respiration.** Murmurs that arise on the right side of the heart become louder during inspiration as this increases venous return and therefore blood flow to the right side of the heart. Left-sided murmurs are either unchanged or become softer. Expiration has the opposite effect. This can be a sensitive and specific way of differentiating right- and left-sided murmurs.
• **Deep expiration.** A routine part of the examination of the heart (Figure 4.33) includes leaning a patient forward in full expiration and listening to the base of the heart for aortic regurgitation, which may otherwise be missed. In this case the manoeuvre brings the base of the heart closer to the chest wall. The scraping sound of a pericardial friction rub is also best heard in this position.

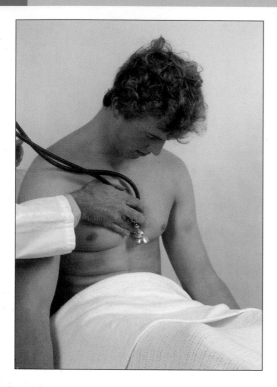

Figure 4.33 Dynamic auscultation for aortic regurgitation or a pericardial friction rub; patient in deep expiration

- **The Valsalva manoeuvre.**[z] This is a forceful expiration against a closed glottis. One should ask the patient to hold his or her nose with the fingers, close the mouth, breathe out hard and completely so as to pop the eardrums, and hold this for as long as possible. Listen over the left sternal edge during this manoeuvre for changes in the systolic murmur of hypertrophic cardiomyopathy, and over the apex for changes when mitral valve prolapse is suspected.

The Valsalva manoeuvre has four phases. In phase 1 (beginning the manoeuvre), a rise in intrathoracic pressure and a transient increase in left ventricular output and blood pressure occurs. In phase 2 (the straining phase), systemic venous return falls, filling of the right and then the left side of the heart is reduced, and stroke volume and blood pressure fall while the heart rate increases. As stroke volume and arterial blood pressure fall, most cardiac murmurs become softer; however,

because the left ventricular volume is reduced, the systolic murmur of hypertrophic cardiomyopathy becomes louder and the systolic click and murmur of mitral valve prolapse begins earlier. In phase 3 (the release of the manoeuvre), first right-sided and then left-sided cardiac murmurs become louder briefly before returning to normal. Blood pressure falls further because of pooling of blood in the pulmonary veins. In phase 4, the blood pressure overshoots as a result of increased sympathetic activity as a response to the previous hypotension. Changes in heart rate are opposite to the blood pressure changes.

The blood pressure responses can be measured by inflating a cuff to 15 mmHg over the systolic pressure before the manoeuvre. Korotkoff sounds will then appear in phases 1 and 4 in a normal patient. Absence of the phase 4 overshoot is a sign of cardiac failure. The left ventricle is unable to increase cardiac output despite increased sympathetic activity.

- **Standing to squatting.** When the patient squats rapidly from the standing position, venous return and systemic arterial resistance increase simultaneously, causing a rise in stroke volume and arterial pressure. This makes most murmurs louder. However, left ventricular size is increased, which reduces the obstruction to outflow and therefore reduces the intensity of the systolic murmur of hypertrophic cardiomyopathy, while the midsystolic click and murmur of mitral valve prolapse are delayed.
- **Squatting to standing.** When the patient stands up quickly after squatting, the opposite changes in the loudness of these murmurs occurs.
- **Isometric exercise.** Sustained hand grip or repeated sit-ups for 20 for 30 seconds increases systemic arterial resistance, blood pressure and heart size. The systolic murmur of aortic stenosis may become softer because of a reduction in the pressure difference across the valve but often remains unchanged. Most other murmurs become louder, except the systolic murmur of hypertrophic cardiomyopathy, which is softer, and the mitral valve prolapse murmur, which is delayed because of an increased ventricular volume.

Auscultation of the neck

This is often performed as a part of dynamic auscultation for valvular heart disease, but certain aspects of the examination may be considered here. Abnormal sounds heard over the arteries are called *bruits*. These sounds are low-pitched and may be more easily heard with the bell of the

[z] Antonio Valsalva (1666–1723), Professor of Anatomy at Bologna, was noted for his studies of the ear. He described his manoeuvre in 1704. Forced expiration against the closed glottis causes discharge of pus into the external auditory canal in cases of chronic otitis media. Friedrich Weber rediscovered the manoeuvre in 1859 and demonstrated that he could slow his pulse at will. He stopped demonstrating this after he caused himself to faint and have convulsions.

stethoscope. Carotid artery bruits are most easily heard over the anterior part of the sternomastoid muscle above the medial end of the clavicle. Ask the patient to stop breathing for a brief period to remove the competing noise of breath sounds. It may be prudent to ask the patient not to speak. The amplified voice is often painfully loud when heard through the stethoscope.

A systolic bruit may be a conducted sound from the heart. The murmur of aortic stenosis is always audible in the neck and a soft carotid bruit is sometimes audible in patients with severe mitral regurgitation or pulmonary stenosis. A bruit due to carotid stenosis will not be audible over the base of the heart. Move the stethoscope from point to point onto the chest wall; if the bruit disappears, it is likely the sound arises from the carotid. It is not possible to exclude a carotid bruit in a patient with a murmur of aortic stenosis that radiates to the neck. Carotid artery stenosis is an important cause of a carotid bruit. More severe stenosis is associated with a noise that is longer and of increased pitch. Total obstruction of the vessel leads to disappearance of the bruit. It is not possible to make a diagnosis of significant (>60% obstruction) carotid stenosis clinically. The bottom line is that a carotid bruit poorly predicts significant carotid stenosis or stroke risk. Thyrotoxicosis can result in a systolic bruit (page 303) due to the increased vascularity of the gland.

A continuous noise is sometimes audible at the base of the neck. This is usually a venous hum, a result of audible venous flow. It disappears if light pressure is applied to the neck just above the stethoscope. Occasionally a loud machinery murmur (page 93) or severe aortic regurgitation (page 86) may cause a similar sound. Haemodialysis patients frequently have an audible bruit transmitted from their arterio-venous fistula.

The back

It is now time to leave the praecordium. Percussion and auscultation of the *lung bases* (Chapter 5) are also part of the cardiovascular examination. Signs of cardiac failure may be detected in the lungs; in particular late or pan-inspiratory crackles or a pleural effusion may be present. The murmur associated with coarctation of the aorta may be prominent over the upper back.

While the patient is sitting up, feel for pitting oedema of the sacrum, which occurs in severe right heart failure, especially in patients who have been in bed. This is because the sacrum then becomes a dependent area and oedema fluid tends to settle under the influence of gravity.

The abdomen

Lay the patient down flat (on one pillow) and examine the abdomen (Chapter 6). You are looking particularly for an enlarged tender *liver* which may be found when the hepatic veins are congested in the presence of right heart failure. Distension of the liver capsule is said to be the cause of liver tenderness in these patients. When tricuspid regurgitation is present the liver may be *pulsatile*, as the right ventricular systolic pressure wave is transmitted to the hepatic veins. Test for hepatojugular reflux.[17,29] *Ascites* may occur with severe right heart failure. *Splenomegaly*, if present, may indicate infective endocarditis.

Feel for the pulsation of the abdominal aorta, to the left of the middle line. It is often palpable in normal thin people but the possibility of an abdominal aortic aneurysm should always be considered when the aorta's pulsations are palpable and expansile (page 173).[30,31]

The lower limbs (Table 4.17)

Palpate behind the medial malleolus of the tibia and the distal shaft of the tibia for *oedema* by compressing the area for at least 15 seconds with the thumb. This latter area is often tender in normal people, and gentleness is necessary. Oedema may be pitting (the skin is indented and only slowly refills—Figure 4.34) or non-pitting. Oedema due to hypoalbuminaemia often refills more quickly.

Pitting oedema occurs in cardiac failure unless the condition has been present for a long time and secondary changes in the lymphatic vessels have occurred. If oedema is present, note its upper level (e.g. 'pitting oedema to mid-calf' or 'pitting oedema to mid-thigh'). Severe oedema can involve

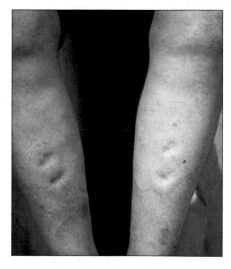

Figure 4.34 Severe pitting oedema of the legs

TABLE 4.17 Lower limb examination

1 Inspection—anterior and lateral surfaces, sole of foot, between toes
- Amputation
- Ulcers
- Erythema
- Varicosities
- Atrophy
- Scars
- Discoloration (e.g. venous staining)
- Loss of hair

2 Palpation
- Temperature: run the dorsum of the hand from the hips to the foot on each side. Note reduction in temperature peripherally and compare left and right
- Test capillary refill: press on great toenail and release. The blanched nail bed should turn pink within 3 seconds
- Test venous filling: occlude the dorsal venous arch of each foot in turn using two fingers; release the distal finger and look for venous refilling. Absence of venous refilling suggests poor arterial supply to the foot
- Pulses: feel for an abdominal aortic aneurysm, feel for a femoral pulse, the popliteal pulses (flex the patient's leg), then feel the posterior tibial and dorsalis pedis pulses

3 Auscultation
- Listen for abdominal, renal, and femoral bruits

4 Perform Buerger's test (see text)

5 Measure the ankle–brachial index

6 Test lower limb sensation. Diabetes may cause sensory loss in a 'stocking' distribution.

7 Test for glucose in the urine

TABLE 4.18 Causes of oedema

Pitting lower limb oedema
Cardiac: congestive cardiac failure, constrictive pericarditis
Drugs: calcium antagonists
Hepatic: cirrhosis causing hypoalbuminaemia
Renal: nephrotic syndrome causing hypoalbuminaemia
Gastrointestinal tract: malabsorption, starvation, protein-losing enteropathy causing hypoalbuminaemia
Beri-beri (wet)
Cyclical oedema

Pitting unilateral lower limb oedema
Deep venous thrombosis
Compression of large veins by tumour or lymph nodes

Non-pitting lower limb oedema
Hypothyroidism
Lymphoedema
- Infectious (e.g. filariasis)
- Malignant (tumour invasion of lymphatics)
- Congenital (lymphatic development arrest)
- Allergy
- Milroy's* disease (unexplained lymphoedema which appears at puberty and is more common in females)

* William Milroy (1855–1914), Professor of Medicine, University of Nebraska, described the disease in 1928.

the skin of the abdominal wall and the scrotum as well as the lower limbs. Causes of oedema are listed in Table 4.18.

Non-pitting oedema suggests chronic lymphoedema which is due to lymphatic obstruction. 'Lipidoedema' is a term used to describe fat deposition in the ankles. It typically spares the feet and affects obese women.

Look for evidence of Achilles[aa] tendon xanthomata due to hyperlipidaemia. Also look for cyanosis and clubbing of the toes (this may occur without finger clubbing in a patient with a patent ductus arteriosus, because a rise in pulmonary artery pressures, sufficient to reverse the direction of flow in the shunt, has occurred).

Peripheral vascular disease

Examine both *femoral arteries* by palpating and then auscultating them. A bruit may be heard if the artery is narrowed. Next palpate the following pulses: *popliteal* (behind the knee—Figure 4.35a: if this is difficult to feel when the patient is supine, try the method shown in Figure 4.35b), *posterior tibial* (under the medial malleolus, Figure 4.36a) and *dorsalis pedis* (on the forefoot, Figure 4.36b) on both sides.[32]

Patients with exertional calf pain (intermittent claudication) are likely to have disease of the peripheral arteries. More severe disease can lead to pain even at rest and to ischaemic changes in the legs and feet (*Good signs guide 4.3*). Look for atrophic skin and loss of hair, colour changes of the feet (blue or red) and ulcers at the lower end of the tibia.[4] Venous and diabetic ulcers can be distinguished from arterial ulcers (Figures 4.37–4.39).

Look for reduced capillary return (compress the toenails—the return of the normal red colour is slow).[33] In such cases, perform *Buerger's test*[bb] to help confirm your diagnosis: elevate the legs to 45 degrees (pallor is rapid if there is a poor arterial

---

aa Achilles, mythical Greek hero, whose body was invulnerable except for his heels, by which he was held when dipped in the River Styx as a baby to make him immortal. He was killed by Paris, who shot an arrow into his heel.

bb Leo Buerger (1879–1943), New York physician, born in Vienna, who described thromboangiitis obliterans. He was obsessed with expensive cars.

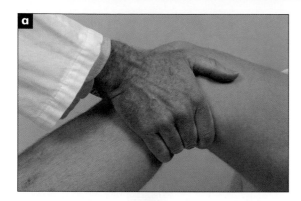

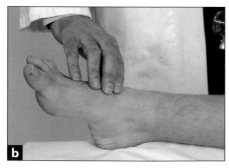

Figure 4.35 Palpating the popliteal artery:
(a) patient supine; (b) patient prone

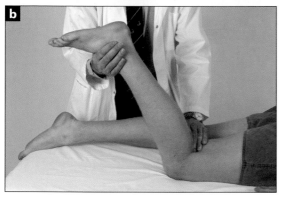

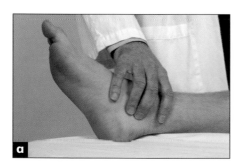

Figure 4.36 Feeling (a) the posterior tibial artery
and (b) the dorsalis pedis artery

GOOD SIGNS GUIDE 4.3 Peripheral vascular
disease

Sign	Positive LR	Negative LR
Sores or ulcers on feet	7.0	NS
Feet pale, red or blue	2.8	0.7
Atrophic skin	1.7	NS
Absent hair	1.7	NS
One foot cooler	6.1	0.9
Absent femoral pulse	6.1	NS
Absent dorsalis pedis and posterior tibial pulses	14.9	0.3
Limb bruit present	7.3	0.7
Capillary refill time >5 seconds	1.9	NS
Capillary refill >20 seconds	3.6	NS

NS = not significant.
From McGee S, *Evidence-based physical diagnosis*, 2nd
   edn. St Louis: Saunders, 2007.

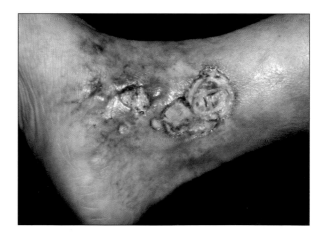

Figure 4.37 Venous ulcer
This venous ulcer has an irregular margin, pale surrounding
neo-epithelium (new skin), and a pink base of granulation
tissue. There is often a history of deep venous thrombosis.
The skin is warm and oedema is often present. (See Table
4.19.)
(From McDonald FS, ed., *Mayo Clinic images in internal
medicine,* with permission. © Mayo Clinic Scientific Press
and CRC Press.)

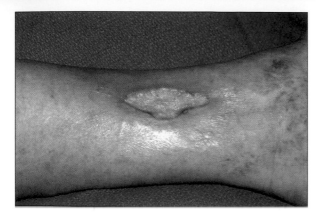

Figure 4.38 Arterial ulcer
This arterial ulcer has a regular margin and 'punched out' appearance. The surrounding skin is cold. The peripheral pulses are absent. (See Table 4.19.)
(From McDonald FS, ed., *Mayo Clinic images in internal medicine,* with permission. © Mayo Clinic Scientific Press and CRC Press.)

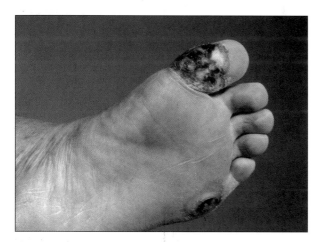

Figure 4.39 Diabetic (neuropathic) ulcer
Neuropathic ulcers are painless and are associated with reduced sensation in the surrounding skin. (See Table 4.19.)
(From McDonald FS, ed., *Mayo Clinic images in internal medicine*, with permission. © Mayo Clinic Scientific Press and CRC Press.)

supply), then place them dependent at 90 degrees over the edge of the bed (cyanosis occurs if the arterial supply is impaired). Normally there is no change in colour in either position.

The **ankle–brachial index** (ABI) is a measure of arterial supply to the lower limbs, and an abnormal index indicates increased cardiovascular risk. The systolic blood pressure in the dorsalis pedis or posterior tibial artery is measured using a Doppler probe and a blood pressure cuff over the calf. This is divided by the systolic blood pressure measured

in the normal way at the brachial artery. An ABI of less than 0.9 indicates significant arterial disease and an ABI of between 0.4 and 0.9 is associated with claudication. ABIs of less than 0.4 are associated with critical limb ischaemia. An ABI greater than 1.3 occurs with a calcified (non-compressible) artery.

Acute arterial occlusion

Acute arterial occlusion of a major peripheral limb artery results in a painful, pulseless, pale, 'paralysed' limb which is perishingly cold and has paraethesiae (the six P's).

It can be the result of embolism, thrombosis or injury. Peripheral arterial embolism usually arises from thrombus in the heart, where it is often secondary to (i) myocardial infarction, (ii) dilated cardiomyopathy, (iii) atrial fibrillation or (iv) infective endocarditis.[34]

Deep venous thrombosis

Deep venous thrombosis is a difficult clinical diagnosis (*Good signs guide 4.4*).[35] The patient may complain of calf pain. On examination, the clinician should look for swelling of the calf and the thigh, and dilated superficial veins. Feel then for increased warmth and squeeze the calf (gently) to determine if the area is tender. Homans' sign[cc] (pain in the calf when the foot is sharply dorsiflexed) is of limited diagnostic value and is theoretically dangerous because of the possibility of dislodgment of loose thrombus.

The causes of thrombosis were described by Virchow[dd] in 1856 under three broad headings (the famous *Virchow's triad*): (i) changes in the vessel wall, (ii) changes in blood flow, and (iii) changes in the constitution of the blood. Deep venous thrombosis is usually caused by prolonged immobilisation, cardiac failure (stasis) or trauma (vessel wall damage), but may also result from occult neoplasm, disseminated intravascular coagulation, the contraceptive pill, pregnancy and a number of inherited defects of coagulation (the *thrombophilias*: e.g. Factor V Leiden, anti-thrombin III deficiency).

cc   John Homans (1877–1954), professor of surgery, Harvard University, Boston. He described his sign in 1941, originally in cases of thrombophlebitis. He later became disenchanted with the sign and is reputed to have asked why if a sign were to be named after him it couldn't be a useful one.
dd   Rudolph Virchow (1821–1902), brilliant German pathologist, regarded as the founder of modern pathology. professor of pathological anatomy in Berlin. He provided the first description of leukaemia. He died at 81 after fracturing his femur jumping from a moving tram.

TABLE 4.19 Causes of leg ulcers

1 Venous stasis ulcer—most common (Figure 4.37)
  Site: around malleoli
  Character: irregular margin, granulation tissue in the floor. Surrounding tissue inflammation and oedema
  Associated pigmentation, stasis eczema

2 Ischaemic ulcer (Figure 4.38)
  • Large-artery disease (atherosclerosis, thromboangiitis obliterans): usually lateral side of leg (pulses absent)
  • Small-vessel disease (e.g. leucocytoclastic vasculitis, palpable purpura)
  Site: over pressure areas, lateral malleolus, dorsum and margins of the feet and toes
  Character: smooth, rounded, 'punched out' pale base which does not bleed

3 Malignant ulcer, e.g. basal cell carcinoma (pearly translucent edge), squamous cell carcinoma (hard everted edge), melanoma, lymphoma, Kaposi's sarcoma

4 Infection, e.g. *Staphylococcus aureus*, syphilitic gumma, tuberculosis, atypical *Mycobacterium*, fungal

5 Neuropathic (painless penetrating ulcer on sole of foot: peripheral neuropathy, e.g. diabetes mellitus, tabes, leprosy) (Figure 4.39)

6 Underlying systemic disease
  • Diabetes mellitus: vascular disease, neuropathy or necrobiosis lipoidica (front of leg)
  • Pyoderma gangrenosum
  • Rheumatoid arthritis
  • Lymphoma
  • Haemolytic anaemia (small ulcers over malleoli), e.g. sickle cell anaemia

GOOD SIGNS GUIDE 4.4 Deep venous thrombosis

Sign	Positive LR	Negative LR
Asymmetrical calf swelling >2 cm difference	2.1	0.6
Thigh swelling	2.5	0.6
Superficial venous dilatation	1.9	NS
Tenderness and erythema	NS	NS
Asymmetrical skin warmth	1.4	NS
Homans' sign	NS	NS

NS = not significant.
From McGee S, *Evidence-based physical diagnosis*, 2nd edn. St Louis: Saunders, 2007.

The following supplementary tests are occasionally helpful (and surgeons like to quiz students on them in examinations).

Trendelenburg test:[ee] with the patient lying down, the leg is elevated. Firm pressure is placed on the saphenous opening in the groin, and the patient is instructed to stand. The sign is positive if the veins stay empty until the groin pressure is released (incompetence at the saphenofemoral valve). If the veins fill despite groin pressure, the incompetent valves are in the thigh or calf, and Perthes' test[ff] is performed.

Perthes' test: repeat the Trendelenburg test, but when the patient stands, allow some blood to be released and then get him or her to stand up and down on the toes a few times. The veins will become less tense if the perforating calf veins are patent and have competent valves (the muscle pump is functioning).

If the pattern of affected veins is unusual (e.g. pubic varices), the clinician should try to exclude secondary varicose veins. These may be due to an intrapelvic neoplasm which has obstructed deep venous return. Rectal and pelvic examinations should then be performed.

Finally, chronic venous stasis is one cause of ulceration of the lower leg. This is often associated with pigmentation and eczema, which are due to venous stasis.

The differential diagnosis of leg ulcers is summarised in Table 4.19.

Varicose veins

If a patient complains of 'varicose veins', ask him or her to *stand* with the legs fully exposed.[36] *Inspect* the front of the whole leg for tortuous, dilated branches of the long saphenous vein (below the femoral vein in the groin to the medial side of the lower leg). Then inspect the back of the calf for varicosities of the short saphenous vein (from the popliteal fossa to the back of the calf and lateral malleolus). Look to see if the leg is inflamed, swollen or pigmented (subcutaneous haemosiderin deposition secondary to venous stasis).

Palpate the veins. Hard leg veins suggest thrombosis, while tenderness indicates thrombophlebitis. Perform the *cough impulse test*. Put the fingers over the long saphenous vein opening in the groin, medial to the femoral vein. (Don't forget the anatomy—femoral vein [medial], artery [your landmark], nerve [lateral].) Ask the patient to cough: a fluid thrill is felt if the saphenofemoral valve is incompetent.

---

ee Friedrich Trendelenburg (1844–1924), professor of surgery, Leipzig.
ff Georg Clemens Perthes (1869–1927), German surgeon, professor of surgery at Tübingen. He was the first to use radiotherapy for the treatment of cancer (in 1903).

Correlation of physical signs and cardiovascular disease

When a disease is named after some author, it is very likely that we don't know much about it.

August Bier (1861–1949)

Cardiac failure

This is one of the commonest syndromes: the signs of cardiac failure should be sought in all patients admitted to hospital, especially if there is a complaint of dyspnoea (see *Questions box 5.2*, page 111).[37] Cardiac failure has been defined as a reduction in cardiac function such that cardiac output is reduced relative to the metabolic demands of the body and compensating mechanisms have occurred. The specific signs depend on whether the left, right or both ventricles are involved. It is important to note that the absence of definite signs of cardiac failure may not exclude the diagnosis. Patients with compensated, chronic cardiac failure may be normal on cardiac examination.

Left ventricular failure (LVF)

- **Symptoms:** exertional dyspnoea, orthopnoea, paroxysmal nocturnal dyspnoea.
- **General signs:** tachypnoea, due to raised pulmonary pressures; central cyanosis, due to pulmonary oedema; Cheyne-Stokes breathing (see Table 5.10, page 112), especially in sedated elderly patients; peripheral cyanosis, due to low cardiac output; hypotension, due to low cardiac output; cardiac cachexia.
- **Arterial pulse:** sinus tachycardia, due to increased sympathetic tone; low pulse pressure (low cardiac output); pulsus alternans (alternate strong and weak beats; it is unlike a bigeminal rhythm caused by regular ectopic beats, in that the beats are regular; see Figure 4.40)—this is an uncommon but specific sign of unknown aetiology.
- **Apex beat:** displaced, with dilatation of the left ventricle; dyskinetic in anterior myocardial infarction or dilated cardiomyopathy; palpable gallop rhythm. The absence of these signs does not exclude left ventricular failure.
- **Auscultation:** left ventricular S3 (an important sign); functional mitral regurgitation (secondary to valve ring dilatation).
- **Lung fields:** signs of pulmonary congestion (basal inspiratory crackles) or pulmonary oedema (crackles and wheezes throughout the lung fields), due to raised venous pressures (increased preload). The typical middle to

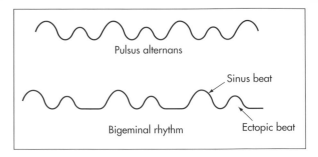

Figure 4.40 Pulsus alternans

late inspiratory crackles at the lung bases may be absent in chronic, compensated heart failure, and there are many other causes of basal inspiratory crackles. This makes crackles a rather non-specific and insensitive sign of heart failure.
- **Other signs:** abnormal Valsalva response, positive abdominojugular reflux test, right ventricular failure may complicate left ventricular failure, especially if this is severe and chronic.
- **Signs of the underlying or precipitating cause:**
  Causes of LVF: (i) myocardial disease (ischaemic heart disease, cardiomyopathy); (ii) volume overload (aortic regurgitation, mitral regurgitation, patent ductus arteriosus); (iii) pressure overload (systolic hypertension, aortic stenosis).
  Signs of a precipitating cause: anaemia, thyrotoxicosis (page 301), rapid arrhythmia (usually atrial fibrillation). (See *Good signs guide 4.5*.)

Right ventricular failure (RVF)

- **Symptoms:** ankle, sacral or abdominal swelling, anorexia, nausea.
- **General signs:** peripheral cyanosis, due to low cardiac output.
- **Arterial pulse:** low volume, due to low cardiac output.
- **Jugular venous pulse:** raised, due to the raised venous pressure (right heart preload); Kussmaul's sign, due to poor right ventricular compliance (e.g. right ventricular myocardial infarction); large *v* waves (functional tricuspid regurgitation secondary to valve ring dilatation).
- **Apex beat:** right ventricular heave.
- **Auscultation:** right ventricular S3; pansystolic murmur of functional tricuspid regurgitation (absence of a murmur does not exclude tricuspid regurgitation).

GOOD SIGNS GUIDE 4.5 Left ventricular failure

General signs	Positive LR	Negative LR
Heart rate >100 beats per minute at rest	5.5	NS
Valsalva manoeuvre abnormal	7.6	0.1
Lungs		
Crackles	NS	NS
Cardiac examination		
JVP elevated	3.9	NS
Abdominojugular test positive	8.0	0.3
Apex displaced lateral to midclavicular line	5.8	NS
S3	5.7	NS
S4	NS	NS
Other findings		
Oedema	NS	NS

NS = not significant.
From McGee S, *Evidence-based physical diagnosis*, 2nd edn. St Louis: Saunders, 2007.

- **Abdomen:** *tender hepatomegaly*, due to increased venous pressure transmitted via the hepatic veins; *pulsatile liver* (a useful sign), if tricuspid regurgitation is present.
- **Oedema:** due to sodium and water retention plus raised venous pressure, may be manifested by pitting ankle and sacral oedema, ascites, or pleural effusions (small).
- **Signs of the underlying cause:**
  Causes of RVF: (i) chronic obstructive pulmonary disease (commonest cause of cor pulmonale); (ii) left ventricular failure (severe chronic LVF causes raised pulmonary pressures resulting in secondary right ventricular failure); (iii) volume overload (atrial septal defect, primary tricuspid regurgitation); (iv) other causes of pressure overload (pulmonary stenosis, idiopathic pulmonary hypertension); (v) myocardial disease (right ventricular myocardial infarction, cardiomyopathy).

Chest pain

Many of the causes of chest pain represent a medical (or surgical) emergency. The appropriate diagnosis or differential diagnosis is often suggested by the history, and urgent investigations (e.g. ECG, chest X-ray, lung scan or pulmonary angiogram) may be indicated. However, a careful and rapid physical examination may add important information in many cases. In all cases the general inspection and measurement of the vital signs will help with the assessment of the severity and urgency of the problem. Certain specific signs may help with the diagnosis.[38,39]

Myocardial infarction

- **General signs:** there are few specific signs of myocardial infarction but many patients appear obviously unwell and in distress from their chest pain. Sweating (often called diaphoresis by accident and emergency staff), an appearance of anxiety (angor animi or sense of impending doom), and restlessness may be obvious. It is important that all this information be recorded so that changes to the patient's condition can be assessed as the infarct evolves.
- **Pulse and blood pressure:** tachycardia and/or hypotension (25% with anterior infarction from sympathetic hyperactivity); bradycardia and/or hypotension (up to 50% with inferior infarction from parasympathetic hyperactivity). Other arrhythmias including atrial fibrillation (due to atrial infarction), ventricular tachycardia and heart block may be present.
- **The JVP:** increased with right ventricular infarction; Kussmaul's sign is a specific and sensitive sign of right ventricular infarction in patients with a recent inferior infarct.
- **Apex beat:** dyskinetic in patients with large anterior infarction.
- **Auscultation:** S4; S3; decreased intensity of heart sounds; transient apical midsystolic or late-systolic murmur (in 25% from mitral regurgitation secondary to papillary muscle dysfunction), or a pericardial friction rub (with transmural infarction).
- **Complications:** arrhythmias (ventricular tachycardia, atrial fibrillation, ventricular fibrillation or heart block); heart failure; cardiogenic shock; rupture of a papillary muscle; perforation of the ventricular septum; ventricular aneurysm; thromboembolism or cardiac rupture. Signs of these complications (which do not usually occur for a few days after the infarct) include the development of a new murmur, recurrent chest pain, dyspnoea, sudden hypotension or sudden death.

The **Killip Class**[gg] can be calculated from the examination. It gives considerable prognostic information.[38]

Killip Class I—no evidence of heart failure
Killip Class II—mild heart failure; crackles over lower third or less of the lungs; systolic BP > 90 mmHg
Killip Class III—pulmonary oedema, crackles more than one-third of chest; systolic BP > 90 mmHg
Killip Class IV—cardiogenic shock, pulmonary oedema, crackles more than one-third of chest, systolic BP < 90 mmHg.

Killip Class III or IV is associated with a >5-fold mortality risk and Class II with a >3-fold risk compared with Class I.

Pulmonary embolism
There may be no physical signs of this condition, but dyspnoea which may be profound and make the patient exhausted is often the most obvious indication of a large pulmonary embolism. There is usually a resting tachycardia. Signs of shock—hypotension and cyanosis—indicate a very large and life-threatening embolus. There may be signs of a DVT in the legs but absence of these by no means excludes the diagnosis.

Acute aortic dissection
This is a difficult diagnosis which cannot usually be excluded on clinical grounds. A tear in the intima leads to blood surging into the aortic media, separating the intima and adventitia; this may present acutely or chronically. There are three different types: *type I* begins in the ascending aorta and extends proximally and distally; *type II* is limited to the ascending aorta and aortic arch (this is particularly associated with Marfan's syndrome); *type III* begins distal to the left subclavian artery and has the best prognosis.
- **Symptoms:** chest pain (typically very severe, it radiates to the back and is maximal in intensity at the time of onset due to either the aortic tear or associated myocardial infarction); stroke; syncope (associated with tamponade); symptoms of left ventricular failure; and, rarely, limb pain (ischaemia), paraplegia (spinal cord ischaemia), or abdominal pain (mesenteric ischaemia).
- **Signs:** the examination can reveal signs that make the diagnosis very likely (specific but not sensitive). There may be signs of a body habitus associated with dissection (e.g. Marfan's, Ehlers-Danlos syndromes). The pulses and blood pressures in the two arms must be assessed. A diminution of the radial pulse on one side or difference in blood pressure of 20 mmHg or more between the two arms is significant and suggests dissection has progressed to involve the origin of the arm vessels. Examine the patient for signs of pericardial tamponade (page 79), which occurs if the aorta ruptures into the pericardial sac. Examine the heart for signs of aortic regurgitation caused by disruption of the aortic valve annulus. A neurological examination may reveal signs of hemiplegia, due to dissection of one of the carotid arteries. Rare signs that have been described include a pulsatile sternoclavicular joint, hoarseness (recurrent laryngeal nerve compression) and dysphagia (oesophageal compression).

Pericardial disease
Acute pericarditis
- **Signs:** fever; dyspnoea; pericardial friction rub—sit the patient up and listen to the heart with the patient holding the breath in deep expiration.
- **Causes of acute pericarditis:** (i) viral infection (coxsackievirus A or B, influenza); (ii) after myocardial infarction—early, or late (10–14 days, termed Dressler's syndrome[hh]); (iii) after pericardiotomy (cardiac surgery); (iv) uraemia; (v) neoplasia—tumour invasion (e.g. bronchus, breast, lymphoma) or after irradiation for tumour; (vi) connective tissue disease (e.g. systemic lupus erythematosus, rheumatoid arthritis); (vii) hypothyroidism; (viii) other infections (e.g. tuberculosis, pyogenic pneumonia or septicaemia); (ix) acute rheumatic fever.

Chronic constrictive pericarditis
- **General signs:** cachexia.
- **Pulse and blood pressure:** pulsus paradoxus (more than the normal 10 mmHg fall in the arterial pulse pressure on inspiration, because increased right ventricular filling compresses the left ventricle); low blood pressure.
- **The JVP:** raised; Kussmaul's sign—lack of a fall or even increased distension on inspiration (50%); prominent *x* and *y* descents (brisk collapse during diastole).

---

99 T. Killip, a New Zealand cardiologist, published his classification in 1967.

hh William Dressler (1890–1969), a New York cardiologist, described this syndrome in 1956.

- **Apex beat:** impalpable.
- **Auscultation:** heart sounds distant, early S3; early pericardial knock (rapid ventricular filling abruptly halted).
- **Abdomen:** hepatomegaly, due to raised venous pressure; splenomegaly, due to raised venous pressure; ascites.
- **Peripheral oedema.**
- **Causes of chronic constrictive pericarditis:** (i) cardiac operation or trauma; (ii) tuberculosis, histoplasmosis or pyogenic infection; (iii) neoplastic disease; (iv) mediastinal irradiation; (v) connective tissue disease (especially rheumatoid arthritis); (vi) chronic renal failure.

Acute cardiac tamponade

- **General signs:** tachypnoea; anxiety and restlessness; syncope. Patients look very ill.
- **Pulse and blood pressure:** rapid pulse rate; pulsus paradoxus; hypotension.
- **The JVP:** raised; prominent x but an absent y descent.
- **Apex beat:** impalpable.
- **Auscultation:** soft heart sounds.
- **Lungs:** dullness and bronchial breathing at the left base, due to lung compression by the distended pericardial sac.

Infective endocarditis

- **General signs:** fever; weight loss; pallor (anaemia).
- **Hands:** splinter haemorrhages; clubbing (within six weeks of onset); Osler's nodes (rare); Janeway lesions (very rare).
- **Arms:** evidence of intravenous drug use (Figure 4.41)—right (and left) heart endocarditis can result from this.
- **Eyes:** pale conjunctivae (anaemia); retinal or conjunctival haemorrhages—Roth's spots[ii] are fundal vasculitic lesions with a yellow centre surrounded by a red ring (Figure 4.42).
- **Heart**—signs of *underlying heart disease*: (i) acquired (mitral regurgitation, mitral stenosis, aortic stenosis, aortic regurgitation); (ii) congenital (patent ductus arteriosus, ventricular septal defect, coarctation of the aorta); (iii) prosthetic valves.
- **Abdomen:** splenomegaly.
- **Peripheral evidence of embolisation** to limbs or central nervous system.
- **Urinalysis:** haematuria (a fresh urine specimen

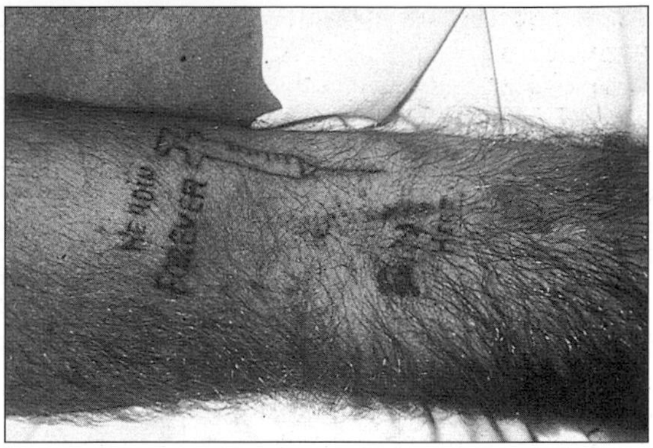

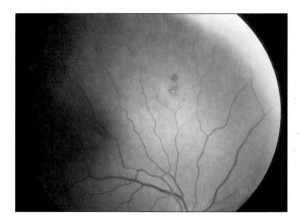

Figure 4.41 Example of an intravenous drug addict's forearm

Figure 4.42 Roth's spot on fundoscopy

will then show dysmorphic red cells and red cell casts on microscopy).

Systemic hypertension

It is important to have in mind a method for the examination of a patient with systemic hypertension. The examination aims to measure the blood pressure level, determine if there is an underlying cause present, and assess the severity as determined by signs of end-organ damage. It is a common clinical problem.

On **general inspection** the signs of the rare causes of secondary hypertension must be sought: for example, Cushing's syndrome,[jj] acromegaly, polycythaemia (page 236) or chronic renal failure.

Take the **blood pressure**, with the patient lying and standing, using an appropriately sized cuff.

[ii] Moritz von Roth (1839–1914), Swiss physician and pathologist, described these changes in 1872.

[jj] Harvey Cushing (1869–1939), professor of surgery, Harvard University, and 'founder of neurosurgery'. Friend of Osler and prize-winning writer of Osler's biography in 1925.

A rise in diastolic pressure on standing occurs typically in essential hypertension; a fall on standing may suggest a secondary cause, but is usually an effect of anti-hypertensive medications. Palpate for radiofemoral delay, and check the blood pressure in the legs if coarctation of the aorta is suspected or if severe hypertension is discovered before 30 years of age.

Next examine the **fundi** for Keith-Wagener retinal changes of hypertension (Figures 4.43 and 4.44) which can be classified from grades 1 to 4:

Grade 1—'silver wiring' of the arteries only (sclerosis of the vessel wall reduces its transparency so that the central light streak becomes broader and shinier)

Grade 2—grade 1 plus arteriovenous nipping or nicking (indentation or deflection of the veins where they are crossed by the arteries)

Grade 3—grade 2 plus haemorrhages (flame-shaped) and exudates (soft—cottonwool spots due to ischaemia, or hard—lipid residues from leaking vessels)

Grade 4—grade 3 plus papilloedema.

It is important to describe the changes present rather than just give a grade.

Now examine the **rest of the cardiovascular system** for signs of left ventricular failure secondary to hypertension, and for coarctation of the aorta. A fourth heart sound is frequently detectable if the blood pressure is greater than 180/110 mmHg.

Then go to the **abdomen** to palpate for renal or adrenal masses (possible causes), and for the presence of an abdominal aortic aneurysm (a possible complication). Auscultate for a renal bruit (page 211) due to renal artery stenosis.[40] Remember that most left-sided abdominal bruits arise from the splenic artery and are of no significance. A bruit is less likely to be significant if it is short, soft and midsystolic. A loud systolic–diastolic bruit that is prominent in the epigastrium is more likely to be associated with renal artery stenosis.

Examine the **central nervous system** for signs of previous cerebrovascular accidents, and palpate and auscultate the **carotid arteries** for bruits (stenosis may be a manifestation of vascular disease, and may be associated with renal artery stenosis). **Urinalysis** should also be performed to look for evidence of renal disease (page 213).

Causes of systemic hypertension

Hypertension may be essential or idiopathic (more than 95% of cases), or secondary (less than 5%). Immoderate alcohol and salt consumption and

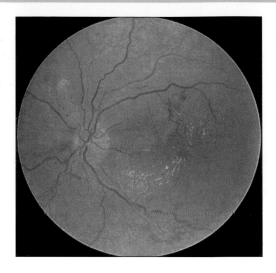

Figure 4.43 Hypertensive retinopathy grade 3
Note flame-shaped haemorrhages and cottonwool spots.

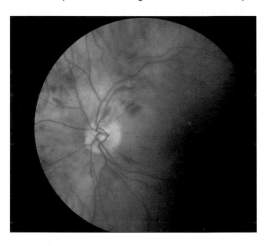

Figure 4.44 Hypertensive retinopathy grade 4
Note AV nipping, silver wiring and papilloedema.

obesity (see *Questions box 4.5*) are associated with hypertension. Obstructive sleep apnoea is also an association.

Secondary causes include: (i) renal disease—renal artery stenosis, chronic pyelonephritis, analgesic nephropathy, connective tissue disease, glomerulonephritis, polycystic disease, diabetic nephropathy, reflux nephropathy; (ii) endocrine disorders—Cushing's syndrome, Conn's syndrome (primary aldosteronism), phaeochromocytoma, acromegaly, thyrotoxicosis, hypothyroidism, hyperparathyroidism; (iii) coarctation of the aorta; and (iv) other, such as the contraceptive pill, polycythaemia rubra vera, toxaemia of pregnancy, neurogenic causes (increased intracranial pressure, lead poisoning, acute porphyria), or hyper-calcaemia.

Complications of hypertension

These include left ventricular failure, cerebrovascular ischaemic events (strokes), renal failure, and eye disease (blindness). Hypertension is also a risk factor for ischaemic heart disease and peripheral vascular disease including abdominal aortic aneurysm and arterial dissections.

Malignant (accelerated) hypertension

This can be defined as the presence of flame-shaped haemorrhages, cottonwool spots and/or papilloedema (≥grade 3 Keith-Wagener retinal changes) as a result of severe hypertension. These patients need admission to hospital for urgent treatment.

Pulmonary hypertension

Systolic pulmonary artery pressures higher than 30 mmHg are abnormal and constitute pulmonary hypertension. Symptoms of pulmonary hypertension do not usually occur until the pressures are about twice normal (i.e. >50 mmHg). Exertional dyspnoea and fatigue are then common, and chest pain probably due to right ventricular ischaemia occurs in up to 50% of patients. It is important to know what signs to look for in a patient who may have pulmonary hypertension.

- **General signs** (usually only in patients with severe hypertension): tachypnoea; peripheral cyanosis and cold extremities, due to low cardiac output; hoarseness (very rare, due to pulmonary artery compression of the left recurrent laryngeal nerve).
- **The pulse:** usually of small volume, due to the low cardiac output (only in severe disease).
- **The JVP:** prominent *a* wave, due to forceful right atrial contraction.
- **Apex beat/praecordium:** right ventricular heave; palpable P2.
- **Auscultation:** systolic ejection click, due to dilatation of the pulmonary artery; loud P2, due to forceful valve closure because of high pulmonary artery pressures; S4; pulmonary ejection murmur, due to dilatation of the pulmonary artery resulting in turbulent blood flow; murmur of pulmonary regurgitation if dilatation of the pulmonary artery occurs.
- **Signs of right ventricular failure** (late: termed *cor pulmonale*).

Causes of pulmonary hypertension

Pulmonary hypertension may be primary (idiopathic) or secondary.

Secondary causes include: (i) pulmonary emboli—e.g. blood clots, tumour particles, fat globules; (ii) lung disease—chronic obstructive pulmonary disease (page 133), obstructive sleep apnoea, interstitial lung disease (e.g. pulmonary fibrosis); (iii) left ventricular failure resulting in back-pressure into the pulmonary circulation; (iv) congenital heart disease causing a left-to-right shunt—atrial septal defect, ventricular septal defect, patent ductus arteriosus; and (v) severe kyphoscoliosis.

Innocent murmurs

The detection of a systolic murmur on routine examination is a common problem. It can cause considerable alarm to both the patient and the examining clinician. These murmurs in asymptomatic people are often the result of normal turbulence within the heart and great vessels. When no structural abnormality of the heart or great vessels is present these are called *innocent, functional* or *organic* murmurs. They probably arise from vibrations within the aortic arch near the origins of the head and neck vessels or from the right ventricular outflow tract. They are more common in children and young adults. They are louder just after exercise and during febrile illnesses (a common time for them to be detected).

Innocent murmurs are always systolic. (A venous hum, which is not really a murmur, has both systolic and diastolic components.) They are usually soft and ejection-systolic in character. Those arising from the aortic arch may radiate to the carotids and be heard in the neck. Those arising from the right ventricular outflow tract are loudest in the pulmonary area and may have a scratchy quality.

These outflow tract murmurs must be distinguished from the pulmonary flow murmur of an atrial septal defect. Therefore it is important to listen carefully for wide or fixed splitting of the second heart sound before pronouncing a murmur innocent (see *Questions box 4.6*).

Valve diseases of the left heart
Mitral stenosis

The normal area of the mitral valve is 4 to 6 cm². Reduction of the valve area to half normal or less causes significant obstruction to left ventricular filling, and blood will flow from the left atrium to the left ventricle only if the left atrial pressure is raised.

- **Symptoms:** dyspnoea, orthopnoea, paroxysmal nocturnal dyspnoea (increased left atrial pressure); haemoptysis (ruptured bronchial veins); ascites, oedema, fatigue (pulmonary hypertension).

Questions box 4.6

Questions to ask the patient with a heart murmur

1 Has anyone noticed this murmur before? Were any tests done?

2 Did you have rheumatic fever as a child?

3 Have you been told you need antibiotics before dental work or surgical operations?

4 Have you become breathless when you exert yourself?

5 Have you had chest tightness during exercise?—Aortic stenosis

6 Have you had dizziness or a blackout during heavy exercise?—Severe aortic stenosis

7 Have you been breathless lying flat?—Heart failure complicating valve disease

- **General signs:** tachypnoea; 'mitral facies'; peripheral cyanosis (severe mitral stenosis).
- **Pulse and blood pressure:** normal or reduced in volume, due to a reduced cardiac output; atrial fibrillation may be present because of left atrial enlargement.
- **The JVP:** normal; prominent *a* wave if pulmonary hypertension is present; loss of the *a* wave if the patient is in atrial fibrillation.
- **Palpation:** tapping quality of the apex beat (palpable S1); right ventricular heave and palpable P2 if pulmonary hypertension is present; diastolic thrill rarely (lay patient on the left side).
- **Auscultation** (Figure 4.45): loud S1 (valve cusps widely apart at the onset of systole)—this also indicates that the valve cusps remain mobile; loud P2 if pulmonary hypertension is present; opening snap (high left atrial pressure forces the valve cusps apart, but the valve cone is halted abruptly); low-pitched rumbling diastolic murmur (best heard with the bell of the stethoscope with the patient in the left lateral position, and quite different in quality and timing from the murmur of aortic regurgitation); a late diastolic accentuation of the diastolic murmur may occur if the patient is in sinus rhythm, but is usually absent if atrial fibrillation has supervened—this is best heard in the left lateral position; exercise accentuates the murmur (ask the patient to sit up and down quickly in bed several times).
- **Signs indicating severe mitral stenosis** (valve area less than 1 cm²): small pulse pressure; soft first heart sound (immobile valve cusps); early opening snap (due to increased left atrial pressure); long diastolic murmur (persists as long as there is a gradient); diastolic thrill at the apex; signs of pulmonary hypertension.
- **Causes of mitral stenosis:** (i) rheumatic (following acute rheumatic fever); (ii) congenital parachute valve (all chordae insert into one papillary muscle—rare).

Mitral regurgitation (chronic)

A regurgitant mitral valve allows part of the left ventricular stroke volume to regurgitate into the left atrium, imposing a volume load on both the left atrium and the left ventricle.

- **Symptoms:** dyspnoea (increased left atrial pressure); fatigue (decreased cardiac output).
- **General signs:** tachypnoea.
- **Pulse:** normal, or sharp upstroke due to rapid left ventricular decompression; atrial fibrillation is relatively common.
- **Palpation:** the apex beat is displaced, diffuse and hyperdynamic; a pansystolic thrill is occasionally present at the apex; a parasternal impulse (due to left atrial enlargement behind the right ventricle—the left atrium is often larger in mitral regurgitation than in mitral stenosis and can be enormous).
- **Auscultation** (Figure 4.46): soft or absent S1 (by the end of diastole, atrial and ventricular pressures have equalised and the valve cusps have drifted back together); left ventricular S3, which is due to rapid left ventricular filling in early diastole and, when soft, does not imply severe regurgitation; pansystolic murmur maximal at the apex and usually radiating towards the axilla.
- **Signs indicating severe chronic mitral regurgitation:** small volume pulse; enlarged left ventricle; loud S3; soft S1; A2 is early, because rapid left ventricular decompression into the left atrium causes the aortic valve to close early; early diastolic rumble; signs of pulmonary hypertension; signs of left ventricular failure (*Good signs guide 4.6*).
- **Causes of chronic mitral regurgitation:** (i) mitral valve prolapse; (ii) 'degenerative'—associated with ageing; (iii) rheumatic; (iv) papillary muscle dysfunction, due to left ventricular failure or ischaemia; (v) cardiomyopathy—hypertrophic, dilated or restrictive cardiomyopathy; (vi) connective tissue disease—e.g. Marfan's syndrome, rheumatoid arthritis, ankylosing spondylitis; (vii) congenital (e.g. atrioventricular canal defect).

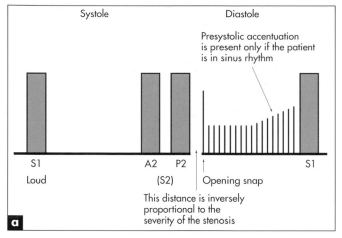
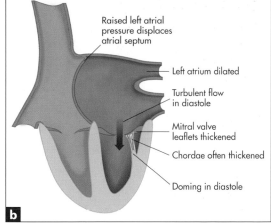

Figure 4.45 Mitral stenosis, at the apex: (a) murmur; (b) anatomy

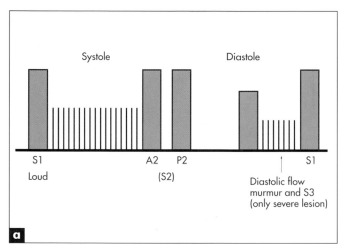
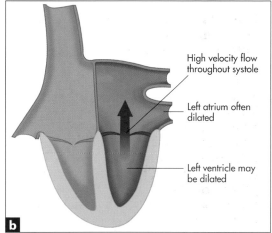

Figure 4.46 Mitral regurgitation: (a) murmur, at the apex; (b) anatomy

Acute mitral regurgitation

In this case patients can present with pulmonary oedema and cardiovascular collapse. There is usually a systolic apical thrill and a loud apical systolic murmur present (it is short because atrial pressure is increased).

With anterior leaflet chordae rupture the murmur radiates to the axilla and back; with posterior leaflet rupture the murmur radiates to the cardiac base and carotids.

- **Causes:** (i) myocardial infarction (dysfunction or rupture of papillary muscles); (ii) infective endocarditis; (iii) trauma or surgery; (iv) spontaneous rupture of a myxomatous chord (sometimes during exercise).

GOOD SIGNS GUIDE 4.6 Moderate to severe mitral regurgitation

	Positive LR	Negative LR
Characteristic murmur grade 3 or more	4.4	0.2
S3 (third heart sound)	1.8	0.8

From McGee S, *Evidence-based physical diagnosis*, 2nd edn. St Louis: Saunders, 2007.

Mitral valve prolapse (systolic-click murmur syndrome)

This syndrome can cause a systolic murmur or click, or both, at the apex. The presence of the murmur indicates that there is some mitral regurgitation present.

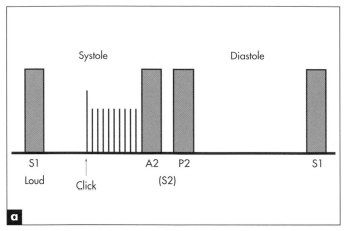

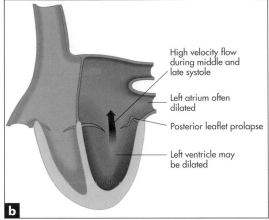

Figure 4.47 Mitral valve prolapse (MVP): (a) murmur, at the apex; (b) anatomy

- **Auscultation** (Figure 4.47): systolic click or clicks at a variable time (usually midsystolic) may be the only abnormality audible, but a click is not always audible; the midsystolic click varies 'all over systole' with changing the position of the patient (unlike the ejection click of aorta or pulmonary stenosis)—when supine the click occurs later than when standing; systolic murmur—high-pitched late systolic murmur, commencing with the click and extending throughout the rest of systole.
- **Dynamic auscultation:** murmur and click occur earlier and may become louder with the Valsalva manoeuvre and with standing, but both occur later and may become softer with squatting and isometric exercise.
- **Causes of mitral valve prolapse:** (i) myxomatous degeneration of the mitral valve tissue—it is very common, especially in women, and the severity may increase with age, particularly in men, so that significant mitral regurgitation may supervene; (ii) may be associated with atrial septal defect (secundum), hypertrophic cardiomyopathy, or Marfan's syndrome.

Aortic stenosis

The normal area of the aortic valve is more than 2 cm². Significant narrowing of this valve restricts left ventricular outflow and imposes a pressure load on the left ventricle.

- **Symptoms:** exertional chest pain (50% do not have coronary artery disease), exertional dyspnoea and exertional syncope.
- **General signs:** usually there is nothing remarkable about the general appearance.

- **The pulse:** there may be a plateau or anacrotic pulse, or the pulse may be late peaking (tardus) and of small volume (parvus).[41]
- **Palpation:** the apex beat is hyperdynamic and may be slightly displaced; systolic thrill at the base of the heart (aortic area).
- **Auscultation** (Figure 4.48): a narrowly split or reversed S2 because of delayed left ventricular ejection; a harsh midsystolic ejection murmur, maximal over the aortic area and extending into the carotid arteries (Figure 4.49), is characteristic. However, it may be heard widely over the praecordium and extend to the apex. The murmur is loudest with the patient sitting up and in full expiration; associated aortic regurgitation is common; in congenital aortic stenosis where the valve cusps remain mobile and the dome of the valve comes to a sudden halt, an ejection click may precede the murmur—the ejection click is absent if the valve is calcified or if the stenosis is not at the valve level but above or below it.
- **Signs indicating severe aortic stenosis** (*Good signs guide 4.7*) (valve area less than 1 cm², or valve gradient greater than 50 mmHg): plateau pulse, carotid pulse reduced in force; thrill in the aortic area; length of the murmur and lateness of the peak of the systolic murmur, soft or absent A2; left ventricular failure (very late sign); pressure-loaded apex beat. These signs are not reliable for distinguishing moderate and severe disease. It is important to remember that the signs of severity of aortic stenosis are less reliable in the elderly.[42]
- **Causes of aortic stenosis:** (i) degenerative calcific aortic stenosis, particularly in elderly

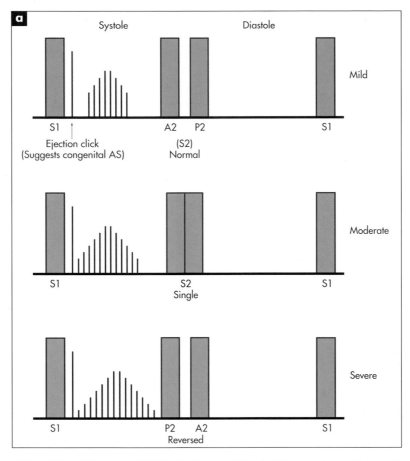

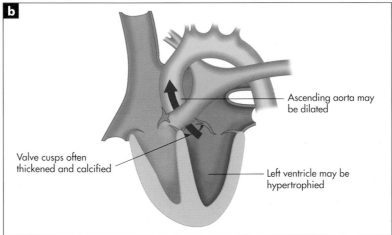

Figure 4.48 Aortic stenosis (AS): (a) murmur, at the aortic area; (b) anatomy

patients; (ii) calcific in younger patients, usually on a congenital bicuspid valve; (iii) rheumatic.

- **Other types of aortic outflow obstruction are also possible:** (i) supravalvular obstruction, where there is narrowing of the ascending aorta or a fibrous diaphragm just above the aortic valve—this is rare and may be associated with a characteristic facies (a broad forehead, widely set eyes and a pointed chin); there is a loud A2 and often a thrill in the area of the sternal notch; (ii) subvalvular obstruction,

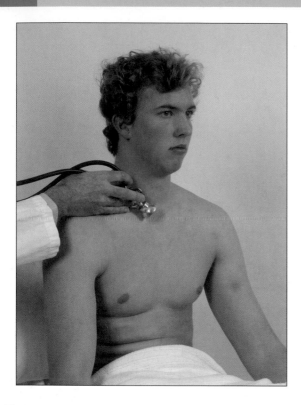

Figure 4.49 Aortic stenosis: listening over the carotid

GOOD SIGNS GUIDE 4.7 Severe aortic stenosis

Sign	Positive LR	Negative LR
Delayed carotid upstroke	3.7	0.4
Diminished carotid pulse on palpation	2.3	0.3
Apical impulse sustained (pressure-loaded)	4.1	0.3
Absent or decreased A2	3.6	0.4
S4 gallop	NS	NS
Late peaking murmur	4.4	0.2
Long murmur	3.9	0.2
Murmur radiates to the neck	1.4	0.1

NS = not significant.
From McGee S, *Evidence-based physical diagnosis*, 2nd edn. St Louis: Saunders, 2007.

where there is a membranous diaphragm or fibrous ridge just below the aortic valve; aortic regurgitation is associated and is due to a jet lesion affecting the coronary cusp of the valve; (iii) dynamic left ventricular outflow tract obstruction may occur in hypertrophic cardiomyopathy; here there may be a double apical impulse. Atrial contraction into a stiff left ventricle may be palpable before the left ventricular impulse (only in the presence of sinus rhythm, of course).

Aortic sclerosis presents in the elderly; there are none of the peripheral signs of aortic stenosis. The diagnosis implies the absence of a gradient across the aortic valve despite some thickening and a murmur.

Aortic regurgitation

The incompetent aortic valve allows regurgitation of blood from the aorta to the left ventricle during diastole for as long as the aortic diastolic pressure exceeds the left ventricular diastolic pressure.[43]

- **Symptoms:** occur in the late stages of disease and include exertional dyspnoea, fatigue, palpitations (hyperdynamic circulation) and exertional angina.

- **General signs:** Marfan's syndrome, ankylosing spondylitis or one of the other seronegative arthropathies or, rarely, Argyll Robertson pupils may be obvious.
- **Pulse and blood pressure:** the pulse is characteristically collapsing, a 'water hammer'[kk] pulse (Table 4.20); there may be a wide pulse pressure. This sign is most obvious if the clinician raises the patient's arm while feeling the radial pulse with the web spaces of the lifting hand. A *bisferiens* pulse (from the Latin, to beat twice) may be a sign of severe aortic regurgitation or of combined aortic regurgitation and aortic stenosis. It is best assessed at the carotid artery, where two beats can be felt in each cardiac cycle. It is probably caused by a Venturi effect in the aorta related to rapid ejection of blood and brief indrawing of the aortic wall, leading to a diminution of the pulse followed by a rebound increase. It was a particular favourite of Galen's.[ll]
- **Neck:** prominent carotid pulsations (Corrigan's sign).

---

kk This Victorian children's toy consisted of a sealed tube half-filled with fluid, with the other half being a vacuum. Inversion of the tube caused the fluid to fall rapidly without air resistance and strike the other end with a noise like a hammer blow. It is not easy to imagine a child today being entertained by this for very long.

ll Claudius Galen (130–200 AD). Born in Pergamum, he worked as a gladiator's surgeon but moved to Rome in 164 AD to become the city's most famous physician. He was the first to describe the cranial nerves. He never performed dissection on human bodies, but his often erroneous anatomical teachings were regarded as infallible for 15 centuries.

TABLE 4.20 Eponymous signs of aortic regurgitation[44]

1 Quincke's sign: capillary pulsation in the nail beds—it is of no value, as this sign occurs normally.

2 Corrigan's sign: prominent carotid pulsations; the Corrigan water hammer pulse sign is present when the patient lies supine with the arms beside the body, the radial pulse is compressed until it disappears, the arm is then lifted perpendicular to the body, the pulse then becomes palpable again even though the same pressure has been maintained on the radial artery.

3 De Musset's sign: head nodding in time with the heartbeat.

4 Hill's sign: increased blood pressure (>20 mmHg) in the legs compared with the arms.

5 Mueller's sign: pulsation of the uvula in time with the heartbeat.

6 Duroziez's sign: systolic and diastolic murmurs over the femoral artery on gradual compression of the vessel.

7 Traube's sign: a double sound heard over the femoral artery on compressing the vessel distally; this is *not* a 'pistol shot' sound that may be heard over the femoral artery with very severe aortic regurgitation.

8 Mayne's sign: a decrease in diastolic pressure of 15 mmHg when the arm is held above the head compared with that when the arm is at the level of the heart.

9 Rosenbach's liver pulsation sign: liver pulsates in time with the heartbeat (in the absence of tricuspid regurgitation).

10 Austin Flint murmur: short rumbling diastolic murmur, thought by Flint to be due to functional mitral stenosis caused by impinging of the aortic regurgitant jet on the anterior mitral valve leaflet.

11 Becker's sign: accentuated retinal artery pulsations.

12 Gerhard's sign: pulsatile spleen.

13 Landolfi's sign: prominent alternating constriction and dilatation of the pupils (hippus, from the Greek *hippos*—'horse'—and its rhythmical galloping).

14 Lincoln's sign: an easily palpable popliteal pulse.

15 Sherman's sign: an easily palpable dorsalis pedis pulse in a patient over the age of 75 years.

16 Watson's water hammer pulse.

17 Ashrafian's sign: pulsatile pseudo proptosis.

Note: These signs are amusing, but not often helpful. The signs were named after the following people: Heinrich Quincke (1842–1922), German neurologist; Dominic Corrigan (1802–80), Edinburgh graduate who worked in Dublin and is credited with discovering aortic regurgitation; Alfred de Musset, 19th century French poet who suffered from aortic regurgitation (the sign was noticed by his brother, a physician); Sir Leonard Hill (1866–1952), English physiologist who also described the physiology of the cerebral circulation; Frederick Von Mueller (1858–1941), German physician who also noted an increase in metabolism in exophthalmic goitre; Paul Duroziez (1826–97), French physician; Ludwig Traube (1818–76), Hungarian physician who worked in Germany; Otto Heinrich Becker (1828–1890), professor of ophthalmology, University of Heidelberg, who also described this sign in patients with Graves' disease; Lincoln's sign is like de Musset's sign in being named after the patient with the condition; Thomas Watson, English physician, described this sign in 1844; Hutan Ashrafian, cardiothoracic surgeon, St Mary's Hospital, London, described this in 2006—proof that the hunt for more signs of aortic regurgitation goes on.

- **Palpation:** the apex beat is characteristically displaced and hyperkinetic. A diastolic thrill may be felt at the left sternal edge when the patient sits up and breathes out.
- **Auscultation** (Figure 4.50): A2 (the aortic component of the second heart sound) may be soft; a decrescendo high-pitched diastolic murmur beginning immediately after the second heart sound and extending for a variable time into diastole—it is loudest at the third and fourth left intercostal spaces; a systolic ejection murmur is usually present (due to associated aortic stenosis or to torrential flow across a normal diameter aortic valve). Aortic stenosis is distinguished from an aortic flow murmur by the presence of the peripheral signs of significant aortic stenosis, such as a plateau pulse. An *Austin Flint murmur*[mm] should also be listened for. This is a low-pitched rumbling mid-diastolic and presystolic murmur audible at the apex (the

---

[mm] Austin Flint (1812–1886), New York physician and professor of medicine at the New Orleans Medical School, described this murmur in 1862. Author of *The principles and practice of medicine*. He was very much opposed to the naming of signs after people.

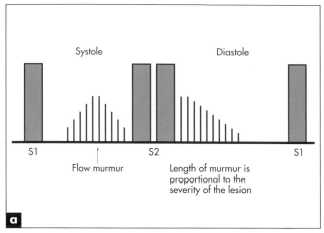

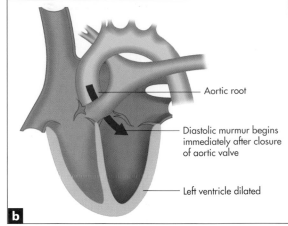

Figure 4.50 Aortic regurgitation: (a) murmur, at the left sternal edge; (b) anatomy

regurgitant jet from the aortic valve causes the anterior mitral valve leaflet to shudder). It can be distinguished from mitral stenosis because S1 (the first heart sound) is not loud and there is no opening snap. Many other signs have been described, but they are interesting rather than helpful (Table 4.20; *Good signs guide 4.8*).

- **Signs indicating severe chronic aortic regurgitation:** collapsing pulse; wide pulse pressure (systolic pressure 80 mmHg more than the diastolic); long decrescendo diastolic murmur; left ventricular S3 (third heart sound); soft A2; Austin Flint murmur; signs of left ventricular failure.
- **Causes of aortic regurgitation:** disease may affect the valvular area or aortic root, and may be acute or chronic.
- **Causes of chronic aortic regurgitation:** (i) valvular—rheumatic (rarely the only murmur in this case), congenital (e.g. bicuspid valve; ventricular septal defect—an associated prolapse of the aortic cusp is not uncommon), seronegative arthropathy, especially ankylosing spondylitis; (ii) aortic root dilatation (murmur may be maximal at the right sternal border)—Marfan's syndrome, aortitis (e.g. seronegative arthropathies, rheumatoid arthritis, tertiary syphilis), dissecting aneurysm.
- **Acute aortic regurgitation:** presents differently—there is no collapsing pulse (blood pressure is low) and the diastolic murmur is short.
- **Causes of acute aortic regurgitation:** (i) valvular—infective endocarditis; (ii) aortic root—Marfan's syndrome, dissecting aneurysm of the aortic root.

GOOD SIGNS GUIDE 4.8 Severity of aortic regurgitation (AR)

Finding	Positive LR	Negative LR
Typical murmur		
Mild AR or worse	9.9	0.3
Moderate to severe AR	4.3	0.1
Murmur grade 3 or more (moderate to severe AR)	8.2	0.6
Pulse pressure		
>80 mmHg	10.9	–
Other signs—moderate to severe AR		
Sustained or displaced apex	2.4	0.1
Duroziez's sign, pistol shot femorals, water hammer pulse	NS	0.7

NS = not significant.
From McGee S, *Evidence-based physical diagnosis*, 2nd edn. St Louis: Saunders, 2007.

Valve diseases of the right heart
Tricuspid stenosis

This is very rare.
- **The JVP:** raised; giant *a* waves with a slow *y* descent may be seen.
- **Auscultation:** a diastolic murmur audible at the left sternal edge, accentuated by inspiration, very similar to the murmur of mitral stenosis except for the site of maximal intensity and the effect of respiration (louder on inspiration);

tricuspid regurgitation and mitral stenosis are often present as well; no signs of pulmonary hypertension.

- **Abdomen:** presystolic pulsation of the liver, caused by forceful atrial systole.
- **Cause of tricuspid stenosis:** rheumatic heart disease.

Tricuspid regurgitation (Figure 4.51)

- **The JVP:** large *v* waves; the JVP is elevated if right ventricular failure has occurred.
- **Palpation:** right ventricular heave.
- **Auscultation:** there may be a pansystolic murmur maximal at the lower end of the sternum that increases on inspiration, but the diagnosis can be made on the basis of the peripheral signs alone.
- **Abdomen:** a pulsatile, large and tender liver is usually present and may cause the right nipple to dance in time with the heart beat; ascites, oedema and pleural effusions may also be present.
- **Legs:** dilated, pulsatile veins.
- **Causes of tricuspid regurgitation:**[nn] (i) functional (no disease of the valve leaflets)—right ventricular failure; (ii) rheumatic—only very rarely does rheumatic tricuspid regurgitation occur alone, usually mitral valve disease is also present; (iii) infective endocarditis (right-sided endocarditis in intravenous drug addicts); (iv) tricuspid valve prolapse; (v) right ventricular papillary muscle infarction; (vi) trauma (usually caused by a

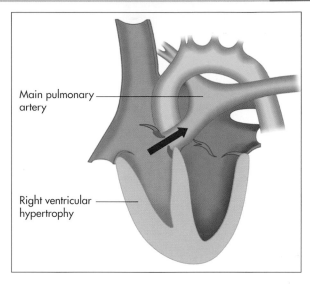

Figure 4.52 Valvar pulmonary stenosis: anatomy

steering wheel injury to the sternum): (vii) congenital—Ebstein's anomaly.[oo]

Pulmonary stenosis (in adults) (Figure 4.52)

- **General signs:** peripheral cyanosis, due to a low cardiac output, but only in severe cases.
- **Pulse:** normal or reduced if cardiac output is low.
- **The JVP:** giant *a* waves because of right atrial hypertrophy; the JVP may be elevated.
- **Palpation:** right ventricular heave; thrill over the pulmonary area.
- **Auscultation:** the murmur may be preceded by an ejection click; a harsh and usually loud ejection systolic murmur, heard best in the pulmonary area and with inspiration, is typically present; right ventricular S4 may be present (due to right atrial hypertrophy). It is not well heard over the carotid arteries.
- **Abdomen:** presystolic pulsation of the liver may be present.
- **Signs of severe pulmonary stenosis:** an ejection systolic murmur peaking late in systole; absence of an ejection click (also absent when the pulmonary stenosis is infundibular—i.e. below the valve level); presence of S4; signs of right ventricular failure.
- **Causes of pulmonary stenosis:** (i) congenital; (ii) carcinoid syndrome (rare).

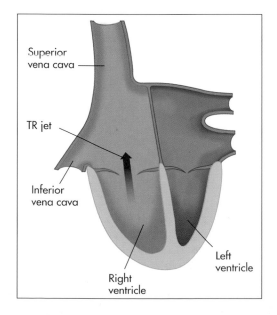

Figure 4.51 Tricuspid regurgitation (TR): anatomy

[nn]   Doppler echocardiography has shown that trivial tricuspid regurgitation is very common and is then considered physiological. Christian Doppler (1803–1853) was an Austrian physicist and mathematician.

[oo]   Wilhelm Ebstein (1836–1912), professor of medicine at Göttingen in Germany, who invented and developed palpation.

TABLE 4.21 Prosthetic heart valves: physical signs

Type	Mitral	Aortic
Ball valve (e.g. Starr-Edwards)*	Sharp mitral opening sound after S2, sharp closing sound at S1 Systolic ejection murmur, no diastolic murmur	Sharp aortic opening sound Systolic ejection murmur (harsh), no diastolic murmur unless a paravalvular leak has occurred, early diastolic murmur indicates AR usually due to a paravalvular leak**
Disc valve (e.g. Bjork-Shiley)†	Sharp closing sound at S1, soft systolic ejection murmur and diastolic rumble (diastolic murmur occasionally)	Sharp closing sound at S2, systolic ejection murmur (soft)
Porcine or bovine pericardial valve‡	Usually sound normal, diastolic rumble mitral opening sound occasionally	Closing sound usually heard, systolic ejection murmur (soft), no diastolic murmur
Bileaflet valve (e.g. St Jude)	–	Aortic valve opening and closing sounds common, soft systolic ejection murmur common
Homograft (human) valve	Normal heart sounds, occasional soft systolic murmur; early diastolic murmur if AR has occurred	

* Modern mechanical valves (e.g. St Jude) make softer opening and closing sounds than older valves. The Starr-Edwards valve is often very noisy and sounds like a ball rattling around in a cage (which is what it is).
** An aortic regurgitation murmur present after aortic valve replacement suggests regurgitation of the valve ring. It is not uncommon. Less often a mitral regurgitation murmur suggests the same problem with a prosthetic mitral valve.
† Severe prosthetic dysfunction causes absence of the opening or closing sounds. Ball and cage valves cause more haemolysis than other types and make the most noise, while disc valves are more thrombogenic.
‡ Bioprosthetic obstruction or patient–prosthetic mismatch cause diastolic rumbling. These valves are used less often in the mitral position because they often have a very limited life there. A degenerated bioprosthetic valve may cause murmurs of regurgitation or stenosis or both.
AR = aortic regurgitation.
(Modified from Smith ND, Raizada V, Abrams J. Auscultation of the normally functioning prosthetic valve. *Ann Intern Med* 1981; 95:594.)

Pulmonary regurgitation

This is an uncommon pathological condition; trivial pulmonary regurgitation is often found at echocardiography and is considered physiological.

- **Auscultation:** a decrescendo diastolic murmur which is high-pitched and audible at the left sternal edge is characteristic—this typically but not always increases on inspiration (unlike the murmur of aortic regurgitation). It is called the Graham Steell murmur[pp] when it occurs secondary to pulmonary artery dilatation caused by pulmonary hypertension. (*Note:* If there are no signs of pulmonary hypertension, a decrescendo diastolic murmur at the left sternal edge is more likely to be due to aortic regurgitation than to pulmonary regurgitation.)

- **Causes of pulmonary regurgitation:** (i) pulmonary hypertension; (ii) infective endocarditis; (iii) following balloon valvotomy for pulmonary stenosis or surgery for pulmonary atresia; (iv) congenital absence of the pulmonary valve.

Prosthetic heart valves

The physical signs with common types of valves are presented in Table 4.21. Mechanical prosthetic valves should have a crisp sound. Muffling of the mechanical sounds may be a sign of thrombotic obstruction of the valve or chronic tissue ingrowth (pannus). After replacement of the aortic valve the presence of audible aortic regurgitation may indicate a *paravalvular leak*, often through a stitching hole in the valve sewing ring. As tissue valves age and degenerate they may develop signs of regurgitation or stenosis, or both.

PP Graham Steell (1851–1942), Manchester physician, described this murmur in 1888.

Cardiomyopathy

Hypertrophic cardiomyopathy (Figure 4.53)

This is abnormal hypertrophy of the muscle in the left ventricular or right ventricular outflow tract, or both. It can obstruct outflow from the left ventricle late in systole when the hypertrophied area contracts. Systolic displacement of the mitral valve apparatus into the left ventricular outflow tract also occurs, causing mitral regurgitation and contributing to the outflow obstruction. Although the outflow tract is narrowed by the hypertrophied septum, the major contribution to the dynamic increase in obstruction comes from the systolic movement of the mitral valve. Variants of hypertrophic cardiomyopathy may involve the mid-ventricle or apex with varying degrees of obstruction.

- **Symptoms:** dyspnoea (increased left ventricular end-diastolic pressure due to abnormal diastolic compliance), angina, syncope or sudden death (secondary to ventricular fibrillation or a sudden increase in outflow obstruction).
- **Pulse:** sharp, rising and jerky. Rapid ejection by the hypertrophied ventricle early in systole is followed by obstruction caused by the displacement of the mitral valve into the outflow tract. This is quite different from the pulse of aortic stenosis.

- **The JVP:** there is usually a prominent *a* wave, due to forceful atrial contraction against a non-compliant right ventricle.
- **Palpation:** double or triple apical impulse, due to presystolic expansion of the ventricle caused by atrial contraction.
- **Auscultation:** late systolic murmur at the lower left sternal edge and apex (due to the obstruction) and a pansystolic murmur at the apex (due to mitral regurgitation); S4.
- **Dynamic manoeuvres:** the outflow murmur is increased by the Valsalva manoeuvre, by standing and by isotonic exercise; it is decreased by squatting and isometric exercise.
- **Causes of hypertrophic cardiomyopathy:** (i) autosomal dominant (sarcomeric heavy chain or troponin gene mutation) with variable expressivity; (ii) idiopathic; (iii) Friedreich's ataxia[qq] (page 396).

Dilated cardiomyopathy

This heart muscle abnormality results in a global reduction in cardiac function. Coronary artery disease is excluded as a cause by definition. (Ischaemic cardiomyopathy is a term often used to describe severe myocardial dysfunction secondary to recurrent ischaemic events.) The signs are those of congestive cardiac failure, including those of mitral and tricuspid regurgitation. The heart sounds themselves may be very quiet. Ventricular arrhythmias are common. It is a common indication for cardiac transplantation.

- **Causes of dilated cardiomyopathy:** (i) idiopathic and familial; (ii) alcohol; (iii) post-viral; (iv) postpartum; (v) drugs (e.g. doxorubicin); (vi) dystrophia myotonica; (vii) haemochromatosis.

Restrictive cardiomyopathy

This causes similar signs to those caused by constrictive pericarditis, but Kussmaul's sign is more common and the apex beat is usually easily palpable.

- **Causes of restrictive cardiomyopathy:** (i) idiopathic; (ii) eosinophilic endomyocardial disease; (iii) endomyocardial fibrosis; (iv) infiltrative disease (e.g. amyloid); (v) granulomas (e.g. sarcoid).

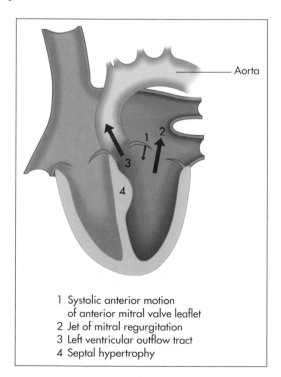

1 Systolic anterior motion
  of anterior mitral valve leaflet
2 Jet of mitral regurgitation
3 Left ventricular outflow tract
4 Septal hypertrophy

Figure 4.53 Hypertrophic pulmonary stenosis: anatomy

[qq] Nikolaus Friedreich (1825–82), German physician, described this disease in 1863. He succeeded Virchow as professor of pathological anatomy at Würzburg at the age of 31.

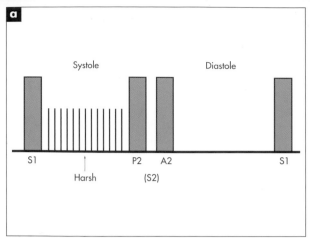

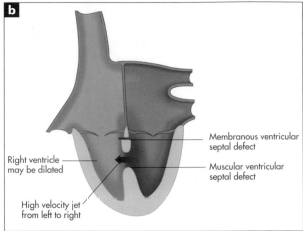

Figure 4.54 Ventricular septal defect (VSD): (a) murmur, at the left sternal edge; (b) anatomy

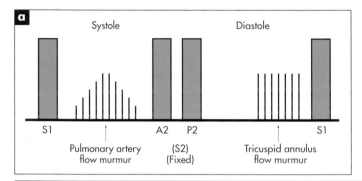

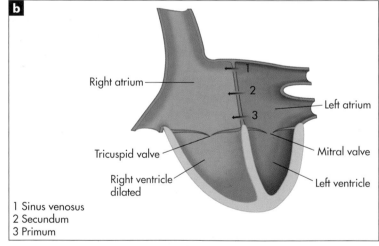

1 Sinus venosus
2 Secundum
3 Primum

Figure 4.55 Atrial septal defect (ASD): (a) murmur, at the left sternal edge; (b) anatomy

Acyanotic congenital heart disease

Ventricular septal defect

In this condition one or more holes are present in the membranous or muscular ventricular septum.

- **Palpation:** hyperkinetic displaced apex if the defect is large; and a thrill at the left sternal edge.
- **Auscultation** (Figure 4.54): a harsh pansystolic murmur maximal at, and almost confined

to, the lower left sternal edge with a third or fourth heart sound—the murmur is louder on expiration; sometimes a mitral regurgitation murmur is associated. There is often a palpable systolic thrill. The murmur is often louder and harsher when the defect is small.

- **Causes of ventricular septal defect:** (i) congenital; (ii) acquired—e.g. myocardial infarction involving the septum.

Atrial septal defect

There are two main types: *ostium secundum* (90%), where there is a defect in the part of the septum which does not involve the atrioventricular valves, and *ostium primum*, where the defect does involve the atrioventricular valves.

- **Palpation:** normal or right ventricular enlargement.
- **Auscultation** (Figure 4.55): fixed splitting of S2; the defect produces no murmur directly, but increased flow through the right side of the heart can produce a low-pitched diastolic tricuspid flow murmur and more often a pulmonary systolic ejection murmur—these are both louder on inspiration.
- **Signs:** The signs of an ostium primum defect are the same as for an ostium secundum defect, but associated mitral regurgitation, tricuspid regurgitation or a ventricular septal defect may be present. The left ventricular impulse is often impalpable.

Patent ductus arteriosus (Figure 4.56)

This is a persistent embryonic vessel which connects the pulmonary artery and the aorta. The shunt is from the aorta to the pulmonary artery unless pulmonary hypertension has supervened.

- **Pulse and blood pressure:** a collapsing pulse with a sharp upstroke (due to ejection of a large volume of blood into the empty aorta with systole); low diastolic blood pressure (due to rapid decompression of the aorta).
- **Palpation:** often there is a hyperkinetic apex beat.
- **Auscultation:** if the shunt is of moderate size a single second heart sound is heard, but if the shunt is of significant size reversed splitting of the second heart sound occurs (due to a

delayed A2 because of an increased volume load in the left ventricle); a continuous loud 'machinery' murmur maximal at the first left intercostal space is usually present; flow murmurs through the left side of the heart, including a mitral mid-diastolic murmur, may be heard.

Coarctation of the aorta (Figure 4.57)

This is congenital narrowing of the aorta usually just distal to the origin of the left subclavian artery. It is more common in males. The underlying cause is uncertain but seems related to abnormal placement of tissue involved in the closing of the ductus arteriosus. There is an association with bicuspid aortic valve and Turner's syndrome.

- **Signs:** the upper body may be better developed than the lower; radiofemoral delay is present, and the femoral pulses are weak; hypertension occurs in the arms but not in the legs; a midsystolic murmur is usually audible over the praecordium and the back, due to blood flow through collateral chest vessels and across the coarct itself.

Ebstein's anomaly

This is a very rare lesion. The abnormality is a downward displacement of the tricuspid valve apparatus into the right ventricle so that the right atrium becomes very large and consists partly of ventricular muscle, while the right ventricle becomes small. An atrial septal defect is commonly associated. Characteristically, multiple clicks occur due to asynchronous closure of the tricuspid valve. Tricuspid regurgitation is usually present.

Cyanotic congenital heart disease

This is a difficult area. The causes are listed in Table

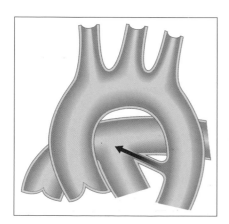

Figure 4.56 Patent ductus arteriosus: anatomy

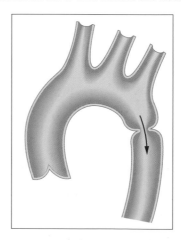

Figure 4.57 Coarctation of the aorta: anatomy

4.22. The important point to determine is whether or not signs of pulmonary hypertension are present. Congenital heart disease in which a shunt from the left to the right side of the circulation occurs leads to an increase in pulmonary blood flow. This can cause reactive pulmonary hypertension so that pulmonary pressures eventually exceed systemic pressures. When that happens, the systemic to pulmonary (left to right) shunt will reverse. This right-to-left shunt leads to deoxygenated blood being mixed in the systemic circulation, resulting in cyanosis. This is called Eisenmenger's syndrome.[rr]

Eisenmenger's syndrome (pulmonary hypertension and a right-to-left shunt)

- **Signs:** central cyanosis; clubbing; polycythaemia; signs of pulmonary hypertension.

It may be possible to decide at what level the shunt occurs by listening to the second heart sound (S2). If there is wide fixed splitting, this suggests an atrial septal defect. If a single second heart sound is present, this suggests truncus arteriosus or a ventricular septal defect. A normal or reversed S2 suggests a patent ductus arteriosus.

Tetralogy of Fallot[ss]

There are four features which are due to a single developmental abnormality: (i) ventricular septal defect (VSD); (ii) right ventricular outflow obstruction, which determines the severity of the condition, and can be at the pulmonary valve or infundibular level; (iii) an aorta which overrides the VSD and is responsible for the cyanosis; and (iv) right ventricular hypertrophy secondary to outflow obstruction.

- **Signs:** central cyanosis—this occurs without pulmonary hypertension because venous mixing is possible at the ventricular level, where pressures are balanced. The aorta overrides both ventricles and so receives right and left ventricular blood. Clubbing and polycythaemia are usually present. There may be evidence of right ventricular enlargement—a parasternal impulse at the left sternal edge. A systolic thrill caused by pulmonary valve or right ventricular outflow obstruction may be present. There is no overall

TABLE 4.22 Classification of congenital heart disease
Acyanotic
With left-to-right shunt Ventricular septal defect Atrial septal defect Patent ductus arteriosus
With no shunt Bicuspid aortic valve, congenital aortic stenosis Coarctation of aorta Dextrocardia Pulmonary stenosis, tricuspid stenosis Ebstein's anomaly
Cyanotic
Eisenmenger's syndrome (pulmonary hypertension and a right-to-left shunt) Tetralogy of Fallot Ebstein's anomaly (if an atrial septal defect and right-to-left shunt are also present) Truncus arteriosus Transposition of the great vessels Tricuspid atresia Total anomalous pulmonary venous drainage

cardiomegaly. On auscultation the second heart sound is single and there are no signs of pulmonary hypertension; a pulmonary systolic ejection murmur is present.

'Grown-up' congenital heart disease

Patients who have been treated for serious congenital cardiac conditions now frequently survive into adult life. Many of the surgical procedures undertaken for these conditions, especially 20 years ago, were palliative rather than curative. The patients present with specific symptoms and signs.

Tetralogy of Fallot

Patients who have had repair of this condition in infancy may present with particular problems. Repair of the right ventricular outflow obstruction and enlargement of the pulmonary valve annulus may leave severe pulmonary regurgitation. This may lead eventually to exertional dyspnoea. The surgery itself has, until recently, required a right ventriculotomy (cutting into the right ventricle). This leaves a scar that can be associated with cardiac rhythm abnormalities in later life. Patients may present with palpitations or syncope.

- **Signs:** may include a median sternotomy scar, a long diastolic murmur of pulmonary regurgitation, and signs of right ventricular enlargement (parasternal impulse) and later of tricuspid regurgitation (big *v* waves in the neck and a pulsatile liver).

[rr] Victor Eisenmenger (1864–1932), German physician. He described this syndrome in 1897.
[ss] Etienne-Louis Fallot (1850–1911), professor of hygiene, Marseilles, described this in 1888.

TABLE 4.23 Features of important valve lesions and congenital abnormalities

	Site	Timing	Radiation	Character	Accentuation and manoeuvres	Other features
Aortic regurgitation	Aortic area	Early diastolic	Lower left sternal edge	Decrescendo	Expiration, patient leaning forward	Wide pulse pressure, eponymous signs
Aortic stenosis	Aortic area	Systolic	Carotids	Ejection	Expiration	Separate from heart sounds, slow-rising pulse
Mitral stenosis	Apex	Middle and late diastolic	—	Low-pitched (use stethoscope bell)	Presystolic accentuation, left lateral position, exercise	Loud S1, opening snap
Mitral regurgitation	Apex	Pansystolic or middle and late systolic (mitral valve prolapse)	Axilla or left sternal edge	Blowing (MVP)	Longer and louder with Valsalva (MVP)	Para-sternal impulse (enlarges left atrium)
Ventricular septal defect	Lower left sternal edge	Pansystolic	None	Localised		Often associated with a thrill
Tricuspid regurgitation	Lower left and right sternal edge	Pansystolic			Louder on inspiration	Big V waves, pulsatile liver
Hypertrophic cardiomyopathy	Apex and left sternal edge	Late systolic at left sternal edge, pan-systolic at apex			Louder with Valsalva, softer with squatting	S4, double-impulse apex beat, jerky carotid pulse

MVP = mitral valve prolapse.

Transposition of the great arteries

Most adults who have had surgery for this abnormality have had a palliative operation called a Mustard procedure. In this abnormality, the pulmonary artery is connected to the left ventricle and the aorta to the right ventricle. Thus the systemic and pulmonary circulations are in parallel. This is not compatible with life unless some connection between the two circulations is present. Neonates with the condition will have an atrial septal defect (ASD) created soon after birth with a catheter-based balloon (balloon septostomy). This allows mixing of the circulations. Later 'baffles' are created surgically in the atria to direct blood returning from the body into the right atrium across the ASD and into the left atrium, where it is pumped into the pulmonary artery and into the lungs. Blood returning from the lungs into the left atrium is directed across into the right atrium and into the morphological right ventricle and on into the aorta. This means that the morphological right ventricle is working as the systemic ventricle. This arrangement works very well, but there are long-term concerns about the ability of the right ventricle to cope with systemic workloads.

- **Symptoms:** symptoms that commonly occur include palpitations caused by supraventricular arrhythmias, dizziness caused by bradycardias and breathlessness related to failure of the systemic ventricle. Occasionally, obstruction of the baffles may occur. The most common problem is with the superior vena caval baffle which leads to facial swelling and flushing.
- **Signs:** include the usual scar, facial flushing and oedema, cyanosis, peripheral oedema from inferior caval baffle obstruction and signs of tricuspid regurgitation. On auscultation there may be a gallop rhythm and the murmurs of mitral and tricuspid regurgitation.

The chest X-ray: a systematic approach

Analysis of the chest X-ray is complementary to the patient's physical examination. It provides much information about the heart and lungs.

The interpretation of the chest X-ray is not easy. It requires knowledge of anatomy and pathology, appreciation of the whole range of normal appearances (Figure 4.58), and knowledge of the likely X-ray changes occurring with pathological processes. The clinician should feel personally responsible for viewing a patient's radiographs.

Most medical students faced with giving their interpretation of a chest X-ray either opt for a 'spot

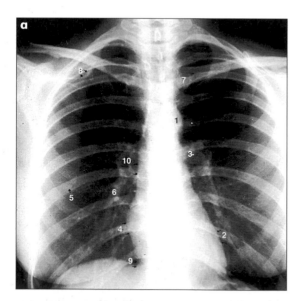
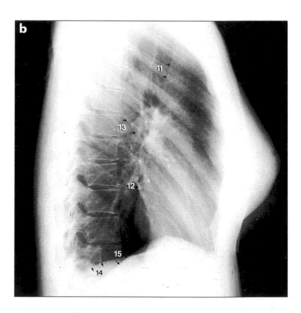

Figure 4.58 Normal chest X-ray

(a) The posteroanterior view shows (1) aortic knuckle; (2) left heart border formed by the lateral border of the left ventricle; (3) left hilum, formed mostly by the left main pulmonary artery and partly by the left upper pulmonary veins; (4) right heart border formed by the right atrium; (5) inferior angle of the scapula; (6) right basal pulmonary artery; (7) medial aspect of the left clavicle; (8) spine of the scapula; (9) right cardiophrenic angle; (10) superimposition of right lateral margins of the superior vena cava and the ascending aorta.

(b) The lateral view shows: (11) anterior border of trachea; (12) pulmonary vein, entering left atrium; (13) oblique fissure; (14) left hemidiaphragm; (15) right hemidiaphragm.

diagnosis' (usually wrong) or raise their eyes to heaven, hoping for divine inspiration. However, a systematic approach is generally more useful! More is missed by not looking than by not knowing.

Frontal film

Name, date and projection

First, it is important to check the name and date, to be sure that it is the correct patient's film. Checking the left or right marker prevents missing dextrocardia. The film markings will also indicate the projection and patient position. The standard frontal film is taken by a posteroanterior (PA; back to front) projection of an erect patient. Anteroposterior (AP) and supine films are only second-best. On a supine film there is distension of all the posterior (gravity-dependent) vessels and thus the lung fields appear more plethoric. A small pleural effusion may not be visible if it is lying posteriorly and the heart often appears large on a supine film.

Centring

The medial ends of the clavicles should be equidistant from the midline spinous processes. If the patient is rotated, this will accentuate the hilum that is turned forwards.

Exposure

The quality of the film is important. There should be enough X-ray penetration for the spine to be just seen through the mediastinum, otherwise the film will be too white. With good radiographic technique, the scapulae are projected outside the lung fields.

The film needs to be exposed on full inspiration so that there is no basal crowding of the pulmonary vessels and so that estimation of the cardiothoracic ratio is accurate.

On full inspiration, the diaphragm lies at the level of the tenth or eleventh rib posteriorly or at the level of the sixth costal cartilage anteriorly. The right hemidiaphragm usually lies about 2 cm higher than the left.

Correct orientation

Do not miss dextrocardia—the heart apex will be to the right and the stomach gas to the left. Do not be misled by left or right markers wrongly placed by a radiographer.

Systematic film interpretation

Mediastinum. The trachea should lie in the midline. It may be deviated by a goitre or mediastinal mass. It is normally deviated a little to the left as it passes the aortic knuckle. (The aortic arch becomes wider and unfolded with age because of loss of elasticity.)

The mediastinum, including the trachea, can be deviated by a large pleural effusion, a tension pneumothorax or pulmonary collapse.

Rotation of the patient may make the mediastinum appear distorted.

Hila. The hila are mostly formed by the pulmonary arteries with the upper lobe veins superimposed. The left hilum is higher than the right. The left has a squarish shape whereas the right has a V shape.

A hilum can be more prominent if the patient is rotated. Lymphadenopathy or a large pulmonary artery will cause hilar enlargement.

Heart. The heart shape is ovoid with the apex pointing to the left. Characteristically, about two-thirds of the heart projects to the left of the spine.

The right heart border is formed by the outer border of the right atrium, and the left heart border by the left ventricle. The left margin of the right ventricle lies about a thumb's breadth in from the left heart border. (On the surface of the heart, this is marked by the left anterior descending coronary artery.)

The cardiothoracic diameter is a rather approximate way of determining whether the heart is enlarged. If the heart size is more than 50% of the transthoracic diameter, enlargement may be present. Apparent slight cardiac enlargement can occur because of a relatively small AP diameter of the chest. A cardiothoracic ratio at the upper limit of normal should not cause alarm if the patient has no reason to have cardiac failure and no symptoms of it.

Valve calcification, if present, is better seen on the lateral view. On the frontal view, the valve calcification cannot be visualised over the spine.

Diaphragm. The hemidiaphragms visualised on the frontal films are the top of the domes seen tangentially. Much lung in the posterior costophrenic angles is not seen on the frontal film.

If the hemidiaphragms are low and flat, emphysema may be present. A critical look must be made beneath the diaphragm to see if there is free peritoneal gas (Figure 6.38, page 193).

Lung fields. On the frontal field, it is convenient to divide the lung fields into zones. It is easy then to compare one zone with another for density differences and the distribution of the vascular 'markings'.

The apices lie above the level of the clavicles. The upper zones include the apices and pass down to the level of the second costal cartilages. The mid-zones lie between the second and fourth costal cartilage levels. The lower zones lie between the fourth and sixth costal cartilages.

The radiolucency of the lung fields is due to the air filling the lung. The 'greyness' is due to blood in the pulmonary vessels.

The upper zones of the lungs are normally less well perfused, resulting in smaller blood vessels. With raised left atrial pressure, there is upper zone blood diversion and the vessels are congested.

An increase in lung radiolucency occurs with pulmonary vessel loss, as also happens with emphysema. Lung radiolucency is lost with an effusion or consolidation.

Terms such as opacity, consolidation and patchy shadowing are used to describe the lung fields. It is usually unwise to attempt to make too precise a diagnosis of the underlying pathology.

The lungs are divided into lobes by reflections of the visceral pleura. The right lung is composed of the upper, middle and lower lobes. On the left, there are only the upper and lower lobes.

The right upper lobe has three segments: anterior, posterior and apical. The right middle lobe has a lateral and medial segment. Apical, medial basal, lateral basal, anterior basal and posterior basal segments compose the lower lobe.

There are three differences in the segmental anatomy of the left lung (Figure 5.15, page 137). The left upper lobe has four segments: an apicoposterior, anterior and two lingular segments. The superior and inferior lingular segments are the equivalent of the right middle lobe. The left lower lobe has four segments: it does not contain a medial basal segment.

The fissures are seen as hairline shadows. The horizontal fissure is at the level of the right fourth costal cartilage. The oblique fissures are not seen on the frontal view.

Bones and soft tissue. Nipple shadows are often seen over the lower zones and are about 5 mm in diameter. They can be confused with a 'coin' lesion. In such a case, nipple markers may be helpful.

Look carefully for a missing breast shadow in a female patient. A mastectomy may provide a diagnostic clue to explain bony or pulmonary metastases, or upper zone postradiation fibrosis.

Soft tissue gas may accompany a pneumothorax or be present after a thoracotomy.

Calcified tuberculous glands in the neck should be looked for in patients with lung scarring or calcified hilar lymph nodes.

Check that there are no rib fractures or space-occupying lesions. Look for rib notching, due to increased blood flow through intercostal vessels (e.g. coarctation of the aorta). Cervical ribs or a thoracic scoliosis should be noted. Erosions or arthritis around the shoulder joints should be looked for.

Review. Certain parts of the film should be double-checked if the radiograph appears normal.

The retrocardiac region should be looked at again. A collapsed left lower lobe will reveal itself as a triangular opacity behind the heart shadow.

Both apices should be rechecked for lesions, especially Pancoast tumours or tuberculosis.

Has the patient a pneumothorax? There will be a difference between the translucency of the two lungs.

Lateral film

The lateral view is used largely for localisation of an already visible lesion on the frontal film. Examine it just as carefully. Sometimes a lesion is seen only on the lateral view. If there is clinical evidence of heart or lung disease, frontal and lateral views should always be obtained.

- **Points to remember:** (i) the retrosternal and retrocardiac triangles are normally of a similar radiodensity; (ii) the thoracic vertebrae become less opaque lower down the spine, unless there is pulmonary or pleural disease; (iii) the posterior costophrenic angle is sharp unless there is fluid or adjacent consolidation.

The hemidiaphragms are well defined unless there is pleural or pulmonary disease.

The oblique fissure placement is '4 to 4'. It passes from approximately 4 cm behind the anterior costophrenic angle, through the hilum to the T4 vertebral body level.

Heart

The right ventricle forms the anterior heart border on the lateral film. The left atrium forms the upper posterior border.

Mitral valve calcification is seen below an imaginary line drawn from the anterior costophrenic angle to the hilum, whereas aortic valve calcification lies above this line.

Examples of chest X-rays in cardiac disease

The radiological changes seen in pulmonary venous congestion, interstitial pulmonary oedema and alveolar pulmonary oedema are shown in Figures 4.59 to 4.61, respectively. Mitral valve disease is shown in Figure 4.62, while a ventricular aneurysm is seen in Figure 4.63. The characteristic notching of the inferior aspects of the ribs, due to hypertrophy of the intercostal arteries, appears in Figure 4.64, while the pulmonary plethora that is characteristic of a left-to-right shunt is obvious in Figure 4.65. A prosthetic aortic valve, which was inserted when a regurgitant valve was replaced in a patient with Marfan's syndrome, is illustrated in Figure 4.66; and a pacemaker and defibrillators are shown in Figure 4.67.

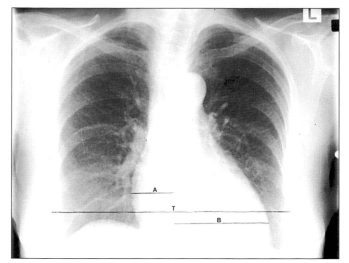

Figure 4.59 Pulmonary venous congestion
The heart is enlarged due to failure. This failure is not severe enough to cause pulmonary oedema. However, the increased pulmonary venous pressure has caused upper zone blood diversion so the vessels above the hilum appear wider than those below. (The mechanism of the blood diversion is not fully understood.) These changes are seen when the pulmonary venous pressure is about 15 to 20 mmHg. The cardiothoracic ratio A + B is a useful indicator of cardiac enlargement if it is greater than 50%. The thoracic measurement (T) is the widest diameter above the costophrenic angles, usually at the level of the right hemidiaphragm. The cardiac diameter is the addition of the two widths A and B.

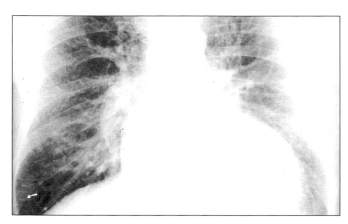

Figure 4.60 Interstitial pulmonary oedema
The heart is moderately enlarged. The interstitial oedema causes fine, diffuse shadowing in the lung fields with blurring of the vessel margins. The escape of fluid into the interstitial tissue occurs when the capillary pressure exceeds the plasma osmotic pressure of 25 mmHg.
The interstitial oedema is characterised by Kerley 'B' lines, which are oedematous interlobular septa. They are best seen peripherally in the right costophrenic angle (arrow), where they lie horizontally, and are about 1 cm long. They contain the engorged lymphatics, which were originally thought by Kerley to be the sole cause of the 'B' lines.
Sternal sutures are present from previous cardiac surgery.

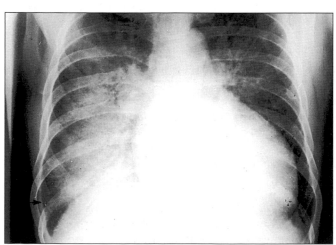

Figure 4.61 Alveolar pulmonary oedema
When the pulmonary venous pressure reaches 30 mmHg, oedema fluid will pass into the alveoli. This causes shadowing (patchy to confluent depending on the extent) in the lung fields. This usually occurs first around the hila and gives a bat's wing appearance. These changes are usually superimposed on the interstitial oedema.
A lamellar pleural effusion (arrow) is seen at the right costophrenic angle where Kerley 'B' lines are also evident.

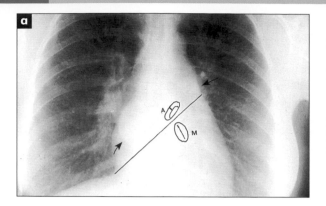
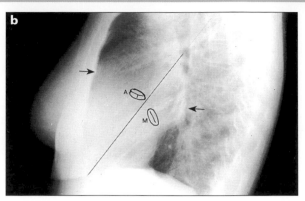

Figure 4.62 Mitral valve disease

The left atrium enlarges because of the pressure and volume load. It bulges posteriorly and to both sides (arrows). The atrial appendage bulges out below the left hilum. The prominent right border of the atrium causes the 'double right heart border' appearance.

To distinguish the valves if calcification is present, draw imaginary lines. On the PA view (a) the line passes from the right cardiophrenic angle to the inferior aspect of the left hilum. The line on the lateral view (b) passes from the antero-inferior angle through the midpoint of the hilum. The aortic valve lies above this line whereas the mitral valve lies below it.

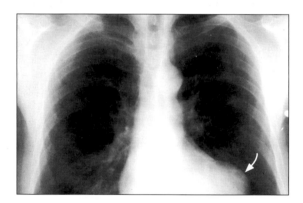

Figure 4.63 Ventricular aneurysm

There is a bulge of the left cardiac border (arrow), which indicates an aneurysm of the left ventricular wall. The most common cause is weakness following myocardial infarction.

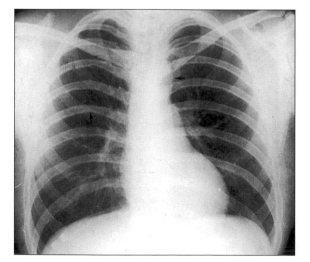

Figure 4.64 Aortic coarctation

The classical sign in aortic coarctation is notching of the inferior aspects of the ribs (arrow on left). This is due to hypertrophy of the intercostal arteries in which retrograde flow from the axillary collaterals is taking blood back to the descending aorta.

Because of the increased resistance to the left heart flow, left ventricular hypertrophy and then failure can occur. Failure causing cardiac enlargement has not yet occurred in this patient. The arrow on the right indicates a smaller than normal aortic knuckle.

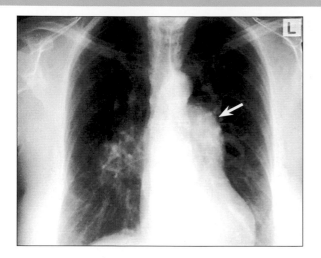

Figure 4.65 Atrial septal defect (ASD)
The most important thing to recognise is that there is pulmonary plethora indicating a left-to-right shunt. Left-to-right shunts occur in ASD, ventricular septal defect (VSD) and patent ductus arteriosus (PDA).
The shunted flow causes enlargement of the main pulmonary artery and its branches. The right hilum is enlarged because of the very dilated right pulmonary artery. The left hilum is hidden by the very dilated main pulmonary artery (arrow).
The ascending aorta is small (in contrast to its enlargement in PDA). The left atrium and ventricle are not enlarged, as they are in VSD and PDA.

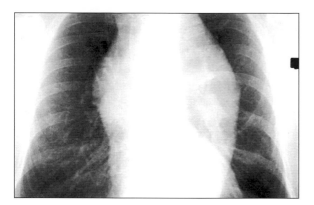

Figure 4.66 Marfan's syndrome
The mediastinum is widened by uniform dilatation of the ascending aorta, the aortic arch and the descending aorta. This patient had Marfan's syndrome. Dissecting aneurysms can also occur and have a similar appearance.

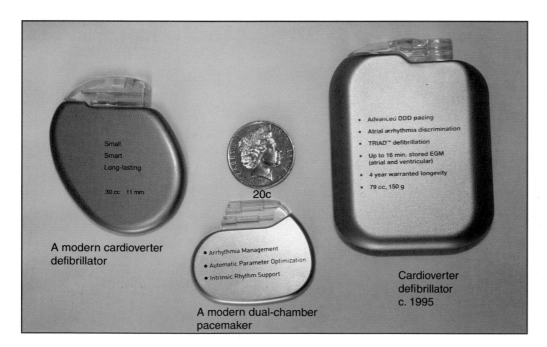

Figure 4.67 Pacemaker and defibrillators
(From Baker T, Nikolić G, O'Connor S, *Practical Cardiology,* 2nd edn. Sydney: Churchill Livingstone, 2008, with permission.)

Summary
The cardiovascular examination: a suggested method (Figure 4.68)

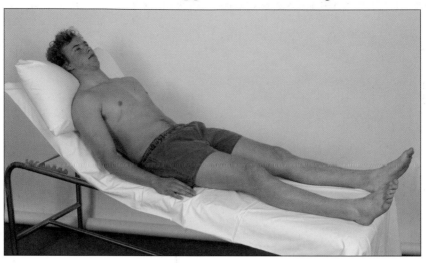

Figure 4.68 Cardiovascular system
Patient lying at 45 degrees

1. **General inspection**
   Marfan's, Turner's, Down syndrome
   Rheumatological disorders, e.g. ankylosing spondylitis (aortic regurgitation)
   Acromegaly etc
   Dyspnoea
2. **Hands**
   Radial pulses—right and left
   Radiofemoral delay
   Clubbing
   Signs of infective endocarditis—splinter haemorrhages etc
   Peripheral cyanosis
   Xanthomata
3. **Blood pressure**
4. **Face**
   Eyes
   • Sclerae—pallor, jaundice
   • Pupils—Argyll Robertson (aortic regurgitation)
   • Xanthelasma
   Malar flush (mitral stenosis, pulmonary stenosis)
   Mouth
   • Cyanosis
   • Palate (high arched—Marfan's)
   • Dentition
5. **Neck**
   Jugular venous pressure
   • Central venous pressure height
   • Wave form (especially large *n* waves)
   Carotids—pulse character
6. **Praecordium**
   Inspect
   • Scars—whole chest, back
   • Deformity
   • Apex beat—position, character
   • Abnormal pulsations

   Palpate
   • Apex beat—position, character
   • Thrills
   • Abnormal impulses
   NB: Beware of dextrocardia
7. **Auscultate**
   Heart sounds
   Murmurs
   Position patient
   • Left lateral position
   • Sitting forward (forced expiratory apnoea)
   NB: Palpate for thrills again after positioning
   Dynamic auscultation
   • Respiratory phases
   • Valsalva
   • Exercise (isometric, e.g. hand grip)
   • Carotids
8. **Back (sitting forward)**
   Scars, deformity
   Sacral oedema
   Pleural effusion (percuss)
   Left ventricular failure (auscultate)
9. **Abdomen (lying flat—1 pillow only)**
   Palpate liver (pulsatile etc.), spleen, aorta
   Percuss for ascites (right heart failure)
   Femoral arteries—palpate, auscultate
10. **Legs**
    Peripheral pulses
    Cyanosis, cold limbs, trophic changes, ulceration (peripheral vascular disease)
    Oedema
    Xanthomata
    Calf tenderness
11. **Other**
    Urine analysis (infective endocarditis)
    Fundi (endocarditis)
    Temperature chart (endocarditis)

Position the patient at 45 degrees and make sure his or her chest and neck are fully exposed. Cover the breasts of a female patient with a towel or loose garment.

Inspect while standing back for the appearance of Marfan's, Turner's or Down syndromes. Also look for dyspnoea, cyanosis, jaundice and cachexia.

Pick up the patient's **hand**. Feel the radial pulse. At the same time inspect the hands for clubbing. Also look for the peripheral stigmata of infective endocarditis: splinter haemorrhages are common (and are also caused by trauma), while Osler's nodes and Janeway lesions are rare. Look quickly, but carefully, at each nail bed, otherwise it is easy to miss these signs. Note any tendon xanthoma (type II hyperlipidaemia).

The **pulse** at the wrist should be timed for rate and rhythm. Feel for radiofemoral delay (which occurs in coarctation of the aorta) and radial–radial inequality. Pulse character is best assessed at the carotids.

Take the **blood pressure** (lying and standing or sitting—postural hypotension).

Next inspect the **face**. Look at the eyes briefly for jaundice (e.g. valve haemolysis) or xanthelasma (type II or type III hyperlipidaemia). You may also notice the classical mitral facies. Then inspect the mouth using a torch for a high arched palate (Marfan's syndrome), petechiae and the state of dentition (endocarditis). Look at the tongue or lips for central cyanosis.

The **neck** is very important. The jugular venous pressure (JVP) must be assessed for height and character. Use the right internal jugular vein for this assessment. Look for a change with inspiration (Kussmaul's sign). Now feel each carotid pulse separately. Assess the pulse character.

Proceed to the **praecordium**. Always begin by inspecting for scars, deformity, site of the apex beat and visible pulsations. Do not forget about pacemaker boxes. Mitral valvotomy scars (usually under the left breast) can be quite lateral and very easily missed.

Palpate for the position of the **apex beat**. Count down the correct number of interspaces. The normal position is the fifth left intercostal space, one centimetre medial to the midclavicular line. The character of the apex beat is important. There are a number of types. A *pressure-loaded* (hyperdynamic, systolic overloaded) apex beat is a forceful and sustained impulse that is not displaced (e.g. aortic stenosis, hypertension). A *volume-loaded* (hyperkinetic, diastolic overloaded) apex beat is a forceful but unsustained impulse that is displaced down and laterally (e.g. aortic regurgitation, mitral regurgitation). A *dyskinetic* apex beat (cardiac failure) is palpable over a larger area than normal and moves in an uncoordinated way under the examiner's hand. Do not miss the tapping apex beat of mitral stenosis (a palpable first heart sound). The double or triple apical impulse of hypertrophic cardiomyopathy is very important too. Feel also for an apical thrill, and time it.

Then palpate with the heel of your hand for a left parasternal impulse (which indicates right ventricular enlargement or left atrial enlargement) and for thrills. Now feel at the base of the heart for a palpable pulmonary component of the second heart sound (P2) and aortic thrills. Percussion may be helpful if there is uncertainty about cardiac enlargement.

Auscultation begins in the mitral area with both the bell and the diaphragm. Listen for each component of the cardiac cycle separately. Identify the first and second heart sounds, and decide if they are of normal intensity and whether the second heart sound is normally split. Now listen for extra heart sounds and for murmurs. Do not be satisfied at having identified one abnormality.

Repeat the approach at the left sternal edge and then the base of the heart (aortic and pulmonary areas). Time each part of the cycle with the carotid pulse. Listen over the carotids.

It is now time to **reposition** the patient. First put him or her in the left lateral position. Again feel the apex beat for character (particularly tapping) and auscultate. Sit the patient up and palpate for thrills (with the patient in full expiration) at the left sternal edge and base. Then listen in those areas, particularly for aortic regurgitation or a pericardial rub.

Dynamic auscultation should always be done if there is any doubt about the diagnosis. The Valsalva manoeuvre should be performed whenever there is a pure systolic murmur. Hypertrophic cardiomyopathy is easily missed otherwise.

The patient is now sitting up. Percuss the **back** quickly to exclude a pleural effusion (e.g. due to left ventricular failure), and auscultate for inspiratory crackles (left ventricular failure). If there is a radiofemoral delay, also listen for a coarctation murmur over the back. Feel for sacral oedema and note any back deformity (e.g. ankylosing spondylitis with aortic regurgitation).

Next lay the patient flat and examine the **abdomen** properly for hepatomegaly (right ventricular failure) and a pulsatile liver (tricuspid regurgitation). Test for the abdomino-jugular reflux sign if relevant. Feel for splenomegaly (endocarditis) and an aortic aneurysm.

Move on to the **legs**. Palpate both femoral arteries and auscultate here for bruits. Go on and examine all the peripheral pulses. Look for signs of peripheral vascular disease, peripheral oedema, clubbing of the toes, Achilles tendon xanthomata and stigmata of infective endocarditis.

Finally, examine the **fundi** (for hypertensive changes, and Roth's spots in endocarditis) and the **urine** (haematuria in endocarditis). Take the **temperature**.

References

1. Albert JS. The patient with angina: the importance of careful listening. *J Am Col Cardiol* 1988; 11:27. The history further distinguishes cardiac events even if a coronary angiogram is available.

2. Panju AA, Hemmegan BR, Guyatt GH, Simel DL. Is this patient having a myocardial infarction? *JAMA* 1995; 273:1211–1218. A focused history and examination (and an ECG) can aid subdivision of patients into those highly likely and those highly unlikely to be having a myocardial infarction.

3. Evan AT. Sensitivity and specificity of the history and physical examination for coronary artery disease. *Ann Intern Med* 1994; 120:344–345.

4. Khan NA, Rahim SA, Avand SS et al. Does the clinical examination predict lower extremity peripheral arterial disease? *JAMA* 2006 Feb 1; 295(5):536–546.

5. Poole-Wilson P. The origin of symptoms in patients with chronic heart failure. *Eur Heart J* 1998; 9 (supplement H):49–53. This article dicusses the lack of correlation between symptoms of heart failure and haemodynamic measurements.

6. McGee S. *Evidence-based physical diagnosis*, 2nd edn. St Louis: Saunders; 2007: 196.

7. Wang CS, FitzGerald JS, Schulzer M et al. Does this dyspneic patient in the emergency department have congestive heart failure? *JAMA* 2005 Oct 19; 294(15):1944–1956.

8. Brugada P, Gursoy S, Brugada J, Ardries E. Investigation of palpitations. *Lancet* 1993; 341:1254–1258. Emphasises the role of history taking and examination as well as the ECG in sorting out the patient presenting with palpitations.

9. Gursoy S, Steurer G, Brugada J et al. The hemodynamic mechanism of pounding in the neck in atrioventricular nodal reentrant tachycardia. *N Engl J Med* 1992; 327:772–774.

10. Calkins H, Shyr Y, Frumin H, Schork A, Morady F. The value of the clinical history in the differentiation of syncope due to ventricular tachycardia, atrioventricular block, and neurocardiogenic syncope. *Am J Med* 1995; 98:365–373. Describes useful historical features in differential diagnosis.

11. Special Writing Group of the Committee on Rheumatic Fever, Endocarditis and Kawasaki Disease of the Council on Cardiovascular Disease in the Young of the American Heart Association. Guidelines for the diagnosis of rheumatic fever. Jones Criteria, 1992 Update. *JAMA* 1992; 268:2069–2073.

12. Myers KA. Does this patient have clubbing? *JAMA* 2001, 286 (3):341–347.

13. Reeves RA. Does this patient have hypertension? *JAMA* 1995; 273:15. An important review of technique and of the errors to avoid.

14. Bellman J, Visintin JM, Salvatore R et al. Osler's manoeuvre: absence of usefulness for the detection of pseudo hypertension in an elderly population. *Am J Med* 1995; 98:42–49. Although it is reproducible, the manoeuvre failed to identify pseudohypertension compared with intra-arterial measurements.

15. Jansen RWMM, Lipsitz LA. Postprandial hypotension: epidemiology, pathophysiology and clinical management. *Ann Intern Med* 1995; 122:186–195. It is important to recognise that blood pressure decreases postprandially and that this can affect interpretation of the blood pressure reading and the management of hypertension.

16. Cook DC. Does this patient have abnormal central venous pressure? *JAMA* 1996; 275:8. A useful review that explains how to examine the veins and conduct the hepatojugular reflux test.

17. Maisel AS, Attwood JE, Goldberger AL. Hepatojugular reflux: useful in the bedside diagnosis of tricuspid regurgitation. *Ann Intern Med* 1984; 101:781–782. This test has excellent sensitivity and specificity.

18. O'Neill TW, Barry M, Smith M, Graham IM. Diagnostic value of the apex beat. *Lancet* 1989; 1:410–411. Palpation of the apex beat beyond the left midclavicular line is specific (59%) for identifying true cardiomegaly.

19. Heckerling PS et al. Accuracy and reproducibility of precordial percussion and palpation for detecting increased left ventricular end-diastolic volume and mass. *JAMA* 1993; 270:16. Percussion has a high sensitivity but low specificity for detecting left ventricular enlargement. Therefore this manoeuvre may have some value despite being previously discredited.

20. Harvey WP. Cardiac pearls. *Disease-a-Month* 1994; 40:41–113. A good review of auscultatory findings that helps demystify the many noises heard when auscultating the heart.

21. Sutton G, Harris A, Leatham A. Second heart sound in pulmonary hypertension. *Br Heart J* 1968; 30:743–756.

22. Timmis AJ. The third heart sound. *BMJ* 1987; 294:326–327.

23. Folland ED et al. Implications of third heart sounds in patients with valvular heart disease. *N Engl J Med* 1992; 327:458–462. An analysis of patients with valvular regurgitation shows that a third heart sound may occur before cardiac failure has supervened.

24. Benchimol A, Desser KB. The fourth heart sound in patients with demonstrable heart disease. *Am Heart J* 1977; 93:298–301. In 60 out of 100

consecutive patients with normal studies, an S4 was heard. An S4 can be a normal finding although a loud sound is more likely to be pathological.

25. Tyberg TI, Goodyer AVN, Langou RA. Genesis of pericardial knock in constrictive pericarditis. *Am J Cardiol* 1980; 46:570–575. Sudden cessation of ventricular filling generates this sound.

26. Smith ND, Raizada V, Abrams J. Auscultation of the normally functioning prosthetic valve. *Ann Intern Med* 1981; 95:594–598. Provides clear information on auscultatory changes with prosthetic valves.

27. Levine SA. Notes on the gradation of the intensity of cardiac murmurs. *JAMA* 1961; 177:261.

28. Lembo NJ et al. Bedside diagnosis of systolic murmurs. *N Engl J Med* 1988; 318:24. This well-conducted study describes the predictive value of bedside manoeuvres during auscultation.

29. Ewy GA. The abdominojugular test. *Ann Intern Med* 1988; 109:56–60. Note that an abnormal abdominal-jugular test can occur as a result of left heart disease (i.e. elevated pulmonary-capillary wedge pressure).

30. Lederle FA, Walker JM, Reinke DB. Selective screening for abdominal aortic aneurysms with physical examination and ultrasound. *Arch Intern Med* 1988; 148:1753–1756. In fat patients, palpation of aneurysms is unlikely but in thin ones the technique is valuable.

31. Lederle FA, Simel DL. Does this patient have an abdominal aortic aneurysm? *JAMA* 1999; 281:77–82. The only clinical sign of definite value is palpation to detect widening of the aorta. The sensitivity of this sign for aneurysms 5 cm or larger is 76%.

32. Magee TR, Stanley P, Mufti R et al. Should we palpate foot pulses? *Ann Roy Coll Surg Eng* 1992; 74:166–168. Elderly patients who do not have a palpable dorsalis pedis pulse will often have adequate perfusion (unless there is clinical evidence of claudication or foot ulcers). Palpation of the dorsalis pedis is more helpful than the posterior tibial.

33. McGee SR, Boyko EJ. Physical examination and chronic lower-extremity ischemia: a critical review. *Arch Intern Med* 1998; 158:1357–1364. The presence of peripheral arterial disease is positively predicted by abnormal pedal pulses, a unilaterally cool extremity, prolonged venous filling time, and a femoral bruit.

34. O'Keefe ST, Woods BO, Breslin DJ, Tsapatsaris NP. Blue toe syndrome. Causes and management. *Arch Intern Med* 1992; 152:2197–2202. Explains how to identify the cause by clinical methods and directed investigations.

35. Anand SS, Wells PS, Hunt D et al. Does this patient have deep venous thrombosis? *JAMA* 1998; 279:1094–1099. The sensitivity of individual symptoms and signs is 60%–96% and the specificity 20%–72%. Patients can be subdivided into those

with a low, intermediate or high pretest probability, based on risk factors and clinical features.

36. Butie A. Clinical examination of varicose veins. *Dermat Surg* 1995; 21:52–56. Techniques are outlined and compared with Doppler ultrasound assessment.

37. Stevenson LW, Perluff JK. The limited reliability of physical signs for estimating hemodynamics in chronic heart failure. *JAMA* 1989; 261:884–888. Physical signs poorly predict haemodynamic changes in heart failure. However, some signs are useful.

38. Khot U, Jia G, Moliterno DJ et al. Prognostic value of physical examination for heart failure in non-ST elevation acute coronary syndromes. *JAMA* 2003; 290: 2174–2181. This analysis of the Killip classification for patients with acute coronary syndromes expands the relevance of the classification from its original use for patients with ST elevation infarction in the pre-thrombolytic era.

39. Klompas M. Does this patient have an acute thoracic dissection? *JAMA* 2002; 287(17): 2262–2272.

40. Turnbull JM. Is listening for abdominal bruits useful in the evaluation of hypertension? The rational clinical examination. *JAMA* 1995; 274:16. If an abdominal bruit extends into diastole, this has a high predictive value for a clinically important bruit. The pitch and intensity are not helpful.

41. Etchells E, Bell C, Robb K. Does this patient have an abnormal systolic murmur? *JAMA* 1997; 277:564–571. The most useful positive predictive features for aortic stenosis appear to be a slow rate of rise of the carotid pulse, a mid-to-late peak intensity of the murmur and a decreased second heart sound; absence of radiation to the right carotid helps rule it out.

42. Aronow WS. Prevalence and severity of valvular aortic stenosis determined by Doppler echocardiography, and its association with echocardiographic and electrocardiographic left ventricular hypertrophy and physical signs of aortic stenosis in elderly patients. *Am J Cardiol* 1991; 67:776–777. Analysis of the signs of severity of aortic stenosis in elderly patients shows that they are less reliable than in younger patients.

43. Choudhry NK, Etchells EE. Does this patient have aortic regurgitation? *JAMA* 1999; 281:2231–2238 (Rational Clinical Examination Series).

44. Babu AN, Kymes SM, Carpenter Fryer SM. Eponyms and the diagnosis of aortic regurgitation: What says the evidence? *Ann Intern Med* 2003: 138:736–745.

Suggested reading

Braunwald E, Zipes DP, Libby P. Heart disease. *A textbook of cardiovascular medicine*, 8th edn. Philadelphia: WB Saunders, 2007.

Crawford MH, DiMarco JP, Paulus WJ. *Cardiology*, 2nd edn. London: Mosby, 2004.

Chapter 5

The respiratory system

A medical chest specialist is long-winded about the short-winded.

Kenneth T Bird (b. 1917)

This chapter deals with common respiratory symptoms, and the examination of the respiratory system.

The respiratory history
Presenting symptoms (Table 5.1)

TABLE 5.1 Respiratory history
Major symptoms
Cough
Sputum
Haemoptysis
Dyspnoea (acute, progressive or paroxysmal)
Wheeze
Chest pain
Fever
Hoarseness
Night sweats

Cough and sputum

Cough is a common presenting respiratory symptom. It occurs when deep inspiration is followed by explosive expiration. Flow rates of air in the trachea approach the speed of sound during a forceful cough. Coughing enables the airways to be cleared of secretions and foreign bodies. The duration of a cough is important.

Find out when the cough first became a problem. A cough of recent origin, particularly if associated with fever and other symptoms of respiratory tract infection, may be due to acute bronchitis or pneumonia. A chronic cough (of more than 8 weeks duration) associated with wheezing may be due to asthma; sometimes asthma can present with just cough alone. A change in the character of a chronic cough may indicate the development of a new and serious underlying problem (e.g. infection or lung cancer).

A differential diagnosis of cough based on its character is shown in Table 5.2 and on its duration is shown in Table 5.3.

A cough associated with a postnasal drip or sinus congestion or headaches may be due to the upper airway cough syndrome, which is the single most common cause of chronic cough. Although patients with this problem often complain of a cough, when asked to demonstrate their cough they do not cough but clear the throat. An irritating, chronic dry cough can result from oesophageal reflux and acid irritation of the lungs. There is some controversy about these as causes of true cough. A similar dry cough may be a feature of late interstitial lung disease or associated with the use of the angiotensin-converting enzyme (ACE) inhibitors—drugs used in the treatment of hypertension and cardiac failure. Cough that wakes a patient from sleep may be a symptom of cardiac failure or of the reflux of acid from the oesophagus into the lungs that can occur when a person lies down. A chronic cough that is productive of large volumes of purulent sputum may be due to bronchiectasis.

Patients' descriptions of their cough may be helpful. In children, a cough associated with inflammation of the epiglottis may have a muffled quality and cough related to viral croup is often described as 'barking'. Cough caused by tracheal compression by a tumour may be loud and brassy. Cough associated with recurrent laryngeal nerve palsy has a hollow sound because the vocal cords

TABLE 5.2 Differential diagnosis of cough based on its character

Origin	Character	Causes
Naso-pharynx/larynx	Throat clearing, chronic	Postnasal drip, acid reflux
Larynx	Barking, painful, acute or persistent	Laryngitis, pertussis (whooping cough), croup
Trachea	Acute, painful	Tracheitis
Bronchi	Intermittent, sometimes productive, worse at night	Asthma
	Worse in morning	Chronic obstructive pulmonary disease (COPD)
	With blood	Bronchial malignancy
Lung parenchyma	Dry then productive	Pneumonia
	Chronic, very productive	Bronchiectasis
	Productive, with blood	Tuberculosis
	Irritating and dry, persistent	Interstitial lung disease
	Worse on lying down, sometimes with frothy sputum	Pulmonary oedema
ACE inhibitors	Dry, scratchy, persistent	Medication-induced

TABLE 5.3 Differential diagnosis of cough based on its duration

Acute cough (<3 weeks duration): differential diagnosis
Upper respiratory tract infection
• Common cold, sinusitis
Lower respiratory tract infection
• Pneumonia, bronchitis, exacerbation of COPD
• Irritation—inhalation of bronchial irritant, e.g. smoke or fumes

Chronic cough: differential diagnosis and clues
COPD—smoking history
Asthma—wheeze, relief with bronchodilators
Gastro-oesophageal reflux—occurs when lying down, burning chest pain
Upper airway cough syndrome —history of rhinitis, postnasal drip, sinus headache and congestion
Bronchiectasis—chronic, very productive
ACE inhibitor medication—drug history
Carcinoma of the lung—smoking, haemoptysis
Cardiac failure—dyspnoea, PND
Psychogenic—variable, prolonged symptoms, usually mild

ACE = angiotensin-converting enzyme.
COPD = chronic obstructive pulmonary disease.
PND = paroxysmal nocturnal dyspnoea.

are unable to close completely; this has been described as a bovine cough. A cough that is worse at night is suggestive of asthma or heart failure, while coughing that comes on immediately after eating or drinking may be due to incoordinate swallowing or oesophageal reflux or, rarely, a tracheo-oesophageal fistula.

It is an important (though perhaps a somewhat unpleasant task) to inquire about the type of sputum produced and then to look at it, if it is available. Be warned that some patients have more interest in their sputum than others and may go into more detail than you really want. A large volume of purulent (yellow or green) sputum suggests the diagnosis of bronchiectasis or lobar pneumonia. Foul-smelling dark-coloured sputum may indicate the presence of a lung abscess with anaerobic organisms. Pink frothy secretions from the trachea, which occur in pulmonary oedema, should not be confused with sputum. It is best to rely on the patient's assessment of the taste of the sputum, which, not unexpectedly, is foul in conditions like bronchiectasis or lung abscess.

Haemoptysis

Haemoptysis (coughing up of blood) can be a sinister sign of lung disease (Table 5.4) and must always be investigated. It must be distinguished from haematemesis (vomiting of blood) and from nasopharyngeal bleeding (Table 5.5).

Ask how much blood has been produced. Mild haemoptysis usually means less than 20 mL in 24 hours. It appears as streaks of blood discolouring sputum. Massive haemoptysis is more than 250 mL of blood in 24 hours and represents a medical emergency. Its most common causes are carcinoma, cystic fibrosis, bronchiectasis and tuberculosis.

TABLE 5.4 Causes (differential diagnosis) of haemoptysis and typical histories

Respiratory

Bronchitis	Small amounts of blood with sputum
Bronchial carcinoma	Frank blood, history of smoking, hoarseness
Bronchiectasis	Large amounts of sputum with blood
Pneumonia	Fever, recent onset of symptoms, dyspnoea

(The above four account for about 80% of cases)

Pulmonary infarction	Pleuritic chest pain, dyspnoea
Cystic fibrosis	Recurrent infections
Lung abscess	Fever, purulent sputum
Tuberculosis (TB)	Previous TB, contact with TB, HIV-positive status
Foreign body	History of inhalation, cough, stridor
Goodpasture's* syndrome	Pulmonary haemorrhage, glomerulonephritis, antibody to basement membrane antigens
Wegener's granulomatosis	History of sinusitis, saddle-nose deformity
Systemic lupus erythematosus	Pulmonary haemorrhage, multi-system involvement
Rupture of a mucosal blood vessel after vigorous coughing	

Cardiovascular

Mitral stenosis (severe)
Acute left ventricular failure

Bleeding diatheses

Note: Exclude spurious causes, such as nasal bleeding or haematemesis.
* Ernest W Goodpasture (1886–1960), pathologist at Johns Hopkins, Baltimore. He described this syndrome in 1919.

Questions box 5.1

Questions to ask the patient with a cough

❗ denotes symptoms for the possible diagnosis of an urgent or dangerous problem.

1 How long have you had the cough?
2 Do you cough up anything? What? How much?
3 Have you had sinus problems?
❗ 4 Is the sputum clear or discoloured? Is there any blood in the sputum?
5 Have you had high temperatures?
6 Does coughing occur particularly at night (acid reflux)?
7 Have you become short of breath?
8 Have you had lung problems in the past?
9 Have you been a smoker? Do you still smoke?
10 Have you noticed wheezing?—Asthma, chronic obstructive pulmonary disease (COPD)?
11 Do you take any tablets?—ACE inhibitors

TABLE 5.5 Features distinguishing haemoptysis from haematemesis and nasopharyngeal bleeding

Favours haemoptysis	Favours haematemesis	Favours naso-pharyngeal bleeding
Mixed with sputum	Follows nausea	Blood appears in mouth
Occurs immediately after coughing	Mixed with vomitus; follows dry retching	

Breathlessness (dyspnoea) (Table 5.6)

The awareness that an abnormal amount of effort is required for breathing is called dyspnoea. It can be due to respiratory or cardiac disease, or lack of physical fitness. Careful questioning about the timing of onset, severity and pattern of dyspnoea is helpful in making the diagnosis (*Questions box 5.2* and Table 5.7).[1] The patient may be aware of this only on heavy exertion or have much more limited exercise tolerance. Dyspnoea can be graded from I to IV based on the New York Heart Association classification:

Class I—disease present but no dyspnoea or dyspnoea only on heavy exertion
Class II—dyspnoea on moderate exertion
Class III—dyspnoea on minimal exertion
Class IV—dyspnoea at rest.

It is more useful, however, to determine the amount of exertion that actually causes dyspnoea—that is, the distance walked or the number of steps climbed.

TABLE 5.6 Causes of dyspnoea

Respiratory

1 Airways disease

Chronic bronchitis and emphysema (chronic obstructive pulmonary disease, COPD)

Asthma

Bronchiectasis

Cystic fibrosis

Laryngeal or pharyngeal tumour

Bilateral cord palsy

Tracheal obstruction or stenosis

Tracheomalacia

Cricoarytenoid rheumatoid arthritis

2 Parenchymal disease

Interstitial lung diseases (diffuse parenchymal lung diseases), e.g. idiopathic pulmonary fibrosis, sarcoidosis, connective tissue disease, inorganic or organic dusts

Diffuse infections

Acute respiratory distress syndrome (ARDS)

Infiltrative and metastatic tumour

Pneumothorax

Pneumoconiosis

3 Pulmonary circulation

Pulmonary embolism

Chronic thromboembolic pulmonary hypertension

Pulmonary arteriovenous malformation

Pulmonary arteritis

4 Chest wall and pleura

Effusion or massive ascites

Pleural tumour

Fractured ribs

Ankylosing spondylitis

Kyphoscoliosis

Neuromuscular diseases

Bilateral diaphragmatic paralysis

Cardiac

Left ventricular failure

Mitral valve disease

Cardiomyopathy

Pericardial effusion or constrictive pericarditis

Intracardiac shunt

Anaemia

Non-cardiorespiratory

Psychogenic

Acidosis (compensatory respiratory alkalosis)

Hypothalamic lesions

The association of dyspnoea with wheeze suggests *airways disease*, which may be due to asthma or chronic obstructive pulmonary disease (COPD) (Table 5.8). The duration and variability of the dyspnoea are important. Dyspnoea that worsens progressively over a period of weeks, months or years may be due to *interstitial lung disease* (ILD). Dyspnoea of more rapid onset may be due to an *acute respiratory infection* (including bronchopneumonia or lobar pneumonia) or to *pneumonitis* (which may be infective or secondary to a hypersensitivity reaction). Dyspnoea that varies from day to day or even from hour to hour suggests a diagnosis of *asthma*. Dyspnoea of very rapid onset associated with sharp chest pain suggests a *pneumothorax* (Table 5.9). Dyspnoea that is described by the patient as inability to take a breath big enough to fill the lungs and associated with sighing suggests *anxiety*. Dyspnoea that occurs on moderate exertion may be due to the combination of *obesity and a lack of physical fitness* (a not uncommon occurrence).

Wheeze

A number of conditions can cause a continuous whistling noise that comes from the chest (rather than the throat) during breathing. These include asthma or COPD, infections such as bronchiolitis and airways obstruction by a foreign body or tumour. Wheeze is usually maximal during expiration and is accompanied by prolonged expiration. This must be differentiated from *stridor* (see below), which can have a similar sound, but is loudest over the trachea and occurs during inspiration.

Chest pain

Chest pain due to respiratory disease is usually different from that associated with myocardial ischaemia (page 35). The pleura and central airways have pain fibres and may be the source of respiratory pain. Pleural pain is characteristically *pleuritic* in nature: sharp and made worse by deep inspiration and coughing. It is typically localised to one area of the chest. It may be of sudden onset in patients with lobar pneumonia, pulmonary embolism and infarction or pneumothorax, and is often associated with dyspnoea. The sudden onset of pleuritic chest pain and dyspnoea is an urgent diagnostic problem, as all three of these conditions may be life-threatening if not treated promptly.

Other presenting symptoms

Bacterial pneumonia is an acute illness in which prodromal symptoms (fever, malaise and myalgia) occur for a short period (hours) before pleuritic pain and dyspnoea begin. *Viral pneumonia* is often preceded by a longer (days) prodromal illness. Patients may occasionally present with episodes of *fever at night*. Tuberculosis, pneumonia and lymphoma should always be considered in these cases. Occasionally patients with tuberculosis present with episodes of *drenching sweating* at night.

Hoarseness or *dysphonia* (an abnormality of the voice) may sometimes be considered a respiratory system symptom. It can be due to transient inflammation of the vocal cords (laryngitis), vocal cord tumour or recurrent laryngeal nerve palsy.

Sleep apnoea is an abnormal increase in the periodic cessation of breathing during sleep. Patients with *obstructive sleep apnoea* (OSA) (where airflow stops during sleep for periods of at least 10 seconds and sometimes for over 2 minutes, despite persistent respiratory efforts) typically present with daytime somnolence, chronic fatigue, morning headaches and personality disturbances. Very loud snoring may be reported by anyone within earshot. These patients are often obese and hypertensive.

Questions box 5.2

Questions to ask the breathless patient

! denotes symptoms for the possible diagnosis of an urgent or dangerous problem.

1 How long have you been short of breath? Has it come on quickly?

2 How much exercise can you do before your shortness of breath stops you or slows you down? Can you walk up a flight of stairs?

! 3 Have you been woken at night by breathlessness or had to sleep sitting up?—Paroxysmal nocturnal dyspnoea (PND), orthopnoea

4 Have you had heart or lung problems in the past?

! 5 Have you had a temperature?

6 Do you smoke?

! 7 Is there a feeling of tightness in the chest when you feel breathless?—Angina

8 Do you get wheezy in the chest? Cough?

9 Is the feeling really one of difficulty getting a satisfying breath?—Anxiety

10 Is it painful to take a big breath?—Pleurisy or pericarditis

! 11 Did the shortness of breath come on very quickly or instantaneously?—Pulmonary embolus (very quick onset) or pneumothorax (instantaneous onset)

TABLE 5.7 Differential diagnosis of dyspnoea based on time course of onset

Seconds to minutes—favours:

Asthma

Pulmonary embolism

Pneumothorax

Pulmonary oedema

Anaphylaxis

Foreign body causing airway obstruction

Hours or days—favours:

Exacerbation of chronic obstructive pulmonary disease (COPD)

Cardiac failure

Asthma

Respiratory infection

Pleural effusion

Metabolic acidosis

Weeks or longer—favours:

Pulmonary fibrosis

COPD

Pleural effusion

Anaemia

TABLE 5.8 Characteristics of chronic obstructive pulmonary disease (COPD)

History

History of smoking

Breathlessness and wheeze

Examination

Increased respiratory rate

Pursed-lips breathing

Cyanosis

Leaning forward—arms on knees

Intercostal and supraclavicular indrawing

Hoover's sign

Tracheal tug

TABLE 5.9 Differential diagnosis of dyspnoea of sudden onset based on other features

Presence of pleuritic chest pain—favours:

Pneumothorax, pleurisy/pneumonia

Pulmonary embolism

Trauma

Absence of chest pain—favours:

Pulmonary oedema

Metabolic acidosis

Pulmonary embolism

Presence of central chest pain—favours:

Myocardial infarction and cardiac failure

Large pulmonary embolism

Presence of cough and wheeze—favours:

Asthma

Bronchial irritant inhalation

Chronic obstructive pulmonary disease (COPD)

TABLE 5.10 The Epworth sleepiness scale

'How easily would you fall asleep in the following circumstances?'*

0 = never
1 = slight chance
2 = moderate chance
3 = high chance

- Sitting reading
- Watching television
- At a meeting or at the theatre
- As a passenger in a car on a drive of more than an hour
- Lying down in the afternoon to rest
- Sitting talking to someone
- Sitting quietly after lunch (no alcohol)
- When driving and stopped at traffic lights

* A normal score is between 0 and 9. Severe sleep apnoea scores from 11 to 20.

TABLE 5.11 Abnormal patterns of breathing

Type of breathing	Cause(s)
1 Sleep apnoea—cessation of airflow for more than 10 seconds more than 10 times a night during sleep	Obstructive (e.g. obesity with upper airway narrowing, enlarged tonsils, pharyngeal soft tissue changes in acromegaly or hypothyroidism)
2 Cheyne-Stokes* breathing—periods of apnoea (associated with reduced level of consciousness) alternate with periods of hyperpnoea (lasts 30 s on average and is associated with agitation). This is due to a delay in the medullary chemoreceptor response to blood gas changes	Left ventricular failure Brain damage (e.g. trauma, cerebral haemorrhage) High altitude
3 Kussmaul's breathing (air hunger)— deep, rapid respiration due to stimulation of the respiratory centre	Metabolic acidosis (e.g. diabetes mellitus, chronic renal failure)
4 Hyperventilation, which results in alkalosis and tetany	Anxiety
5 Ataxic (Biot†) breathing—irregular in timing and depth	Brainstem damage
6 Apneustic breathing—a post-inspiratory pause in breathing	Brain (pontine) damage
7 Paradoxical respiration—the abdomen sucks inwards with inspiration (it normally pouches outwards due to diaphragmatic descent)	Diaphragmatic paralysis

* John Cheyne (1777–1836), Scottish physician who worked in Dublin, described this in 1818. William Stokes (1804–1878), Irish physician, described it in 1854.
† Camille Biot (b. 1878), French physician.

The Epworth sleepiness scale is a way of quantifying the severity of sleep apnoea (Table 5.10).

Patients with *central sleep apnoea* (where there is cessation of inspiratory muscle activity) may also present with somnolence but do not snore excessively (Table 5.11).

Some patients respond to anxiety by increasing the rate and depth of their breathing. This is called *hyperventilation*. The result is an increase in CO_2 excretion and the development of alkalosis—a rise in the pH of the blood. These patients may complain of variable dyspnoea; they have more difficulty breathing in than out. The alkalosis results in paraesthesiae of the fingers and around the mouth, light-headedness, chest pain and a feeling of impending collapse.

Treatment

It is important to find out what drugs the patient is using (Table 5.12), how often they are taken and

TABLE 5.12 Drugs and the lungs

Cough

ACE inhibitors

Beta-blockers

Wheeze

Beta-blockers

Aspirin (aspirin sensitivity)

Other non-steroidal anti-inflammatory drugs (NSAIDs)

Tamoxifen, dipyridamole (idiosyncratic)

Morphine sulfate

Succinylcholine

Interstitial lung disease (pulmonary fibrosis)

Amiodarone

Hydralazine

Gold salts

Bleomycin

Nitrofurantoin

Methotrexate

Pulmonary embolism

Oestrogens

Tamoxifen

Raloxifene

Non-cardiogenic pulmonary oedema

Hydrochlorothiazide

Pleural disease/effusion

Nitrofurantoin

Phenytoin, hydralazine (induction of systemic lupus
    erythematosus)

Methotrexate

Methysergide

whether they are inhaled or swallowed. The patient's previous and current medications may give a clue to the current diagnosis. Bronchodilators and inhaled steroids are prescribed for COPD and asthma. A patient's increased use of bronchodilators suggests poor control of asthma and the need for review of treatment. Chronic respiratory disease, including sarcoidosis, hypersensitivity pneumonias and asthma, may have been treated with oral steroids. Oral steroid use may predispose to tuberculosis or pneumocystis pneumonia. Patients with chronic lung conditions like cystic fibrosis or bronchiectasis will often be very knowledgeable about their treatment and can describe the various forms of physiotherapy that are essential for keeping their airways clear.

Almost every class of drug can produce lung toxicity. Examples include pulmonary embolism from use of the oral contraceptive pill, interstitial lung disease from cytotoxic agents (e.g. methotrexate, cyclophosphamide, bleomycin), bronchospasm from beta-blockers or non-steroidal anti-inflammatory drugs (NSAIDs), and cough from ACE inhibitors. Some medications known to cause lung disease may not be mentioned by the patient because they are illegal (e.g. cocaine), are used sporadically (e.g. hydrochlorothiazide), can be obtained over the counter (e.g. tryptophan) or are not taken orally (e.g. timolol; beta-blocker eye drops for glaucoma). The clinician therefore needs to ask about these types of drug specifically.

Past history

One should always ask about previous respiratory illness, including pneumonia, tuberculosis or chronic bronchitis, or abnormalities of the chest X-ray that have previously been reported to the patient. Many previous respiratory investigations may have been memorable, such as bronchoscopy, lung biopsy and video-assisted thoracoscopy. Spirometry, with or without challenge testing for asthma, may have been performed. Many severe asthmatics perform their own regular peak flow testing (page 128). Ask about the results of any of these investigations. Patients with the acquired immunodeficiency syndrome (AIDS) have a high risk of developing *Pneumocystis jiroveci (carinii)* pneumonia and indeed other chest infections, including tuberculosis.

Occupational history

In no system are the patient's present and previous occupations of more importance (Table 5.13).[2] A detailed occupational history is essential. The occupational lung diseases or pneumoconioses cause interstitial lung disease by damaging the alveoli and small airways. Prolonged exposure to substances whose use is now heavily restricted is usually required. Cigarette smoking has an additive effect for these patients. These occupational conditions are now rare, and the most common occupational lung disease is asthma.

One must ask about exposure to dusts in mining industries and factories (e.g. asbestos, coal, silica, iron oxide, tin oxide, cotton, beryllium, titanium oxide, silver, nitrogen dioxide, anhydrides). Heavy exposure to asbestos can lead to asbestosis (Table 5.14), but even trivial exposure can result in pleural plaques or mesothelioma (malignant disease of the pleura). The patient may be unaware that his or her occupation involved exposure to dangerous substances; for example, factories making insulating cables and boards very often used asbestos until 25 years ago. Asbestos exposure can result in

TABLE 5.13 Occupational lung disease (pneumoconioses)

Substance	Disease
Coal	Coal worker's pneumoconiosis
Silica	Silicosis
Asbestos	Asbestosis
Talc	Talcosis

TABLE 5.14 Possible occupational exposure to asbestos

Asbestos mining, including relatives of miners

Naval dockyard workers and sailors—lagging of pipes

Builders—asbestos in fibreboard (particles are released during cutting or drilling)

Factory workers—manufacture of fibro-sheets, brake linings, some textiles

Building maintenance workers—asbestos insulation

Building demolition workers

Home renovation

TABLE 5.15 Allergic alveolitis—sources

Bird fancier's lung	Bird feathers and excreta
Farmer's lung	Mouldy hay or straw (*Aspergillus fumigatus*)
Byssinosis	Cotton or hemp dust
Cheese worker's lung	Mouldy cheese (*Aspergillus clavatus*)
Malt worker's lung	Mouldy malt (*Aspergillus clavatus*)
Humidifier fever	Air-conditioning (thermophilic *Actinomycetes*)

the development of asbestosis, mesothelioma or carcinoma of the lung up to 30 years later. Relatives of people working with asbestos may be exposed when handling work clothes.

Work or household exposure to animals, including birds, is also relevant (e.g. Q fever or psittacosis which are infectious diseases caught from animals).

Exposure to organic dusts can cause a local immune response to organic antigens and result in *allergic alveolitis*. Within a few hours of exposure, patients develop flu-like symptoms. These often include fever, headache, muscle pains, dyspnoea without wheeze and dry cough. The culprit antigens may come from mouldy hay, humidifiers or air conditioners, among others (Table 5.15).

It is most important to find out what the patient actually does when at work, the duration of any exposure, use of protective devices and whether other workers have become ill. An improvement in symptoms over the weekend is a valuable clue to the presence of occupational lung disease, particularly occupational asthma. This can occur as a result of exposure to spray paints or plastic or soldering fumes.

Social history

A smoking history must be routine, as it is the major cause of COPD and lung cancer (see Table 1.2, page 6). It also increases the risk of spontaneous pneumothorax and of Goodpasture's syndrome. It is necessary to ask how many packets of cigarettes a day a patient has smoked and how many years the patient has smoked. An estimate should be made of the number of packet-years of smoking. Remember that this is based on 20-cigarette packets and that packets of cigarettes are getting larger; curiously, most manufacturers now make packets of 30 or 35. More recently, giant packets of 50 have appeared. These are too large to fit into pockets and must be carried in the hands as a constant reminder to the patient of his or her addiction. Occupation may further affect cigarette smokers; for example, asbestos workers who smoke are at an especially high risk of lung cancer. Passive smoking is now regarded as a significant risk for lung disease and the patient should be asked about exposure to other people's cigarette smoke at home and at work.

Many respiratory conditions are chronic, and may interfere with the ability to work and exercise and interfere with normal family life. In some cases involving occupational lung disease there may be compensation matters affecting the patient. Ask about these problems and whether the patient has been involved in a pulmonary rehabilitation programme. Housing conditions may be inappropriate for a person with a limited exercise tolerance or an infectious disease. An inquiry about the patient's alcohol consumption is important. The drinking of large amounts of alcohol in binges can sometimes result in aspiration pneumonia, and alcoholics are more likely to develop pneumococcal or *Klebsiella* pneumonia. Intravenous drug users are at risk of lung abscess and drug-related pulmonary oedema. Sexual orientation or history of intravenous drug use may be related to an increased risk of HIV infection and susceptibility to infection. Such information may influence the decision about whether to advise treatment at home or in hospital.

Family history

A family history of asthma or other atopic diseases, cystic fibrosis, lung cancer or emphysema should be sought. Alpha$_1$-antitrypsin deficiency, for example, is an inherited disease, and those affected are extremely susceptible to the development of emphysema. A family history of infection with tuberculosis is also important. A number of pulmonary diseases may have a familial or genetic association. These include carcinoma of the lung and pulmonary hypertension.

The respiratory examination

Examination anatomy

The **lungs** are paired asymmetrical organs protected by the cylinder composed of the ribs, vertebrae and diaphragm. The surface of the lungs is covered by the visceral **pleura**, a thin membrane, and a similar outer layer (the parietal pleura) lines the rib cage. These membranes are separated by a thin layer of fluid and enable the lungs to move freely during breathing. Various diseases of the lungs and of the pleura themselves, including infection and malignancy, can cause accumulation of fluid within the pleural cavity (a pleural effusion).

The heart, trachea, oesophagus and the great blood vessels and nerves sit between the lungs and make up the structure called the **mediastinum**. The left and right pulmonary arteries supply their respective lung. Gas exchange occurs in the pulmonary capillaries which surround the alveoli, the tiny air sacs which lie beyond the terminal bronchioles. Oxygenated blood is returned via the pulmonary veins to the left atrium. Abnormalities of the pulmonary circulation such as raised pulmonary venous pressure resulting from heart failure or pulmonary hypertension can interfere with gas exchange.

The position of the heart with its apex pointing to the left means that the **left lung** is smaller than the right and has only two lobes, which are separated by the oblique fissure. The **right lung** has both horizontal (upper) and oblique (lower) fissures dividing it into three lobes (Figure 5.1).

The muscles of respiration are the **diaphragm** upon which the bases of the lungs rest and the **intercostal muscles**. During inspiration the diaphragm flattens and the intercostal muscles contract to elevate the ribs. Intrathoracic pressure falls as air is forced under atmospheric pressure into the lungs. Expiration is a passive process resulting from elastic recoil of the muscles. Abnormalities of lung function or structure may change the normal anatomy and physiology of respiration, for example as a result of over-inflation of the lungs (COPD, page 133). Muscle and neurological diseases can also affect muscle function adversely, and abnormalities of the control of breathing in the respiratory centres of the brain in the pons and medulla can interfere with normal breathing patterns.

During the respiratory examination, keep in mind the **surface anatomy** (Figure 5.1) of the lungs and try to decide which lobes are affected.

Positioning the patient

The patient should be undressed to the waist.[3] Women should wear a gown or have a towel or some clothing to cover their breasts when the front of the chest is not being examined. If the patient is not acutely ill, the examination is easiest to perform with him or her sitting over the edge of the bed or on a chair.

General appearance

If the patient is an inpatient in hospital, look around the bed for oxygen masks, metered dose inhalers (puffers) and other medications, and the presence of a sputum mug. Then make a deliberate point of looking for the following signs before beginning the detailed examination.

Dyspnoea

Watch the patient for signs of dyspnoea at rest. Count the respiratory rate; the normal rate at rest should not exceed 25 breaths per minute (range 16–25). The frequently quoted normal value of 14 breaths per minute is probably too low; normal people can have a respiratory rate of up to 25, and the average is 20 breaths per minute. It is traditional to count the respiratory rate surreptitiously while affecting to count the pulse. The respiratory rate is the only vital sign that is under direct voluntary control. *Tachypnoea* refers to a rapid respiratory rate of greater than 25. *Bradypnoea* is defined as a rate below 8, a level associated with sedation and adverse prognosis. In normal relaxed breathing, the diaphragm is the only active muscle and is active only in inspiration; expiration is a passive process.

Characteristic signs of chronic obstructive pulmonary disease (COPD)[a]

Look to see whether the accessory muscles of respiration are being used. This is a sign of an

---

[a]   This condition has undergone many changes in nomenclature, and it is pleasing to think that chest physicians have something to keep them occupied. The term COPD encompasses emphysema, chronic bronchitis, chronic obstructive lung disease (COLD) and chronic airflow limitation (CAL). It now seems quite firmly established. The diagnosis of COPD depends on clinical, radiographic and lung function assessment. There may be components of what used to be called chronic bronchitis and emphysema.

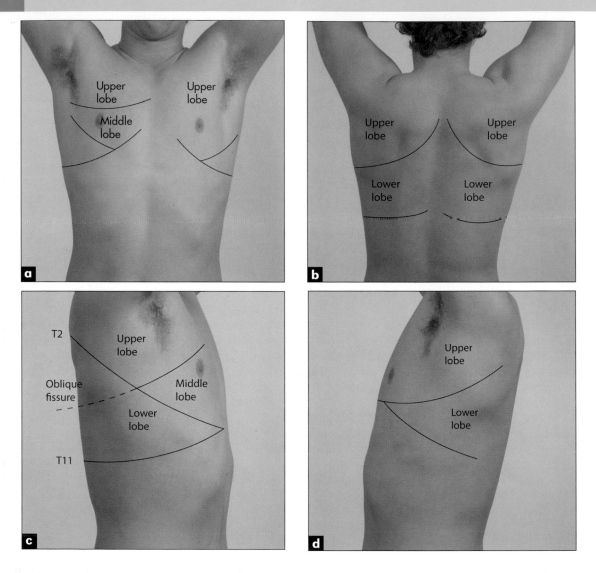

Figure 5.1 Lobes of the lung
(a) Anterior. (b) Posterior. (c) Lobes of the right lung. (d) Lobes of the left lung. Refer to Figure 5.15, page 137, for a list of the segments in each lobe.

increase in the work of breathing, and COPD is an important cause. These muscles include the sternomastoids, the platysma and the strap muscles of the neck. Characteristically the accessory muscles cause elevation of the shoulders with inspiration, and aid respiration by increasing chest expansion. Contraction of the abdominal muscles may occur in expiration in patients with obstructed airways. Patients with severe COPD often have indrawing of the intercostal and supraclavicular spaces during inspiration. This is due to a delayed increase in lung volume despite the generation of large negative pleural pressures.

In some cases, the pattern of breathing is diagnostically helpful (Table 5.11). Look for pursed-lips breathing, which is characteristic of patients with severe COPD. This manoeuvre reduces the patient's breathlessness, possibly by providing continuous positive airways pressure and helping to prevent airways collapse during expiration. Patients with severe COPD may feel more comfortable leaning forward with their arms on their knees. This position compresses the abdomen and pushes the diaphragm upwards. This partly restores its normal domed shape and improves its effectiveness during inspiration. Increased diaphragmatic movements may cause downward displacement of the trachea during inspiration—tracheal tug.

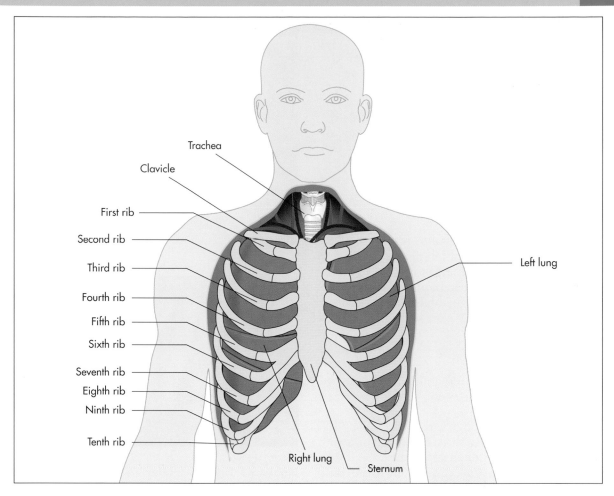

Figure 5.2 Basic anatomy of the lungs

Cyanosis

Central cyanosis is best detected by inspecting the tongue. Examination of the tongue differentiates central from peripheral cyanosis. Lung disease severe enough to result in significant ventilation–perfusion imbalance, such as pneumonia, COPD and pulmonary embolism, may cause reduced arterial oxygen saturation and central cyanosis. Cyanosis becomes evident when the absolute concentration of deoxygenated haemoglobin is 50 g/L of capillary blood. Cyanosis is usually obvious when the arterial oxygen saturation falls below 90% in a person with a normal haemoglobin level. Central cyanosis is therefore a sign of severe hypoxaemia. In patients with anaemia, cyanosis does not occur until even greater levels of arterial desaturation are reached. The absence of obvious cyanosis does not exclude hypoxia. The detection of cyanosis is much easier in good (especially fluorescent) lighting conditions and is said to be more difficult if the patient's bed is surrounded by cheerful pink curtains.

Character of the cough

Coughing is a protective response to irritation of sensory receptors in the submucosa of the upper airways or bronchi. Ask the patient to cough several times. *Lack of the usual explosive beginning* may indicate vocal cord paralysis (the 'bovine' cough). A *muffled, wheezy, ineffective cough* suggests obstructive pulmonary disease. A *very loose productive cough* suggests excessive bronchial secretions due to chronic bronchitis, pneumonia or bronchiectasis. A *dry, irritating cough* may occur with chest infection, asthma or carcinoma of the bronchus and sometimes with left ventricular failure or interstitial lung disease. It is also typical of the cough produced by ACE inhibitor drugs. A *barking* or *croupy cough* may suggest a problem with the upper airway—the pharynx and larynx, or pertussis infection.

Sputum

Sputum should be inspected. Careful study of

the sputum is an essential part of the physical examination. The colour, volume and type (purulent, mucoid or mucopurulent), and the presence or absence of blood, should be recorded.

Stridor

Obstruction of the larynx or trachea (the extra-thoracic airways) may cause stridor, a rasping or croaking noise loudest on inspiration. This can be due to a foreign body, a tumour, infection (e.g. epiglottitis) or inflammation (Table 5.16). It is a sign that requires urgent attention.

Hoarseness

Listen to the voice for hoarseness (dysphonia), as this may indicate recurrent laryngeal nerve palsy associated with carcinoma of the lung (usually left-sided), or laryngeal carcinoma. However, the commonest cause is laryngitis and the use of inhaled corticosteroids for asthma. Non-respiratory causes include hypothyroidism.

The hands

As usual, examination in detail begins with the hands.

Clubbing

Look for clubbing, which is due to respiratory disease in up to 80% of cases (Figure 5.3, Table 4.9 on page 51). An uncommon but important association with clubbing is *hypertrophic pulmonary osteoarthropathy* (HPO). HPO is characterised by the presence of periosteal inflammation at the distal ends of long bones, the wrists, the ankles, the metacarpal and the metatarsal bones. There is swelling and tenderness over the wrists and other involved areas. Rarely HPO may occur without clubbing. The causes of HPO include primary lung carcinoma and pleural fibromas. Remember, chronic bronchitis and emphysema do not cause clubbing. It is important to note that clubbing does not occur as a result of COPD.

Staining

Look for staining of the fingers (actually caused by tar, as nicotine is colourless); a sign of cigarette smoking. The density of staining does not indicate the number of cigarettes smoked, but depends rather on the way the cigarette is held in the hand.

Wasting and weakness

Compression and infiltration by a peripheral lung tumour of a lower trunk of the T1 nerve root results in wasting of the small muscles of the hand and weakness of finger abduction.

TABLE 5.16 Some causes of stridor in adults
Sudden onset (minutes)
Anaphylaxis
Toxic gas inhalation
Acute epiglottitis
Inhaled foreign body
Gradual onset (days, weeks)
Laryngeal or pharyngeal tumours
Cricoarytenoid rheumatoid arthritis
Bilateral vocal cord palsy
Tracheal carcinoma
Paratracheal compression by lymph nodes
Post-tracheostomy or intubation granulomata

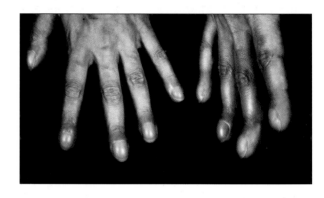

Figure 5.3 Finger clubbing

Pulse rate

Tachycardia and pulsus paradoxus are important signs of severe asthma. Tachycardia is a common side-effect of the treatment of asthma with β-agonist drugs, and accompanies dyspnoea or hypoxia of any cause.

Flapping tremor (asterixis)

Ask the patient to dorsiflex the wrists with the arms outstretched and to spread out the fingers. A flapping tremor with a 2- to 3-second cycle may occur with severe carbon dioxide retention, usually due to severe COPD.[4] The problem is an inability to maintain a posture. Asterixis[b] can also be demonstrated by asking the patient to protrude the tongue or lift the leg and keep the foot dorsiflexed. However, this is a late and unreliable sign and can also occur in patients with liver or renal failure. Patients with severe carbon dioxide retention may be confused, and typically have warm peripheries and a bounding pulse.

---

b   The word is derived from the Greek word *sterigma* which means *to support*, and refers to a flapping tremor.

The face

The *nose* is sited conveniently in the centre of the face. In this position it may readily be inspected inside and out. Get the patient to tilt the head back. It may be necessary to use a nasal speculum to open the nostrils, and a torch. Look for polyps (associated with asthma), engorged turbinates (various allergic conditions) and a deviated septum (nasal obstruction).

As already discussed, look at the *tongue* for central cyanosis. Look in the *mouth* for evidence of an upper respiratory tract infection (a reddened pharynx and tonsillar enlargement, with or without a coating of pus). A broken tooth or a rotten tooth stump may predispose to lung abscess or pneumonia. Patients with sleep apnoea may have 'crowding' of the pharynx. This means a reduction in the size of the *velopharyngeal lumen*, which is the space between the soft palate, tonsils and the back of the tongue. Those who use a sleep apnoea mask at night often have marks from the mask on the face and puffiness around the eyes. They tend to be obese and have a short thick neck and a small pharynx; sometimes the maxilla and mandible appear retracted (receding chin).

Sinusitis is suggested by tenderness over the *sinuses* on palpation. If acute sinusitis is suspected, a torch can be used to transilluminate the frontal and maxillary sinuses.[5] A torch is placed in the patient's mouth and the sinuses examined in a dark room. Normal transillumination generally excludes sinusitis. Complete opacification suggests sinusitis but partial opacification is less helpful. The torch should then be used to look for purulent discharge in the pharynx.

Look at the patient's *face* for the red, leathery, wrinkled skin of the smoker.[6] There may be facial plethora or cyanosis if superior vena caval obstruction is present. Look for the characteristics of obstructive sleep apnoea (see above).

Inspect the *eyes* for evidence of the rare Horner's[c] syndrome (a constricted pupil, partial ptosis and loss of sweating), which can be due to an apical lung carcinoma (Pancoast[d] tumour) compressing the sympathetic nerves in the neck. There may be skin changes on the face that suggest scleroderma or connective tissue disease.

The trachea

The position of the trachea is most important, and time should be spent establishing it accurately. From in front of the patient the forefinger of the right hand is pushed up and backwards from the suprasternal notch until the trachea is felt (Figure 5.4). If the trachea is displaced to one side, its edge

TABLE 5.17 Causes of tracheal displacement
1 Towards the side of the lung lesion
Upper lobe collapse
Upper lobe fibrosis
Pneumonectomy
2 Away from the side of the lung lesion (uncommon)
Massive pleural effusion
Tension pneumothorax
3 Upper mediastinal masses, such as retrosternal goitre

rather than its middle will be felt and a larger space will be present on one side than the other. Slight displacement to the right is fairly common in normal people. This examination is uncomfortable for the patient, so you must be gentle.

Significant displacement of the trachea suggests, but is not specific for, disease of the upper lobes of the lung (Table 5.17).

A tracheal tug is demonstrated when the finger resting on the trachea feels it move inferiorly with each inspiration. This is a sign of gross overexpansion of the chest because of airflow obstruction. This movement of the trachea may be visible, and it is worth spending time inspecting the trachea when COPD is suspected.

If the patient appears dyspnoeic and use of the accessory muscles of respiration is suspected, the examiner's fingers should be placed in the supraclavicular fossae. When the scalene muscles are recruited, they can be felt to contract under the fingers. Even more severe dyspnoea will result in use of the sternomastoid muscles. Their contraction is also easily felt with inspiration. Use of these muscles for long periods is exhausting and a sign of impending respiratory failure.

The chest

The chest should be examined anteriorly and posteriorly by inspection, palpation, percussion and auscultation.[3] Compare the right and left sides during each part of the examination.

Inspection

Shape and symmetry of chest. When the antero-posterior (AP) diameter is increased compared with the lateral diameter, the chest is described as barrel-shaped (Figure 5.5). An increase in the AP diameter compared with the lateral diameter (the

---

c Johann Horner (1831–1886), professor of ophthalmology in Zurich, described this syndrome in 1869.
d Henry Khunrath Pancoast (1875–1939), professor of roentgenology, University of Pennsylvania, described this in 1932.

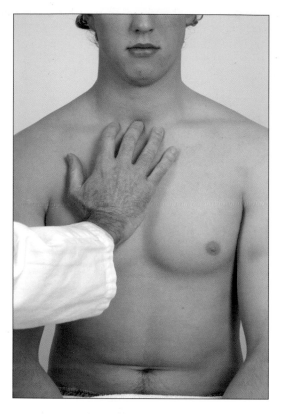

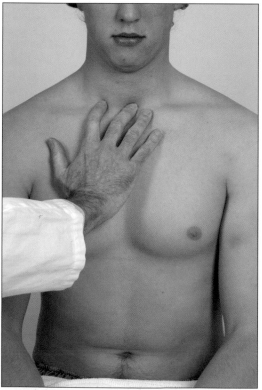

Figure 5.4 Feeling for the position of the trachea—a similar gap should be palpable on each side

thoracic ratio) beyond 0.9 is abnormal and is seen often in patients with severe asthma or emphysema. It is not always a reliable guide to the severity of the underlying lung disease and may be present in normal elderly people. Severe kyphoscoliosis is a cause of asymmetrical chest deformity.

A **pigeon chest (pectus carinatum)** is a localised prominence (an outward bowing of the sternum and costal cartilages)(Figure 5.6). It may be a manifestation of chronic childhood respiratory illness, in which case it is thought to result from repeated strong contractions of the diaphragm while the thorax is still pliable. It also occurs in rickets.

A **funnel chest (pectus excavatum)** is a developmental defect involving a localised depression of the lower end of the sternum (Figure 5.6). The problem is usually an aesthetic one, but in severe cases lung capacity may be restricted.

Harrison's sulcus[e] is a linear depression of the lower ribs just above the costal margins at the site of attachment of the diaphragm. It can result from severe asthma in childhood, or rickets.

Kyphosis refers to an exaggerated forward curvature of the spine, while scoliosis is lateral bowing. **Kyphoscoliosis** may be idiopathic (80%), secondary to poliomyelitis, or associated with Marfan's syndrome. Severe thoracic kyphoscoliosis may reduce the lung capacity and increase the work of breathing.

Lesions of the chest wall may be obvious. Look for *scars* from previous thoracic operations, or from chest drains for a previous pneumothorax or pleural effusion. Surgical removal of a lung (pneumonectomy) or of the lobe of a lung (lobectomy) leaves a long diagonal posterior scar on the thorax. The presence of three 2–3 cm scars suggests previous video-assisted thoracoscopic surgery, which can be performed to biopsy lymph nodes or carry out lung reduction surgery or pleurodesis. Thoracoplasty causes severe chest deformity; this operation was performed for tuberculosis and involved removal of a large number of ribs on one side of the chest to achieve permanent collapse of the affected lung. It is no longer performed because of the availability of effective antituberculous chemotherapy.[f] *Radiotherapy* may cause erythema and thickening of the skin over the irradiated area. There is sharp demarcation between abnormal and normal skin.

---

e   Edward Harrison (1766–1838), British general practitioner in Lincolnshire, described this deformity in rickets in 1798. The sign has also been ascribed to Edwin Harrison (1779–1847), a London physician.

f   It also probably didn't help!

There may be small tattoo marks indicating the limits of the irradiated area. Signs of radiotherapy usually indicate that the patient has been treated for carcinoma of the lung, breast or, less often, for lymphoma.

Subcutaneous emphysema is a crackling sensation felt on palpating the skin of the chest or neck. On inspection, there is often diffuse swelling of the chest wall and neck. It is caused by air tracking from the lungs and is usually due to a pneumothorax; less commonly it can follow rupture of the oesophagus or a pneumomediastinum (air in the mediastinal space).

Prominent veins may be seen in patients with superior vena caval obstruction. It is important to determine the direction of blood flow (page 166).

Movement of the chest wall should be noted. Look for asymmetry of chest wall movement anteriorly and posteriorly. Assessment of expansion of the upper lobes is best achieved by inspection from behind the patient, looking down at the clavicles during moderate respiration (Figure 5.7). Diminished movement indicates underlying lung disease. The affected side will show delayed or decreased movement. For assessment of lower lobe expansion, the chest should be inspected posteriorly.

Reduced chest wall movement on one side may be due to localised lung fibrosis, consolidation, collapse, pleural effusion or pneumothorax.

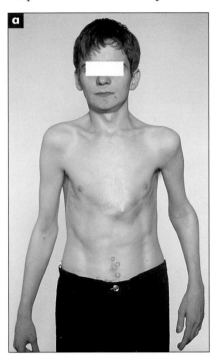

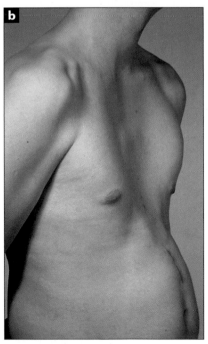

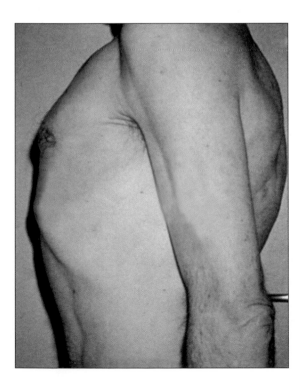

Figure 5.5 Barrel chest
(From McDonald FS, ed., *Mayo Clinic images in internal medicine*, with permission. © Mayo Clinic Scientific Press and CRC Press.)

Figure 5.6 (a) Pigeon chest (pectus carinatum); (b) Funnel chest (pectus excavatum)
(From Mir MA, *Atlas of Clinical Diagnosis*, 2nd edn. Edinburgh: Saunders, 2003, with permission.)

Bilateral reduction of chest wall movement indicates a diffuse abnormality such as COPD or diffuse interstitial lung disease. Unilateral reduced chest excursion or *splinting* may be present when patients have pleuritic chest pain or injuries such as rib fractures.

Look for paradoxical inward motion of the abdomen during inspiration when the patient is supine (indicating diaphragmatic paralysis).

Palpation

Chest expansion. Place the hands firmly on the chest wall with the fingers extending around the sides of the chest. The thumbs should almost meet in the middle line and should be lifted slightly off the chest so that they are free to move with respiration (Figure 5.8). As the patient takes a big breath in, the thumbs should move symmetrically apart at least 5 cm. Reduced expansion on one side indicates a lesion on that side. The causes have been discussed above.

If COPD is suspected, Hoover's sign[g] may be sought (Figure 5.9). The examiner places the hands along the costal margins with the thumbs close to the xiphisternum. Normally inspiration causes them to separate, but the overinflated chest of the COPD patient cannot expand in this way and the diaphragm pulls the ribs and the examiner's thumbs closer together[7] (positive LR 4.2).[8]

Lower lobe expansion is assessed from the back in this way. Some idea of upper and middle lobe expansion is possible when the manoeuvre is repeated on the front of the chest, but this is better gauged by inspection.

---

g Charles Hoover (1865–1927), professor of medicine in Cleveland from 1907. He also described Hoover's test for non-organic limb weakness.

Apex beat. When the patient is lying down, establishing the position of the apex beat may be helpful (page 60), as displacement towards the side of the lesion can be caused by collapse of the lower lobe or by localised interstitial lung disease (ILD). Movement of the apex beat away from the side of the lung lesion can be caused by pleural effusion or tension pneumothorax. The apex beat is often impalpable in a chest which is hyperexpanded secondary to chronic obstructive pulmonary disease.

Vocal (tactile) fremitus. Palpate the chest wall with the palm of the hand while the patient repeats 'ninety-nine'. The front and back of the chest are each palpated in two comparable positions, with the palm of one hand on each side of the chest. In this way differences in vibration on the chest wall can be detected. This can be a difficult sign to interpret, with considerable inter-observer variability, and it is no longer a routine part of the examination. It depends on the recognition of changes in vibration conducted to the examiner's hands while the patient speaks. Practice is needed to appreciate the difference between normal and abnormal. Vocal fremitus is more obvious in men because of their lower-pitched voices. It may be absent in normal people (high-pitched voice or thick chest wall). It is only abnormal if different on one side from the other. The causes of change in vocal fremitus are the same as those for vocal resonance (page 127).

Ribs. Gently compress the chest wall antero-posteriorly and laterally. Localised pain suggests a rib fracture, which may be secondary to trauma or may be spontaneous as a result of tumour deposition, bone disease or sometimes the result

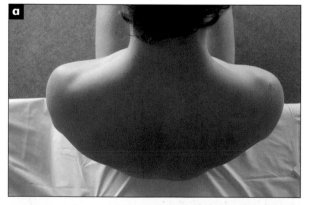
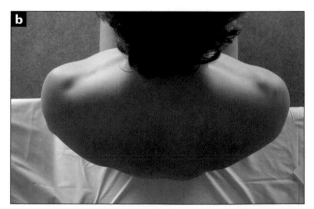

Figure 5.7 Inspecting upper lobe expansion: (a) expiration; (b) inspiration—note symmetrical elevation of the clavicles

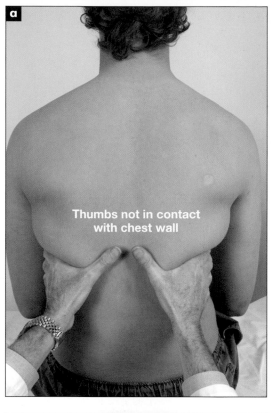

Thumbs not in contact
with chest wall

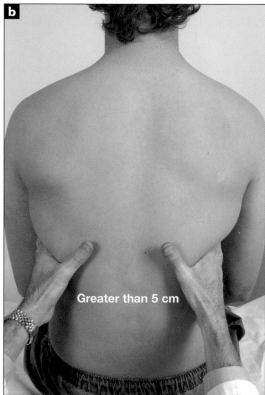

Greater than 5 cm

Figure 5.8 Palpation for lower lobe expansion:
(a) expiration; (b) inspiration

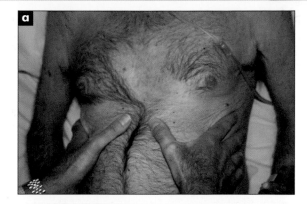

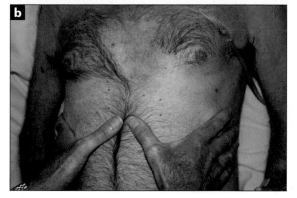

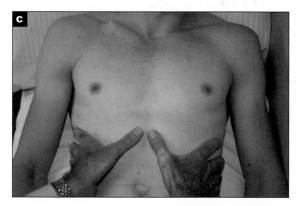

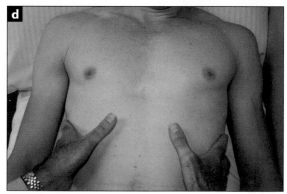

Figure 5.9 Hoover's sign
(a) Expiration; (b) inspiration. (c) Normal expiration;
(d) normal inspiration.

of severe and prolonged coughing. Tenderness over the costochondral junctions suggests the diagnosis of costochondritis as the cause of chest pain.

Regional lymph nodes. The axillary and cervical and supraclavicular nodes must be examined (pages 227, 228); they may be enlarged in lung malignancies and some infections.

Percussion

With the left hand on the chest wall and the fingers slightly separated and aligned with the ribs, the middle finger is pressed firmly against the chest. Then the pad of the right middle finger (the *plexor*) is used to strike firmly the middle phalanx of the middle finger of the left hand (the *pleximeter*); this was often a piece of wood, ivory or a coin in the 19th century but is now always the examiner's finger. The percussing finger (plexor) is quickly removed so that the note generated is not dampened (this may be less important if the pleximeter finger is held firmly on the chest wall, as it should be). The percussing finger must be held partly flexed and a loose swinging movement should come from the wrist and not from the forearm. Medical students will soon learn to keep the right middle fingernail short.

Percussion of symmetrical areas of the anterior, posterior and axillary regions is necessary (Figure 5.10). Percussion in the supraclavicular fossa over the apex of the lung and direct percussion of the clavicle with the percussing finger are a traditional part of the examination. For percussion posteriorly, the scapulae should be moved out of the way by asking the patient to move the elbows forward across the front of the chest; this rotates the scapulae anteriorly.

The feel of the percussion note is as important as its sound. The note is affected by the thickness of the chest wall, as well as by underlying structures. Percussion over a solid structure, such as the liver or a consolidated or collapsed area of lung, produces a dull note. Percussion over a fluid-filled area, such as a pleural effusion, produces an extremely dull (stony dull) note. Percussion over the normal lung produces a resonant note and percussion over hollow structures, such as the bowel or a pneumothorax, produces a hyperresonant note (*Good signs guide 5.1*).

Considerable practice is required before expert percussion can be performed, particularly in front of an audience. The ability to percuss well is usually obvious in clinical examinations and counts in a student's favour, as it indicates a reasonable amount of experience in the wards.

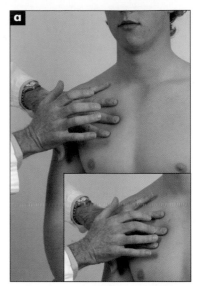

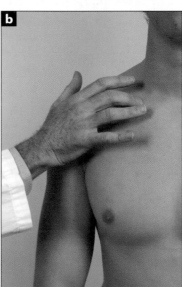

Figure 5.10 Percussion of the chest
(a) Percussing (plexor) finger poised. Inset: plexor finger strikes pleximeter finger. (b) Direct percussion of the clavicle for upper lobe resonance.

Liver dullness. The upper level of liver dullness is determined by percussing down the anterior chest in the midclavicular line. Normally, the upper level of the liver dullness is the fifth rib in the right midclavicular line. If the chest is resonant below this level, it is a sign of hyperinflation, usually due to emphysema or asthma. This is a sign with considerable inter-observer variability.

Cardiac dullness. The area of cardiac dullness usually present on the left side of the chest may be decreased in emphysema or asthma.

GOOD SIGNS GUIDE 5.1 Comparative percussion of the chest

Sign	Positive LR	Negative LR
Dullness—pneumonia	3.0	NS
Hyperresonance—COPD	5.1	NS

NS = not significant.
COPD = chronic obstructive pulmonary disease.
From McGee S, *Evidence-based physical diagnosis*, 2nd edn. St Louis: Saunders, 2007.

TABLE 5.18 Causes of bronchial breath sounds

Common
Lung consolidation (lobar pneumonia)

Uncommon
Localised pulmonary fibrosis
Pleural effusion (above the fluid)
Collapsed lung (e.g. adjacent to a pleural effusion)

Note: The large airways must be patent.

Auscultation

Breath sounds. Using the diaphragm of the stethoscope, one should listen to the breath sounds in the areas shown in Figure 5.11.[9–11] It is important to compare each side with the other. Remember to listen high up into the axillae and, using the bell of the stethoscope applied above the clavicles, to listen to the lung apices. A number of observations must be made while auscultating and, as with auscultation of the heart, different parts of the cycle must be considered. Listen for the quality of the breath sounds, the intensity of the breath sounds, and the presence of additional (adventitious) sounds.

Quality of breath sounds. *Normal breath sounds* are heard with the stethoscope over nearly all parts of the chest. The patient should be asked to breathe through the mouth so that added sounds from the nasopharynx do not interfere. These sounds are produced in the airways rather than the alveoli. They had once been thought to arise in the alveoli (vesicles) of the lungs and are therefore called vesicular sounds. They have rather fancifully been compared by Laënnec to the sound of wind rustling in leaves. Their intensity is related to total airflow at the mouth and to regional airflow. Normal (vesicular) breath sounds are louder and longer on inspiration than on expiration and there is no gap between the inspiratory and expiratory sounds. They are due to the transmission of air turbulence in the large airways filtered through the normal lung to the chest wall.

Bronchial breath sounds are present when turbulence in the large airways is heard without being filtered by the alveoli, producing a different quality. Bronchial breath sounds have a hollow, blowing quality. They are audible throughout expiration and there is often a gap between inspiration and expiration. The expiratory sound has a higher intensity and pitch than the inspiratory sound. Bronchial breath sounds are more easily remembered than described. They are audible in normal people, posteriorly over the right upper chest where the trachea is contiguous with the right upper bronchus. They are heard over areas of consolidation, as solid lung conducts the sound of turbulence in main airways to peripheral areas without filtering. Causes of bronchial breath sounds are shown in Table 5.18.

Occasionally breath sounds over a large cavity have an exaggerated bronchial quality. This very hollow or *amphoric* sound has been likened to that

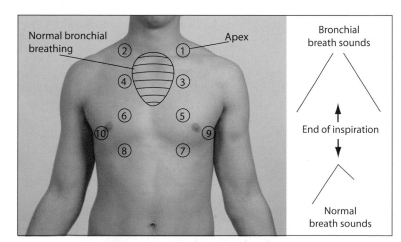

Figure 5.11 Normal and bronchial breath sounds
Auscultate in each area shown (the numbers represent a suggested order). Distinguish normal breath sounds from bronchial breathing.

heard when air passes over the top of a hollow jar (Greek *amphoreus*).

Intensity of the breath sounds. It is better to describe breath sounds as being of normal or reduced intensity than to speak about air entry. The entry of air into parts of the lung cannot be directly gauged from the breath sounds. Asymmetrical reduction of breath sounds is a sign of bronchial obstruction, for example by carcinoma or a foreign body on the side where breath sounds are reduced.

Causes of reduced breath sounds include COPD (especially emphysema), pleural effusion, pneumothorax, pneumonia, a large neoplasm and pulmonary collapse.

Added (adventitious) sounds. There are two types of added sounds—continuous (wheezes) and interrupted (crackles).

Continuous sounds are called *wheezes*. They are abnormal findings and have a musical quality. The wheezes must be timed in relation to the respiratory cycle. They may be heard in expiration or inspiration, or both. Wheezes are due to continuous oscillation of opposing airway walls and imply significant airway narrowing. Wheezes tend to be louder on expiration. This is because the airways normally dilate during inspiration and are narrower during expiration. An inspiratory wheeze implies severe airway narrowing.

The pitch (frequency) of wheezes varies. It is determined only by the velocity of the air jet and is not related to the length of the airway. High-pitched wheezes are produced in the smaller bronchi and have a whistling quality, whereas low-pitched wheezes (sometimes called rhonchi) arise from the larger bronchi.

Wheezes are usually the result of acute or chronic airflow obstruction due to asthma (often high-pitched) or COPD (often low-pitched), secondary to a combination of bronchial muscle spasm, mucosal oedema and excessive secretions. Wheezes are a poor guide to the severity of airflow obstruction. In severe airways obstruction, wheeze can be absent because ventilation is so reduced that the velocity of the air jet is reduced below a critical level necessary to produce the sound.

A fixed bronchial obstruction, usually due to a carcinoma of the lung, tends to cause a localised wheeze, which has a single musical note (monophonic) and does not clear with coughing.

Wheezes must be distinguished from *stridor* (page 118), which sounds very similar to wheeze but is louder over the trachea and is always inspiratory (wheezes usually occur in expiration—the majority—but can occur in both inspiration and expiration).

Interrupted non-musical sounds are best called *crackles*.[12,13] There is a lot of confusion about the naming of these sounds, perhaps as a result of mistranslations of Laënnec. Some authors describe low-pitched crackles as rales and high-pitched ones as crepitations, but others do not make this distinction. The simplest approach is to call all these sounds crackles, but also to describe their timing and pitch. Crackles are sometimes present in normal people but these crackles will always clear with coughing.

Crackles are probably the result of loss of stability of peripheral airways that collapse on expiration. With high inspiratory pressures, there is rapid air entry into the distal airways. This causes the abrupt opening of alveoli and of small- or medium-sized bronchi containing secretions in regions of the lung deflated to residual volume. More compliant (distensible) areas open up first, followed by the increasingly stiff areas. Fine- and medium-pitched crackles are not caused by air moving through secretions as was once thought, but by the opening and closing of small airways.

The timing of crackles is of great importance. *Early inspiratory crackles* (cease before the middle of inspiration) suggest disease of the small airways, and are characteristic of COPD.[12] The crackles are heard only in early inspiration and are of medium coarseness. They are different from those heard in left ventricular failure, which occur later in the respiratory cycle.

Late or *pan-inspiratory crackles* suggest disease confined to the alveoli. They may be fine, medium or coarse in quality. *Fine crackles* have been likened to the sound of hair rubbed between the fingers, or to the sound Velcro makes when pulled apart—they are typically caused by interstitial lung disease (pulmonary fibrosis). Characteristically, more crackles are heard in each inspiration when they are due to fibrosis—up to 14 compared with 1 to 4 for COPD and 4 to 9 for cardiac failure. As ILD becomes more severe the crackles extend earlier into inspiration and are heard further up the chest.[h] *Medium crackles* are usually due to left ventricular failure. Here the presence of alveolar fluid disrupts the function of the normally secreted surfactant. *Coarse crackles* are characteristic of pools of retained secretions and have an unpleasant gurgling quality. They tend to change with coughing, which also has an unpleasant gurgling quality. Bronchiectasis is a common cause, but any disease that leads to

---

h   Expiratory crackles may also occur with lung fibrosis.[13]

GOOD SIGNS GUIDE 5.2 Crackles and wheezes

Sign	Positive LR	Negative LR
Crackles		
Pulmonary fibrosis in asbestos workers	5.9	0.2
Pneumonia patients with cough and fever	2.0	0.8
Early inspiratory crackles		
Detecting COPD	14.6	NS
Severe COPD	20.8	0.1
Unforced (audible during breathing at rest) **wheezing**		
Detecting COPD	6.0	NS

NS = not significant. COPD = chronic obstructive pulmonary disease.
From McGee S, *Evidence-based physical diagnosis*, 2nd edn. St Louis: Saunders, 2007.

retention of secretions may produce these features. (See *Good signs guide 5.2*.)

Pleural friction rub: when thickened, roughened pleural surfaces rub together as the lungs expand and contract, a continuous or intermittent grating sound may be audible. A pleural rub indicates pleurisy, which may be secondary to pulmonary infarction or pneumonia. Rarely, malignant involvement of the pleura, a spontaneous pneumothorax or pleurodynia may cause a rub.

Vocal resonance. Auscultation over the chest while a patient speaks gives further information about the lungs' ability to transmit sounds. Over normal lung, the low-pitched components of speech are heard with a booming quality and high-pitched components are attenuated. Consolidated lung, however, tends to transmit high frequencies so that speech heard through the stethoscope takes on a bleating quality (called *aegophony* by Laënnec[14]—from Greek *aix* 'goat', *phone* 'voice'). When a patient with aegophony says 'e' as in 'bee' it sounds like 'a' as in 'bay'.

Increased vocal resonance is a helpful sign in confirming consolidation but may not be necessary as a routine. Ask the patient to say 'ninety-nine' while you listen over each part of the chest. Over consolidated lung the numbers will become clearly audible, while over normal lung the sound is muffled. If vocal resonance is present, bronchial breathing is likely to be heard (Table 5.18). Sometimes vocal resonance is increased to such an extent that whispered speech is distinctly heard; this is called whispering pectoriloquy.

If a very localised abnormality is found at auscultation, try to determine the lobe and approximately which segment or segments are involved (Figure 5.1, page 116).

The heart
Cardiac examination is an essential part of the respiratory assessment and vice versa. These two systems are intimately related.

Lay the patient down at 45 degrees and measure the jugular venous pressure for evidence of right heart failure (page 58). Next examine the praecordium. It is important to pay close attention to the pulmonary component of the second heart sound (P2). This is best heard at the second intercostal space on the left. It should not be louder than the aortic component, best heard at the right second inter-costal space. If the P2 is louder (and especially if it is palpable), pulmonary hypertension should be strongly suspected. There may be signs of right ventricular failure or hypertension. Pulmonary hypertensive heart disease (cor pulmonale) may be due to COPD, ILD, pulmonary thromboembolism, marked obesity, sleep apnoea or severe kyphoscoliosis.

The abdomen
Palpate the liver for ptosis,[i] due to emphysema, or for enlargement from secondary deposits of tumour in cases of lung carcinoma.

Other
Pemberton's[j] sign
Ask the patient to lift the arms over the head and wait for one minute.[15] Note the development of facial plethora, cyanosis, inspiratory stridor and non-pulsatile elevation of the jugular venous pressure. This occurs in superior vena caval obstruction.

---

i From the Greek word for falling, this was once mostly applied to the eyelid but now seems accepted as a description of the displacement of any organ.
j Hugh Pemberton (1891–1956), physician, Liverpool, UK.

Legs

Inspect for swelling (oedema) or cyanosis, which may be clues to cor pulmonale, and look for evidence of deep venous thrombosis.

Respiratory rate on exercise

Patients complaining of dyspnoea should have their respiratory rate measured at rest, at maximal tolerated exertion (e.g. after climbing one or two flights of stairs or during a treadmill exercise test), and supine. If dyspnoea is not accompanied by tachypnoea when a patient climbs stairs, one should consider the possibility of anxiety or malingering

Temperature

Fever may occur with any acute or chronic chest infection.

Bedside assessment of lung function

Forced expiratory time

Physical examination can be complemented with an estimate of the forced expiratory time (FET).[16] Measure the time taken by a patient to exhale forcefully and completely through the open mouth after taking a maximum inspiration. The normal forced expiratory time is 3 seconds or less. Note any audible wheeze or cough. An increased FET indicates airways obstruction. The combination of a significant smoking history and an FET of 9 seconds or more is predictive of COPD (positive LR 9.6).[8] A peak flow meter or spirometer, however, will provide a more accurate measurement of lung function.

Peak flow meter

A peak flow meter is a simple gauge that is used to measure the maximum flow rate of expired air. Again the patient is asked to take a full breath in, but rather than a prolonged expiration, a rapid forced maximal expiratory puff is made through the mouth. The value obtained (the peak expiratory flow, PEF) depends largely on airways diameter. Normal values for young men are approximately 600 litres a minute and for women 400 litres a minute. The value depends on age, sex and height, so tables of normal values should be consulted. Airways obstruction, such as that caused by asthma or COPD, results in a reduced and variable PEF. It is a simple way of assessing and following patients with airways obstruction, but is rather effort-dependent. The PEF is most useful when used for serial estimates of lung function.

Spirometry (Figure 5.12)

The spirometer records graphically or numerically the forced expiratory volume and the forced vital capacity. The *forced expiratory volume* (FEV) is the volume of air expelled from the lungs after maximum inspiration using maximum forced effort, and is measured in a given time. Usually this is 1 second (FEV_1). The *forced vital capacity* (FVC) is the total volume of air expelled from the lungs after maximum inspiratory effort followed by maximum forced expiration. The FVC is often nearly the same as the vital capacity, but in airways obstruction it may be less because of premature airways closure. It is usual to record the best of three attempts and calculate the FEV_1/FVC ratio as a percentage. In healthy youth, the normal value is 80%, but this may decline to as little as 60% in old age. Normal values also vary with sex, age, height and race.

Reversibility of a reduced FEV_1/FVC after the use of bronchodilators is an important test for distinguishing asthma from COPD.

Obstructive ventilatory defect. When the FEV_1/FVC ratio is reduced (<0.7) this is referred to as an obstructive defect. Both values tend to be reduced, but the FEV_1 is disproportionately low. The causes are loss of elastic recoil or airways narrowing, as in asthma or COPD.

Restrictive ventilatory defect. When the FEV_1/FVC ratio is normal or higher than normal, but both values are reduced, the pattern is described as a restrictive defect. This occurs in parenchymal lung disease, such as ILD, sarcoidosis, or when lung expansion is reduced by pneumonia or chest wall abnormalities.

Flow volume curve

As a part of spirometric assessment, the flow volume curve may be measured using a portable electronic device. This measures expiratory and inspiratory flow as a function of exhaled volume rather than against time. It is a simple and reproducible test easily performed in the respiratory laboratory or at the bedside. The FVC, FEV_1 and various flow measurements (e.g. peak flow) can be calculated from the curve (Figure 5.13).

Correlation of physical signs and respiratory disease (Table 5.19)

Consolidation (lobar pneumonia)

Pneumonia is defined as inflammation of the lung which is characterised by exudation into the alveoli. X-ray changes of new shadowing in one or more lung segments (lobes) are present. Pneumonia is

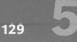

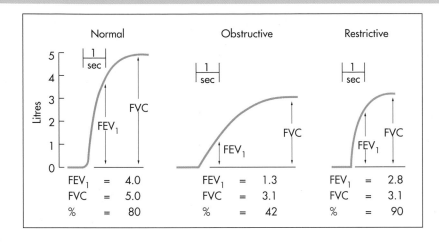

Figure 5.12 Spirometry tracings

now classified as:

1 community-acquired (CAP)
2 hospital-acquired
3 occurring in a damaged lung, e.g. as a result of aspiration; or
4 occurring in an immuno-compromised host.

This classification allows prediction of the likely pathogens and assists in the choice of antibiotics for treatment. The signs of lobar pneumonia are characteristic and are referred to clinically as *consolidation*.[17]

There may be a history of the sudden onset of malaise, chest pain, dyspnoea and fever. Patients may appear very ill and the vital signs, including the temperature, respiratory rate and blood pressure, must be recorded. There may be signs of cyanosis and exhaustion in sick patients. The term *bronchopneumonia* refers to lung infection characterised by more patchy X-ray changes which often affect both lower lobes. The clinical signs of consolidation may be absent.

Symptoms

- Cough (painful and dry at first).
- Fever and rigors (shivers).
- Pleuritic chest pain.
- Dyspnoea.
- Tachycardia.
- Confusion.

Signs

- **Expansion:** reduced on the affected side.
- **Vocal fremitus:** increased on the affected side (in other chest disease this sign is of very little use!).
- **Percussion:** dull, but not stony dull.
- **Breath sounds:** bronchial.
- **Additional sounds:** medium, late or pan-inspiratory crackles as the pneumonia resolves.

- **Vocal resonance:** increased.
- **Pleural rub:** may be present.

See also *Good signs guide 5.3*.

Causes of community-acquired pneumonia

- *Streptococcus pneumoniae* (>30%).
- *Chlamydia pneumoniae* (10%).
- *Mycoplasma pneumoniae* (10%).
- *Legionella pneumoniae* (5%).

Atelectasis (Collapse)

If a bronchus is obstructed by a tumour mass, retained secretions or a prolonged presence of a foreign body, the air in the part of the lung supplied by the bronchus is absorbed and the affected part of the lung collapses.

Signs

- **Trachea:** displaced towards the collapsed side.
- **Expansion:** reduced on the affected side with flattening of the chest wall on the same side.
- **Percussion:** dull over the collapsed area.
- **Breath sounds:** reduced, often without bronchial breathing above the area of atelectasis when a tumour is the cause, because the airways are not patent.

Note: (i) There may be no signs with complete lobar collapse. (ii) The early changes after the inhalation of a foreign body may be over-inflation of the affected side.

Causes

- **Intraluminal:** mucus (e.g. postoperative, asthma, cystic fibrosis), foreign body, aspiration.
- **Mural:** bronchial carcinoma.
- **Extramural:** peribronchial lymphadenopathy, aortic aneurysm.

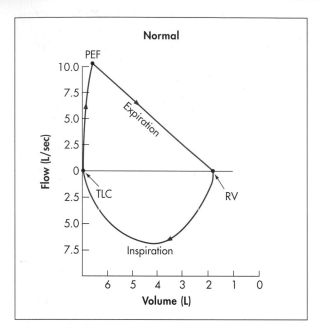

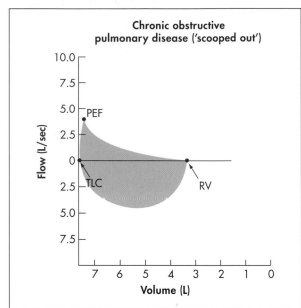

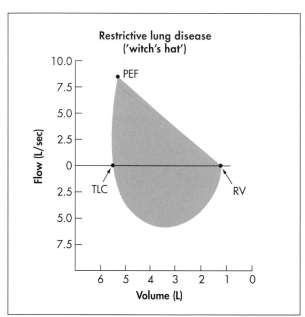

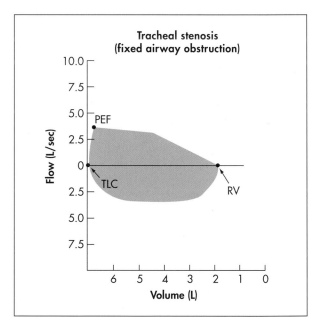

Figure 5.13 Flow volume curves
Look at the shape of the loop in each case. A normal flow volume curve is convex and symmetrical. In chronic obstructive lung disease (COPD), all flow routes are reduced and there is prolonged expiration (creating a 'scooped out' shape). In restrictive lung disease (e.g. pulmonary fibrosis), the loop is narrow but the shape normal (like a 'witch's hat'). In fixed airway obstruction (e.g. tracheal stenosis), the loops look flattened as both expiration and inspiration are limited.
PEF = peak expiratory flow
TLC = total lung capacity
RV = residual volume

Pleural effusion

This is a collection of fluid in the pleural space. Note that pleural collections consisting of blood (haemothorax), chyle (chylothorax) or pus (empyema) have specific names, and are not called pleural effusions although the physical signs are similar.

TABLE 5.19 Comparison of the chest signs in common respiratory disorders

Disorder	Mediastinal displacement	Chest wall movement	Percussion note	Breath sounds	Added sounds
Consolidation	None	Reduced over affected area	Dull	Bronchial	Crackles
Collapse	Ipsilateral shift	Decreased over affected area	Dull	Absent or reduced	Absent
Pleural effusion	Heart displaced to opposite side (trachea displaced only if massive)	Reduced over affected area	Stony dull	Absent over fluid; may be bronchial at upper border	Absent; pleural rub may be found above effusion
Pneumothorax	Tracheal deviation to opposite side if under tension	Decreased over affected area	Resonant	Absent or greatly reduced	Absent
Bronchial asthma	None	Decreased symmetrically	Normal or decreased	Normal or reduced	Wheeze
Interstitial pulmonary fibrosis	None	Decreased symmetrically (minimal)	Normal unaffected by cough or posture	Normal	Fine, late or pan-inspiratory crackles over affected lobes

Signs

- **Trachea and apex beat:** displaced away from a massive effusion.
- **Expansion:** reduced on the affected side.
- **Percussion:** stony dullness over the fluid.
- **Breath sounds:** reduced or absent. There may be an area of bronchial breathing audible above the effusion due to compression of overlying lung.
- **Vocal resonance:** reduced.

Causes

- **Transudate** (Light's criteria): (i) cardiac failure; (ii) hypoalbuminaemia from the nephrotic syndrome or chronic liver disease; (iii) hypothyroidism; (iv) Meigs syndrome[k] (ovarian fibroma causing pleural effusion and ascites).
- **Exudate** (Light's criteria[l]): (i) pneumonia; (ii) neoplasm—bronchial carcinoma, metastatic carcinoma, mesothelioma; (iii) tuberculosis; (iv) pulmonary infarction; (v) subphrenic abscess; (vi) acute pancreatitis; (vii) connective tissue disease such as rheumatoid arthritis, systemic lupus erythematosus; (viii) drugs such

GOOD SIGNS GUIDE 5.3 Pneumonia

Sign	Positive LR	Negative LR
General appearance		
Cachexia	4.0	NS
Abnormal mental state	2.2	NS
Vital signs		
Temperature >37.8°C	2.2	0.7
Respiratory rate >28/minute	2.2	0.8
Heart rate >100 beats/minute	1.6	0.7
Lung findings		
Percussion dullness	3.0	NS
Reduced breath sounds	2.3	0.8
Bronchial breath sounds	3.3	NS
Aegophony	4.1	NS
Crackles	2.0	0.8
Wheezes	NS	NS

NS = not significant.
From McGee S, *Evidence-based physical diagnosis*, 2nd edn. St Louis: Saunders, 2007.

---

k   Joe Vincent Meigs (1892–1963), Professor of Gynaecology at Harvard, described this in 1937.

l   The formal definition of an exudate is that the fluid has at least one of the following (Light's) criteria; 1. fluid protein/serum protein >0.5, 2. pleural fluid LDH/serum LDH >0.6, 3. pleural fluid LDH >2/3 normal upper limit of LDH in serum. The fluid is otherwise a transudate.

as methysergide, cytotoxics; (ix) irradiation; (x) trauma.

- **Haemothorax** (blood in the pleural space): (i) severe trauma to the chest; (ii) rupture of a pleural adhesion containing a blood vessel.
- **Chylothorax** (milky-appearing pleural fluid due to leakage of lymph): (i) trauma or surgery to the thoracic duct; (ii) carcinoma or lymphoma involving the thoracic duct.
- **Empyema** (pus in the pleural space): (i) pneumonia; (ii) lung abscess; (iii) bronchiectasis; (iv) tuberculosis; (v) penetrating chest wound.

Yellow nail syndrome

This is a rare condition which is caused by hypoplasia of the lymphatic system. The nails are thickened and yellow (Figure 5.14) and there is separation of the distal nail plate from the nail bed (onycholysis). It may be associated with a pleural effusion and bronchiectasis, and usually with lymphoedema of the legs.

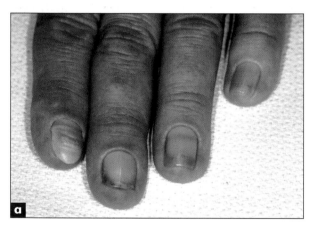

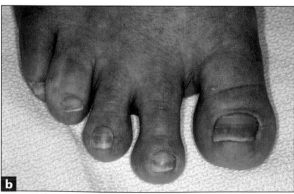

Figure 5.14 Yellow nail syndrome: (a) hands; (b) feet
(From McDonald FS, ed., *Mayo Clinic images in internal medicine*, with permission. © Mayo Clinic Scientific Press and CRC Press.)

Pneumothorax

Leakage of air from the lung or a chest wall puncture into the pleural space causes a pneumothorax.

Signs

- **Expansion:** reduced on the affected side.
- **Percussion:** hyperresonance if the pneumothorax is large.
- **Breath sounds:** greatly reduced or absent.
- There may be subcutaneous emphysema.
- There may be no signs if the pneumothorax is small (less than 30%).

Causes

Primary

- 'Spontaneous': subpleural bullae rupture, usually in tall, healthy young males.

Secondary

- Traumatic: rib fracture, penetrating chest wall injury, or during pleural or pericardial aspiration.
- Iatrogenic (caused by medical intervention): following the insertion of a central venous catheter.
- Emphysema with rupture of bullae, usually in middle-aged or elderly patients with generalised emphysema.
- Rarer causes include asthma, lung abscess, bronchial carcinoma, eosinophilic granuloma lymphangioleiomyomatosis (LAM—premenopausal women), end-stage fibrosis or Marfan's syndrome.

Tension pneumothorax

This occurs when there is a communication between the lung and the pleural space, with a flap of tissue acting as a valve, allowing air to enter the pleural space during inspiration and preventing it from leaving during expiration. A tension pneumothorax results from air accumulating under increasing pressure in the pleural space; it causes considerable displacement of the mediastinum with obstruction and kinking of the great vessels, and represents a medical emergency.

Signs

- The patient is often tachypnoeic and cyanosed, and may be hypotensive.
- **Trachea and apex beat:** displaced away from the affected side.
- **Expansion:** reduced or absent on affected side.
- **Percussion:** hyperresonant over the affected side.
- **Breath sounds:** absent.
- **Vocal resonance:** absent.

Causes
- Trauma.
- Mechanical ventilation at high pressure.
- Spontaneous (rare cause of tension pneumothorax).

Bronchiectasis
This is a pathological dilatation of the bronchi, resulting in impaired clearance of mucus, and chronic infection. A history of chronic cough and purulent sputum since childhood is virtually diagnostic.

Signs
Most likely during an exacerbation of the condition.
- **Systemic signs:** fever, cachexia; sinusitis (70%).
- Clubbing and cyanosis (if disease is severe).
- **Sputum:** voluminous, purulent, foul-smelling, sometimes bloodstained.
- Coarse pan-inspiratory or late inspiratory crackles over the affected lobe.
- **Signs of severe bronchiectasis:** very copious sputum and haemoptysis, clubbing, widespread crackles, signs of airways obstruction, signs of respiratory failure and cor pulmonale, signs of secondary amyloidosis (e.g. oedema from proteinuria, cardiac failure, enlarged liver and spleen, carpal tunnel syndrome).

Causes
- **Congenital:** (i) primary ciliary dyskinesia (including the immotile cilia syndrome); (ii) cystic fibrosis; (iii) congenital hypogammaglobulinaemia.
- **Acquired:** (i) infections in childhood, such as whooping cough, pneumonia or measles; (ii) localised disease such as a foreign body, a bronchial adenoma or tuberculosis; (iii) allergic bronchopulmonary aspergillosis—this causes proximal bronchiectasis.

Bronchial asthma
This may be defined as paroxysmal recurrent attacks of wheezing (or in childhood of cough) due to airways narrowing which changes in severity over short periods of time.

Signs
- Wheezing.
- Dry or productive cough.
- Tachypnoea.
- Tachycardia.
- Prolonged expiration.
- Prolonged forced expiratory time (decreased peak flow, decreased FEV_1).
- Use of accessory muscles of respiration.
- Hyperinflated chest (increased anteroposterior diameter with high shoulders and, on percussion, decreased liver dullness).
- Inspiratory and expiratory wheezes.
- **Signs of severe asthma:** appearance of exhaustion and fear, inability to speak because of breathlessness, drowsiness due to hypercapnia (preterminal), cyanosis (a very sinister sign), tachycardia (pulse above 130/minute correlates with significant hypoxaemia), pulsus paradoxus (more than 20 mmHg), reduced breath sounds or a 'silent' chest.

Chronic obstructive pulmonary disease (COPD, chronic airflow limitation)
This represents a spectrum of abnormalities: from predominantly emphysema, where there is pathologically an increase beyond normal in the size of the air spaces distal to the terminal bronchioles, to chronic bronchitis, where there is mucous gland hypertrophy, increased numbers of goblet cells and hypersecretion of mucus in the bronchial tree resulting in a chronic cough and sputum. Chronic obstructive pulmonary disease limitation does not cause clubbing or haemoptysis. Fifty per cent of patients with chronic bronchitis have emphysema, so there is often considerable overlapping of signs.[18]

The diagnosis can often be made on the basis of three findings:
1 A history of heavy smoking (more than 70 packet-years).
2 Reduced breath sounds.
3 Previous diagnosis of emphysema or COPD.
If two or three of these are present, the positive LR of COPD is 25.7.

Signs
The patients are usually not cyanosed but are dyspnoeic, and used to be called 'pink puffers'. The signs result from hyperinflation.
- Barrel-shaped chest with increased anteroposterior diameter.
- Pursed-lip breathing (this occurs in emphysema and not in chronic bronchitis): expiration through partly closed lips increases the end-expiratory pressure and keeps airways open, helping to minimise air trapping.
- Use of accessory muscles of respiration and drawing in of the lower intercostal muscles with inspiration.
- **Palpation:** reduced expansion and a hyperinflated chest, Hoover's sign, tracheal tug.

GOOD SIGNS GUIDE 5.4 Chronic obstructive pulmonary disease

Sign	Positive LR	Negative LR
Hoover's sign	4.2	0.5
Absent cardiac dullness, left sternal border	11.8	NS
Early inspiratory crackles	14.6	NS
Unforced wheeze	2.8	0.8
Greatly reduced breath sounds	10.2	—
Forced expiratory time:		
<3s	0.2	—
3–9s	NS	—
>9s	4.1	—

From McGee, S, *Evidence-based physical diagnosis*, 2nd edn. St Louis: Saunders, 2007.

- **Percussion:** hyperresonant with decreased liver dullness.
- **Breath sounds:** decreased, early inspiratory crackles.
- Wheeze is often absent.
- Signs of right heart failure may occur, but only late in the course of the disease.

Causes of generalised emphysema

- Usually, smoking.
- Occasionally, alpha$_1$-antitrypsin deficiency.

Chronic bronchitis

This is defined clinically as the daily production of sputum for three months a year for at least two consecutive years. It is not now diagnosed as a separate entity from COPD and is probably now of mostly historical interest.

Signs

The signs are the result of bronchial hypersecretion and airways obstruction.

- Loose cough and sputum (mucoid or mucopurulent), particularly in the morning shortly after wakening, and lessening as the day progresses.
- **Cyanosis:** these patients were sometimes called 'blue bloaters' because of cyanosis present in the latter stages, and because of associated oedema from right ventricular failure.
- **Palpation:** hyperinflated chest with reduced expansion.
- **Percussion:** increased resonance.
- **Breath sounds:** reduced with end-expiratory

high or low-pitched wheezes and early inspiratory crackles.
- Signs of right ventricular failure.

Causes

Smoking is the major cause, but recurrent bronchial infection may cause progression of the disease.

Interstitial lung disease (ILD)

Diffuse fibrosis of the lung parenchyma impairs gas transfer and causes ventilation–perfusion mismatching. This fibrosis may be the result of inflammation (alveolitis and interstitial inflammation) or granulomatous disease (Table 5.20). It has often no known cause (idiopathic interstitial fibrosis) or is secondary to a disease of unknown aetiology (e.g. sarcoidosis, connective tissue disease). It can result from inhalation of mineral dusts (focal fibrosis), replacement of lung tissue following disease which damages the lungs (e.g. aspiration pneumonia, tuberculosis). Collagen diseases and vasculitis are important causes.

Remember the three Cs:
Cough (dry)
Clubbing
Crackles.

Signs

- **General:** dyspnoea, cyanosis and clubbing may be present.
- **Palpation:** expansion is slightly reduced.
- **Auscultation:** fine (Velcro-like) late inspiratory or pan-inspiratory crackles heard over the affected lobes.
- **Signs of associated connective tissue disease:** rheumatoid arthritis, systemic lupus erythematosus, scleroderma, Sjögren's[m] syndrome, polymyositis and dermatomyositis.

Causes

- **Upper lobe predominant:** SCART. S = silicosis (progressive massive fibrosis), sarcoidosis; C = coal workers' pneumoconiosis (progressive massive fibrosis); A = ankylosing spondylitis, allergic bronchopulmonary aspergillosis; R = radiation; T = tuberculosis. Also cystic fibrosis, alveolar haemorrhage syndromes, chronic allergic alveolitis, chronic eosinophilic pneumonitis.
- **Lower lobe predominant:** RASIO. R =

---

m   Henrik Samuel Conrad Sjögren (1899–1986), Stockholm ophthalmologist. He described the syndrome in 1933.

TABLE 5.20 Interstitial lung disease

Secondary to alveolitis (previously called fibrosing alveolitis)

Unknown cause
- Idiopathic pulmonary fibrosis
- Connective tissue disease (e.g. SLE, rheumatoid arthritis, ankylosing spondylitis, systemic sclerosis)
- Pulmonary haemorrhage syndromes (e.g. Goodpasture's syndrome)
- Graft versus host disease
- Gastrointestinal or liver diseases (Crohn's disease, primary biliary cirrhosis, chronic active hepatitis)

Known cause
- Asbestosis
- Radiation injury
- Aspiration pneumonia
- Drugs (e.g. amiodarone)
- Exposure to gases or fumes

Secondary to granulomatous disease

Unknown cause
- Sarcoidosis
- Wegener's disease, Churg-Strauss disease

Known cause
- Hypersensitivity pneumonitis to organic or inorganic dusts (silica, beryllium)

SLE = systemic lupus erythematosus.

rheumatoid arthritis; A = asbestosis; S = scleroderma (systemic sclerosis); I = idiopathic interstitial fibrosis ; O = other (drugs, e.g. busulfan, bleomycin, nitrofurantoin, hydralazine, methotrexate, amiodarone). Also other collagen vascular diseases, acute allergic alveolitis, acute eosinophilic pneumonitis.

Tuberculosis

Primary tuberculosis

A Ghon[n] focus with hilar lymphadenopathy occurs usually in children.

Usually no abnormal chest signs are found, but segmental collapse, due to bronchial obstruction by the hilar lymph nodes, occasionally occurs. Erythema nodosum (page 191) is an important associated sign, but is rare.

Post-primary tuberculosis

Reactivation of a primary lesion or occasionally reinfection are the causes of post-primary or adult tuberculosis. Immune suppression and malnutrition predispose to reactivation of tuberculosis.

There are often no chest signs. The clues to the diagnosis are the classical symptoms of cough, haemoptysis, weight loss, night sweats and malaise.

Miliary tuberculosis

Widespread haematogenous dissemination of tubercle bacilli causes multiple millet-seed tuberculous nodules in various organs—spleen, liver, lymph nodes, kidneys, brain or joints. Miliary tuberculosis may complicate both childhood and adult tuberculosis.

Fever, anaemia and cachexia are the general signs. The patient may also be dyspnoeic, and pleural effusions, lymphadenopathy, hepatosplenomegaly or signs of meningitis may be present.

Mediastinal compression

Mediastinal structures may be compressed by a variety of pathological masses, including carcinoma of the lung (90%), other tumours (lymphoma, thymoma, dermoid cyst), a large retrosternal goitre or rarely an aortic aneurysm.

Signs

- **Superior vena caval obstruction:**[o] the face is plethoric and cyanosed with periorbital oedema; the eyes may show exophthalmos, conjunctival injection, and venous dilatation in the fundi; in the neck the jugular venous pressure is raised but not pulsatile, the thyroid may be enlarged, there may be supraclavicular lymphadenopathy and a positive Pemberton's sign; the chest may show dilated collateral vessels, or signs of lung carcinoma.
- **Tracheal compression:** stridor, usually accompanied by respiratory distress.
- **Recurrent laryngeal nerve involvement:** hoarseness of the voice.
- **Horner's syndrome.**
- **Paralysis of the phrenic nerve:** dullness to percussion at the affected base, which does not change with deep inspiration (abnormal tidal percussion), and absent breath sounds suggest a paralysed diaphragm due to phrenic nerve involvement.

Carcinoma of the lung

Many patients have no signs.

---

[n] Anton Ghon (1866–1936), Austrian pathologist and Professor of Anatomical Pathology in Prague. He described the lesion in 1912.

[o] First described by William Hunter (1718–83; brother of John Hunter) in a patient with a syphilitic aortic aneurysm.

Respiratory and chest signs

- Haemoptysis.
- Clubbing, sometimes with hypertrophic pulmonary osteoarthropathy (usually not small cell carcinoma).
- Lobar collapse or volume loss.
- Pneumonia.
- Pleural effusion.
- Fixed inspiratory wheeze.
- Tender ribs (secondary deposits of tumour in the ribs).
- Mediastinal compression, including signs of nerve involvement.
- Supraclavicular or axillary lymphadenopathy.

Apical (Pancoast) tumour

Horner's syndrome, recurrent laryngeal nerve palsy (hoarseness), C8/T1 nerve root lesion.

Distant metastases

Brain, liver and bone are the most commonly affected organs.

Non-metastatic extrapulmonary manifestations

- Anorexia, weight loss, cachexia, fever.
- **Endocrine changes:** (i) hypercalcaemia, due to secretion of parathyroid hormone-like substances, occurs in squamous cell carcinoma; (ii) hyponatraemia—antidiuretic hormone is released by small (oat) cell carcinomas; (iii) ectopic adrenocorticotrophic hormone (ACTH) syndrome (small cell carcinoma); (iv) carcinoid syndrome (small cell carcinoma); (v) gynaecomastia (gonadotrophins—rare; more often squamous cell); (vi) hypoglycaemia (insulin-like peptide from squamous cell carcinoma).
- **Neurological manifestations:** Eaton-Lambert[p] syndrome (progressive muscle weakness) and retinal blindness (small cell carcinoma), peripheral neuropathy, subacute cerebellar degeneration, polymyositis, cortical degeneration.
- **Haematological features:** migrating venous thrombophlebitis, disseminated intravascular coagulation, anaemia.
- **Skin:** acanthosis nigricans, dermatomyositis (rare).
- **Renal:** nephrotic syndrome due to membranous glomerulonephritis (rare).

Sarcoidosis

This is a systemic disease, characterised by the presence of non-caseating granulomas which commonly affect the lungs, skin, eyes, lymph nodes, liver and spleen, and the nervous system. The aetiology is unknown. There may be no pulmonary signs.

Pulmonary signs

- **Lungs:** no signs usually, although 80% of patients have lung involvement. In severe disease there may be signs of ILD.

Extrapulmonary signs

- **Skin:** lupus pernio (violaceous patches on the face, especially the nose, fingers or toes), pink nodules and plaques (granulomata) in old scars, erythema nodosum on the shins.
- **Eyes:** ciliary injection, anterior uveitis.
- **Lymph nodes:** generalised lymphadenopathy.
- **Liver and spleen:** enlarged (uncommon).
- **Parotids:** gland enlargement (uncommon) (page 161).
- **Central nervous system:** cranial nerve lesions, peripheral neuropathy (uncommon).
- **Musculoskeletal system:** arthralgia, swollen fingers, bone cysts (rare).
- **Heart:** heart block presenting as syncope, cor pulmonale (both rare).
- Signs of hypercalcaemia.

Pulmonary embolism (PE)

Embolism to the lungs often occurs without symptoms or signs. One should always entertain this diagnosis if there has been sudden and unexplained dyspnoea when a patient has risk factors for embolism (Table 5.21). Pleuritic chest pain and haemoptysis occur only when there is infarction. Syncope or the sudden onset of severe substernal pain can occur with massive embolism.

- **General signs:** tachycardia, tachypnoea, fever (with infarction).
- **Lungs:** pleural friction rub if infarction has occurred.

TABLE 5.21 Risk factors for pulmonary embolism (PE)
1 Previous PE
2 Immobilisation (long aeroplane flight or especially after surgery)
3 Known clotting-factor abnormalities
4 Known malignancy

---

p ML Eaton, 20th century American physician, and EH Lambert (b. 1915), American neurologist.

- **Massive embolism:** elevated jugular venous pressure, right ventricular gallop, right ventricular heave, tricuspid regurgitation murmur, palpable pulmonary component of the second heart sound (P2), gallop (S3 and/or S4).
- **Signs of deep venous thrombosis:** fewer than 50% of patients have clinical evidence of a source.

Note: A firm diagnosis cannot be made on the symptoms and signs alone.

The chest X-ray

The radiological appearance of a normal lung, with the lung segments labelled, is shown in Figure 5.15.

The radiological changes of consolidation, pleural effusion, pneumothorax and hydropneumothorax are shown in Figures 5.16 to 5.19.

A pulmonary mass is obvious in Figure 5.20, while multiple metastases are seen in Figure 5.21. Primary tuberculosis is shown in Figure 5.22, and Figure 5.23 illustrates the features of emphysema.

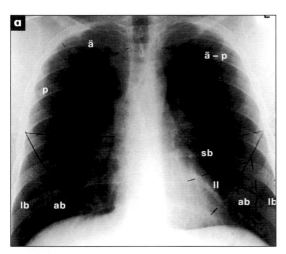

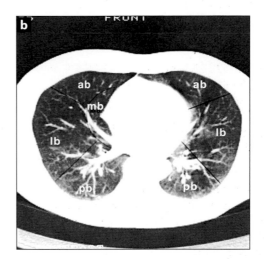

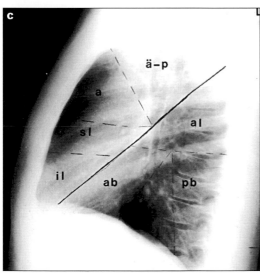

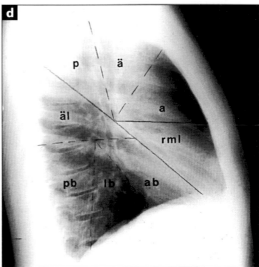

Figure 5.15 Lung segments

(a) Posteroanterior view. (b) CT scan through lung bases. (c) Left lateral view. (d) Right lateral view.

Right upper lobe: ä = apical segment; a = anterior segment, p = posterior segment.

Left upper lobe: ä-p = apico-posterior segment, s = anterior segment, sl = superior lingular segment, il = inferior lingular segment.

Right middle lobe (rml): m = medial segment, l = lateral segment.

Right lower lobe: äl = apical segment, mb = medial basal segment, lb = lateral basal segment, ab = anterior basal segment, pb = posterior basal segment.

Left lower lobe: äl = apical segment, lb = lateral basal segment, ab = anterior basal segment, pb = posterior basal segment.

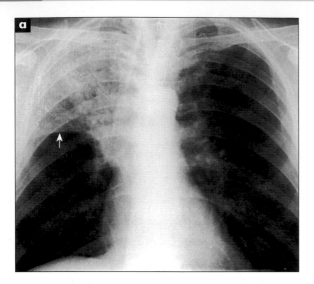 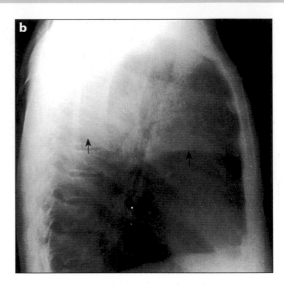

Figure 5.16 Right upper lobe consolidation
The right upper lobe is opacified and is limited inferiorly by the horizontal fissure (arrows). There must be some collapse as well, as the fissure shows some elevation. These changes could be due to a bacterial lobar pneumonia per se, but a central bronchostenotic lesion should be considered. If the pneumonia persists, a bronchoscopy is indicated to search for a central carcinoma.

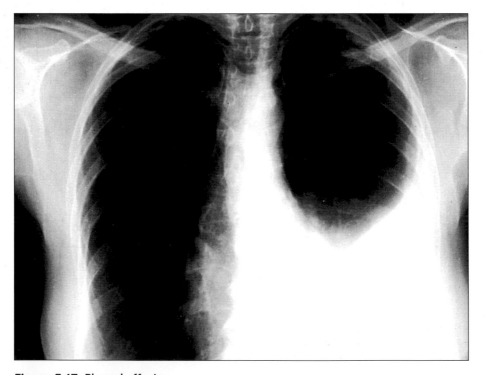

Figure 5.17 Pleural effusion
The upper margin of the effusion is curved ('meniscus sign'). The left hemidiaphragm is not seen because there is no adjacent aerated lung for contrast. The heart shows some deviation to the right. It is unlikely that this is caused by an effusion of this size. It is probably related to the lower thoracic scoliosis.

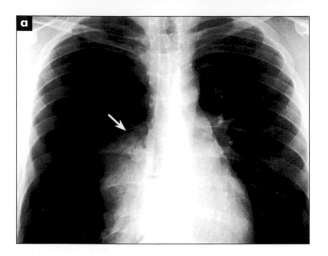

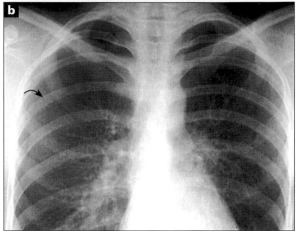

Figure 5.18 Pneumothorax

(a) There is a massive right pneumothorax with collapsed lung seen against the hilum (arrow). There is increased translucency because of the absence of vascular shadows. (b) Different patient with a smaller pneumothorax. Small pneumothoraces are easier to see on an expiratory film as the pneumothorax volume remains constant, surrounding the partly deflated lung. The visceral pleural surface is marked (arrow).

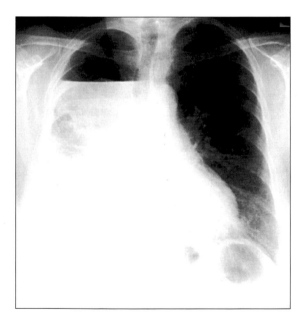

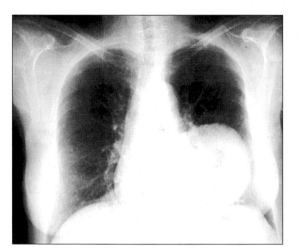

Figure 5.20 A pulmonary mass

There is a large solitary mass lesion in the left lower zone. The differential diagnosis is primary or secondary neoplasm, hydatid cyst or large abscess. No air–fluid level is seen within it to indicate cavitation.

Figure 5.19 Hydropneumothorax

An air–fluid level is seen in the upper portion of the right hemithorax. When air and fluid are present in the pleural space, the fluid no longer forms a meniscus at its upper margin. Some aerated lung is seen deep to the fluid.

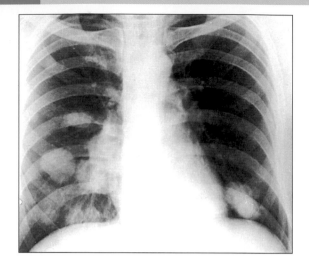

Figure 5.21 Pulmonary metastases
Multiple rounded opacities are seen in both lung fields, mainly at the left base and around the right hilum. The most likely cause is multiple pulmonary metastases. Other rare possibilities are hydatid cysts, large sarcoid nodules or large rheumatoid nodules. Multiple abscesses are extremely unlikely in the absence of cavitation.

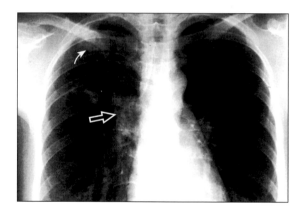

Figure 5.22 Primary tuberculosis
Two small rounded areas of shadowing are seen in the right upper zone (solid arrow). The right hilum is enlarged by the enlarged draining lymph nodes (open arrow). This combination of focal shadowing and enlarged lymph nodes is the primary (Ghon) complex of tuberculosis. With healing, calcification may occur in the parenchymal and nodal lesions. In contrast, in tuberculosis reactivation or reinfection, cavitation may occur and there is no lymphadenopathy.

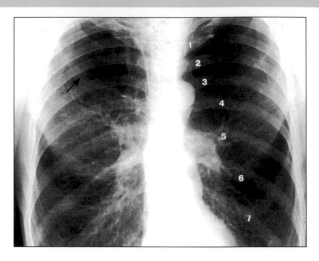

Figure 5.23 Emphysema
The lungs are overinflated with low, flat hemidiaphragms. The level of the hemidiaphragms is well below the anterior aspects of the sixth ribs. The diaphragm normally projects over the sixth rib anteriorly and the tenth intercostal space posteriorly. Count the ribs anteriorly (1–6). There is increased translucency of both upper zones with loss of the vascular markings due to bulla formation (arrow). This increased translucency is not due to overexposure. The hila are prominent because of the enlarged central pulmonary arteries. In contrast, the smaller peripheral pulmonary arteries (the lung markings) are decreased in size and number. This is due to actual destruction, displacement around bullae, and decreased perfusion through emphysematous areas.

Chest X-ray checklist

A—Airway (midline, no obvious deformities, no paratracheal masses).

B—Bones and soft tissue (no fractures, subcutaneous emphysema).

C—Cardiac size, silhouette and retrocardiac density normal.

D—Diaphragms (right above left by 1–3 cm, costophrenic angles sharp, diaphragmatic contrast with lung sharp).

E—Equal volume (count ribs, look for mediastinal shift).

F—Fine detail (pleura and lung parenchyma).

G—Gastric bubble (above the air bubble one shouldn't see an opacity of any more than 0.5 cm width).

H—Hilum (left normally above right by up to 3 cm, no larger than a thumb), hardware (especially in the intensive care unit: endotracheal tube, central venous catheters, pacemaker).

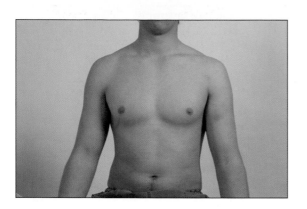 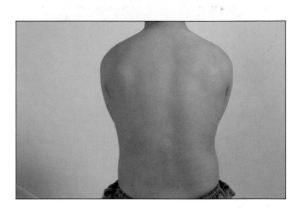

Figure 5.24   Respiratory system
SVC = superior vena cava.

Sitting up (if not acutely ill)

1. **General inspection**
   Sputum mug contents (blood, pus etc)
   Type of cough
   Rate and depth of respiration, and breathing pattern
   at rest
   Accessory muscles of respiration
2. **Hands**
   Clubbing
   Cyanosis (peripheral)
   Nicotine staining
   Wasting, weakness—finger abduction and adduction
   (lung cancer involving the brachial plexus)
   Wrist tenderness (hypertrophic pulmonary
   osteoarthropathy)
   Pulse (tachycardia, pulsus paradoxus)
   Flapping tremor (CO_2 narcosis)
3. **Face**
   Eyes—Horner's syndrome (apical lung cancer),
   anaemia
   Mouth—central cyanosis
   Voice—hoarseness (recurrent laryngeal nerve palsy)
   Facial plethora—smoker, SVC obstruction
4. **Trachea**
5. **Chest posteriorly**
   Inspect
   • Shape of chest and spine
   • Scars
   • Prominent veins (determine direction of flow)
   Palpate
   • Cervical lymph nodes
   • Expansion
   • Vocal fremitus

Percuss
• Supraclavicular region
• Back
• Axillae
• Tidal percussion (diaphragm paralysis)
Auscultate
• Breath sounds
• Adventitious sounds
• Vocal resonance

6. **Chest anteriorly**
   Inspect
   • Radiotherapy marks, other signs as noted above
   Palpate
   • Supraclavicular nodes
   • Expansion
   • Vocal fremitus
   • Apex beat
   Percuss
   Auscultate
   Pemberton's sign (SVC obstruction)
7. **Cardiovascular system (lying at 45°)**
   Jugular venous pressure (SVC obstruction etc)
   Cor pulmonale
8. **Forced expiratory time**
9. **Other**
   Lower limbs—oedema, cyanosis
   Breasts
   Temperature chart (infection)
   Evidence of malignancy or pleural effusion: examine
   the breasts, abdomen, rectum, lymph nodes etc
   Respiratory rate after exercise

Summary

The respiratory examination: a suggested method (Figure 5.24)

Ask the patient to undress to the waist (provide women with a gown), and to sit over the side of the bed. In the clinic or surgery the examination can often be performed with the patient sitting on a chair. While standing back to make your usual **inspection** (does the patient appear breathless while walking into the room or undressing?), ask if sputum is available for inspection. Purulent sputum always indicates respiratory infection, and a large volume of purulent sputum is an important clue to bronchiectasis. Haemoptysis is also an important sign. Look for dyspnoea at rest and count the respiratory rate. Note any paradoxical inward motion of the abdomen during inspiration (diaphragmatic paralysis). Look for use of the accessory muscles of respiration, and any intercostal indrawing of the lower ribs anteriorly (a sign of emphysema). General cachexia should also be noted.

Pick up the **hands**. Look for clubbing, peripheral cyanosis, tar staining and anaemia. Note any wasting of the small muscles of the hands and weakness of finger abduction (lung cancer involving the brachial plexus). Palpate the wrists for tenderness (hypertrophic pulmonary osteoarthropathy). While holding the hand, palpate the radial pulse for obvious pulsus paradoxus. Take the blood pressure if indicated.

Go on to the **face**. Look closely at the eyes for constriction of one of the pupils and for ptosis (Horner's syndrome from an apical lung cancer). Inspect the tongue for central cyanosis.

Palpate the position of the **trachea**. This is an important sign, so spend time on it. If the trachea is displaced, you must concentrate on the upper lobes for physical signs. Also look and feel for a tracheal tug, which indicates severe airflow obstruction, and feel for the use of the accessory muscles. Now ask the patient to speak (hoarseness) and then cough, and note whether this is a loose cough, a dry cough or a bovine cough. Next measure the forced expiratory time (FET). Tell the patient to take a maximal inspiration and blow out as rapidly and forcefully as possible while you listen. Note audible wheeze and prolongation of the time beyond 3 seconds as evidence of chronic obstructive pulmonary disease.

The next step is to examine the **chest**. You may wish to examine the front first, or go to the back to start. The advantage of the latter is that there are often more signs there, unless the trachea is obviously displaced.

Inspect the **back**. Look for kyphoscoliosis. Do not miss ankylosing spondylitis, which causes decreased chest expansion and upper lobe fibrosis. Look for thoracotomy scars and prominent veins. Also note any skin changes from radiotherapy.

Palpate first from behind for the cervical nodes. Then examine for expansion—first upper lobe expansion, which is best seen by looking over the patient's shoulders at clavicular movement during moderate respiration. The affected side will show a delay or decreased movement. Then examine lower lobe expansion by palpation. Note asymmetry and reduction of movement.

Now ask the patient to bring his or her elbows together in the front to move the scapulae out of the way. Examine for vocal fremitus, then **percuss** the back of the chest.

Auscultate the chest. Note breath sounds (whether normal or bronchial) and their intensity (normal or reduced). Listen for adventitious sounds (crackles and wheezes). Finally examine for vocal resonance. If a localised abnormality is found, try to determine the abnormal lobe and segment.

Return to the **front of the chest**. Inspect again for chest deformity, distended veins, radiotherapy changes and scars. Palpate the supraclavicular nodes carefully. Then proceed with percussion and auscultation as before. Listen high up in the axillae too. Before leaving the chest feel the axillary nodes and examine the breasts (Chapter 14).

Lay the patient down at 45 degrees and measure the jugular venous pressure. Then examine the praecordium and lower limbs for signs of cor pulmonale. Finally examine the **liver** and take the **temperature**.

Remember that most respiratory examinations are 'targeted'. Not every part of the examination is necessary for every patient.

References

1. Schmitt BP, Kushner MS, Wiener SL. The diagnostic usefulness of the history of the patient with dyspnea. *J Gen Intern Med* 1986; 1:386–393. History alone was correct three out of four times when deciding the cause of dyspnoea in defined circumstances.

2. Anonymous. Obtaining an exposure history. Agency for Toxic Substances and Disease Registry. United States Department of Health and Human Services, Public Health Service, Atlanta, Georgia. *Am Fam Phys* 1993; 48:483–491.

3. Mulrow CD, Dolmatch BL, Delong ER et al. Observer variability in the pulmonary examination. *J Gen Intern Med* 1986; 1:364–367. Documents the poor reliability of many respiratory signs.

4. Conn HO. Asterixis: Its occurrence in chronic obstructive pulmonary disease, with a . commentary on its general mechanism. *N Engl J Med* 1958; 259:564–569.

5. Williams JW Jnr, Simel DL, Roberts LR, Samsa GP. Clinical evaluation for sinusitis; making the diagnosis by history and physical examination. *Ann Intern Med* 1992; 117:705–710. The doctor's impression of the likelihood of sinusitis was superior to findings of a purulent nasal discharge, history of maxillary toothache, poor response to nasal decongestants and abnormal transillumination.

6. Model D. Smokers' face: an underrated clinical sign? *BMJ* 1985; 291:1760–1762. A red face with

leathery skin and excessive wrinkling, associated with a gaunt look, may help identify up to half of chronic smokers.

7. Garcia-Pachon E. Paradoxical movement of the lateral rib margin (Hoover sign) for detecting obstructive airway disease. *Chest* 2002; 12:651–655

8. McGee S. *Evidence-based physical diagnosis*, 2nd edn. St Louis: Saunders, 2007.

9. Kraman SS. Lung sounds for the clinician. *Arch Intern Med* 1986; 146:411–412. Describes the physiological evidence for many auscultatory findings.

10. Earis J. Lung sounds. *Thorax* 1992; 47:671–672.

11. Forgacs P. The functional basis of lung sounds. *Chest* 1978; 73:399–405.

12. Nath AR, Caple LH. Respiratory crackles: early and late. *Thorax* 1974; 29:223–227. Severe airways obstruction causes crackles in the first half of inspiration. In contrast, late crackles are not associated with airways obstruction.

13. Walshaw MJ, Nissa M, Pearson MG et al. Expiratory lung crackles in patients with fibrosing alveolitis. *Chest* 1990; 97:407–409. Inspiratory crackles are usually considered more important, but this report suggests that expiratory crackles occur intermittently in fibrosing alveolitis, usually in mid-expiration.

14. Shapira JD. About egophony. *Chest* 1995; 108:865–867.

15. Wallace C, Siminoski K. The Pemberton sign. *Ann Intern Med* 1996; 125:568–569. Discusses the mechanism of this useful sign, which is present when a large retrosternal goitre compresses the thoracic inlet.

16. Schapira RM, Schapira MM et al. The value of the forced expiratory time in the physical diagnosis of obstructive airways disease. *JAMA* 1993; 270:731–736. In patients with chronic obstructive airways who have a low pretest probability, an appropriate low-end cut-off is required (e.g. 3 seconds).

17. Metlay JP, Kappor WN, Fine MJ. Does this patient have community-acquired pneumonia? Diagnosing pneumonia by history and physical examination. *Jama* 1997; 278:1440–1445. Normal vital signs and normal chest auscultation substantially reduce the likelihood of pneumonia, but a chest X-ray is required for a firm diagnosis.

18. Holloman DR, Simmel DL, Goldberg JS. Diagnosis of obstructive airways disease from the clinical examination. *J Gen Intern Med* 1993; 8:63–68. A history of smoking, self-reported wheezing and wheezing detected at auscultation combined had a high predictive value for chronic obstructive airways disease. The forced expiratory time added little additional information to these predictors.

Suggested reading

Bourke SJ. *Lecture notes on respiratory disease*, 6th edn. Oxford: Blackwell, 2003.

Forgacs P. The functional basis of pulmonary sounds. *Chest* 1978; 73:399–405.

Hansen-Flaschen J, Nordberg J. Clubbing and hypertrophic osteoarthropathy. *Clin Chest Med* 1987; 8:287–298.

James DG, Studdy PR. *Color atlas of respiratory diseases*, 2nd edn. Chicago: Mosby-Year Book, 1992.

Light RW. Pleural effusion. *N Eng J Med* 2002; 346:1971–1977.

Chapter 6
The gastrointestinal system

To study the phenomena of disease without books is to sail an uncharted sea, while to study books without patients is not to go to sea at all.

Sir William Osler (1849–1919)

This lord wears his wit in his belly, and his guts in his head.

William Shakespeare, Troilus and Cressida

Gastroenterologists and gastrointestinal surgeons concern themselves with the entire length of the gut, the liver, the exocrine pancreas and the peripheral effects of alimentary disease.

The gastrointestinal history
Presenting symptoms (Table 6.1)

Abdominal pain

There are many causes of abdominal pain, and careful history taking will often lead to the correct diagnosis. The following should be considered.

Frequency and duration. Try to determine whether the pain is acute or chronic, when it began and how often it occurs.

Site and radiation. The site of pain is important. Ask the patient to point to the area affected by pain and to the point of maximum intensity. Parietal peritoneal inflammation that causes pain usually does so in a localised area. Ask about radiation of pain. Pain often radiates through to the back with pancreatic disease or a penetrating peptic ulcer. It may radiate to the shoulder with diaphragmatic irritation or to the neck with oesophageal reflux.

Character and pattern. The pain may be colicky (coming and going in waves and related to peristaltic

TABLE 6.1 Gastrointestinal history
Major symptoms
Abdominal pain
Appetite and/or weight change
Postprandial fullness or early satiation, or both
Nausea and/or vomiting
Heartburn and/or acid regurgitation
Waterbrash
Dysphagia
Disturbed defecation (diarrhoea, constipation, faecal incontinence)
Bloating or visible distension, or both
Bleeding (haematemesis, melaena, rectal bleeding)
Jaundice
Dark urine, pale stools
Pruritus
Lethargy
Fever

movements) or steady. Colicky pain comes from obstruction of the bowel or the ureters. If the pain is chronic, ask about the daily pattern of pain.

Aggravating and relieving factors. Pain due to peptic ulceration may or may not be related to meals. Eating may precipitate ischaemic pain in the gut. Antacids or vomiting may relieve peptic ulcer pain or that of gastro-oesophageal reflux. Defaecation or passage of flatus may relieve the pain of colonic disease temporarily. Patients who get some relief by rolling around vigorously are more likely to have a colicky pain, while those who lie perfectly still are more likely to have peritonitis.

Patterns of pain

Peptic ulcer disease. This is classically a dull or burning pain in the epigastrium that is relieved to a degree by food or antacids. It is typically episodic and may occur at night, waking the patient from sleep. This combination of symptoms is suggestive of the diagnosis. The pain is often unrelated to meals, despite classical teaching to the contrary. It is not possible to distinguish duodenal ulceration from gastric ulceration clinically.

Pancreatic pain. This is a steady epigastric pain that may be partly relieved by sitting up and leaning forwards. There is often radiation of the pain to the back, and vomiting is common.

Biliary pain. Although usually called 'biliary colic', this pain is rarely colicky. With cystic duct obstruction there is often epigastric pain. It is usually a severe, constant pain that can last for hours. There may be a history of episodes of similar pain in the past. If cholecystitis develops, the pain typically shifts to the right upper quadrant and becomes more severe.

Renal colic. This is a colicky pain superimposed on a background of constant pain in the renal angle, often with radiation towards the groin. It can be very severe indeed.

Bowel obstruction. This is colicky pain. Periumbilical pain suggests a small bowel origin but colonic pain can occur anywhere in the abdomen. Small bowel obstruction tends to cause more frequent colicky pain (with a cycle every 2–3 minutes) than large bowel obstruction (every 10–15 minutes). Obstruction is often associated with vomiting, constipation and abdominal distension.

Appetite and weight change

Loss of appetite (anorexia) and weight loss are important gastrointestinal symptoms. The presence of both anorexia and weight loss should make one suspicious of an underlying malignancy, but may also occur with depression and in other diseases. The combination of weight loss with an increased appetite suggests malabsorption of nutrients or a hypermetabolic state (e.g. thyrotoxicosis). It is important to document when the symptoms began and how much weight loss has occurred over this period. Liver disease can sometimes cause disturbance of taste. This may cause smokers with acute hepatitis and jaundice to give up smoking.

Early satiation and postprandial fullness

Inability to finish a normal meal (early satiation) may be a symptom of gastric diseases, including gastric cancer and peptic ulcer. A feeling of inappropriate fullness after eating can also be a symptom of functional (unexplained) gastrointestinal disease.

Nausea and vomiting

Nausea is the sensation of wanting to vomit. Heaving and retching may occur but there is no expulsion of gastric contents. There are many possible causes for these complaints. Gastrointestinal tract infections (e.g. from food poisoning by *Staphylococcus aureus*) or small bowel obstruction can cause acute symptoms. In patients with chronic symptoms, pregnancy and drugs (e.g. digoxin, opiates, dopamine agonists, chemotherapy) should always be ruled out. In the gastrointestinal tract, peptic ulcer disease with gastric outlet obstruction, motor disorders (e.g. gastroparesis from diabetes mellitus, or after gastric surgery), acute hepatobiliary disease and alcoholism are important causes. Finally, psychogenic vomiting, eating disorders (e.g. bulimia) and, rarely, increased intracranial pressure should be considered in patients with chronic unexplained nausea and vomiting.

The timing of the vomiting can be helpful; vomiting delayed more than 1 hour after the meal is typical of gastric outlet obstruction or gastroparesis, while early morning vomiting before eating is characteristic of pregnancy, alcoholism and raised intracranial pressure. Also ask about the contents of the vomitus (e.g. bile indicates an open connection between the duodenum and stomach, old food suggests gastric outlet obstruction, while blood suggests ulceration).

Heartburn and acid regurgitation

Heartburn refers to the presence of a burning pain or discomfort in the retrosternal area. Typically, this sensation travels up towards the throat and occurs after meals or is aggravated by bending, stooping or lying supine. Antacids usually relieve the pain, at least transiently. This symptom is due to regurgitation of stomach contents into the oesophagus. Usually these contents are acidic, although occasionally alkaline reflux can induce similar problems. Associated with gastro-oesophageal reflux may be *acid regurgitation*, in which the patient experiences a sour or bitter-tasting fluid coming up into the mouth. This symptom strongly suggests that reflux is occurring. Some patients complain of a cough that troubles them when they lie down. In patients with gastro-

Questions box 6.1

Questions to ask a patient presenting with recurrent vomiting

! denotes symptoms for the possible diagnosis of an urgent or dangerous problem.

1. How long have you been having attacks of vomiting (distinguish acute from chronic)?
2. Does the vomiting occur with nausea preceding it, or does it occur without any warning?
3. Is the vomiting usually immediately after a meal or hours after a meal?
4. Do you have vomiting early in the morning or late in the evening?
5. **!** What does the vomit look like? Is it bloodstained, bile-stained or faeculent?—Gastro-intestinal bleeding or bowel obstruction
6. Do you have specific vomiting episodes followed by feeling completely well for long periods before the vomiting episode occurs again?—Cyclical vomiting syndrome
7. Is there any abdominal pain associated with the vomiting?
8. **!** Have you been losing weight?
9. What medications are you taking?
10. Do you have worsening headaches?—Neurological symptoms suggest a central cause

Questions box 6.2

Questions to ask the patient with acid reflux or suspected gastro-oesophageal reflux disease (GORD)

! denotes symptoms for the possible diagnosis of an urgent or dangerous problem.

1. Do you have heartburn (a burning pain under the sternum radiating up towards the throat)? How often does this occur?—More than once a week suggests GORD
2. Does your heartburn occur after meals or when you lean forward or lie flat in bed (typical of acid reflux)?
3. **!** Does the pain radiate across the chest down the left arm or into the jaw?—Suggests myocardial ischaemia
4. Is the pain relieved by antacids or over-the-counter acid-suppressing medicines?
5. Do you experience suddenly feeling bitter tasting fluid in the mouth?—Acid regurgitation
6. Have you experienced the sudden appearance of a salty tasting or tasteless fluid in the mouth?—Waterbrash
7. **!** Have you had trouble swallowing?—Dysphagia (see *Questions box 6.3*)
8. Have you been troubled by a cough when you lie down?

oesophageal reflux disease, the lower oesophageal sphincter muscle relaxes inappropriately. Reflux symptoms may be aggravated by alcohol, chocolate, caffeine, a fatty meal, theophylline, calcium channel blockers and anticholinergic drugs, as these lower the oesophageal sphincter pressure.

Waterbrash refers to excessive secretion of saliva into the mouth and should not be confused with regurgitation; it may occur, uncommonly, in patients with peptic ulcer disease or oesophagitis.

Dysphagia

Dysphagia is difficulty in swallowing. Such difficulty may occur with solids or liquids. The causes of dysphagia are listed in Table 6.2. If a patient complains of difficulty swallowing, it is important to differentiate painful swallowing from actual difficulty.[1] Painful swallowing is termed *odynophagia* and occurs with any severe inflammatory process involving the oesophagus. Causes include infectious oesophagitis (e.g. *Candida*, herpes simplex), peptic ulceration of the

oesophagus, caustic damage to the oesophagus or oesophageal perforation.

If the patient complains of difficulty initiating swallowing, fluid regurgitating into the nose or choking on trying to swallow, this suggests that the cause of the dysphagia is in the pharynx (pharyngeal dysphagia). Causes of pharyngeal dysphagia can include neurological disease (e.g. motor neurone disease, resulting in bulbar or pseudobulbar palsy).

If the patient complains of food sticking in the oesophagus, it is important to consider a number of anatomical causes of oesophageal blockage.[1] Ask the patient to point to the site where the solids stick. If there is a mechanical obstruction at the lower end of the oesophagus, most often the patient will localise the dysphagia to the lower retrosternal area. However, obstruction higher in the oesophagus may be felt anywhere in the retrosternal area. If heartburn is also present, for example, this suggests that gastro-oesophageal reflux with or without stricture formation may

TABLE 6.2 Causes of dysphagia

Mechanical obstruction

Intrinsic (within oesophagus)
Reflux oesophagitis with stricture formation
Carcinoma of oesophagus or gastric cardia
Pharyngeal or oesophageal web
Pharyngeal pouch
Schatzki (lower oesophageal) ring
Foreign body

Extrinsic (outside oesophagus)
Goitre with retrosternal extension
Mediastinal tumours, bronchial carcinoma, vascular
  compression (rare)

Neuromuscular motility disorders (hints from the
  history: solids and liquids equally difficult, symptoms
  intermittent)
Achalasia
Diffuse oesophageal spasm
Scleroderma

Pharyngeal dysphagia (hints: aspiration, fluid
  regurgitation into the nose)
Cricopharyngeal dysfunction—Zenker's diverticulum
Neurological diseases: bulbar or pseudobulbar palsy,
  myasthenia gravis, polymyositis, myotonic dystrophy

Questions box 6.3

Questions to ask a patient who reports difficulty swallowing

! denotes symptoms for the possible diagnosis of an urgent or dangerous problem.

1 Do you have trouble swallowing solids, liquid or both?—Solids and liquids suggests a motor problem, e.g. achalasia

2 Where does the hold-up occur (please point to the area)?—Oesophageal carcinoma

3 Is the trouble swallowing intermittent or persistent?—Intermittent suggests eosinophilic oesophagitis

4 Has the problem been getting progressively worse?

5 Do you cough or choke on starting to swallow (oropharyngeal dysphagia)?

6 Is it painful to swallow (odynophagia)?

7 Do you have any heartburn or acid regurgitation?

! 8 Have you been losing weight?

be the cause of the dysphagia. The actual course of the dysphagia is also a very important part of the history to obtain. If the patient states that the dysphagia is intermittent or is present only with the first few swallows of food, this suggests either a lower oesophageal ring or oesophageal spasm. However, if the patient complains of progressive difficulty swallowing, this suggests a stricture, carcinoma or achalasia. If the patient states that both solids and liquids stick, then a motor disorder of the oesophagus is more likely, such as achalasia or diffuse oesophageal spasm.

Diarrhoea

The symptom diarrhoea can be defined in a number of different ways. Patients may complain of frequent stools (more than three per day being abnormal) or they may complain of a change in the consistency of the stools, which have become loose or watery. There are a large number of possible causes of diarrhoea.

Some patients pass small amounts of formed stool more than three times a day because of an increased desire to defecate. The stools are not loose and stool volume is not increased. This is not true diarrhoea. It can occur because of local rectal pathology, incomplete rectal emptying, or because of a psychological disturbance that leads to an increased interest in defaecation.

When a history of diarrhoea is obtained, it is also important to determine if this has occurred acutely or whether it is a chronic problem. Acute diarrhoea is more likely to be infectious in nature, while chronic diarrhoea has a large number of causes.

Clinically, diarrhoea can be divided into a number of different groups based on the likely disturbance of physiology.[2]

1 *Secretory diarrhoea* is likely if the diarrhoea is of high volume (commonly more than 1 litre per day) and persists when the patient fasts; there is no pus or blood, and the stools are not excessively fatty. Secretory diarrhoea occurs when net secretion in the colon or small bowel exceeds absorption; some of the causes include infections (e.g. *E. coli*, *Staphylococcus aureus*, *Vibrio cholerae*), hormonal conditions (e.g. vasoactive intestinal polypeptide-secreting tumour, Zollinger-Ellison[a] syndrome, carcinoid syndrome) and villous adenoma.

2 *Osmotic diarrhoea* is characterised by its

---

a Robert Milton Zollinger (b. 1903), American surgeon, and Edwin H Ellison (b. 1918), American physician. This syndrome is characterised by gastric acid hypersecretion, peptic ulceration and in 40% of cases diarrhoea, due to a gastrinoma (gastrin-secreting tumour). It was described in 1955.

Questions box 6.4

Questions to ask the patient presenting with diarrhoea

! denotes symptoms for the possible diagnosis of an urgent or dangerous problem.

1 How many stools a day do you pass now normally?

2 What do the stools look like (stool form e.g. loose and watery)?

3 Do you have to race to the bathroom to have a bowel movement?—Urgency in colonic disease

4 Have you been woken from sleep during the night by diarrhoea?—Organic cause more likely

! 5 Have you seen any bright-red blood in the stools or mucus or pus?—Suggests colonic disease

6 Are you passing large volumes of stool every day?—Suggests small bowel disease

7 Are your stools pale, greasy, smelly and difficult to flush away (steatorrhoea)? Have you seen oil droplets in the stool?—Pancreatic disease

8 Have you had problems with leakage of stool (faecal incontinence)?

! 9 Have you lost weight?—e.g. cancer, malabsorption

10 Have you had any abdominal pain or vomiting?

11 Have you had treatment with antibiotics recently?

12 Have you had any recent travel? Where to?

13 Have you a personal history of inflammatory bowel disease or prior gastrointestinal surgery?

14 Have you any history in the family of coeliac disease or inflammatory bowel disease?

15 Have you had any problems with arthritis?—Inflammatory bowel disease, Whipple's disease

! 16 Have you had recent fever, rigors, or chills (e.g. infection, lymphoma)? Have you had frequent infections?—Immunoglobulin deficiency

deficiency), magnesium antacids or gastric surgery.

3 *Abnormal intestinal motility* (e.g. thyrotoxicosis, the irritable bowel syndrome) can also cause diarrhoea.

4 *Exudative diarrhoea* occurs when there is inflammation in the colon. Typically the stools are of small volume but frequent, and there may be associated blood or mucus (e.g. inflammatory bowel disease, colon cancer).

5 *Malabsorption* of nutrients can result in steatorrhoea. Here the stools are fatty, pale coloured, extremely smelly, float in the toilet bowel and are difficult to flush away. Steatorrhoea is defined as the presence of more than 7 g of fat in a 24-hour stool collection. There are many causes of steatorrhoea (page 190).

Constipation

It is important to determine what patients mean if they say they are constipated.[3] Constipation is a common symptom and can refer to the passage of infrequent stools (fewer than three times per week), hard stools or stools that are difficult to evacuate. This symptom may occur acutely or may be a chronic problem. In many patients, chronic constipation arises because of habitual neglect of the impulse to defecate, leading to the accumulation of large, dry faecal masses. With constant rectal distension from faeces, the patient may grow less aware of rectal fullness, leading to chronic constipation. Constipation may arise from ingestion of drugs (e.g. codeine, antidepressants and aluminium or calcium antacids), and with various metabolic or endocrine diseases (e.g. hypothyroidism, hypercalcaemia, diabetes mellitus, phaeochromocytoma, porphyria, hypokalaemia) and neurological disorders (e.g. aganglionosis, Hirschsprung's[b] disease, autonomic neuropathy, spinal cord injury, multiple sclerosis). Constipation can also arise after partial colonic obstruction from carcinoma; it is, therefore, very important to determine whether there has been a recent change in bowel habit, as this may indicate development of a malignancy. Patients with very severe constipation in the absence of structural disease may be found on a transit study to have slow colonic transit; such slow-transit constipation is most common in young women.

Constipation is common in the later stages of pregnancy.

disappearance with fasting and by large-volume stools related to the ingestion of food. Osmotic diarrhoea occurs due to excessive solute drag; causes include lactose intolerance (disaccharidase

b Harold Hirschsprung (1830–1916), physician, Queen Louise Hospital for Children, Copenhagen, described this disease in 1888. It had previously been described by Caleb Parry, English physician, in 1825.

Difficulty with evacuation of faeces may occur with disorders of the pelvic floor muscles or nerves, or anorectal disease (e.g. fissure, or stricture). Patients with this problem may complain of straining, a feeling of anal blockage or even the need to self-digitate to perform manual evacuation of faeces.

A chronic but erratic disturbance in defaecation (typically alternating constipation and diarrhoea) associated with abdominal pain, in the absence of any structural or biochemical abnormality, is very common; such patients are classified as having the *irritable bowel syndrome*.[4] Patients who report abdominal pain plus two or more of the following symptoms—abdominal pain relieved by defaecation, looser or more frequent stools with the onset of abdominal pain, passage of mucus per rectum, a feeling of incomplete emptying of the rectum following defaecation and visible abdominal distension—are more likely to have the irritable bowel syndrome than organic disease.

Mucus

The passage of mucus (white slime) may occur because of a solitary rectal ulcer, fistula or villous adenoma, or in the irritable bowel syndrome.

Bleeding

Patients may present with the problem of haematemesis (vomiting blood), melaena (passage of jet-black stools) or haematochezia (passage of bright-red blood per rectum). Sometimes patients may present because routine testing for occult blood in the stools is positive (page 183). It is important to ensure that if vomiting of blood is reported, this is not the result of bleeding from a tooth socket or the nose, or coughing up of blood.

Haematemesis indicates that the site of the bleeding is proximal to or at the duodenum. Ask about symptoms of peptic ulceration; haematemesis is commonly due to bleeding chronic peptic ulceration, particularly from a duodenal ulcer. Acute peptic ulcers often bleed without abdominal pain. A Mallory-Weiss tear usually occurs with repeated vomiting; typically the patient reports first the vomiting of clear gastric contents and then the vomiting of blood. Less-common causes of upper gastrointestinal bleeding are presented in Table 6.3.

Haemorrhoids and local anorectal diseases such as fissures will commonly present with passing small amounts of bright-red blood per rectum. The blood is normally not mixed in the stools but is on the toilet paper, on top of the stools or in the toilet bowl. Melaena usually results from bleeding

---

Questions box 6.5

Questions to ask a patient presenting with constipation

❗ denotes symptoms for the possible diagnosis of an urgent or dangerous problem.

1 How often do you have a bowel movement?

2 Are your stools hard or difficult to pass?

3 What do the stools look like (stool form e.g. small pellets)?

4 Do you strain excessively on passing stool?

5 Do you feel there may be a blockage at the anus area when you try to pass stool?

6 Do you ever press your finger in around the anus (or vagina) to help stool pass?

❗ 7 Has your bowel habit changed recently?

8 Any recent change in your medications?

❗ 9 Any blood in the stools?

10 Any abdominal pain?

❗ 11 Recent weight loss?

12 Do you ever have diarrhoea?

❗ 13 Do you have a history of colon polyps or cancer? Any family history of colon cancer?

Questions box 6.6

Questions to ask the patient who presents with vomiting blood (haematemesis)

❗ denotes symptoms for the possible diagnosis of an urgent or dangerous problem.

❗ 1 Was there fresh blood in the vomitus? Or was the vomitus coffee-grain stained?

❗ 2 Have you passed any black stools or blood in the stools?

3 Before any blood was seen in the vomitus, did you experience intense retching or vomiting?—Mallory-Weiss tear

4 Have you been taking aspirin, non-steroidal anti-inflammatory drugs or steroids?

5 Do you drink alcohol?

6 Have you ever had a peptic ulcer?

❗ 7 Have you lost weight?

---

from the upper gastrointestinal tract, although right-sided colonic and small bowel lesions can occasionally be responsible. Massive rectal bleeding can occur from the distal colon or rectum, or from a major bleeding site higher in the gastrointestinal tract. With substantial lower gastrointestinal tract

TABLE 6.3 Causes of acute gastrointestinal bleeding

Upper gastrointestinal tract

More common

1 Chronic peptic ulcer: duodenal ulcer, gastric ulcer
2 Acute peptic ulcer (erosions)

Less common

3 Mallory-Weiss* syndrome (tear at the gastro-oesophageal junction)
4 Oesophageal and/or gastric varices
5 Erosive or ulcerative oesophagitis
6 Gastric carcinoma, polyp, other tumours
7 Dieulafoy's[†] ulcer (single defect that involves an ectatic submucosal artery)
8 Watermelon stomach (antral vascular ectasias)
9 Aortoenteric fistula (usually aortoduodenal and after aortic surgery)
10 Vascular anomalies—angiodysplasia, arteriovenous malformations, blue rubber bleb naevus syndrome, hereditary haemorrhagic telangiectasia, CRST syndrome
11 Pseudoxanthoma elasticum, Ehlers-Danlos[‡] syndrome
12 Amyloidosis
13 Vasculitis
14 Ménétrier's[§] disease
15 Bleeding diathesis
16 Pseudohaematemesis (nasopharyngeal origin)

Lower gastrointestinal tract

More common

1 Angiodysplasia
2 Diverticular disease
3 Colonic carcinoma or polyp
4 Haemorrhoids or anal fissure

Less common

5 Massive upper gastrointestinal bleeding
6 Inflammatory bowel disease
7 Ischaemic colitis
8 Meckel's[#] diverticulum
9 Small bowel disease, e.g. tumour, diverticula, intussusception
10 Haemobilia (bleeding from the gallbladder)
11 Solitary colonic ulcer

---

* George Kenneth Mallory (b. 1900), professor of pathology, Boston, and Soma Weiss (1898–1942), professor of medicine, Boston City Hospital described this syndrome in 1929.
† Georges Dieulafoy (1839–1911), Paris physician.
‡ Edvard Ehlers (1863–1937), German dermatologist, described the syndrome in 1901, and Henri Alexandre Danlos (1844–1912), French dermatologist, described the syndrome in 1908.
§ Pierre Ménétrier (1859–1935), French physician.
# Johann Friedrich Meckel the younger (1781–1833), Professor of Surgery and Anatomy at Halle. His father and grandfather were also professors of anatomy.
CRST = calcinosis, Raynaud's phenomenon, sclerodactyly and telangiectasia.

---

bleeding, it is important to consider the presence of angiodysplasia or diverticular disease (where bleeding more often occurs from the right rather than the left colon, even though diverticula are more common in the left colon). Less-common causes of lower gastrointestinal bleeding are presented in Table 6.3.

Spontaneous bleeding into the skin, or from the nose or mouth, can be a problem for patients with coagulopathy resulting from liver disease.

Jaundice

Usually the relatives notice a yellow discoloration of the sclerae or skin before the patient does. Jaundice is due to the presence of excess bilirubin being deposited in the sclerae and skin. The causes of jaundice are described on page 185. If there is jaundice, ask about the colour of the urine and stools; pale stools and dark urine occur with obstructive or cholestatic jaundice because urobilinogen is unable to reach the intestine. Also ask about abdominal pain; gallstones, for example, can cause biliary pain and jaundice.[5]

Pruritus

This symptom means itching of the skin, and may be either generalised or localised. Cholestatic liver disease can cause pruritus which tends to be worse over the extremities. Other causes of pruritus are discussed on page 445.

Abdominal bloating and swelling

A feeling of swelling (bloating) may be a result of excess gas or a hypersensitive intestinal tract (as occurs in the irritable bowel syndrome). Persistent swelling can be due to ascitic fluid accumulation; this is discussed on page 175. It may be associated with ankle oedema.

Lethargy

Tiredness and easy fatiguability are common symptoms for patients with acute or chronic liver disease, but the mechanism is not known. This can also occur because of anaemia due to gastrointestinal or chronic inflammatory disease. Lethargy is also very common in the general population and is not a specific symptom.

Treatment

The treatment history is very important. Traditional non-steroidal anti-inflammatory drugs (NSAIDs), including aspirin, can induce bleeding from acute or chronic damage to the gastrointestinal tract. As described above, many drugs can result in disturbed defaecation. A large number of drugs are also known to affect the liver. For example, acute hepatitis can occur with halothane, phenytoin or chlorothiazide. Cholestasis may occur from a

hypersensitivity reaction to chlorpromazine or other phenothiazines, sulfonamides, sulfonylureas, phenylbutazone, rifampicin or nitrofurantoin. Anabolic steroids and the contraceptive pill can cause dose-related cholestasis. Fatty liver can occur with alcohol use, tetracycline, valproic acid or amiodarone. Large blood-filled cavities in the liver called peliosis hepatis can occur with anabolic steroid use or the contraceptive pill. Acute liver cell necrosis can occur if an overdose of paracetamol (acetaminophen) is taken.

Past history

Surgical procedures can result in jaundice from the anaesthesia (e.g. multiple uses of halothane), hypoxaemia of liver cells (hypotension during the operative or postoperative period) or direct damage to the bile duct during abdominal surgery. A history of relapsing and remitting epigastric pain in a patient who presents with severe abdominal pain may indicate that a peptic ulcer has perforated. A past history of inflammatory bowel disease (either ulcerative colitis or Crohn's disease) is important as these are chronic diseases that tend to flare up.

Social history

The patient's occupation may be relevant (e.g. healthcare workers may be exposed to hepatitis). Toxin exposure can also be important in chronic liver disease (e.g. carbon tetrachloride, vinyl chloride). If a patient has symptoms suggestive of liver disease, ask about recent travel to countries where hepatitis is endemic.

The alcohol history is very important, particularly as alcoholics often deny or understate the amount they consume (see Table 1.3, page 7).[6] Contact with anybody who has been jaundiced should always be noted. The sexual history should be obtained. A history of any injections (e.g. intravenous drugs, plasma transfusions, dental treatment or tattooing) in a patient who presents with symptoms of liver disease is important, particularly as hepatitis B or C may be transferred in this way.

Family history

A family history of colon cancer, especially of familial polyps, or inflammatory bowel disease is important. Ask about coeliac disease in the family. A positive family history of jaundice, anaemia, splenectomy or cholecystectomy may occur in patients with haemolytic anaemia (due to haemoglobin abnormalities or auto-immune disease) or congenital or familial hyperbilirubinaemia.

Questions box 6.7

Questions to ask the patient presenting with jaundice

! denotes symptoms for the possible diagnosis of an urgent or dangerous problem.

1. Is your urine dark? Are your stools pale?—Obstructive jaundice
2. Do you have any skin itching (pruritus)?
3. Have you had any fever?
! 4. Have you had a change in your appetite or weight?—Malignancy
5. Have you had any abdominal pain or change in bowel habit?
! 6. Have you had any vomiting of blood or passage of dark stools?
7. Do you drink alcohol? How much? How long? (CAGE questions, page 7)
8. Have you ever used intravenous drugs?
9. Have you ever had a blood transfusion?
10. Have you started any new medications recently?
11. Have you had any recent contact with patients with jaundice or liver problems?
12. Any history of recent high-risk sexual behaviours?
13. Have you travelled overseas to areas where hepatitis A is endemic?
14. Have you been immunised against hepatitis B?
15. Any history of inflammatory bowel disease?
16. What is your occupation (contact with hepatotoxins)?
17. Is there any family history of liver disease?

The gastrointestinal examination

Examination of the gastrointestinal system includes a complete examination of the abdomen. It is also important to search for the peripheral signs of gastrointestinal and liver disease. Some signs are more useful than others.[7]

Examination anatomy

An understanding of the structure and function of the gastrointestinal tract and abdominal organs is critical for the diagnosis of gastrointestinal disease (Figure 6.1). The mouth is the gateway to the gastrointestinal tract. It and the anus and rectum are readily accessible to the examiner, and both must be examined carefully in any patient with suspected abdominal disease. The position of the abdominal organs can be quite variable, but there are important surface markings which should be kept in mind during the examination.

The **liver** is the largest organ in the abdomen; it comprises a large right lobe and smaller left lobe divided into eight segments, including the caudate lobe (segment I) squeezed in between. The lower border of the liver extends from the tip of the right tenth rib to just below the left nipple. Normally the liver is not palpable but it may just be possible to feel the lower edge in healthy people.

The **spleen** is a lymphoid organ that underlies the ninth, tenth and eleventh ribs posteriorly on the left. It is usually not palpable in health.

The **kidneys** lie anteriorly 4 finger-breadths from the midline and posteriorly under the twelfth rib. Normally, the right kidney extends 2.5 cm lower than the left. In thin patients, the lower pole of the right kidney may be palpable in health.

The **gallbladder** is a pear-shaped organ and the fundus (top) is at the tip of the right ninth costal cartilage; it cannot be felt in health. The **pancreas** is situated in the retroperitoneum (behind the peritoneum), with the head tucked into the C-shaped duodenum and the tail snuggling into the spleen. A huge pancreatic mass may rarely be large enough to be palpable.

The **aorta** lies in the midline and terminates just to the left of the midline at the level of the iliac crest. A pulsatile mass in the middle of the abdomen is likely to be arising from the aorta and may indicate an aneurysm.

The **stomach** is usually J-shaped and lies in the left upper part of the abdomen over the spleen and pancreas; it connects with the duodenum. The **small intestine** ranges from 3 to 10 metres in length and comprises the upper half (duodenum and jejunum) and the lower half (ileum). The small intestine lies over the middle section of the abdomen but is usually impalpable.

The **colon** is approximately 1.5 metres in length, and from right to left consists of the caecum, ascending colon, hepatic flexure, transverse colon, splenic flexure, descending colon, sigmoid colon, rectum and anal canal (anorectum). The **appendix** usually lies in the right lower abdominal area, arising posterior-medially from the caecum. The caecum and ascending colon lie on the right side of the abdomen, the transverse colon runs across the upper abdomen from right to left, and then the descending colon and sigmoid and rectum lie on the left side of the abdomen. Rarely, masses arising from the colon will be felt in the abdomen.

Other important anatomical areas include the **inguinal canal** and the **anorectum** which will be described later in this chapter in relation to examination of hernias and the rectal examination.

Positioning the patient

For the proper examination of the abdomen it is important that the patient be lying flat with the head resting on a single pillow (Figure 6.2). This relaxes the abdominal muscles and facilitates

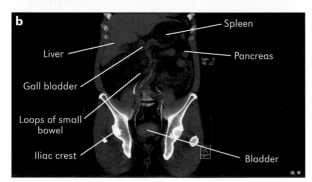

Figure 6.1 MRI scans of the abdomen
(a) Front. (b) Back.
(Courtesy M Thomson, National Capital Diagnostic Imaging, Canberra.)

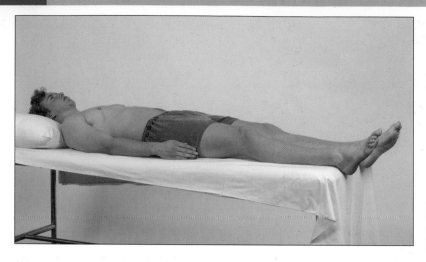

Figure 6.2 Gastrointestinal examination: positioning the patient

abdominal palpation. Helping the patient into this position affords the opportunity to make a general inspection.

General appearance
Jaundice

The yellow discoloration of the sclerae (conjunctivae) and the skin that results from hyperbilirubinaemia is best observed in natural daylight (page 185). Whatever the underlying cause, the depth of jaundice can be quite variable.

Weight and wasting

The patient's weight must be recorded. Failure of the gastrointestinal tract to absorb food normally may lead to loss of weight and cachexia. This may also be the result of gastrointestinal malignancy or alcoholic cirrhosis. Folds of loose skin may be visible hanging from the abdomen and limbs. These suggest recent weight loss. Obesity can cause fatty infiltration of the liver (non-alcoholic steatohepatitis) and result in abnormal liver function tests. Anabolic steroid use can induce increase in muscle bulk (sometimes considered desirable) and various liver tumours, including adenomas or hepatocellular carcinomas.

Skin

The gastrointestinal tract and the skin have a common origin from the embryoblast. A number of diseases can present with both skin and gut involvement (Figures 6.3–6.8, Table 6.4).[8]

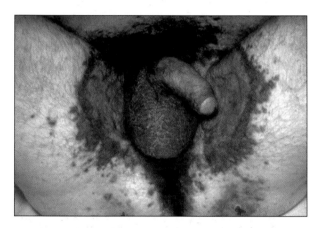

Figure 6.3 (above) Glucagonoma: migratory rash involving the groin
(From McDonald FS, ed., *Mayo Clinic images in internal medicine*, with permission. © Mayo Clinic Scientific Press and CRC Press.)

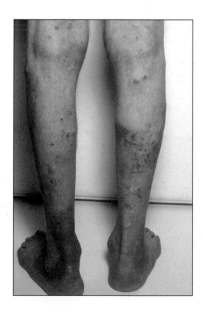

Figure 6.4 (right) **Dermatitis herpetiformis**
(From McDonald FS, ed., *Mayo Clinic images in internal medicine*, with permission. © Mayo Clinic Scientific Press and CRC Press.)

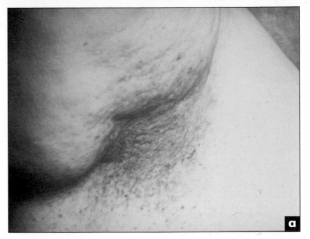

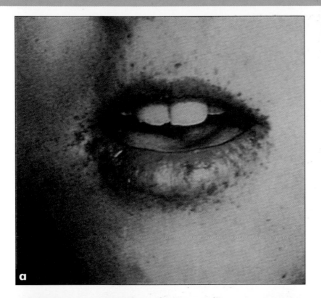

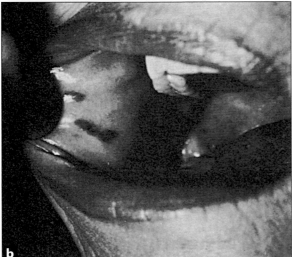

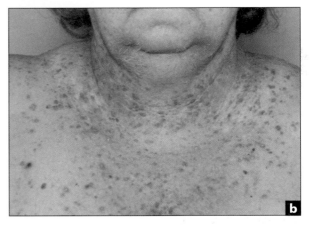

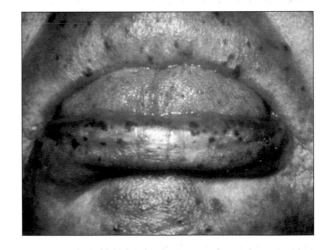

Figure 6.6 Acanthosis nigricans: (a) axilla; (b) chest wall
(From McDonald FS, ed., *Mayo Clinic images in internal medicine*, with permission. © Mayo Clinic Scientific Press and CRC Press.)

Figure 6.5 Peutz-Jeghers syndrome, with discrete brown-black lesions of the lips
(Figure (a) from Jones DV et al, in Feldman M et al, *Sleisenger & Fordtran's gastrointestinal disease*, 6th edn, Chapter 112. Philadelphia: WB Saunders, 1998, with permission. Figure (b) from McDonald FS, ed., *Mayo Clinic images in internal medicine*, with permission. © Mayo Clinic Scientific Press and CRC Press.)

Figure 6.7 (right) Hereditary haemorrhagic telangiectasia involving the lips
(From McDonald FS, ed., *Mayo Clinic images in internal medicine*, with permission. © Mayo Clinic Scientific Press and CRC Press.)

TABLE 6.4 The skin and the gut

Disease	Skin	Gut	Other associations
Gastrointestinal polyposis syndromes			
Peutz-Jeghers syndrome (autosomal dominant)	Pigmented macules on hands, feet, lips	Hamartomatous polyps (rarely adenocarcinoma) in stomach, small bowel, large bowel	
Gardner's* syndrome (autosomal dominant)	Cysts, fibromas, lipomas (multiple)	Polyps, adenocarcinoma in large bowel	Bone osteomata
Cronkhite-Canada syndrome	Alopecia, hyperpigmentation, glossitis, dystrophic nails	Hamartomatous polyps, diarrhoea, exocrine pancreatic insufficiency	
Hormone-secreting tumours			
Carcinoid syndrome	Flushing, telangiectases	Watery diarrhoea, hepatomegaly	Wheeze, right heart murmurs
Systemic mastocytosis (due to mast cell proliferation and histamine release)	Telangiectases, flushing, pigmented papules, pruritus, dermographism, Darier's† sign (rub skin lesion with the blunt end of a pen: a palpable red wheal occurs minutes later)	Peptic ulcer, diarrhoea, malabsorption	Asthma, headache, tachycardia
Glucagonoma (glucagon-secreting tumour)	Migratory necrolytic rash (on flexural and friction areas)	Glossitis, weight loss, diabetes mellitus	
Vascular disorders			
Hereditary haemorrhagic telangiectasia (autosomal dominant)	Telangiectases (especially nail beds, palms, feet)	Gastrointestinal bleeding	Nasopharyngeal bleeding, pulmonary arteriovenous fistulas, high output cardiac failure
Pseudoxanthoma elasticum (autosomal recessive)	Yellow plaques/papules in flexural areas	Bowel bleeding, ischaemia	Angioid streaks in fundus
Blue rubber bleb syndrome	Hemangiomas (e.g. tongue)	Bleeding into bowel or liver	
Degos' disease (malignant atrophic papulosis)	Dome-shaped red papules (early), small porcelain white atrophic scars (late)	Intestinal perforation, infarction (primarily in young men—very rare)	

TABLE 6.4 The skin and the gut (continued)

Disease	Skin	Gut	Other associations
Vascular disorders (continued)			
Acanthosis nigricans	Brown to black skin papillomas (usually axillae)	Carcinoma	Acromegaly, diabetes mellitus
Dermatitis herpetiformis	Pruritic vesicles—typically on knees, elbows, buttocks	Coeliac disease	
Zinc deficiency	Red, scaly, crusting lesions around mouth, eyes, genitalia; white patches on tongue	Diarrhoea (zinc deficiency occurs particularly in setting of Crohn's disease with fistulas, cirrhosis, parenteral nutrition, pancreatitis)	
Porphyria cutanea tarda	Vesicles on exposed skin (e.g. hands)	Alcoholic liver disease	
Inflammatory bowel disease	Pyoderma gangrenosum		
	Erythema nodosum		
	Clubbing		
	Mouth ulcers		
Haemochromatosis (autosomal recessive)	Skin pigmentation (bronze)	Hepatomegaly, signs of chronic liver disease	Diabetes mellitus, heart failure (cardiomyopathy), arthropathy, testicular atrophy
Systemic sclerosis	Skin that is thick and bound down, calcinosis, Raynaud's[‡] phenomenon, sclerodactyly, telangiectases	Gastro-oesophageal reflux, oesophageal dysmotility, small bowel bacterial overgrowth with malabsorption	

* Eldon John Gardner (b. 1909), American geneticist.
[†] Ferdinand Jean Darier (1856–1938), Paris dermatologist.
[‡] Maurice Raynaud (1834–1881), Paris physician.

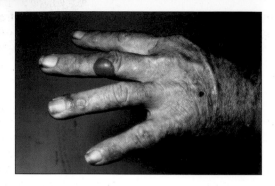

Figure 6.8 Porphyria cutanea tarda—scarring from photosensitivity

Pigmentation. Generalised skin pigmentation can result from chronic liver disease, especially in haemochromatosis (due to haemosiderin-stimulating melanocytes, to produce melanin). Malabsorption may result in Addisonian-type pigmentation ('sunkissed' pigmentation) of the nipples, palmar creases, pressure areas and mouth (page 311).

Peutz-Jeghers[c] **syndrome.** Freckle-like spots (discrete, brown-black lesions) around the mouth and on the buccal mucosa (Figure 6.5) and on the fingers and toes, are associated with hamartomas of the small bowel (50%) and colon (30%), which can present with bleeding or intussusception. In this autosomal dominant condition the incidence of gastrointestinal adenocarcinoma is increased.

Acanthosis nigricans. These are brown-to-black velvety elevations of the epidermis due to confluent papillomas and are usually found in the axillae and nape of the neck (Figure 6.6). Acanthosis nigricans is associated rarely with gastrointestinal carcinoma (particularly stomach) and lymphoma, as well as with acromegaly, diabetes mellitus and other endocrinopathies.

Hereditary haemorrhagic telangiectasia (Rendu-Osler-Weber syndrome[d]). Multiple small telangiectasia occur in this disease. They are often present on the lips and tongue (Figure 6.7), but may be found anywhere on the skin. When they are present in the gastrointestinal tract they can cause chronic blood loss or even, occasionally, torrential bleeding. An associated arteriovenous malform-

ation in the liver may be present. This is an autosomal dominant condition and is uncommon.

Porphyria cutanea tarda. Fragile vesicles appear on exposed areas of the skin and heal with scarring (Figure 6.8). The urine is dark in this chronic disorder of porphyrin metabolism associated with alcoholism, liver disease and hepatitis C.

Systemic sclerosis. Tense tethering of the skin in systemic sclerosis is often associated with gastro-oesophageal reflux and gastrointestinal motility disorders (page 285).

Mental state

Assess orientation (page 380). The syndrome of hepatic encephalopathy, due to decompensated advanced cirrhosis (chronic liver failure) or fulminant hepatitis (acute liver failure), is an organic neurological disturbance. The features depend on the aetiology and the precipitating factors (page 188). Patients eventually become stuporous and then comatose. The combination of hepatocellular damage and portosystemic shunting due to disturbed hepatic structure (both extrahepatic and intrahepatic) causes this syndrome. It is probably related to the liver's failure to remove toxic metabolites from the portal blood. These toxic metabolites may include ammonia, mercaptans, short-chain fatty acids and amines.

The hands

Even the experienced gastroenterologist must restrain his or her excitement and begin the examination of the gastrointestinal tract with the hands. The signs that may be elicited here give a clue to the presence of chronic liver disease. Whatever its aetiology, permanent diffuse liver damage results in similar peripheral signs. However, none of these signs alone is specific for chronic liver disease.

Nails

Leuconychia. When chronic liver or other disease results in hypoalbuminaemia, the nail beds opacify (the abnormality is of the nail bed and not of the nail), often leaving only a rim of pink nail bed at the top of the nail (Terry's nails;[e] Figure 6.9). The thumb and index nails are most often involved. The exact mechanism is uncertain. It may be that

c   John Peutz (1886–1957), physician at St John's Hospital, The Hague, Holland, first described this condition in 1921. Harold Jeghers (b. 1904), professor of medicine, Boston City Hospital, USA, described it in 1949.
d   Henri Rendu (1844–1902), French physician. Frederick Weber (1863–1962), English physician. The condition was described in 1907.

e   These changes were first described by Terry in 1954 in association with cirrhosis. They are also found in patients with cardiac failure and become more common in normal people with age. In a patient under the age of 50, their presence indicates cirrhosis, heart failure or diabetes, with a likelihood ratio of 5.3.

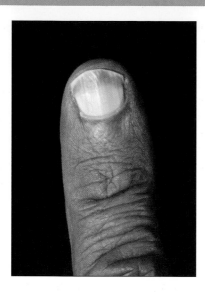

Figure 6.9 Leuconychia—Terry's nails
(From McDonald FS, ed., *Mayo Clinic images in internal medicine*, with permission. © Mayo Clinic Scientific Press and CRC Press.)

the explanation is compression of capillary flow by extracellular fluid.

Muehrcke's lines (transverse white lines) can also occur in hypoalbuminaemic states, including cirrhosis. Blue lunulae may be seen in patients with Wilson's disease (hepatolenticular degeneration).

Clubbing. Up to one-third of patients with cirrhosis may have finger clubbing. In at least some cases, this may be related to arteriovenous (AV) shunting in the lungs, resulting in arterial oxygen desaturation. Cyanosis may be associated with severe long-standing chronic liver disease. The cause of this pulmonary AV shunting is unknown. Conditions such as inflammatory bowel disease and coeliac disease, which cause long-standing nutritional depletion, can also cause clubbing.

The palms

Palmar erythema ('liver palms'). This is reddening of the palms of the hands affecting the thenar and hypothenar eminences. Often the soles of the feet are also affected. This can be a feature of chronic liver disease. While the finding has been attributed to raised oestrogen levels, it has not been shown to be related to plasma oestradiol levels, so the aetiology remains uncertain. Palmar erythema can also occur with pregnancy, thyrotoxicosis, rheumatoid arthritis, polycythaemia and rarely with chronic febrile diseases or chronic leukaemia. It may also be a normal finding, especially in women, and like spider naevi can occur in pregnancy.

Anaemia. Inspect the palmar creases for pallor suggesting anaemia, which may result from gastrointestinal blood loss, malabsorption (folate, vitamin B_{12}), haemolysis (e.g. hypersplenism) or chronic disease.

Dupuytren's contracture.[f] This is a visible and palpable thickening and contraction of the palmar fascia causing permanent flexion, most often of the ring finger. It is often bilateral and occasionally affects the feet. It is associated with alcoholism (not liver disease), but is also found in some manual workers; it may be familial. The palmar fascia of these patients contains abnormally large amounts of xanthine, and this may be related to the pathogenesis.

Hepatic flap (asterixis[g])

Before leaving the hands one should ask the patient to stretch out the arms in front, separate the fingers and extend the wrists for 15 seconds. Jerky, irregular flexion–extension movement at the wrist and metacarpophalangeal joints, often accompanied by lateral movements of the fingers, constitute the flapping of hepatic encephalopathy. It is thought to be due to interference with the inflow of joint position sense information to the reticular formation in the brainstem. This results in rhythmical lapses of postural muscle tone. Occasionally the arms, neck, tongue, jaws and eyelids can also be involved. It can be demonstrated if the patient is asked to close the eyes forcefully or to protrude the tongue. The flap is usually bilateral, tends to be absent at rest, and is brought on by sustained posture. The rhythmic movements are not synchronous on each side and the flap is absent when coma supervenes.

Although this flap is a characteristic and early sign of liver failure, it is not diagnostic: it can also occur in cardiac, respiratory and renal failure, as well as in hypoglycaemia, hypokalaemia, hypomagnesaemia or barbiturate intoxication.

An apparent tremor (really a form of choreoathetosis, page 399) may occur in Wilson's disease. A fine resting tremor is common in alcoholism.

The arms

Inspect the upper limbs for *bruising*. Large bruises (ecchymoses) may be due to clotting abnormalities. Hepatocellular damage can interfere with protein

---

[f] Baron Guillaume Dupuytren (1777–1835), Surgeon-in-Chief at the Hotel-Dieu in Paris. A cold, rude, ambitious and arrogant man, he was called 'the Napoleon of surgery'. He saw 10,000 private patients a year.

[g] From Greek *a*, 'not' and *sterixis*, 'fixed position'.

synthesis and therefore the production of all the clotting factors (except factor VIII, which is made elsewhere in the reticuloendothelial system). Obstructive jaundice results in a shortage of bile acids in the intestine, and therefore may reduce absorption of vitamin K (a fat-soluble vitamin), which is essential for the production of clotting factors II (prothrombin), VII, IX and X.

Petechiae (pinhead-sized bruises) may also be present. Chronic excessive alcohol consumption can sometimes result in bone marrow depression, causing thrombocytopenia, which may be responsible for petechiae. In addition, splenomegaly secondary to portal hypertension can cause hypersplenism, with resultant excessive destruction of platelets in the spleen; in severe liver disease (especially acute hepatic necrosis), diffuse intravascular coagulation can occur.

Look for muscle wasting, which is often a late manifestation of malnutrition in alcoholic patients. Alcohol can also cause a proximal myopathy (page 391).

Scratch marks due to severe itch (pruritus) are often prominent in patients with obstructive or cholestatic jaundice. This is commonly the presenting feature of primary biliary cirrhosis[h] before other signs are apparent. The mechanism of pruritus is thought to be retention of an unknown substance normally excreted in the bile, rather than bile salt deposition in the skin as was earlier thought.

Spider naevi[i] (Figure 6.10) consist of a central arteriole from which radiate numerous small vessels which look like spiders' legs. They range in size from just visible to half a centimetre in diameter. Their usual distribution is in the area drained by the superior vena cava, so they are found on the arms, neck and chest wall. They can occasionally bleed profusely. Pressure applied with a pointed object to the central arteriole causes blanching of the whole lesion. Rapid refilling from the centre to the legs occurs on release of the pressure.

The finding of more than two or three spider naevi anywhere on the body is likely to be abnormal. Spider naevi can be caused by cirrhosis, most frequently due to alcohol. In patients with cirrhosis the number of spider naevi may increase or decrease as the patient's condition changes, as does palmar erythema. They may occur transiently

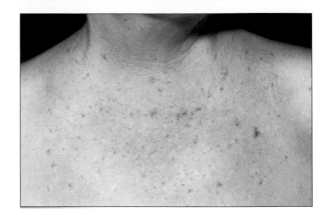

Figure 6.10 A large crop of spider naevi

with viral hepatitis. During the second to fifth months of pregnancy, spider naevi frequently appear, only to disappear again within days of delivery. It is not known why they occur only in the upper part of the body, but it may be related to the fact that this is the part of the body where flushing usually occurs. Like palmar erythema they are traditionally attributed to oestrogen excess. Part of the normal hepatic function is the inactivation of oestrogens, which is impaired in chronic liver disease. Oestrogens are known to have a dilating effect on the spiral arterioles of the endometrium, and this has been used to explain the presence of spider naevi, but changes in plasma oestradiol levels have not been found to correlate with the appearance and disappearance of spider naevi.

The differential diagnosis of spider naevi includes *Campbell de Morgan*[j] *spots,* venous stars and hereditary haemorrhagic telangiectasia. Campbell de Morgan spots are flat or slightly elevated red circular lesions that occur on the abdomen or the front of the chest. They do not blanch on pressure and are very common. *Venous stars* are 2- to 3-cm lesions that can occur on the dorsum of the feet, legs, back and the lower chest. They are due to elevated venous pressure and are found overlying the main tributary to a large vein. They are not obliterated by pressure. The blood flow is from the periphery to the centre of the lesion, which is the opposite of the flow in the spider naevus. Lesions of *hereditary haemorrhagic telangiectasia* (page 228) occasionally resemble spider naevi.

h   Primary biliary cirrhosis (PBC) is an uncommon chronic non-suppurative destructive cholangitis of unknown aetiology; 90% of affected patients are female.
i   Spider naevi were first described in 1867 by Erasmus Wilson, an English physician.

j   Campbell de Morgan (1811–76), London surgeon. He was one of the 300 original Fellows of the Royal College of Surgeons. He described his spots in 1872 and believed them to be a sign of cancer (which they are not).

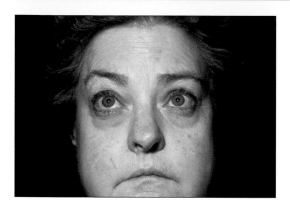

Figure 6.11 Scleral icterus

Palpate the axillae for *lymphadenopathy* (page 229). Look in the axillae for acanthosis nigricans.

The face
Eyes

Look first at the sclerae for signs of *jaundice* (Figure 6.11) or *anaemia*. Bitot's[k] spots are yellow keratinised areas on the sclera (Figure 6.12). They are the result of severe vitamin A deficiency due to malabsorption or malnutrition. Retinal damage and blindness may occur as a later development. *Kayser-Fleischer rings*[l] (Figure 6.13) are brownish green rings occurring at the periphery of the cornea, affecting the upper pole more than the lower. They are due to deposits of excess copper in Descemet's membrane[m] of the cornea. Slit-lamp examination is often necessary to show them. They are typically found in Wilson's disease,[n] a copper storage disease that causes cirrhosis and neurological disturbances. The Kayser-Fleischer rings are usually present by the time neurological signs have appeared. Patients with other cholestatic liver diseases, however, can also have these rings. *Iritis* may be seen in inflammatory bowel disease (page 191).

Xanthelasma are yellowish plaques in the subcutaneous tissues in the periorbital region and are due to deposits of lipids (see Figure 4.19, page 57). They may indicate protracted elevation of the serum cholesterol. In patients with cholestasis, an abnormal lipoprotein (lipoprotein X) is found in

---

[k]   Pierre Bitot (1822–88) described this in 1863.
[l]   Bernhard Kayser (1869–1954), German ophthalmologist, described these rings in 1902. Bruno Fleischer (1848–1904), German ophthalmologist, described them in 1903.
[m] Jean Descemet (1732–1810), professor of surgery and anatomy, Paris. He described the membrane in 1785.
[n]   Samuel Alexander Wilson (1878–1937), London neurologist at Queen Square. His colleagues there included Gowers and Hughlings Jackson. He described his disease in 1912 in his MD thesis. He also described the glabellar tap sign in Parkinson's disease, which is sometimes called Wilson's sign. He did not, however, describe the Kayser-Fleischer rings.

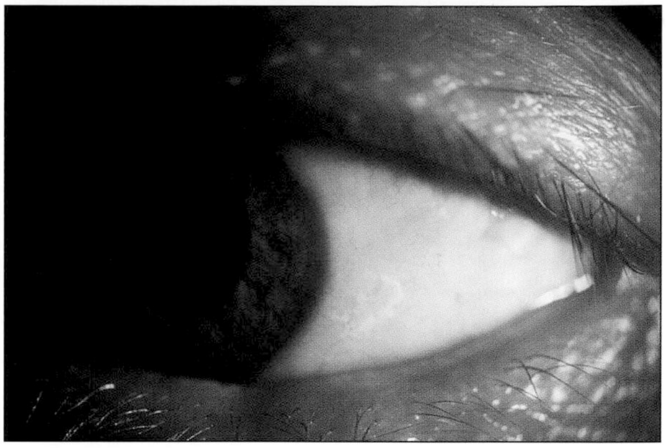

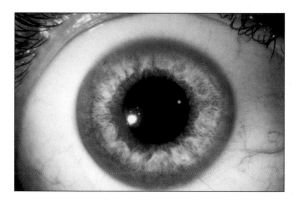

Figure 6.12 Bitot spot: focal area of conjunctival xerosis with a foamy appearance
(From Mir MA, *Atlas of Clinical Diagnosis*, 2nd edn. Edinburgh: Saunders, 2003, with permission.)

Figure 6.13 Kayser-Fleischer rings
(From McDonald FS, ed., *Mayo Clinic images in internal medicine*, with permission. © Mayo Clinic Scientific Press and CRC Press.)

the plasma and is associated with elevation of the serum cholesterol. Xanthelasma are common in patients with primary biliary cirrhosis.

Periorbital purpura following proctosigmoidoscopy ('black eye syndrome') is a characteristic sign of amyloidosis (perhaps related to factor X deficiency) but is exceedingly rare (Figure 6.14).

Salivary glands

Next inspect and palpate the cheeks over the parotid area for *parotid enlargement* (Table 6.5). Ask the patient to clench the teeth so that the masseter muscle is palpable; the normal parotid gland is impalpable but the enlarged gland is best felt behind the masseter muscle and in front of the ear. Parotidomegaly that is bilateral is associated with alcoholism rather than liver disease per se. It is due to fatty infiltration, perhaps secondary to alcohol toxicity with or without malnutrition. A tender,

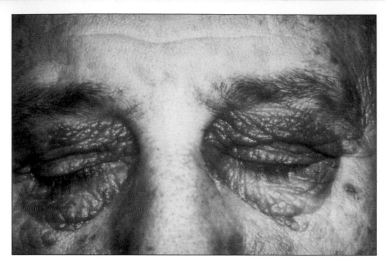

Figure 6.14 Amyloidosis causing periorbital purpura
Note the periorbital purpura that followed a proctoscopic examination, a characteristic (albeit rare) sign.
(From McDonald FS, ed., *Mayo Clinic images in internal medicine*, with permission. © Mayo Clinic Scientific Press and CRC Press.)

warm, swollen parotid suggests the diagnosis of parotiditis following an acute illness or surgery. A mixed parotid tumour (a pleomorphic adenoma) is the commonest cause of a lump. Parotid carcinoma may cause a facial nerve palsy (page 343). Feel in the mouth for a parotid calculus, which may be present at the parotid duct orifice (opposite the upper second molar). Mumps also causes acute parotid enlargement which is usually bilateral.

Submandibular gland enlargement is most often due to a calculus. This may be palpable bimanually (Figure 6.15). The examiner's gloved index finger is placed on the floor of the mouth beside the tongue, feeling between it and fingers placed behind the body of the mandible. It may also be enlarged in chronic liver disease.

The mouth

The teeth and breath. The very beginning of the gastrointestinal tract is, like the very end of the tract, accessible to inspection without elaborate equipment.[9] Look first briefly at the state of the teeth and note whether they are real or false. False teeth will have to be removed for a complete examination of the mouth. Note whether there is gum hypertrophy (Table 6.6) or pigmentation (Table 6.7). Loose-fitting false teeth may be responsible for ulcers and decayed teeth may be responsible for fetor (bad breath).

Other causes of fetor are listed in Table 6.8. These must be distinguished from *fetor hepaticus* which is a rather sweet smell of the breath. It is

---

TABLE 6.5 Causes of parotid enlargement

Bilateral

1 Mumps (can be unilateral)

2 Sarcoidosis or lymphoma, which may cause painless bilateral enlargement

3 Mikulicz* syndrome: bilateral painless enlargement of all three salivary glands. This disease is probably an early stage of Sjögren's syndrome

5 Alcohol-associated parotitis

6 Malnutrition

7 Severe dehydration: as occurs in renal failure, terminal carcinomatosis and severe infections

Unilateral

1 Mixed parotid tumour (occasionally bilateral)

2 Tumour infiltration, which usually causes painless unilateral enlargement and may cause facial nerve palsy

3 Duct blockage, e.g. salivary calculus

* Johann von Mikulicz-Radecki (1850–1905), professor of surgery, Breslau. He described this condition in 1892.

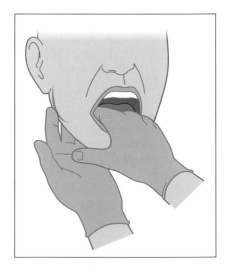

Figure 6.15 Examination of the submandibular gland

an indication of severe hepatocellular disease and may be due to methylmercaptans. These substances are known to be exhaled in the breath and may be derived from methionine when this amino acid is not demethylated by a diseased liver. Severe fetor hepaticus that fills the patient's room is a bad sign and indicates a precomatose condition in many cases. The presence of fetor hepaticus in a patient with a coma of unknown cause may be a helpful clue to the diagnosis.

Unless the smell is obvious one should get a patient to exhale through the mouth while one sniffs a little of the exhaled air.

The tongue. Thickened epithelium with bacterial debris and food particles commonly causes a *coating* over the tongue, especially in smokers. It is rarely a sign of disease and is more marked on the posterior part of the tongue where there is less mobility and the papillae desquamate more slowly. It occurs frequently in respiratory tract infections, but is in no way related to constipation or any serious abdominal disorder.

Lingua nigra (black tongue) is due to elongation of papillae over the posterior part of the tongue, which appears dark brown because of the accumulation of keratin. There is no known cause and apart from its aesthetic problems it is symptomless. Bismuth compounds may also cause a black tongue.

Geographical tongue is a term used to describe slowly changing red rings and lines that occur on the surface of the tongue. It is not painful, and the condition tends to come and go. It is not usually of any significance, but can be a sign of riboflavin (vitamin B_2) deficiency.

Leucoplakia is white-coloured thickening of the mucosa of the tongue and mouth; the condition is premalignant. Most of the causes of leucoplakia begin with 'S': sore teeth (poor dental hygiene), smoking, spirits, sepsis or syphilis, but often no cause is apparent. Leucoplakia may also occur on the larynx, anus and vulva.

The term *glossitis* is generally used to describe a smooth appearance of the tongue which may also be erythematous. The appearance is due to atrophy of the papillae, and in later stages there may be shallow ulceration. These changes occur in the tongue often as a result of nutritional deficiencies to which the tongue is sensitive because of the rapid turnover of mucosal cells. Deficiencies of iron, folate and the vitamin B group, especially vitamin B_{12}, are common causes. Glossitis is common in alcoholics and can also occur in the rare carcinoid syndrome. However, many cases,

especially those in elderly people, are impossible to explain.

Enlargement of the tongue (*macroglossia*) may occur in congenital conditions such as Down syndrome (page 314) or in endocrine disease, including acromegaly (page 307). Tumour infiltration (e.g. haemangioma or lymphangioma)

TABLE 6.6 Causes of gum hypertrophy
1 Phenytoin
2 Pregnancy
3 Scurvy (vitamin C deficiency: the gums become spongy, red, bleed easily and are swollen and irregular)
4 Gingivitis, e.g. from smoking, calculus, plaque, Vincent's* angina (fusobacterial membranous tonsillitis)
5 Leukaemia (usually monocytic)
* Jean Hyacinthe Vincent (1862–1950), professor of forensic medicine and French Army bacteriologist, described this in 1898.

TABLE 6.7 Causes of pigmented lesions in the mouth
1 Heavy metals: lead or bismuth (blue-black line on the gingival margin), iron (haemochromatosis—blue-grey pigmentation of the hard palate)
2 Drugs: antimalarials, the oral contraceptive pill (brown or black areas of pigmentation anywhere in the mouth)
3 Addison's disease (blotches of dark brown pigment anywhere in the mouth)
4 Peutz-Jeghers syndrome (lips, buccal mucosa or palate)
5 Malignant melanoma (raised, painless black lesions anywhere in the mouth)

TABLE 6.8 Causes of fetor (bad breath)
1 Faulty oral hygiene
2 Fetor hepaticus (a sweet smell)
3 Ketosis (diabetic ketoacidosis results in excretion of ketones in exhaled air, causing a sickly sweet smell)
4 Uraemia (fish breath: an ammoniacal odour)
5 Alcohol (distinctive)
6 Paraldehyde
7 Putrid (due to anaerobic chest infections with large amounts of sputum)
8 Cigarettes

TABLE 6.9 Causes of mouth ulcers
Common
Aphthous
Drugs (e.g. gold, steroids)
Trauma
Uncommon
Gastrointestinal disease: Crohn's disease, ulcerative colitis, coeliac disease
Rheumatological disease: Behçet's* syndrome, Reiter's[†] syndrome
Erythema multiforme
Infection: viral—herpes zoster, herpes simplex; bacterial—syphilis (primary chancre, secondary snail track ulcers, mucous patches), tuberculosis
Self-inflicted

* Halusi Behçet (1889–1948), Turkish dermatologist. He described the disease in 1937.
[†] Hans Reiter (1881–1969), Berlin bacteriologist, described this in 1916.

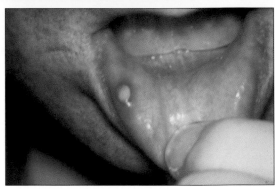

Figure 6.16 Aphthous ulceration
(From McDonald FS, ed., *Mayo Clinic images in internal medicine*, with permission. © Mayo Clinic Scientific Press and CRC Press.)

or infiltration of the tongue with amyloid material in amyloidosis can also be responsible for macroglossia.

Mouth ulcers. This is an important topic because a number of systemic diseases can present with ulcers in the mouth (Table 6.9). *Aphthous ulceration* is the commonest type seen (Figure 6.16). This begins as a small painful vesicle on the tongue or mucosal surface of the mouth, which may break down to form a painful, shallow ulcer. These ulcers heal without scarring. The cause is completely unknown. They usually do not indicate any serious underlying systemic disease, but may occur in Crohn's[o] disease or coeliac disease. HIV infection may be associated with a number of mouth lesions (page 457). *Angular stomatitis* refers to cracks at the corners of the mouth; causes include deficiencies in vitamin B_6, vitamin B_{12}, folate and iron.

Candidiasis (moniliasis). Fungal infection with *Candida albicans* (thrush) causes creamy white curd-like patches in the mouth which are removed only with difficulty and leave a bleeding surface. The infection may spread to involve the oesophagus, causing dysphagia or odynophagia. Moniliasis is associated with immunosuppression (steroids, tumour chemotherapy, alcoholism or an underlying immunological abnormality such as HIV infection,

or haematological malignancy), where it is due to decreased host resistance. Broad-spectrum antibiotics, which inhibit the normal oral flora, are also a common cause, because fungal overgrowth is permitted. Faulty oral hygiene, iron deficiency and diabetes mellitus can also be responsible. Rarely, chronic mucocutaneous candidiasis, a distinct syndrome comprising recurrent or persistent oral thrush, fingernail or toenail bed infection and skin involvement, occurs; in some of these patients, endocrine diseases such as hypoparathyroidism, hypothyroidism or Addison's disease are associated (page 305).

The neck and chest

Palpate the cervical lymph nodes. It is particularly important to feel for the supraclavicular nodes, especially on the left side. These may be involved

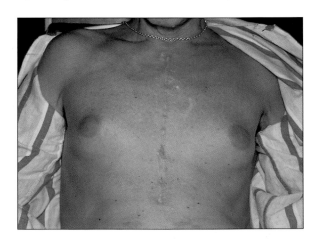

Figure 6.17 Gynaecomastia with prominent breasts and unassociated with confounding obesity
(From Mir MA, *Atlas of Clinical Diagnosis*, 2nd edn. Edinburgh: Saunders, 2003, with permission.)

---

o   Burrill Bernard Crohn (1884–1983), American gastroenterologist at Mount Sinai Hospital, New York, described this disease in 1932. It had previously been described by Morgagni (1682–1771) in 1769.

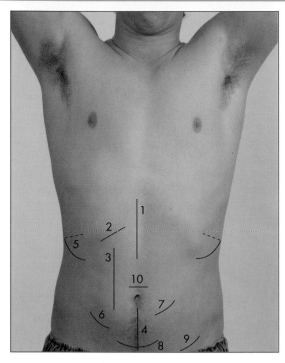

Figure 6.18 Abdominal scars
Note: Laparoscopic surgical scars are now common. Most of these procedures include a port about 2 cm in length, just above the umbilicus.

1. Upper midline
2. Right subcostal (Kocher's)
3. Right paramedian
4. Lower midline
5. Nephrectomy
6. Appendicectomy (Gridiron)
7. Transplanted kidney
8. Suprapubic (Pfannensteil)
9. Left inguinal
10. Umbilical port—laparoscopic surgery

with advanced gastric or other gastrointestinal malignancy, or with lung cancer. The presence of a large left supraclavicular node (Virchow's node) in combination with carcinoma of the stomach is called Troisier's sign.[p] Look for spider naevi.

In males, *gynaecomastia* may be a sign of chronic liver disease. Gynaecomastia may be unilateral or bilateral and the breasts may be tender (Figure 6.17). This may be a sign of cirrhosis, particularly alcoholic cirrhosis, or of chronic autoimmune hepatitis. In chronic liver disease, changes in the oestradiol-to-testosterone ratio may be responsible. In cirrhotic patients, spironolactone, used to treat ascites, is also a common cause. Gynaecomastia may also occur in alcoholics without liver disease because of damage to the Leydig cells[q] of the testis from alcohol. A number of drugs may rarely cause gynaecomastia (e.g. digoxin, cimetidine).

The abdomen

Self-restraint is no longer required and it is now time to examine the abdomen itself.

Inspection

The patient should lie flat, with one pillow under the head and the abdomen exposed from the nipples to the pubic symphysis (see Figure 6.2). It may be preferable to expose this area in stages to preserve the patient's dignity.

Does the patient appear unwell? The patient with an *acute abdomen* may be lying very still and have shallow breathing (page 186).

Inspection begins with a careful look for abdominal *scars,* which may indicate previous surgery or trauma (Figure 6.18). Look in the area around the umbilicus for laparoscopic surgical scars. Older scars are white and recent scars are pink because the tissue remains vascular. Note the presence of stomata (end-colostomy, loop colostomy, ileostomy or ileal conduit) or fistulae. There may be visible abdominal striae following weight loss.

Generalised abdominal *distension* (Figure 6.19) may be present. All the causes of this sound as if they begin with the letter 'F': fat (gross obesity), fluid (ascites), fetus, flatus (gaseous distension due to bowel obstruction), faeces, 'filthy' big tumour (e.g. ovarian tumour or hydatid cyst) or 'phantom' pregnancy. Look at the shape of the umbilicus, which may give a clue to the underlying cause. An umbilicus buried in fat suggests that the patient eats too much. However, when the peritoneal cavity is filled with large volumes of fluid (ascites) from whatever cause, the abdominal flanks and wall appear tense and the umbilicus is shallow or everted and points downwards. In pregnancy the umbilicus is pushed upwards by the uterus enlarging from

---

p   Charles Émile Troisier (1844–1919), professor of pathology in Paris, described this sign in 1886.
q   Franz von Leydig (1821–1908), Bonn anatomist and zoologist, Germany.

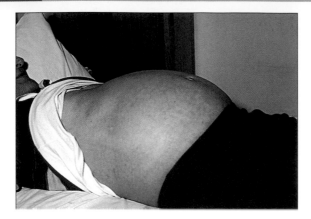

Figure 6.19 Abdomen distended with ascites: umbilicus points downwards, unlike cases of distension due to a pelvic mass

the pelvis. This appearance may also result from a huge ovarian cyst.

Local *swellings* may indicate enlargement of one of the abdominal or pelvic organs. A hernia is a protrusion of an intra-abdominal structure through an abnormal opening; this may occur because of weakening of the abdominal wall by previous surgery (incisional hernia), a congenital abdominal wall defect, or chronically increased intra-abdominal pressure.

Prominent *veins* may be obvious on the abdominal wall. If these are present, the direction of venous flow should be elicited at this stage. A finger is used to occlude the vein and blood is then emptied from the vein below the occluding finger with a second finger. The second finger is removed and, if the vein refills, flow is occurring towards the occluding finger (Figure 6.20). Flow should be tested separately in veins above and below the umbilicus.

In patients with severe portal hypertension, portal to systemic flow occurs through the umbilical veins, which may become engorged and distended (Figure 6.21). The direction of flow then is away from the umbilicus. Because of their engorged appearance they have been likened to the mythical Medusa's hair after Minerva had turned it into snakes; this sign is called a *caput Medusae* (head of Medusa) but is very rare (Figure 6.22). Usually only one or two veins (often epigastric) are visible. Engorgement can also occur because of inferior vena caval obstruction, usually due to a tumour or thrombosis but sometimes because of tense ascites. In this case the abdominal veins enlarge to provide collateral blood flow from the legs, avoiding the blocked inferior vena cava. The direction of flow is then upwards towards the heart. Therefore, to distinguish caput Medusae from inferior vena caval obstruction, determine the direction of flow *below* the umbilicus; it will be towards the legs in the former and towards the head in the latter. Prominent superficial veins can occasionally be congenital.

Pulsations may be visible. An expanding central pulsation in the epigastrium suggests an abdominal aortic aneurysm. However, the abdominal aorta can often be seen to pulsate in normal thin people.

Visible peristalsis may occur occasionally in very thin normal people; however, it usually suggests intestinal obstruction. Pyloric obstruction due to peptic ulceration or tumour may cause visible peristalsis, seen as a slow wave of movement passing across the upper abdomen from left to right. Obstruction of the distal small bowel can cause similar movements in a ladder pattern in the centre of the abdomen.

Skin lesions should also be noted on the abdominal wall. These include the vesicles of

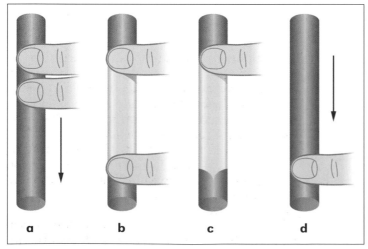

Figure 6.20 Detecting the direction of flow of a vein
(a) Place two fingers firmly on the vein. (b) The second finger is moved along the vein to empty it of blood and keep it occluded. (c) The second finger is removed but the vein does not refill. (d) At repeat testing and removing the first finger, filling occurs, indicating the direction of flow. (Adapted from Swash M, ed. *Hutchison's clinical methods,* 20th edn. Philadelphia: Baillière Tindall, 1995, with permission.)

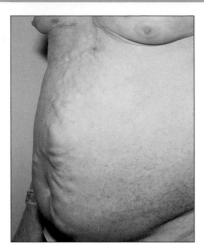

Figure 6.21 Distended abdominal veins in a patient with portal hypertension
(From Mir MA, *Atlas of Clinical Diagnosis,* 2nd edn. Edinburgh: Saunders, 2003, with permission.)

herpes zoster, which occur in a radicular pattern (they are localised to only one side of the abdomen in the distribution of a single nerve root). Herpes zoster may be responsible for severe abdominal pain that is of mysterious origin until the rash appears. The Sister Joseph[r] nodule is a metastatic tumour deposit in the umbilicus, the anatomical region where the peritoneum is closest to the skin. Discoloration of the umbilicus where a faintly bluish hue is present is found rarely, in cases of extensive haemoperitoneum and acute pancreatitis (Cullen's sign[s]—the umbilical 'black eye'). Skin discoloration may also rarely occur in the flanks in severe cases of acute pancreatitis (Grey-Turner's sign[t]).

Stretching of the abdominal wall severe enough to cause rupture of the elastic fibres in the skin produces pink linear marks with a wrinkled appearance, which are called *striae*. When these are wide and purple-coloured, Cushing's syndrome may be the cause (page 309). Ascites, pregnancy or recent weight gain are much more common causes of striae.

Next, squat down beside the bed so that the patient's abdomen is at eye level. Ask him or her to take slow deep breaths through the mouth and watch for evidence of asymmetrical movement, indicating the presence of a mass. In particular

---

[r] Sister Joseph of St Mary's Hospital, Rochester, Minnesota, described this sign to Dr William Mayo (1861–1939) of the Mayo Clinic.
[s] Thomas S Cullen (1869–1953), professor of gynaecology at Johns Hopkins University, Baltimore, originally described this sign as an indication of a ruptured ectopic pregnancy.
[t] George Grey-Turner (1877–1951), surgeon, Royal Victoria Infirmary, Newcastle-on-Tyne, England.

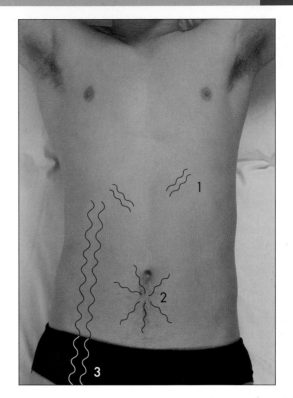

Figure 6.22 Prominent veins on the abdominal wall
1 = thin veins over the costal margin—not of clinical relevance. 2 = caput Medusae. 3 = inferior vena caval obstruction.
(Based on Swash M, ed. *Hutchison's clinical methods*, 20th edn. Philadelphia: Baillière Tindall, 1995.)

a large liver may be seen to move below the right costal margin or a large spleen below the left costal margin.

Palpation

This part of the examination often reveals the most information. Successful palpation requires relaxed abdominal muscles. To this end, reassure the patient that the examination will not be painful and use warm hands. Ask the patient if any particular area is tender and examine this area last. Encourage the patient to breathe gently through the mouth. If necessary, ask the patient to bend the knees to relax the abdominal wall muscles.

For descriptive purposes the abdomen has been divided into nine areas or regions (Figure 6.23). Palpation in each region is performed with the palmar surface of the fingers acting together. For the palpation of the edges of organs or masses, the lateral surface of the forefinger is the most sensitive part of the hand.

Palpation should begin with *light pressure* in each region. All the movements of the hand should occur

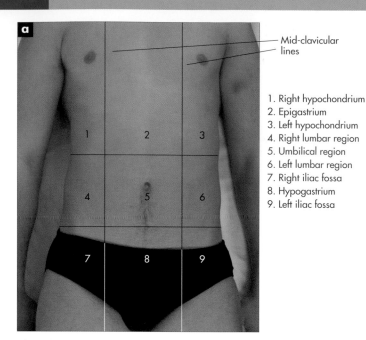

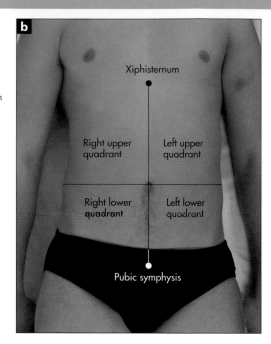

1. Right hypochondrium
2. Epigastrium
3. Left hypochondrium
4. Right lumbar region
5. Umbilical region
6. Left lumbar region
7. Right iliac fossa
8. Hypogastrium
9. Left iliac fossa

Figure 6.23 (a) Regions of the abdomen (b) Quadrants of the abdomen

at the metacarpophalangeal joints and the hand should be moulded to the shape of the abdominal wall. Note the presence of any tenderness or lumps in each region. As the hand moves over each region, the mind should be considering the anatomical structures that underlie it. *Deep palpation* of the abdomen is performed next, though care should be taken to avoid the tender areas until the end of the examination. Deep palpation is used to detect deeper masses and to define those already discovered. Any mass must be carefully characterised and described (Table 6.10).

Guarding of the abdomen (when resistance to palpation occurs due to contraction of the abdominal muscles) may result from tenderness or anxiety, and may be voluntary or involuntary. The latter suggests peritonitis. *Rigidity* is a constant involuntary contraction of the abdominal muscles always associated with tenderness and indicates peritoneal irritation. *Rebound tenderness* is said to be present when the abdominal wall, having been compressed slowly, is released rapidly and a sudden stab of pain results. This may make the patient wince, so the face should be watched while this manoeuvre is performed. It strongly suggests the presence of peritonitis and should be performed if there is doubt about the presence of localised or generalised peritonitis. The patient with a confirmed acute abdomen should not be subjected to repeated testing of rebound tenderness because of the distress this can cause. Be careful not

to surprise your patient by a sudden jabbing and release movement: rebound tenderness should be elicited slowly. If you suspect the patient may be feigning a tender abdomen, test for rebound with your stethoscope after telling the patient to lie still and quiet so that you can hear.

The liver. Feel for hepatomegaly (Figure 6.24).[10] With the examining hand aligned parallel to the right costal margin, and beginning in the right iliac fossa, ask the patient to breathe in and out slowly through the mouth. With each expiration the hand is advanced by 1 or 2 cm closer to the right

TABLE 6.10 Descriptive features of intra-abdominal masses
For any abdominal mass all the following should be determined:
1 Site: the region involved
2 Tenderness
3 Size (which must be measured) and shape
4 Surface, which may be regular or irregular
5 Edge, which may be regular or irregular
6 Consistency, which may be hard or soft
7 Mobility and movement with inspiration
8 Whether it is pulsatile or not
9 Whether one can get above the mass

costal margin. During inspiration the hand is kept still and the lateral margin of the forefinger waits expectantly for the liver edge to strike it.

If the liver edge has been identified, an attempt

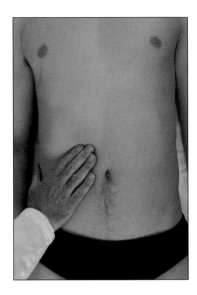

Figure 6.24 Abdominal examination: the liver

should be made to feel the surface of the liver. The edge of the liver and the surface itself may be hard or soft, tender or non-tender, regular or irregular, and pulsatile or non-pulsatile. The normal liver edge may be just palpable below the right costal margin on deep inspiration, especially in thin people. The edge is then felt to be soft and regular with a fairly sharply defined border and the surface of the liver itself is smooth. Sometimes only the left lobe of the liver may be palpable (to the left of the midline) in patients with cirrhosis.

If the liver edge is palpable the total *liver span* can be measured. Remember that the liver span varies with height and is greater in men than women, and that inter-observer error is quite large for this measurement. The normal upper border of the liver is level with the sixth rib in the midclavicular line. At this point the percussion note over the chest changes from resonant to dull (Figure 6.25a). To estimate the liver span (Figure 6.25b), percuss down along the right midclavicular line until the liver dullness is encountered and measure from here to the palpable liver edge. Careful assessment of the position of the midclavicular line will improve the accuracy of this measurement. The normal span is

Figure 6.25 Percussing the liver span: (a) upper border; (b) lower border

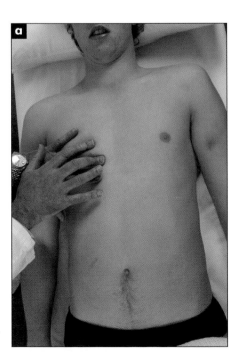
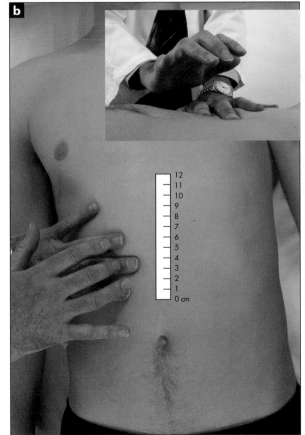

less than 13 cm. Note that the clinical estimate of the liver span usually underestimates its actual size by 2 to 5 cm.

Other causes of a normal but palpable liver include ptosis due to emphysema, asthma or a subdiaphragmatic collection, or a Riedel's lobe.[u] The Riedel's lobe is a tongue-like projection of the liver from the right lobe's inferior surface; it can be quite large and rarely extends as far as the right iliac fossa. It can be confused with an enlarged gallbladder or right kidney.

Many diseases cause hepatic enlargement and these are listed in Table 6.11. Detecting the liver edge below the costal margin clinically is highly specific (100%) but insensitive (48%)—positive LR 2.5, negative LR 0.5.[10,11] Remember, the diseased liver is not always enlarged; a small liver is common in advanced cirrhosis, and the liver shrinks rapidly with acute hepatic necrosis (due to liver cell death and collapse of the reticulin framework).

The gallbladder. The gallbladder is occasionally palpable below the right costal margin where this crosses the lateral border of the rectus muscles. If biliary obstruction or acute cholecystitis is suspected, the examining hand should be oriented perpendicular to the costal margin, feeling from medial to lateral. Unlike the liver edge, the gallbladder, if palpable, will be a bulbous, focal, rounded mass which moves downwards on inspiration. The causes of an enlarged gallbladder are listed in Table 6.12.

Murphy's sign[v] should be sought if cholecystitis is suspected (*Good signs guide 6.1*). On taking a deep breath, the patient catches his or her breath when an inflamed gallbladder presses on the examiner's hand, which is lying at the costal margin. Other signs are less helpful.

The clinician examining for an enlarged gallbladder must always be mindful of *Courvoisier's law*,[w] which states that, if the gallbladder is enlarged and the patient is jaundiced, the cause is unlikely to be gallstones. Rather, carcinoma of the pancreas or lower biliary tree resulting in obstructive jaundice is likely to be present. This is because the gallbladder with stones is usually chronically fibrosed and therefore incapable of enlargement. Note that if the gallbladder is not palpable, and the patient is jaundiced, some cause other than gallstones is still

---

[u] Bernhard Riedel (1846–1916), German surgeon, described this in 1888.
[v] John Murphy (1857–1916), American surgeon, professor of surgery at Rush Medical College, Chicago, described this in 1912.
[w] Ludwig Courvoisier (1843–1918), professor of surgery, Switzerland, described this principle in 1890. He was a keen natural historian and wrote 21 papers on entomology.

TABLE 6.11 Differential diagnosis in liver palpation

Hepatomegaly

1 Massive
- Metastases
- Alcoholic liver disease with fatty infiltration
- Myeloproliferative disease
- Right heart failure
- Hepatocellular cancer

2 Moderate
- The above causes
- Haemochromatosis
- Haematological disease—e.g. chronic leukaemia, lymphoma
- Fatty liver—secondary to e.g. diabetes mellitus, obesity, toxins
- Infiltration—e.g. amyloid

3 Mild
- The above causes
- Hepatitis
- Biliary obstruction
- Hydatid disease
- Human immunodeficiency virus (HIV) infection

Firm and irregular liver

Hepatocellular carcinoma

Metastatic disease

Cirrhosis

Hydatid disease, granuloma (e.g. sarcoid), amyloid, cysts, lipoidoses

Tender liver

Hepatitis

Rapid liver enlargement—e.g. right heart failure, Budd-Chiari* syndrome (hepatic vein thrombosis)

Hepatocellular cancer

Hepatic abscess

Biliary obstruction/cholangitis

Pulsatile liver

Tricuspid regurgitation

Hepatocellular cancer

Vascular abnormalities

---

* George Budd (1808–1882), professor of medicine, King's College Hospital, London, described this in 1845. Hans Chiari (1851–1916), professor of pathology, Prague, described it in 1898.

possible, as at least 50% of dilated gallbladders are impalpable (*Good signs guide 6.2*).

The spleen. The spleen enlarges inferiorly and medially (Figure 6.26). Its edge should be sought below the umbilicus in the midline initially. A two-handed technique is recommended. The left hand is placed posterolaterally over the left lower ribs

TABLE 6.12 Gallbladder enlargement

With jaundice

1 Carcinoma of the head of the pancreas
2 Carcinoma of the ampulla of Vater*
3 In-situ gallstone formation in the common bile duct
4 Mucocele of the gallbladder due to a stone in Hartmann's[†] pouch and a stone in the common bile duct (very rare)

Without jaundice

1 Mucocele or empyema of the gallbladder.
2 Carcinoma of the gallbladder (stone hard, irregular swelling)
3 Acute cholecystitis

* Abraham Vater (1684–1751), Wittenberg anatomist and botanist.
† Henri Hartmann (1860–1952), professor of surgery, Paris.

GOOD SIGNS GUIDE 6.1 Cholecystitis

Sign	Positive LR	Negative LR
Murphy's sign	2.0	NS
Back tenderness	0.4	2.0
Right upper quadrant mass	NS	NS

NS = not significant.
From McGee S, *Evidence-based physical diagnosis*, 2nd edn. St Louis: Saunders, 2007.

GOOD SIGNS GUIDE 6.2 Gallbladder

Sign	Positive LR	Negative LR
Detecting obstructed bile duct in jaundiced patient		
Palpable gallbladder	26.0	0.7
Malignant obstruction in patient with obstructive jaundice	2.6	0.7

From McGee S, *Evidence-based physical diagnosis*, 2nd edn. St Louis: Saunders, 2007.

and the right hand is placed on the abdomen below the umbilicus, parallel to the left costal margin (Figure 6.27a). Don't start palpation too near the costal margin or a large spleen will be missed. As the right hand is advanced closer to the left costal margin, the left hand compresses firmly over the rib cage so as to produce a loose fold of skin (Figure 6.27b); this removes tension from the abdominal wall and enables a slightly enlarged soft spleen to be felt as it moves down towards the right iliac fossa at the end of inspiration (Figure 6.27c).

If the spleen is not palpable, the patient must be rolled onto the right side towards the examiner (the right lateral decubitus position) and palpation repeated. Here one begins close to the left costal margin (Figure 6.27d). As a general rule, splenomegaly becomes just detectable if the spleen is one-and-a-half to two times enlarged. Palpation for splenomegaly is only moderately sensitive but highly specific. The positive LR of splenomegaly when the spleen is palpable is 9.6 and the negative LR of splenomegaly if the spleen is not palpable is 0.6.[11] The causes of splenomegaly are listed in Table 8.8 (page 230). The causes of hepatosplenomegaly are listed in Table 6.13.

The kidneys. The first important differential diagnosis to consider, if a right or left subcostal mass is palpable, must be a kidney. An attempt to palpate the kidney should be a routine part of the examination. The bimanual method is the best. The patient lies flat on his or her back. To palpate the right kidney, the examiner's left hand slides underneath the back to rest with the heel of the hand under the right loin. The fingers remain free to flex at the metacarpophalangeal joints in the area of the renal angle. The flexing fingers can push the contents of the abdomen anteriorly. The examiner's right hand is placed over the right upper quadrant.

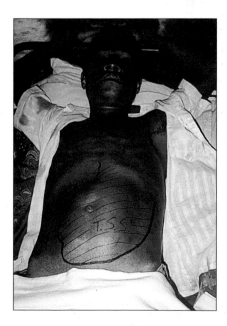

Figure 6.26 Massive splenomegaly: note the splenic notch

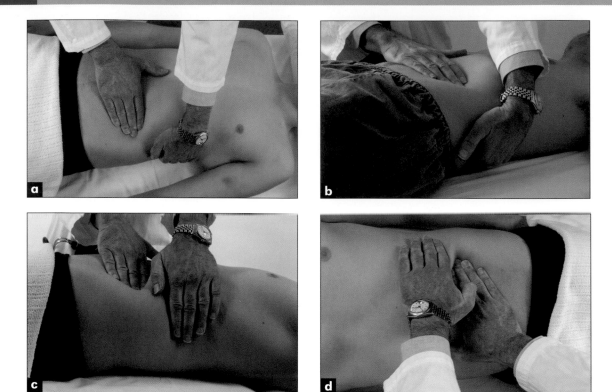

Figure 6.27 Palpation of the spleen
(a) Palpation begins in the lower mid-abdomen and finishes up under the left costal margin.
(b) The examiner's hand supports the patient's side...
(c) ...and then rests over the lower costal margin to reduce skin resistance.
(d) If the spleen is not palpable when the patient is flat, he or she should be rolled towards the examiner.

First an attempt should be made to capture the kidney between the two hands. It is more often possible to feel a kidney by bimanual palpation (this is traditionally called *ballotting*, although this term should probably be reserved for the palpation of an organ or mass in a fluid medium). In this case the renal angle is pressed sharply by the flexing fingers of the posterior hand. The kidney can be felt to float upwards and strike the anterior hand. The opposite hands are used to palpate the left kidney.

When palpable, the kidney feels like a swelling with a rounded lower pole and a medial dent (the hilum). However, it is unusual for a normal kidney to be felt as clearly as this. The lower pole of the right kidney may be palpable in thin, normal persons. Both kidneys move downwards with inspiration. The causes of kidney enlargement are listed in Table 7.8 (page 210).

It is particularly common to confuse a large left kidney with splenomegaly. The major distinguishing features are: (i) the spleen has no palpable upper border—the space between the spleen and the costal margin, which is present in renal enlargement, cannot be felt; (ii) the spleen, unlike the kidney, has a notch that may be palpable; (iii) the spleen moves inferomedially on inspiration while the kidney moves inferiorly; (iv) the spleen is not usually ballottable unless gross ascites is present, but the kidney is, again because of its retroperitoneal position; (v) the percussion note is dull over the spleen but is usually resonant over the kidney, as the latter lies posterior to loops of gas-

TABLE 6.13 Causes of hepatosplenomegaly
Chronic liver disease with portal hypertension
Haematological disease, e.g. myeloproliferative disease, lymphoma, leukaemia, pernicious anaemia, sickle cell anaemia
Infection, e.g. acute viral hepatitis, infectious mononucleosis, cytomegalovirus
Infiltration, e.g. amyloid, sarcoid
Connective tissue disease, e.g. systemic lupus erythematosus
Acromegaly
Thyrotoxicosis

filled bowel; (vi) a friction rub may occasionally be heard over the spleen, but never over the kidney because it is too posterior.

Other abdominal masses. The causes of a mass in the abdomen, excluding the liver, spleen and kidneys, are summarised in Table 6.14.

Stomach and duodenum. Although many clinicians palpate the epigastrium to elicit tenderness in patients with suspected peptic ulcer, the presence or absence of tenderness is not helpful in making this diagnosis. With gastric outlet obstruction due to a peptic ulcer or gastric carcinoma (page 194), the 'succussion splash' (the sign of Hippocrates) may occasionally be present but unfortunately this entertaining sign is more of historical interest than practical use now. In a case of suspected gastric outlet obstruction, after warning the patient what is to come, grasp one iliac crest with each hand, place your stethoscope close to the epigastrium and shake the patient vigorously from side to side. The listening ears eagerly await a splashing noise due to excessive fluid retained in an obstructed stomach. The test is not useful if the patient has just drunk a large amount of milk or other fluid for his or her ulcer; the clinician must then return 4 hours later, having forbidden the patient to drink anything further.

Pancreas. A pancreatic pseudocyst following acute pancreatitis may, if large, be palpable as a rounded swelling above the umbilicus. It is characteristically tense, does not descend with inspiration and feels fixed. Occasionally a pancreatic carcinoma may be palpable in thin patients.

Aorta. Arterial pulsation from the abdominal aorta may be present, usually in the epigastrium, in thin normal people. The problem is to determine whether such a pulsation represents an aortic aneurysm (usually due to atherosclerosis) or not. Measure the width of the pulsation gently with two fingers by aligning these parallel to the aorta and placing them at the outermost palpable margins. With an aortic aneurysm, the pulsation is expansile (i.e. it enlarges appreciably with systole) (Figure 6.28). If an abdominal aortic aneurysm is larger than 5 cm in diameter, it usually merits surgical repair. The sensitivity of examination for finding an aneurysm of 5 cm or larger is 82%.[12,13] The sensitivity of the examination for detecting an aneurysm increases *pari passu* with the size of the aneurysm. The overall LR for a significant aneurysm when one is suspected on palpation is 2.7, with a negative LR of 0.43 if the examination is normal.[11]

Bowel. Particularly in severely constipated patients with soft abdominal walls and retained

TABLE 6.14 Causes of abdominal masses
Right iliac fossa
Appendiceal abscess or mucocele of the appendix
Carcinoma of the caecum or caecal distension due to distal obstruction
Crohn's disease (usually when complicated by an abscess)
Ovarian tumour or cyst
Carcinoid tumour
Amoebiasis
Psoas abscess
Ileocaecal tuberculosis
Hernia
Transplanted kidney
Left iliac fossa
Faeces (NB: Can often be indented)
Carcinoma of sigmoid or descending colon
Diverticular abscess
Ovarian tumour or cyst
Psoas abscess
Hernia
Transplanted kidney
Upper abdomen
Retroperitoneal lymphadenopathy (e.g. lymphoma, teratoma)
Left lobe of the liver
Abdominal aortic aneurysm (expansile)
Carcinoma of the stomach
Pancreatic pseudocyst or tumour
Gastric dilatation (e.g. pyloric stenosis, acute dilatation in diabetic ketoacidosis or after surgery)
Carcinoma of the transverse colon
Omental mass (e.g. metastatic tumour)
Small bowel obstruction
Pelvis
Bladder
Ovarian tumour or cyst
Uterus (e.g. pregnancy, tumour, fibroids)
Small bowel obstruction

faeces, the sigmoid colon is often palpable. Unlike other masses, faeces can usually be indented by the examiner's finger. Rarely, carcinoma of the bowel may be palpable, particularly in the caecum where masses can grow to a large size before they cause obstruction. Such a mass does not move on respiration. In the examination of children or adults with chronic constipation and a megarectum, the enlarged rectum containing impacted stool may be felt above the symphysis pubis, filling a variable part of the pelvis in the midline.

Bladder. An empty bladder is impalpable. If there is urinary retention, the full bladder may be palpable above the pubic symphysis. It forms part

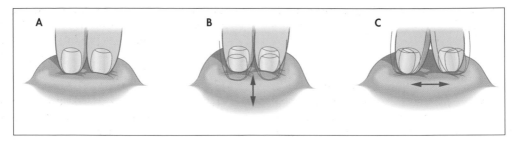

Figure 6.28 Detecting an expansile impulse
A = no impulse; B = transmitted pulsation from a neighbouring artery; C = expansile impulse, the sign of an aneurysm.
(Adapted from Clain A, ed. *Hamilton Bailey's Physical signs in clinical surgery*, 17th edn. John Wright & Sons, 1986.)

of the differential diagnosis of any swelling arising out of the pelvis. It is characteristically impossible to feel the bladder's lower border. The swelling is typically regular, smooth, firm and oval-shaped. The bladder may sometimes reach as high as the umbilicus. It is unwise to make a definite diagnosis concerning a swelling coming out of the pelvis until you are sure the bladder is empty. This may require the insertion of a urinary catheter.

Inguinal lymph nodes. These are described on page 229.

Testes. Palpation of the testes should be considered if indicated during the abdominal examination (page 215). Testicular atrophy occurs in chronic liver disease (e.g. alcoholic liver disease, haemochromatosis); its mechanism is believed to be similar to that responsible for gynaecomastia.

Anterior abdominal wall. The skin and muscles of the anterior abdominal wall are prone to the same sorts of lumps that occur anywhere on the surface of the body (Table 6.15). So to avoid embarrassment it is important not to confuse these with intra-abdominal lumps. To determine whether a mass is in the abdominal wall, ask the patient to fold the arms across the upper chest and sit halfway up. An intra-abdominal mass disappears or decreases in size, but one within the layers of the abdominal wall will remain unchanged.

Pain can arise from the abdominal wall; this can cause confusion with intra-abdominal causes of pain. To test for *abdominal wall pain*, feel for an area of localised tenderness that reproduces the pain while the patient is supine. If this is found, ask the patient to fold the arms across the upper chest and sit halfway up, then palpate again (Carnett's test: described by JB Carnett in 1926). If the tenderness disappears, this suggests that the pain is in the abdominal cavity (as tensed abdominal muscles are protecting the viscera), but if the tenderness

persists or is greater, this suggests that the pain is arising from the abdominal wall (e.g. muscle strain, nerve entrapment, myositis).[14-16] However, the Carnett test may occasionally be positive when there is visceral disease with involvement of the parietal peritoneum producing inflammation of the overlying muscle (e.g. appendicitis).

Percussion

Percussion is used to define the size and nature of organs and masses, but is most useful for detecting fluid in the peritoneal cavity, and for eliciting tenderness in patients with peritonitis.

Liver. The liver borders should be percussed routinely to determine the liver span. If the liver edge is not palpable and there is no ascites, the right side of the abdomen should be percussed in the midclavicular line up to the right costal margin until dullness is encountered. This defines the liver's lower border even when it is not palpable. The upper border of the liver must always be defined by percussing down the midclavicular line. Loss of

TABLE 6.15 Some causes of anterior abdominal wall masses
Lipoma
Sebaceous cyst
Dermal fibroma
Malignant deposits—e.g. melanoma, carcinoma
Epigastric hernia
Umbilical or paraumbilical hernia
Incisional hernia
Rectus sheath divarication
Rectus sheath haematoma

normal liver dullness may occur in massive hepatic necrosis, or with free gas in the peritoneal cavity (e.g. perforated bowel).

Spleen. Percussion over the left costal margin may be more sensitive than palpation for detection of enlargement of the spleen. Percuss over the lowest intercostal space in the left anterior axillary line in both inspiration and expiration with the patient supine (Figure 6.29). Splenomegaly should be suspected if the percussion note is dull or becomes *dull on complete inspiration*. Percussion appears to be more sensitive than palpation for the detection of splenomegaly. If the percussion note is dull, palpation should be repeated.

Kidneys. Percussion over a right or left subcostal mass can help distinguish hepatic or splenic from renal masses: in the latter case there will usually be a resonant area because of overlying bowel (be warned, however, that sometimes a very large renal mass may displace overlying bowel).

Bladder. An area of suprapubic dullness may indicate the upper border of an enlarged bladder or pelvic mass.

Ascites. The percussion note over most of the abdomen is resonant, due to air in the intestines.[17] The resonance is detectable out to the flanks. When peritoneal fluid (ascites) collects, the influence of gravity causes this to accumulate first in the flanks in a supine patient. Thus, a relatively early sign of ascites (when at least 2 litres of fluid have accumulated) is a dull percussion note in the flanks (*Good signs guide 6.3*). With gross ascites, the abdomen distends, the flanks bulge, umbilical eversion occurs (see Figure 6.19) and dullness is

detectable closer to the midline. However, an area of central resonance will always persist. Routine abdominal examination should include percussion starting in the midline with the finger pointing towards the feet; the percussion note is tested out towards the flanks on each side.

If (and only if) dullness is detected in the flanks, the sign of **shifting dullness** should be sought.[17] To detect this sign, while standing on the right side of the bed percuss out to the left flank until dullness is reached (Figure 6.30a). This point should be marked and the patient rolled towards the examiner. Ideally 30 seconds to 1 minute should then pass so that fluid can move inside the abdominal cavity and then percussion is repeated over the marked point (Figure 6.30b).

Shifting dullness is present if the area of dullness has changed to become resonant. This is because peritoneal fluid moves under the influence of gravity to the right side of the abdomen when this is the lowermost point. Very occasionally, fluid and air in dilated small bowel in small intestinal obstruction, or a massive ovarian cyst filling the whole abdomen, can cause confusion.

To detect a **fluid thrill** (or wave) the clinician asks an assistant (or the patient) to place the medial edges of both palms firmly on the centre of the abdomen with the fingers pointing towards each other. The examiner flicks the side of the abdominal wall, and a pulsation (thrill) is felt by the hand placed on the other abdominal wall. A fluid thrill is of more value when there is massive ascites. Interestingly, it may also occur when there is a massive ovarian cyst or a pregnancy with hydramnios.

The presence of bulging in the flanks has good sensitivity and specificity for the detection of ascites. Shifting dullness has both good sensitivity and specificity. The presence of ankle oedema

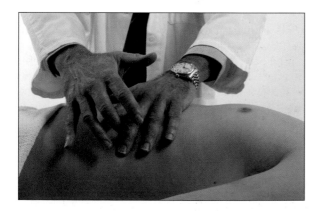

Figure 6.29 Percussion of the spleen

GOOD SIGNS GUIDE 6.3 Ascites

Sign	Positive LR	Negative LR
Inspection		
Bulging flanks	1.9	0.4
Oedema	3.8	0.2
Palpation and percussion		
Flank dullness	NS	0.3
Shifting dullness	2.3	0.4
Fluid wave	5.0	0.5

NS = not significant.
From McGee S, *Evidence-based physical diagnosis*, 2nd edn. St Louis: Saunders, 2007.

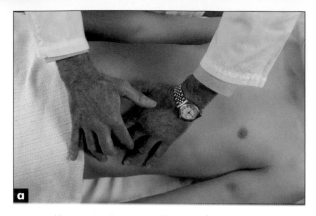

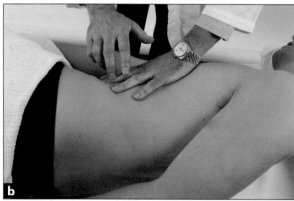

Figure 6.30 Shifting dullness
(a) Percuss out to the left flank until the percussion note becomes dull. Mark this spot with your finger.
(b) Roll the patient towards you, wait 30 seconds. Shifting dullness is present if the left lateral dull area is now resonant.

TABLE 6.16 Classification of ascites by the serum ascites to albumin concentration gradient

High gradient (>11g/L)

1 Cirrhosis*

2 Alcoholic hepatitis

3 Budd-Chiari syndrome (hepatic vein thrombosis) or veno-occlusive disease

4 Fulminant hepatic failure

5 Congestive heart failure, constrictive pericarditis (cardiac ascites)

6 Myxoedema (rare)

Low gradient (<11g/L)

1 Peritoneal carcinomatosis

2 Tuberculosis

3 Pancreatic ascites

4 Nephrotic syndrome

* Patients with a high serum-to-ascites albumin gradient most often have portal hypertension (97% accuracy).

increases the likelihood of ascites. (See *Good signs guide 6.3*.)

The causes of ascites are listed in Table 6.16.

When significant ascites is present, abdominal masses may be difficult to feel by direct palpation. Here is the opportunity to practise *dipping*. Using the hand placed flat on the abdomen, the fingers are flexed at the metacarpophalangeal joints rapidly so as to displace the underlying fluid. This enables the fingers to reach a mass covered in ascitic fluid. In particular, this should be attempted to palpate an enlarged liver or spleen. The liver and spleen may become ballottable when gross ascites is present.

Auscultation

While some cardiologists believe that the sounds produced in the abdominal cavity are not as varied or as interesting as those one hears in the chest, they have some value.

Bowel sounds. Place the diaphragm of the stethoscope just below the umbilicus. Bowel sounds can be heard over all parts of the abdomen in normal healthy people. They are poorly localised and there is little point in listening for them in more than one place. Most bowel sounds originate in the stomach, some from the large bowel and the rest from the small bowel. They have a soft gurgling character and occur only intermittently. Bowel sounds should be described as either present or absent; the terms 'decreased' or 'increased' are meaningless because the sounds vary, depending on when a meal was last eaten.

Complete absence of any bowel sounds over a 4-minute period indicates paralytic ileus (this is complete absence of peristalsis in a paralysed bowel). As only liquid is present in the gut, the heart sounds may be audible over the abdomen, transmitted by the dilated bowel.

The bowel that is obstructed produces a louder and higher-pitched sound with a tinkling quality due to the presence of air and liquid ('obstructed bowel sounds'). The presence of normal bowel sounds makes obstruction unlikely. Intestinal hurry or rush, which occurs in diarrhoeal states, causes loud gurgling sounds, often audible without the stethoscope. These bowel sounds are called *borborygmi*.

Friction rubs. These indicate an abnormality of the parietal and visceral peritoneum due to inflammation, but are very rare and non-specific.

They may be audible over the liver or spleen. A rough creaking or grating noise is heard as the patient breathes. Hepatic causes include a tumour within the liver (hepatocellular cancer or metastases), a liver abscess, a recent liver biopsy, a liver infarct, or gonococcal or chlamydial perihepatitis due to inflammation of the liver capsule (Fitz-Hugh-Curtis syndrome[x]). A splenic rub indicates a splenic infarct.

Venous hums. A venous hum is a continuous, low-pitched, soft murmur that may become louder with inspiration and diminish when more pressure is applied to the stethoscope. Typically it is heard between the xiphisternum and the umbilicus in cases of portal hypertension, but is rare. It may radiate to the chest or over to the liver. Large volumes of blood flowing in the umbilical or para-umbilical veins in the falciform ligament are responsible. These channel blood from the left portal vein to the epigastric or internal mammary veins in the abdominal wall. A venous hum may occasionally be heard over the large vessels such as the inferior mesenteric vein or after portacaval shunting. Sometimes a thrill is detectable over the site of maximum intensity of the hum. The Cruveilhier-Baumgarten[y] syndrome is the association of a venous hum at the umbilicus and dilated abdominal wall veins. It is almost always due to cirrhosis of the liver. It occurs when patients have a patent umbilical vein, which allows portal-to-systemic shunting at this site. The presence of a venous hum or of prominent central abdominal veins suggests that the site of portal obstruction is intrahepatic rather than in the portal vein itself.

Bruits. Uncommonly, an arterial systolic bruit can be heard over the liver. This sound is higher pitched than a venous hum, is not continuous and is well localised. This is usually due to a hepatocellular cancer but may occur in acute alcoholic hepatitis, with an arteriovenous malformation, or transiently after a liver biopsy. Auscultation for renal bruits on either side of the midline above the umbilicus is indicated if renal artery stenosis is suspected. A bruit in the epigastrium may be heard in patients with chronic intestinal ischaemia from mesenteric arterial stenosis, but may also occur in the absence of pathology. A bruit may occasionally be audible over the spleen when there is a tumour of the body of the pancreas or a splenic arteriovenous fistula.

Hernias

Hernias are of surgical importance and should not be missed during an abdominal examination. They are very frequently the focus of student assessment examinations. This section will be restricted to examination of groin hernias, which comprise inguinal and femoral hernias.

The principal sign of a hernia is that of a lump in the groin region. Naturally, not all lumps in the region are hernias (Table 6.17). A lump that is present on standing or during manoeuvres that raise intra-abdominal pressure (such as coughing or straining), and that disappears on recumbency, is easily identified as a hernia. Some hernias, however, are *irreducible*. Another term used for irreducible is incarcerated, but this term is probably best avoided. Some irreducible hernias contain bowel, which may become *obstructed*, giving rise to symptoms of small bowel obstruction in addition to the irreducible lump. Sometimes the bowel contents' blood supply becomes jeopardised, and these are known as *strangulated* hernias; they are usually painful, red, tense and tender.

Examination technique

A thorough examination for a hernia should be commenced with the patient standing if possible. The patient should be asked to stand with full exposure from the thigh to the upper abdomen.

Inspection is carried out initially. Pay careful attention to scars from previous surgery, which

TABLE 6.17 Differential diagnosis of a solitary groin lump
Above the inguinal ligament
Inguinal hernia
Undescended testis
Cyst of the canal of Nuck
Encysted hydrocele or lipoma of the cord
Iliac node
Large femoral hernia (rare)
Below the inguinal ligament
Femoral hernia
Lymph node
Saphena varix (sensation of a 'jet of water' on palpation, disappears when supine)
Femoral aneurysm (pulsatile)
Psoas abscess (associated with fever, flank pain and flexion deformity)

---

[x] AH Curtis described hepatic adhesions associated with pelvic inflammatory disease in 1930, while T Fitz-Hugh described right upper abdominal acute gonococcal peritonitis in 1934. However, this syndrome was actually first described by C Stajano in 1920.

[y] Jean Cruveilhier (1791–1874), professor of pathological anatomy, Paris, who had been Dupuytren's registrar, and Paul von Baumgarten (1848–1928), German pathologist.

may be difficult to see. Look for obvious lumps and swellings. Before palpation is commenced the patient is asked to turn the head away from the examiner and to cough. The examiner's eyes should be fixed in the region of the pubic tubercle (see below) and note the presence of a visible cough impulse. The patient is then asked to cough again with the examiner inspecting the opposite side.

Of key importance is the position of a hernia in relation to the *pubic tubercle*, which can usually easily be felt *lateral to the symphysis pubis* (2–3 cm from the midline). In the obese individual, it may be difficult to locate the pubic tubercle and in such situations if the thigh is flexed and abducted, the adductor longus muscle can be traced proximally, leading the examiner to the pubic tubercle.

Palpation is commenced with the gloved fingers being placed over the region of the pubic tubercle. Once again the patient is asked to cough and a palpable expansile impulse is sought. If a hernia is present, attempts at reduction should *not* be performed while the patient is erect, as it is more difficult and painful than when the patient is placed supine.

The patient is then asked to lie supine on the examination couch. The procedure of inspection and palpation is performed in the same manner again. The exact position of any hernia is usually easier to define with the patient lying supine.

If a lump or cough impulse is present, it must be determined whether this is a hernia and, if so, what sort of hernia. Identify the pubic tubercle. If an inguinal hernia is large, the pubic tubercle may be obscured by the hernia (especially by an irreducible inguinal hernia) and its position may be less distinct, but an accurate indication can usually be made by comparing the lump with the pubic tubercle on the opposite side.

Inguinal hernias

Inguinal hernias typically bulge above the crease of the groin. They arise from a deficiency *above* the inguinal ligament and this is where they are usually felt (Figure 6.31). The inguinal ligament lies between the anterior superior iliac spine and the pubic tubercle. The pubic tubercle is just above the attachment of the adductor longus tendon to the pubic bone (feel the upper medial aspect of the thigh to palpate the tendon). The internal inguinal ring lies 2 cm above the midpoint of the inguinal ligament.

An *indirect* inguinal hernia protrudes through the deep inguinal ring. The best surface marking for this point is just above the midpoint of the inguinal ligament, which is halfway between the pubic tubercle and the anterior superior iliac spine (it is the position where the spermatic cord structures enter the inguinal canal). This is lateral to the inferior epigastric vessels. A *direct* hernia, on the other hand, pushes into the inguinal canal posteriorly through a region of weakness known as Hesselbach's triangle.[z] This triangle is bounded inferiorly by the inguinal ligament, laterally by the inferior epigastric vessels and medially by the lateral border of the rectus sheath.

The student may be asked to differentiate between direct and indirect inguinal hernias. However, clinically this is difficult and the true nature of an inguinal hernia can often be determined only at the time of operation. The muscular defect in a direct hernia is usually larger than that of an indirect hernia, and as such direct hernias are typically easier to demonstrate and usually reduce

---

[z] Franz Hesselbach (1759–1816), professor of surgery, Würzburg, described this triangle bounded by the inguinal ligament, the inferior epigastric artery and the rectus abdominis.

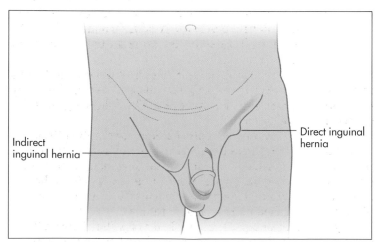

Indirect inguinal hernia

Direct inguinal hernia

Figure 6.31 Note the elliptical swelling of an indirect inguinal hernia descending into the scrotum on the right side. Also note the globular swelling of a direct inguinal hernia on the left side

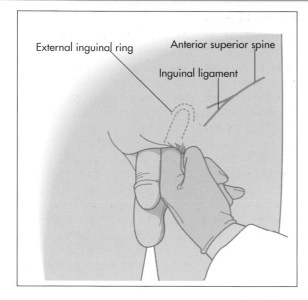

Figure 6.32 To examine the inguinal canal in a male, the scrotum can be invaginated as shown (always wear gloves)

immediately and spontaneously. An indirect hernia may often be felt on palpation to slide along the direction of the inguinal canal under the examining fingers.

A large inguinal hernia may descend through the external ring immediately above the pubic tubercle into the scrotum. Gentle invagination of the scrotum with the tip of the gloved little finger in the external ring may be performed to confirm an indirect hernia in men but this can be difficult to interpret without substantial experience (Figure 6.32). A maldescended testis can be confused with an inguinal hernia; always confirm that there is a testis in each scrotum. A large inguinal hernia may present as a lump in the scrotum. It is important initially in this situation to ascertain whether one can get above the lump. If so, the lump is of primary intrascrotal pathology and is not a hernia.

Femoral hernias
Femoral hernias typically bulge into the groin crease at its medial end. Hence they occur lateral to and below the pubic tubercle, just medial to the femoral pulse (about 2 cm away) (Table 6.17). They are less common than inguinal hernias and are not related to the inguinal canal. They are usually smaller and firmer than inguinal hernias and quite commonly do not exhibit a cough impulse. They are frequently irreducible. As such, they are commonly mistaken for an enlarged inguinal lymph node. A cough impulse is rare from a femoral hernia and needs to be distinguished from the thrill produced by a saphena varix when a patient coughs.

Remember that hernias are often bilateral and that two different types may occur on the one side. Sometimes there is also a hydrocele (Figure 7.11, page 217)—one can get above a hydrocele in the inguinal canal but not a hernia.

Incisional hernias
Any abdominal scar may be the site of a hernia because of abdominal wall weakness. Assess this by asking the patient to cough while you look for abnormal bulges. Next have the patient lift the head and shoulders off the bed while the examiner's hand rests on the forehead and resists this movement. If a bulge is seen, the examiner's other hand should palpate for a fascial layer defect in the muscle.

Rectal examination (Figure 6.33)

The examining physician often hesitates to make the necessary examination because it involves soiling the finger.

William Mayo (1861–1939)

The abdominal examination is not complete without the performance of a rectal examination.[18,19] It should be considered in all patients admitted to hospital who are over the age of 40, unless the examiner has no fingers, the patient no anus, or acute illness such as myocardial infarction presents a temporary contraindication.

The patient's permission must be obtained and if indicated a chaperone introduced to the patient. Privacy must be ensured for the patient throughout the examination. Following an explanation as to what is to happen and why, the patient lies on his or her left side with the knees drawn up and back to the examiner. This is called the left lateral position. The examination can be performed with the patient standing and in the bent-over position. This may help provide good information about the prostate, but makes assessment of rectal function more difficult.

The examiner dons a pair of gloves and begins the inspection of the anus and perianal area by separating the buttocks. The following must be looked for:
1 **Thrombosed external haemorrhoids (piles).** Small (less than 1 cm), tense bluish swellings may be seen on one side of the anal margin. They are painful and are due to rupture of a vein in the external haemorrhoidal plexus. They are also called perianal haematomas.
2 **Skin tags.** These look like tags elsewhere on the body and can be an incidental finding or occur

with haemorrhoids or Crohn's disease.

3 **Rectal prolapse.** Circumferential folds of red mucosa are visible protruding from the anus. These may become apparent only when the patient is asked to strain as if to pass stool. A gaping anus suggests loss of internal and external sphincter tone. This may coexist with prolapse.

4 **Anal fissure (fissure-in-ano).** This is a crack in the anal wall which may be painful enough to prevent rectal examination with the finger. Fissures-in-ano usually occur directly posteriorly and in the midline. A tag of skin may be present at the base: this is called a sentinel pile. It indicates that the fissure is chronic. It may be necessary to get the patient to bear down for a fissure to become visible. Multiple or broad-based fissures may be present in patients with inflammatory bowel disease, malignancy or sexually transmitted disease.

5 **Fistula-in-ano.** The entrance of this tract may be visible, usually within 4 cm of the anus. The mouth has a red pouting appearance caused by granulation tissue. This may occur with Crohn's disease or perianal abscess (page 191).

6 **Condylomata acuminata (anal warts)** may be confused with skin tags, but are in fact pedunculated papillomas with a white surface and red base. They may surround the anus.

7 **Carcinoma of the anus.** This may be visible as a fungating mass at the anal verge.

8 **Pruritus ani.** The appearance of this irritating anal condition varies from weeping red dermatitis to a thickened white skin. It is usually caused by faecal soiling.

9 **Excoriation** as a result of inflammation or **contact dermatitis** caused by faeces—diarrhoea.

Next ask the patient to strain and watch the perineum: look for incontinence and leakage of faeces or mucus, abnormal descent of the perineum or the presence of a patulous anus. The presence of a gaping anus often correlates with lower resting pressures on anorectal manometry. Internal haemorrhoids can prolapse in the right anterior, right posterior and left lateral positions.

If there is rectal prolapse, straining may cause a dark red mass to appear at the anal verge; mucosal prolapse causes the appearance of radial folds and concentric folds are a sign of complete prolapse. This mass is continuous with the perianal skin and is usually painless. In cases of mucosal rectal prolapse, the prolapsed mucosa can be felt between the examiner's thumb and forefinger.

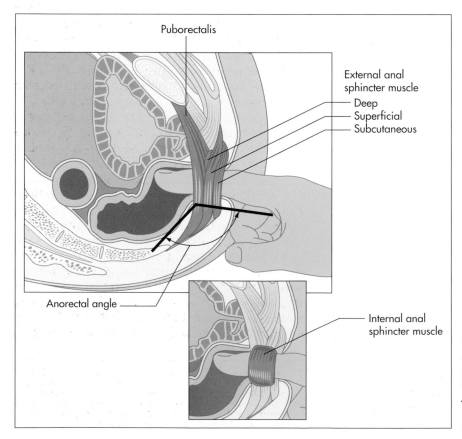

Figure 6.33 The rectal examination: regional anatomy
(From Talley NJ, *American Journal of Gastroenterology*. 2008; 108: 802–803, with permission.)

Now test the anal wink. Stroke a cotton pad in all four quadrants around the anus. Usually you will see a brisk anal contraction which indicates the sacral nerve pathways are intact. Sometimes the response is weak in healthy people. However, the complete absence of an anal wink, particularly in the setting of faecal incontinence, suggests that there is a spinal cord problem and indicates the need to perform a more detailed neurological examination and consider further investigations accordingly.

Now the time for action has come. The tip of the gloved right index finger is lubricated and placed over the anus. Ask the patient to breathe in and out quietly through the mouth, as a distraction and to aid relaxation. If there is excruciating pain at the start of the examination, this strongly suggests that there is an anal fissure and the remainder of the rectal examination should be abandoned. Often the fissure can be seen on inspection. An anal fissure can precipitate constipation but may be secondary to constipation itself. By liberally lubricating the rectum with lignocaine jelly, it may still be possible to complete the rest of the examination, but usually it is better to perform anoscopy under appropriate sedation for these patients. Other causes of significant anal pain during palpation include recently thrombosed external haemorrhoids, an ischiorectal abscess, active proctitis, or anal ulceration from another cause.

TABLE 6.18 Causes of a palpable mass in the rectum
Rectal carcinoma
Rectal polyp
Hypertrophied anal papilla
Diverticular phlegmon (recent or old)
Sigmoid colon carcinoma (prolapsing into the pouch of Douglas*)
Metastatic deposits in the pelvis (Blumer's shelf)
Uterine or ovarian malignancy
Prostatic or cervical malignancy (direct extension)
Endometriosis
Pelvic abscess or sarcoma
Amoebic granuloma
Foreign body

Note: Faeces, while palpable, also indent.
* James Douglas (1675–1742), Scottish anatomist and male midwife, physician to Queen Caroline (wife of George II) in London.

Slowly increasing pressure is applied with the pulp of the finger until the sphincter is felt to relax slightly. At this stage the finger is advanced into the rectum slowly. During entry, sphincter tone should be assessed as normal or reduced. The accuracy of this assessment has been questioned in the past, but more recently has been shown to correlate well with anorectal manometry measurements.[20] This resting tone is predominantly (70%–80%) attributable to the internal anal sphincter muscle. Reduced sphincter tone may indicate a sphincter tear. A high anal resting tone may contribute to difficulties with evacuation.

Palpation of the anterior wall of the rectum for the *prostate gland* in the male and for the *cervix* in the female is performed first. The normal prostate is a firm, rubbery bilobed mass with a central furrow. It becomes firmer with age. With prostatic enlargement, the sulcus becomes obliterated and the gland is often asymmetrical. A very hard nodule is apparent when a carcinoma of the prostate is present. The prostate is boggy and tender in prostatitis. A mass above the prostate or cervix may indicate a metastatic deposit on Blumer's shelf.[aa]

The finger is then rotated clockwise so that the left lateral wall, posterior wall and right lateral wall of the rectum can be palpated in turn. Then the finger is advanced as high as possible into the rectum and slowly withdrawn along the rectal wall. A soft lesion, such as a small rectal carcinoma or polyp, is more likely to be felt this way[bb] (Table 6.18). Ask the patient to squeeze your finger with the anal muscles as a further test of anal tone.

Ask the patient to strain again when the examiner's finger is rotated anteriorly. In this position a *rectocele* (a defect in the anterior wall of the rectum) may be palpable.

The pelvic floor—special tests for pelvic floor dysfunction. The first test is simple: ask the patient to strain and try to push out your finger. Normally, the anal sphincter and puborectalis should relax and the perineum should descend by 1–3.5 cm. If the muscles seem to tighten, particularly when there is no perineal descent, this suggests paradoxical external anal sphincter and puborectalis contraction, which in fact are blocking normal defaecation (pelvic floor dyssynergia).

aa George Blumer (1858–1940), professor of medicine at Yale, in 1909 described cancer in the pouch of Douglas forming a shelf-like structure.
bb It can be useful to perform the rectal examination with the patient supine and the head of the bed elevated; this allows the intra-abdominal contents to descend and a bimanual examination (using the opposite hand to compress the lower abdomen) is possible.

Second, press on the posterior rectal wall and ask if this causes pain; this suggests puborectalis muscle tenderness, which can also occur in pelvic floor dyssynergia. Third, assess whether the anal sphincter and the puborectalis contract when you ask your patient to contract or squeeze the pelvic floor muscles. Puborectalis contraction is perceived as a 'lift'; that is, the muscle lifts the examining finger toward the umbilicus. Many patients with faecal incontinence cannot augment anal pressure when asked to squeeze. Finally, place your other hand on the anterior abdominal wall while asking the patient to strain again. This provides some information on whether the patient is excessively contracting the abdominal wall (e.g. by performing an inappropriate Valsalva manoeuvre) and perhaps also the pelvic floor muscles while attempting to defaecate, which may impede evacuation. However, the exact value of this test is unclear.

Constipation that is due to pelvic floor dysfunction responds to biofeedback in about 70% of cases, and this treatment can result in a laxative-free existence for patients with troubling outlet constipation; the diagnosis should be entertained in all patients with chronic constipation, and a good rectal examination can help guide you as to whether anorectal manometry testing is warranted.

After the finger has been withdrawn, the glove is inspected for bright blood or melaena, mucus or pus, and the colour of the faeces is noted. Haemorrhoids are not palpable unless thrombosed. Persistent gaping of the anal canal after withdrawal of the examining finger may indicate external anal sphincter denervation.

Proctosigmoidoscopy

The examination of the rectum with a sigmoidoscope is an essential part of the physical examination of any patient with symptoms referable to the anorectal region or large bowel. The principal indications include rectal bleeding, chronic diarrhoea, constipation or change in bowel habit. It should also be performed in some patients with abdominal pain, before treatment is begun for any anorectal condition, and before a barium enema is ordered for any reason.

The examination can be performed without anaesthesia, except in patients who have a very painful anal condition.

Procedure

Begin by inspecting the anal area as outlined earlier. Then a digital examination of the rectum is performed.

Explain to the patient what is about to happen. Warn him or her that there will be a feeling of fullness and the desire to defecate, and possibly cramps in the rectal region. The patient is then placed in the left lateral position and asked to relax and breathe quietly through the mouth.

If a rigid sigmoidoscope is to be used, it is warmed slightly and, with the obturator in place, is inserted into the rectum in the direction of the umbilicus until the rectal ampulla is reached (4–5 cm). This is the only part of the examination that is performed blind. The obturator is then removed. The tip of the sigmoidoscope is gently swung posteriorly under direct vision to follow the curve of the sacrum. The important landmarks to note during sigmoidoscopy are the anal verge, the dentate line, the anorectal junction, the lowest and middle rectal valves, and finally the rectosigmoid junction. Small amounts of air may be insufflated to assist with this. At about 12–15 cm, smooth rectal mucosa gives way to the concentric rugae of the distal sigmoid. It is possible to advance the rigid instrument into the distal sigmoid in the majority of men and in many women. The flexible sigmoidoscope usually can examine the entire left colon in skilled hands. The instrument must *never* be advanced unless the lumen is clearly visible and the patient is not experiencing pain.

Once the sigmoidoscope has been advanced as far as possible, it should be withdrawn gradually while the circumference of the mucosa is inspected carefully. Look behind for the valves of Houston.[cc] It is possible to sample faeces from areas away from the anal margin, which can be tested for occult blood and subjected to microbiological examination. Mucosal lesions can also be biopsied.

Common abnormalities seen on sigmoidoscopy

1 Blood, seen to be arising from above the highest level examined, indicates that a total examination of the colon by colonoscopy is essential.
2 Erythematous and ulcerated areas indicating inflammation, which may be local or diffuse.
3 Mucosal oedema, where there is loss of the normal vascular pattern of the colon, may be seen in mild inflammatory bowel disease.
4 Polyps, which may be sessile or pedunculated, solitary or multiple.
5 Carcinoma.
6 Strictures, which may be due to carcinoma, Crohn's disease, trauma, ischaemia, radiation or (very rarely) tuberculosis.

---

cc The middle one of three transverse folds of mucous membrane in the rectum, described in 1830 by John Houston (1802–45), Irish surgeon.

7 The orifices of diverticula.
8 Fissures.

If an abnormality of the anal canal is suspected, this is best seen using *anoscopy*, which can be carried out after sigmoidoscopy. Lesions to look for in the anal canal include swellings, masses, fissures, the internal openings of fistulae, squamous metaplasia and haemorrhoids. Haemorrhoids appear as swellings at the site of the normal anal cushions at 3, 7 and 11 o'clock, and they descend on straining. Remember that haemorrhoids are common and may coexist with more sinister bowel disease.

Testing of the stools for blood

Testing of the stools for blood may be considered in the assessment of anaemia, iron deficiency, gastrointestinal bleeding or symptoms suggesting colonic cancer. In the guaiac test, stool is placed on a guaiac-impregnated paper; blood results in phenolytic oxidation, causing a blue colour. Newer tests can quantify the amount of blood in the stool.

Unfortunately, both false-positive and false-negative results occur with the occult blood tests. Peroxidase and catalase, present in various foods (e.g. fresh fruit, uncooked vegetables), and haem in red meat can cause false-positive results, as can aspirin, anticoagulants or oral iron. Vitamin C can reduce the sensitivity of guaiac results, and should not be taken before testing.

False-negative results are not uncommon with colorectal neoplasms because they bleed intermittently. Hence, testing for faecal occult blood from the glove after a rectal examination is of little value,[21] and more sensitive and specific testing (e.g. colonoscopy) is required, depending on the clinical setting.

Other

Examine the legs for bruising or oedema, which may be the result of liver disease. Neurological signs of alcoholism (e.g. a coarse tremor) or evidence of thiamine deficiency (peripheral neuropathy or memory loss) may also be present.

Examination of the cardiovascular system may be helpful in patients with hepatomegaly. Cardiac failure is a common cause of liver enlargement and can even cause cirrhosis. Measurement of the patient's temperature is important, especially in an acute abdominal case or if there is any suggestion of infection.

Examine with particular care all lymph node groups, the breasts and chest if there is any evidence of malignant disease such as firm, irregular hepatomegaly (see Table 8.9, page 230).

Examination of the gastrointestinal contents
Faeces

Never miss an opportunity to inspect a patient's faeces, because considerable information about the gastrointestinal tract can be obtained in this way.

Melaena

Melaena stools are poorly formed, black and have a tarry appearance. They have a very characteristic and offensive smell. The cause is the presence of blood digested by gastric acid and colonic bacteria. Melaena usually indicates bleeding from the oesophagus, stomach or duodenum. The most common cause is acute or chronic peptic ulceration. Less often, right-sided colonic bleeding and (rarely) small-bowel bleeding can cause melaena. The differential diagnosis of dark stools includes ingestion of iron tablets, bismuth, liquorice or charcoal. However, these tend to result in small well-formed non-tarry stools and the offensive smell is absent.

Bright-red blood (haematochezia)

This appearance usually results from haemorrhage from the rectum or left colon. Beetroot ingestion can sometimes cause confusion. Blood loss may result from a carcinoma or polyp, an arteriovenous malformation, inflammatory bowel disease or diverticular disease. It can occasionally occur with massive upper gastrointestinal bleeding. The blood is mixed in with the bowel motion if it comes from above the anorectum, but if blood appears on the surface of the motion or only on the toilet paper this suggests, but does not guarantee, that bleeding is from a local rectal cause, such as internal haemorrhoids or a fissure. Dark red jelly-like stools may be seen with ischaemic bowel.

Steatorrhoea

The stools are usually very pale, offensive, smelly and bulky. They float and are difficult to flush away. However, the commonest cause of floating stools is gas and water rather than fat.

Steatorrhoea results from malabsorption of fat. In severe pancreatic disease, oil (triglycerides) may be passed per rectum and this is virtually pathognomonic of pancreatic steatorrhoea (lipase deficiency).

'Toothpaste' stools

Here the faeces are expressed like toothpaste from a tube: the condition is usually due to severe constipation with overflow diarrhoea. It may, however, also occur in the irritable bowel syndrome, with a stricture, or in Hirschsprung's disease.

Rice-water stools

Cholera causes massive excretion of fluid and electrolytes from the bowel, which results in a severe secretory diarrhoea. The pale watery stools are of enormous volume and contain mucous debris.

Vomitus

The clinician who is fortunate enough to have vomitus available for inspection (ill-informed staff may throw out this valuable substance) should not lose the opportunity of a detailed examination. There are a number of interesting types of vomitus.

'Coffee grounds'

An old blood clot in vomitus has the appearance of the dregs of a good cup of espresso coffee. Unfortunately, darker vomitus is often described as having this appearance. This emphasises the need for personal inspection. Iron tablets and red wine, not to mention coffee ingestion, can have the same effect on the vomitus.

Bright-red blood (haematemesis)

Look for the presence of fresh clot. It usually indicates fresh bleeding from the upper gastrointestinal tract.

Yellow-green vomitus

This results from the vomiting of bile and upper small bowel contents, often when there is obstruction.

Faeculent vomiting

Here brown offensive material from the small bowel is vomited. It is a late sign of small intestinal obstruction. Recently ingested tea can have the same appearance but lacks the smell.

Brownish-black fluid in large volumes may be vomited in cases of acute dilatation of the stomach. A succussion splash will usually be present. Acute dilatation may occur in association with diabetic ketoacidosis or following abdominal surgery. It represents a medical emergency because of the risk of aspiration; there is a need for urgent placement of a nasogastric tube (see Figure 6.42, page 194).

Projectile vomiting

This term describes the act of vomiting itself and may indicate pyloric stenosis (a paediatric illness). It may also occur with raised intracranial pressure.

Urinalysis

Note that testing of the urine can be very helpful in diagnosing liver disease.

Strip colour tests can detect the presence of bilirubin and urobilinogen in the urine. False-positive or false-negative results can occur with vitamin C or even exposure to sunlight.

An understanding of the reasons for the presence of bilirubin or urobilinogen in the urine necessitates an explanation of the metabolism of these substances (Figure 6.34).

Red blood cells are broken down by the reticuloendothelial system, causing the release of haem, which is converted to biliverdin and then *unconjugated bilirubin*, a water-insoluble compound. For this reason, unconjugated bilirubin released with haemolytic anaemia will not appear in the urine (termed *acholuric jaundice*).

Unconjugated bilirubin is transported in the blood bound largely to albumin but also to other plasma proteins. Unconjugated bilirubin is then taken up by the liver cells and transported to the endoplasmic reticulum, where glucuronyl transferases conjugate bilirubin with glucuronide. This results in the formation of *conjugated bilirubin*, which is water-soluble. Conjugated bilirubin is then concentrated and excreted by the liver cell into the canaliculus.

Conjugated bilirubin is virtually all excreted into the small bowel; it is converted in the terminal ileum and colon to *urobilinogen*, and then to *stercobilin*. Stercobilin is responsible for the normal colour of the stools with other non-bilirubinoid dietary pigments. Up to 20% of urobilinogen is reabsorbed by the bowel, and small amounts are excreted in the urine as urinary urobilinogen. This can often be normally detected by reagent strips.

Total biliary obstruction, from whatever cause, results in absence of urinary urobilinogen, as no conjugated bilirubin reaches the bowel, resulting in pale stools (absence of stercobilin). The conjugated bilirubin, unable to be excreted (the rate-limiting step), leaks from the hepatocytes into the blood and from there is excreted into the urine (normally there is no bilirubin detected in urine). This results in dark urine (excess conjugated bilirubin). Acute liver damage, as in viral hepatitis, may sometimes initially result in excessive urinary urobilinogen, because the liver is

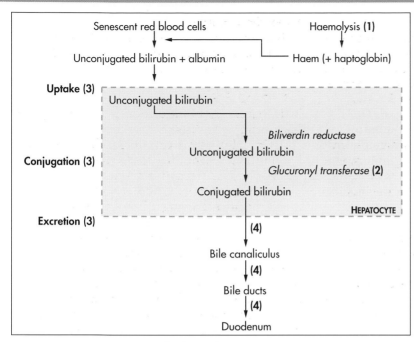

Figure 6.34 Schematic representation of the bilirubin pathway
Increased haemolysis (1) overwhelms the hepatocytes' ability to conjugate bilirubin and excrete the conjugated form, leading to increased serum levels of unconjugated bilirubin. Low levels of glucuronyl transferase (2) (e.g. Gilbert's disease) cause decreased conjugation. Hepatocellular dysfunction (3) causes decreased uptake, conjugation and excretion with increases of unconjugated bilirubin and conjugated bilirubin. Post-hepatic obstruction (4) from stones or tumour prevents passage of bilirubin through the bile ducts into the bowel, leading to increased serum levels of conjugated bilirubin.

TABLE 6.19 Changes in urine and faeces with jaundice

Substance and site	Cause of jaundice:		
	Haemolysis	**Obstruction or cholestasis**	**Hepatocellular liver disease**
Urine			
Bilirubin (conjugated)	Normal*	Raised	Normal or raised
Urobilinogen	Raised	Absent or decreased	Normal or raised
Faeces			
Stercobilinogen	Raised	Absent or decreased	Normal
Causes	Haemolytic anaemia	Extrahepatic biliary obstruction (e.g. gallstones, carcinoma of pancreas or bile duct, strictures of the bile duct), intrahepatic cholestasis (e.g. drugs, recurrent jaundice of pregnancy)	Hepatitis, cirrhosis, drugs, venous obstruction

* Unconjugated bilirubin levels are elevated in the serum.

unable to re-excrete the urobilinogen reabsorbed from the bowel. These changes are summarised in Table 6.19.

Examination of the acute abdomen

It is very important to try to determine whether a patient who presents with acute abdominal pain requires an urgent operation or whether careful observation with reassessment is the best course of action.[22,23] First, take note of the *general appearance* of the patient. The patient who is obviously distressed with pain or who looks unwell often is, and conversely some reassurance can be gained if a patient does not look sick and appears comfortable.

Assess the patient's *vital signs* immediately and recheck these at frequent intervals. Signs of reduced circulating blood volume and dehydration, including tachycardia, postural hypotension, tachypnoea, vasoconstriction and sweating, are of great concern. These signs associated with abdominal pain are usually an indication of substantial intra-abdominal blood loss (such as a ruptured aortic aneurysm), or of substantial fluid losses (e.g. due to acute pancreatitis), or of septic shock (as with a perforated viscus or abscess). Take the patient's temperature.

Inspect the abdomen. Look particularly for lack of movement with respiration, with splinting of the abdominal wall muscles. Note any abdominal distension, visible peristalsis or other lumps and masses, without forgetting the groin region and hernias. Note also any abdominal scars and inquire as to their nature and age.

Palpate very gently. The presence or absence of peritonism is first assessed. Peritonism is an inflammation that causes pain when peritoneal surfaces are moved relative to each other (Table 6.20; see also *Good signs guide 6.4*). Traditionally, rebound tenderness is used to assess whether peritonism is present or not. However, if peritonism is present, this test is far more uncomfortable (and cruel) than eliciting tenderness to light percussion. If the patient is extremely apprehensive, ask him or her first to cough; the reaction will be a guide to the degree of peritonism and also its location. Palpation is then continued slowly, but more deeply if possible and if masses are sought. Do not forget to palpate for the pulsatile mass of a ruptured aneurysm. This may be quite indistinct.

Then perform light percussion over areas of tenderness. If generalised peritonitis is present, this almost invariably necessitates a surgical approach, with the notable exception of acute pancreatitis.

Examine for hernias. The presence of a hernia does not necessarily mean that this is the cause of pathology, as they are quite common. However, a tender or irreducible hernia is more likely to be of significance, particularly if this has only very recently been noticed by the patient or has recently become tender.

Auscultation is now performed. In the presence of a bowel obstruction (*Good signs guide 6.5*), bowel sounds will be louder, more frequent and high-pitched. In an ileus from any cause, bowel sounds are usually reduced or absent.

Rectal and vaginal examinations may be very important but the findings are not helpful for the diagnosis of appendicitis or obstruction; note any tenderness (and its location), masses or blood loss. Per rectal blood should make the examiner think of acute colitis (e.g. Crohn's disease, ulcerative colitis, ischaemic colitis or infectious colitis), or of mesenteric ischaemia. A purulent vaginal discharge suggests salpingitis.

Urinalysis may show glycosuria and ketonuria

in diabetic ketoacidosis (which can cause acute abdominal pain), haematuria in renal colic, bilirubinuria in cholangitis or proteinuria in pyelonephritis (page 200).

Examine the *respiratory system* for signs of

TABLE 6.20 Differential diagnosis of the acute abdomen

Severe abdominal pain with rigidity of the entire abdominal wall and prostration
Perforated peptic ulcer
Perforation of other intra-abdominal organs
Dissecting aneurysm
Severe pancreatitis

Tenderness and rigidity in the right hypochondrium
Acute cholecystitis
Appendicitis in a high appendix
Perforated or penetrating duodenal ulcer
Pleurisy, pneumonitis
Subphrenic abscess
Acute pyelonephritis
Cholangitis
Bleed into an hepatic tumour

Tenderness and rigidity in the left hypochondrium
Pancreatitis
Subphrenic abscess
Diverticulitis
Ruptured spleen
Acute pyelonephritis
Leaking aneurysm of the splenic artery
Acute gastric distension

Tenderness and rigidity in the right iliac fossa
Appendicitis
Perforated or penetrating duodenal ulcer
Crohn's disease or inflamed ileocaecal glands
Inflamed Meckel's diverticulum
Cholecystitis with a low gallbladder

Tenderness and rigidity in the left iliac fossa
Diverticulitis
Colitis
Colonic cancer
Pelvic peritonitis, ruptured ovarian cyst

Periumbilical pain without abdominal signs
Acute mesenteric ischaemia/infarction
Acute appendicitis
Acute small bowel obstruction
Acute pancreatitis

Obstetric and gynaecological causes
Ectopic pregnancy
Torsion of, or haemorrhage into, an ovarian cyst
Acute salpingitis
Ruptured uterus

GOOD SIGNS GUIDE 6.4 Peritonitis

Sign	Positive LR	Negative LR
Abdominal examination		
Guarding	2.6	0.6
Rigidity	5.1	NS
Rebound tenderness	2.1	0.5
Abnormal bowel sounds	NS	0.8
Rectal examination		
Rectal tenderness	NS	NS
Other tests		
Positive abdominal wall tenderness test	0.1	NS

NS = not significant.
From McGee S, *Evidence-based physical diagnosis*, 2nd edn. St Louis: Saunders, 2007.

GOOD SIGNS GUIDE 6.5 Acute bowel obstruction

Sign	Positive LR	Negative LR
Inspection of the abdomen		
Visible peristalsis	18.8	NS
Abdominal distension	9.6	0.4
Palpation		
Guarding	NS	NS
Rigidity	NS	NS
Rebound tenderness	NS	NS
Auscultation		
Increased (obstructed) bowel sounds	5.0	0.6
Abnormal bowel sounds	3.2	0.4
Rectal examination		
Rectal tenderness	NS	NS

NS = not significant.
From McGee S, *Evidence-based physical diagnosis*, 2nd edn. St Louis: Saunders, 2007.

consolidation, a pleural rub or pleural effusion, and examine the *cardiovascular system* for atrial fibrillation (a major cause of embolism to a mesenteric artery) or for signs of a myocardial infarction. Examine the *back* for evidence of spinal disease that may radiate to the abdomen. Remember that herpes zoster may cause abdominal pain before the typical vesicles erupt.

Consider the symptoms and signs of appendicitis.[22] Malaise and fever is usually associated with abdominal pain, which is at first worst in the hypogastrium and then moves to the right iliac fossa. The examination will often reveal tenderness and guarding in the right iliac fossa. The pain and tenderness are usually maximum over *McBurney's point*.[dd] He described this point as $1^{1}/_{2}$ to 2 in (3.8 to 5.0 cm) along a line from the anterior superior iliac spine to the umbilicus. *Rovsing's sign*[ee] is another way of testing rebound tenderness. Press over the patient's left lower quadrant, then release quickly; this causes pain in the right iliac fossa. The *psoas sign* is positive when the patient lies on the left side and the clinician attempts to extend the right hip. If this is painful and resisted, the sign is positive. When the appendix causes pelvic inflammation, rectal examination evokes tenderness on the right side. These signs are of variable usefulness (*Good signs guide 6.6*).

Remember that in elderly patients these signs may be reduced or absent.[23]

Correlation of physical signs and gastrointestinal disease
Liver disease
Signs
- **Hands:** leuconychia, clubbing, palmar erythema, bruising, asterixis.
- **Face:** jaundice, scratch marks, spider naevi, fetor hepaticus.
- **Chest:** gynaecomastia, loss of body hair, spider naevi, bruising, pectoral muscle wasting.
- **Abdomen:** hepatosplenomegaly, ascites, signs of portal hypertension, testicular atrophy.
- **Legs:** oedema, muscle wasting, bruising.
- **Fever:** may occur in up to one-third of patients with advanced cirrhosis (particularly when this is secondary to alcohol) or if there is infected ascites.

The presence of two or more of the following signs suggests cirrhosis: (i) spider naevi; (ii) palmar erythema; (iii) splenomegaly or ascites; (iv) abnormal collateral veins on the abdomen; (v) ascites. See also *Good signs guide 6.7*.

Portal hypertension
Signs
- **Splenomegaly:** correlates poorly with the degree of portal hypertension.
- **Collateral veins:** haematemesis (from oesophageal or gastric varices).
- **Ascites.**

---

dd Charles McBurney (1845-1913), New York surgeon described his sign to the New York Surgical Society in 1889.
ee Thorkild Rovsing (1862–1937), professor of surgery, Copenhagen.

GOOD SIGNS GUIDE 6.6 Appendicitis		
Sign	Positive LR	Negative LR
Vital signs		
Fever	1.8	0.5
Abdominal examination		
Severe right lower quadrant tenderness	NS	0.2
McBurney's point tenderness	3.4	0.4
Rovsing's sign	2.5	0.7
Rectal examination		
Rectal tenderness	NS	NS
Others		
Psoas sign	NS	NS

NS = not significant.
From McGee S, *Evidence-based physical diagnosis*, 2nd edn. St Louis: Saunders, 2007.

GOOD SIGNS GUIDE 6.7 Jaundice due to hepatocellular disease		
Sign	Positive LR	Negative LR
General appearance		
Weight loss	NS	NS
Skin		
Spider naevi	4.7	0.6
Palmar erythema	9.8	0.5
Distended abdominal veins	17.5	0.6
Abdomen		
Ascites	4.4	0.6
Palpable spleen	2.9	0.7
Palpable gallbladder	0.04	1.4
(Courvoisier's law)		
Palpable liver	NS	NS
Liver tenderness	NS	NS

NS = not significant.
From McGee S, *Evidence-based physical diagnosis*, 2nd edn. St Louis: Saunders, 2007.

Causes

1 **Cirrhosis** of the liver.
2 **Other causes:**
  (a) *Presinusoidal:* (i) portal vein compression (e.g. lymphoma, carcinoma); (ii) intravascular clotting (e.g. in polycythaemia); (iii) umbilical vein phlebitis.
  (b) *Intrahepatic:* (i) sarcoid, lymphoma or leukaemic infiltrates; (ii) congenital hepatic fibrosis.
  (c) *Postsinusoidal:* (i) hepatic vein outflow obstruction (Budd-Chiari syndrome) may be idiopathic, or caused by myeloproliferative disease, cancer (kidney, pancreas, liver), the contraceptive pill or pregnancy, paroxysmal nocturnal haemoglobinuria (PNH), fibrous membrane, trauma, schistosomiasis; (ii) veno-occlusive disease; (iii) constrictive pericarditis; (iv) chronic cardiac failure.

Hepatic encephalopathy
Grading
Grade 0—normal mental state
Grade 1—mental changes (lack of awareness, anxiety, euphoria, reduced attention span, impaired ability to add and subtract)
Grade 2—lethargy, disorientation (for time), personality changes, inappropriate behaviour
Grade 3—stupor, but responsive to stimuli; gross disorientation, confusion
Grade 4—coma.

Causes
These include:
• Acute liver failure (e.g. postviral hepatitis, alcoholic hepatitis).
• Cirrhosis.
• Chronic portosystemic encephalopathy (e.g. from a portocaval shunt).

Encephalopathy may be precipitated by:
• Diarrhoea, diuretics or vomiting (resulting in hypokalaemia which may increase renal ammonia and other toxin production, or alkalosis which may increase the amount of ammonia and other toxins that cross the blood–brain barrier).
• Gastrointestinal bleeding or a relatively high-protein diet (causing an acute increase in nitrogenous contents in the bowel).
• Infection (e.g. urinary tract, chest or spontaneous bacterial peritonitis).
• Acute liver cell decompensation (e.g. from an alcoholic binge or a hepatoma).
• Sedatives.
• Metabolic disturbances such as hypoglycaemia.

Dysphagia
Dysphagia (difficulty in swallowing) and odynophagia (pain on swallowing) are important

symptoms of underlying organic disease. It is important to examine such patients carefully for likely causes (see Table 6.2, page 148).

Signs

- **General inspection.** Note weight loss, due to decreased food intake or oesophageal cancer per se.
- **The hands.** Inspect the nails for koilonychia (page 208), and the palmar creases for pallor indicative of anaemia. Iron deficiency anaemia can be associated with an upper oesophageal web, which is a thin structure consisting of mucosa and submucosa but not muscle. Iron deficiency anaemia and dysphagia due to an upper oesophageal web is called the Plummer-Vinson[ff] (or sometimes the Paterson–Brown-Kelly[gg] syndrome). Also examine the hands for signs of scleroderma.
- **The mouth.** Inspect the mucosa for ulceration or infection (e.g. candidiasis), which can cause odynophagia; examine the lower cranial nerves for evidence of bulbar or pseudobulbar palsy.
- **The neck.** Palpate the supraclavicular nodes, which may occasionally be involved with oesophageal cancer; examine for evidence of retrosternal thyroid enlargement. A mass on the left side of the neck that is accompanied by gurgling sounds may rarely be caused by a Zenker's diverticulum,[hh] an outpouching of the posterior hypopharyngeal wall.
- **The lungs.** Examine for evidence of aspiration into the lungs (due to overflow of retained material, gastro-oesophageal reflux or, rarely, the development of a tracheo-oesophageal reflux from oesophageal cancer).
- **The abdomen.** Feel for hepatomegaly due to secondary deposits from oesophageal cancer and for an epigastric mass from a gastric cancer; perform a rectal examination to exclude melaena (albeit uncommon with oesophageal disease).

Assessment of gastrointestinal bleeding

Haematemesis, melaena or massive rectal bleeding are dramatic signs of gastrointestinal haemorrhage. It is important in such a case to assess the amount of blood loss and attempt to determine the likely site of bleeding. Haematemesis indicates bleeding from a site proximal to, or in, the duodenum.

Assessing degree of blood loss

First take the pulse rate and the blood pressure lying and sitting. As a general rule, loss of 1.5 litres or more of blood volume over a few hours results in a fall in cardiac output, causing hypotension and tachycardia. A pulse rate of more than 100 a minute or a systolic blood pressure of less than 100 mmHg, or a 15 mmHg postural fall in systolic blood pressure, suggests significant recent blood loss. These are indications for blood transfusion. The signs depend to some extent on the state of the patient's cardiovascular system. Those who have pre-existing cardiovascular disease will become shocked much earlier than young fit patients with a normal cardiovascular system.

Once signs of shock are present, massive blood loss has occurred. These signs include peripheral cyanosis with cold extremities, clammy skin, dyspnoea and air hunger; the patients are anxious. The blood pressure is low, with a compensating tachycardia, and the urine output is reduced or absent. These are ominous signs in patients with gastrointestinal haemorrhage. Urgent resuscitative measures must be instituted.

Determining the possible bleeding site

The causes of acute gastrointestinal haemorrhage are listed in Table 6.3, page 151.

Examine the patient with *acute upper gastro-intestinal bleeding* for signs of chronic liver disease and portal hypertension. Part of the assessment should include inspection of the vomitus and stools (pages 183–184) and a rectal examination. Remember that, of patients with chronic liver disease and upper gastrointestinal bleeding, only about half are bleeding from varices. The others are usually bleeding from peptic ulceration (either acute or chronic). Look for evidence of a bleeding diathesis.

Finally, examine the patient for any evidence of skin lesions that can be associated with vascular anomalies in the gastrointestinal tract, although these are rare (Tables 6.3, 6.4). For example, pseudoxanthoma elasticum is an autosomal recessive disorder of elastic fibres that results in xanthoma-like yellowish nodules, particularly in the axillae or neck. These patients may also have angioid streaks of the optic fundus and angiomatous malformations of blood vessels that can bleed into the gastrointestinal tract. Ehlers-Danlos syndrome is a group of connective tissue disorders resulting

---

[ff] Henry Plummer (1874–1936), physician at the Mayo Clinic, described the syndrome in 1912; Porter Vinson (1890–1959), physician, Medical College Virginia, described the syndrome in 1919.

[gg] Donald Paterson (1863–1939), Cardiff otolaryngologist, and Adam Brown-Kelly (1865–1941), Glasgow otolaryngologist, described this syndrome in 1919.

[hh] Friedrich Albert Zenker (1825–1898), Munich pathologist.

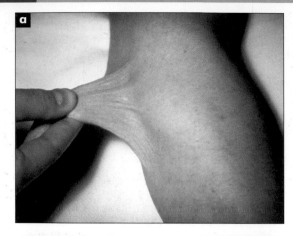

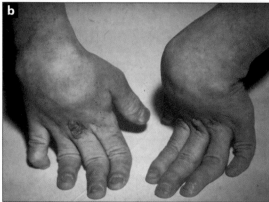

Figure 6.35 Ehlers-Danlos syndrome: (a) arms; (b) hands
Abnormal elasticity of the skin is typical of the Ehlers-Danlos syndrome. The skin may be greatly stretched and takes much longer than normal to return to its normal position. It is also more fragile than normal. Joint hypermobility occurs in type III Ehlers-Danlos syndrome.

in fragile and hyperextensible skin (Figure 6.35). In a number of types, blood vessels are involved. Type IV is characterised by gastrointestinal tract bleeding, spontaneous bowel perforation, minimal skin hyperelasticity and minimal joint hyperextension.

Examine the patient with *acute lower gastrointestinal bleeding* as described above, paying close attention to the abdominal examination and the rectal examination. Inspect the stools and test them for blood. Colonoscopy is a key test for all these patients.

Malabsorption

Numerous diseases can cause maldigestion or malabsorption of food. Fat, protein and/or carbohydrate absorption may be affected.

Signs

- **General:** wasting (protein and fat malabsorption), folds of loose skin (recent weight loss), pallor (anaemia) or pigmentation (e.g. as in Whipple's disease[ii]).
- **Stools:** steatorrhoea (pale, bulky and offensive stools).
- **Mouth:** glossitis and angular stomatitis (deficiency in vitamin B_2, vitamin B_6, vitamin B_{12}, folate or niacin), intraoral purpura (vitamin K deficiency) or hyperkeratotic white patches (vitamin A deficiency).
- **Limbs:** bruising (vitamin K deficiency), oedema (protein deficiency), peripheral neuropathy (vitamin B_{12} or thiamine deficiency), bone pain (vitamin D deficiency).
- **Signs suggesting the underlying cause:** in the abdomen these include scars from previous surgery, such as a gastrectomy, operations for Crohn's disease or massive small bowel resection; on the skin dermatitis herpetiformis (itchy red lumps on the extensor surfaces) may be found—this condition is strongly associated with coeliac disease and the histocompatibility antigen HLA-B8; there may be *signs of chronic liver disease*, or *signs of inflammatory bowel disease*.

Causes

Common causes include coeliac disease, chronic pancreatitis and a previous gastrectomy.

Classification of malabsorption

- **Lipolytic phase defects** (pancreatic enzyme deficiency): (i) chronic pancreatitis; (ii) cystic fibrosis.
- **Micellar phase defects** (bile salt deficiency): (i) extrahepatic biliary obstruction; (ii) chronic liver disease; (iii) bacterial overgrowth; (iv) terminal ileal disease, such as Crohn's disease or resection.
- **Mucosal defects** (diseased epithelial lining): (i) coeliac disease; (ii) tropical sprue; (iii) lymphoma; (iv) Whipple's disease; (v) bowel ischaemia or resection; (vi) amyloidosis; (vii) hypogammaglobulinaemia; (viii) HIV infection.
- **Delivery phase defects** (inability to transport fat out of cells to lymphatics): (i) intestinal lymphangiectasia; (ii) abetalipoproteinaemia;

ii George Hoyt Whipple (1878–1976), Baltimore pathologist, described this rare disease characterised by diarrhoea, arthralgia, central nervous system signs and pigmentation. He shared the 1934 Nobel Prize for work on liver treatment in anaemia and coined the word *thalassaemia*.

(iii) carcinomatous infiltration of lymphatics.

Inflammatory bowel disease

Inflammatory bowel disease refers to two chronic idiopathic diseases of the gastrointestinal tract: ulcerative colitis and Crohn's disease.

Ulcerative colitis

In the gastrointestinal tract only the large bowel is affected. Occasionally the terminal ileum can be secondarily involved (backwash ileitis). The disease almost always involves the rectum and may extend, without skip areas, to involve a variable part of the colon.

- **Abdominal signs:** if there is proctitis only, there are usually no abnormal external findings (except at sigmoidoscopy and biopsy); occasionally, anal fissures are present; with colitis, in the uncomplicated case the abdominal examination may be normal or there may be tenderness and guarding over the affected colon.
- **Signs of complications:** local signs include the following: (i) *toxic dilatation (megacolon)*—one of the most feared complications in which there are signs of distension, generalised guarding and rigidity (peritonism), pyrexia and tachycardia; (ii) *massive bleeding or perforation*; (iii) *carcinoma*—there is an increased incidence of colonic cancer in extensive, long-standing ulcerative colitis.
- **Systemic signs include:** (i) *chronic liver disease*—primary sclerosing cholangitis or cirrhosis; (ii) *anaemia*—due to chronic disease per se, or blood loss, or autoimmune haemolysis; (iii) *arthritis*—there may be a peripheral non-deforming arthropathy affecting particularly the knees, ankles and wrists (10%), and there may be signs of ankylosing spondylitis in 3%; (iv) *skin manifestations*: erythema nodosum (2%) consists of tender red nodules usually on the shins (Figure 6.36); pyoderma gangrenosum (rare) starts as a tender, red raised area which becomes bullous and ulcerates (Figure 6.37)—it may occur anywhere but is often on the anterior aspects of the legs; mouth ulcers are common and are due to aphthous ulceration (5%); finger clubbing may be present; (v) *ocular changes* include conjunctivitis, iritis and episcleritis, which are strongly associated with arthritis and skin rash. (*Conjunctivitis* is an inflammation of the conjunctiva which then appears red and swollen: the eye itself is not tender. *Iritis* is an inflammation of the iris with

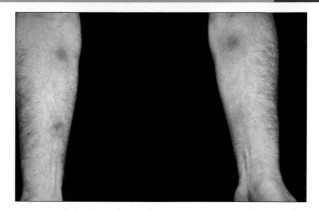

Figure 6.36 Erythema nodosum
(From McDonald FS, ed., *Mayo Clinic images in internal medicine*, with permission. © Mayo Clinic Scientific Press and CRC Press.)

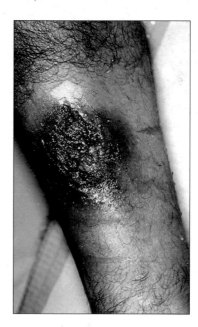

Figure 6.37 Pyoderma gangrenosum
(From Misiewicz JJ, Bantrum CI, Cotton PB et al, *Slide atlas of gastroenterology*. London: Gower Medical Publishing, 1985, with permission.)

central scleral injection, which radiates out from the pupil: the eye is tender. *Episcleritis* is a nodule of inflammation on the scleral surface.)

Crohn's disease

The whole of the gastrointestinal tract may be affected from the mouth to the anus. However, most commonly the terminal ileum, with or without the colon, is involved.

- **Abdominal signs:** if the condition affects only the terminal ileum there are often no abnormal findings, although tenderness, fullness or a mass (either soft or firm) in the right iliac fossa may be present. Occasionally there may be signs of an abdominal abscess: these patients may have a high swinging fever, localised tenderness, a palpable mass and evidence of bowel obstruction (pain, vomiting and constipation with dehydration, abdominal distension and tenderness, and an empty rectum). Anal disease is common, including skin tags, fissures, fistulae and abscesses. Colonic involvement produces the same signs as ulcerative colitis.

- **Signs of complications:** these are similar to those of ulcerative colitis with the following exceptions: (i) *liver disease*—primary sclerosing cholangitis is less common; (ii) *osteomalacia* and *osteoporosis*, which may occur in patients with extensive terminal ileal involvement, results in bone tenderness and fracture; (iii) *signs of malabsorption;* (iv) *finger clubbing* is more common; (v) *signs of gastrointestinal malignancy* (small bowel or colonic carcinoma) are uncommon but the incidence is increased; (vi) the incidence of *gallstones and renal stones* is increased; (vii) *renal disease* due to pyelonephritis, hydronephrosis or very rarely secondary amyloidosis may occur.

The abdominal X-ray: a systematic approach

Interpretation of the plain radiograph requires knowledge of basic anatomy and pathological processes.

The soft-tissue density of the abdominal organs is similar to that of water. Therefore they are usually not visible unless outlined by fat or adjacent gas. For example, fluid-filled bowel is not visible, but the bowel walls are outlined by the contained gas.

Because of this intrinsic lack of contrast in the abdomen, radio-opaque contrast media are introduced to show up various organs. Barium meals, barium enemas, intravenous urograms and arteriograms are contrast studies.

Radiography

As with the chest X-ray, the name and date should be checked. The left and right sides should be easily distinguished by the stomach gas on the left and the triangular bulky soft tissue of the liver seen in the right hypochondrium.

Review of an abdominal X-ray

- **Boundaries:** diaphragm, psoas muscles, the extraperitoneal fat ('flank lines').
- **Bones:** lower ribs and costal cartilages, lumbar spine, pelvis.
- **Hollow viscera gas:** check gas outlining the stomach, small bowel and large bowel.
- **Solid organs:** size of liver, spleen and kidneys.
- **Pelvic organs:** bladder size.
- **Vascular:** aortic calcification.
- **Abnormalities:** renal or biliary calculi, dilated bowel, free peritoneal gas (Figure 6.38).

Bowel gas pattern

Supine films are taken in most conditions to show the distribution of the bowel gas. In patients with an acute abdomen, a horizontal beam film, usually an erect view, is also taken to show air–fluid levels.

With obstruction, there is an accumulation of fluid and gas proximally.

In inflammatory or ischaemic colitis, the swollen bowel mucosa will be outlined by gas ('thumb-printing').

Bowel dilatation

When an ileus (Figure 6.39) or obstruction (Figures 6.40 and 6.41) is present, it is possible to distinguish small- from large-bowel dilatation. The *large-bowel loops* are peripheral, few in number, have diameters greater than 5 cm, contain faeces, and have haustral margins that do not extend across the bowel lumen. In contrast, the *small-bowel loops* are central, multiple, between 3 and 5 cm in diameter, and do not contain faeces. Valvulae conniventes which extend completely across the bowel lumen are seen in the jejunal loops.

With gastric dilatation, the stomach may be massively enlarged and distended with air (Figure 6.42).

Calcification

Calcification shows up well against the grey, soft-tissue densities.

About 90% of renal stones are calcified (Figure 7.4, page 203), whereas only 10% of gallstones are calcified. To identify radiolucent gallstones, an ultrasound examination is the test of choice.

Calcification may be seen in the pancreas in chronic pancreatitis (Figure 6.43).

Costal cartilage calcification is commonly seen in elderly patients, projected over the hypochondrial regions.

Calcification in the walls of an abdominal aortic aneurysm may be seen on a lateral abdominal film. Splenic and renal artery aneurysms are also often calcified.

Vascular calcification is often seen in the elderly.

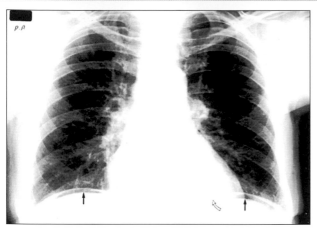

Figure 6.38 Free peritoneal gas
The erect chest X-ray is superior to an erect abdominal film for the demonstration of free gas. On the erect chest X-ray, free peritoneal gas is seen below the hemidiaphragm (black arrows). The free gas on the left must be distinguished from gas in the gastric fundus (open arrow). This free gas (black arrow) on the left is crescentic in shape because it outlines the spleen and lies at the apex of the hemidiaphragm. It indicates a perforation of a hollow abdominal viscus unless there has been recent surgery or penetrating trauma.

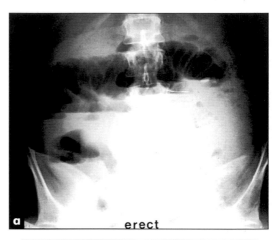

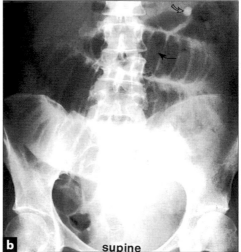

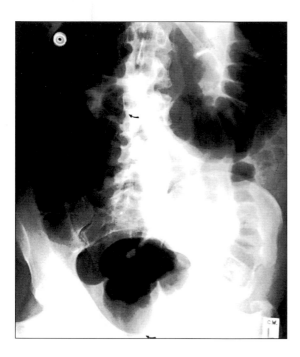

Figure 6.39 Generalised ileus
The large bowel is filled with gas and is dilated, except in the descending colon. Dilated small bowel is also seen in the right hypochondrium (arrow). As gas is seen around to the rectum (arrow), mechanical obstruction is excluded.

Ascites

With accumulation of peritoneal fluid within the peritoneal cavity, the film looks generally grey and lacks detail. On the supine film the bowel loops float towards the middle of the abdomen.

Figure 6.40 Small bowel obstruction
There is gross dilatation of the small bowel. It is recognised as small bowel from its central position and its transverse mucosal bands—the valvulae conniventes (black arrow). Air–fluid levels are seen on the erect view (a). The supine view (b) gives a better view of the distribution of the dilated loops. From the number and position of the displayed dilated loops, the obstruction would be at the level of the mid-small bowel. The round radio-opaque shadow in the left hypochondrium is a tablet (open arrow).

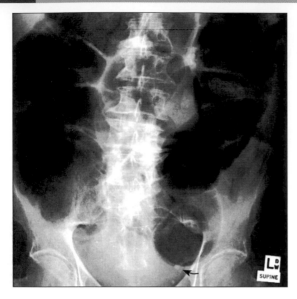

Figure 6.41 Large bowel obstruction
The large bowel is markedly distended around to the sigmoid colon, where it abruptly stops (arrow). The common causes of obstruction are carcinoma or diverticular stricture. The increased peristalsis occurring at the onset of obstruction can remove the gas and faeces distal to the obstruction. Therefore no gas is seen in this patient.

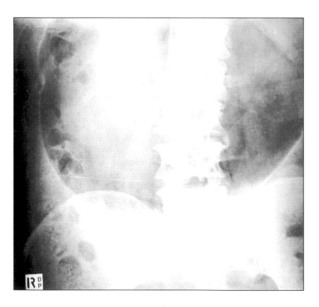

Figure 6.42 Gastric dilatation
The stomach is massively enlarged and distended with air. When this occurs acutely, prompt nasogastric aspiration is necessary. Mechanical obstruction due to a pyloric ulcer or carcinoma needs exclusion. Atonic dilatation is usually a postoperative complication, but may occur with diabetic coma, trauma, pancreatitis or hypokalaemia.

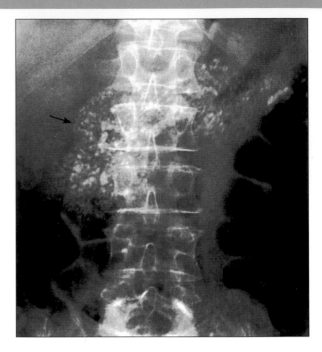

Figure 6.43 Pancreatic calcification
Stippled calcification is seen in the region of the pancreas (arrow), indicating chronic calcific pancreatitis. The most likely cause is alcohol excess.

Summary
The gastrointestinal examination: a suggested method (Figure 6.44)

As with the other systems this examination will usually be targeted. However it cannot be performed properly, even in a busy clinic, unless the patient lies down and removes sufficient clothing—if necessary in stages and with a chaperone.

Position the patient correctly with one pillow for the head and complete exposure of the abdomen. Look briefly at the **general appearance** and inspect particularly for signs of chronic liver disease.

Examine the **hands**. Ask the patient to extend his or her arms and hands and look for the hepatic flap. Look also at the nails for clubbing and for white nails, and note any palmar erythema or Dupuytren's contractures. The arthropathy of haemochromatosis may also be present. Look now at the **arms** for bruising, scratch marks and spider naevi.

Then go to the **face**. Note any scleral abnormality (jaundice, anaemia or iritis). Look at the corneas for Kayser-Fleischer rings. Feel for parotid enlargement; then inspect the mouth with a torch and spatula for angular stomatitis, ulceration, telangiectasiae and atrophic glossitis. Smell the breath for fetor hepaticus. Now look at the chest for spider naevi and in men for gynaecomastia and loss of body hair.

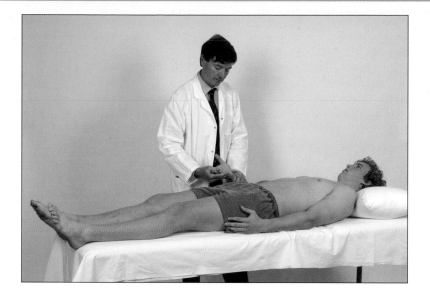

Figure 6.44 Gastrointestinal system
Lying flat (1 pillow)

1. **General inspection**
   Jaundice (liver disease)
   Pigmentation (haemochromatosis, Whipple's disease)
   Xanthomata (chronic cholestasis)
   Mental state (encephalopathy)
2. **Hands**
3. **Nails**
   • Clubbing
   • Leuconychia
   Palmar erythema
   Dupuytren's contractures (alcohol)
   Arthropathy
   Hepatic flap
4. **Arms**
   Spider naevi
   Bruising
   Wasting
   Scratch marks (chronic cholestasis)
5. **Face**
   Eyes
   • Sclerae: jaundice, anaemia, iritis
   • Cornea: Kayser-Fleischer rings (Wilson's disease)
   Parotids (alcohol)
   Mouth
   • *Breath:* fetor hepaticus
   • *Lips:* stomatitis, leucoplakia, ulceration, localised
     pigmentation (Peutz-Jeghers syndrome),
     telangiectasia (hereditary haemorrhagic
     telangiectasia)
   • *Gums:* gingivitis, bleeding, hypertrophy,
     pigmentation, *Monilia*
   • *Tongue:* atrophic glossitis, leucoplakia, ulceration
6. **Cervical/axillary lymph nodes**
7. **Chest**
   Gynaecomastia
   Spider naevi
   Body hair

8. **Abdomen**
   Inspect
   • Scars
   • Distension
   • Prominent veins—determine direction of flow
     (caput Medusae; inferior vena cava obstruction)
   • Striae
   • Bruising
   • Pigmentation
   • Localised masses
   • Visible peristalsis
   Palpate
   • Superficial palpation—tenderness, rigidity, outline
     of any mass
   • Deep palpation—organomegaly (liver, spleen,
     kidney), abnormal masses
   Roll onto right side (spleen)
   Percuss
   • Liver, spleen
   • Ascites—shifting dullness
   Auscultate
   • Bowel sounds
   • Bruits, hums, rubs
9. **Groin**
   Testes
   Lymph nodes
   Hernial orifices (standing up)
10. **Legs**
    Bruising
    Oedema
    Neurological signs (alcohol)
11. **Other**
    Rectal examination—inspect (fistulae, tags, blood,
       mucus), palpate (masses)
    Urine analysis (bile)
    Cardiovascular system (cardiomyopathy, cardiac
       failure, constrictive pericarditis)
    Temperature chart (infection)

Inspect the **abdomen** from the side, squatting to the patient's level. Large masses may be visible. Ask the patient to take slow deep breaths and look especially for the hepatic, splenic and gallbladder outlines. Now stand up and look for scars, distension, prominent veins, striae, hernia, bruising and pigmentation.

Palpate lightly in each region for masses, having asked first if any area is particularly tender. This will avoid causing the patient pain and may also provide a clue to a site of possible pathology. Next palpate each region more deeply; then feel specifically for hepatomegaly and splenomegaly. If there is hepatomegaly, confirm this with percussion and estimate the span. If no spleen is felt, percuss over the left costal margin in the left anterior axillary line during complete expiration (dullness suggests splenomegaly). Always **roll** the patient onto the right side and palpate again if the spleen is not felt initially. Attempt now to feel the kidneys bimanually. Remember the important distinguishing features of a spleen as opposed to a kidney.

Percuss routinely for ascites. If the abdomen is resonant right out to the flanks, do not roll the patient over. Otherwise test for shifting dullness. This is performed by percussing away from your side of the bed until you reach a dull note. Then **roll** the patient towards you and, after waiting a minute or so, begin percussing again for resonance.

By **auscultation** note the presence of bowel sounds. Next auscultate briefly over the liver, spleen and renal areas, listening for bruits, hums and rubs.

Examine the **groin** next. Palpate for inguinal lymphadenopathy. Examine for hernias by asking the patient to stand and then cough. The testes must always be palpated. Now look at the legs for oedema and bruising. Neurological examination of the **legs** may be indicated if there are signs of chronic liver disease.

If the **liver** is enlarged or cirrhosis is suspected ask the patient to sit up to 45 degrees and estimate the jugular venous pressure. This will avoid missing constrictive pericarditis or chronic cardiac failure as a cause of liver disease, or haemochromatosis, which can cause a dilated cardiomyopathy. While the patient is sitting up, palpate in the supraclavicular fossae for **lymph nodes** and feel at the back for **sacral oedema**. If ascites is present, it is necessary to examine the chest for a pleural effusion. If malignant disease is suspected, examine all lymph node groups, the breasts and the lungs.

A **rectal** examination should always be considered and specimens of the patient's vomitus or faeces should be inspected, if available. Perform a **urinalysis** (for bilirubin and urobilinogen, and glucose) and check the **temperature**.

References

1. Hendrix TR. Art and science of history taking in the patient with difficulty swallowing. *Dysphagia* 1993; 8:69–73. A very good review of the key historical features that must be obtained when a patient presents with trouble swallowing.
2. Talley NJ. Chronic unexplained diarrhea: what to do when the initial workup is negative? *Rev Gastroenterol Disord* 2008; 8(3):178–85.
3. Talley NJ, Lasch KL, Baum CL. A gap in our understanding: chronic constipation and its comorbid conditions. *Clin Gastroenterol Hepatol* 2009 Jan; 7(1):9–19.
4. Ford AC, Talley NJ, Veldhuyzen van Zanten SJ, Vakil NB, Simel DL, Moayyedi P. Will the history and physical examination help establish that irritable bowel syndrome is causing this patient's lower gastrointestinal tract symptoms? *JAMA* 2008; 300(15):1793–1805.
5. Theodossi A, Knill-Jones RP, Skene A. Interobserver variation of symptoms and signs in jaundice. *Liver* 1981; 1:21–32. The history and examination permitted a correct clinical diagnosis in jaundiced patients two-thirds of the time.
6. Patten A, Saunders JB. The ABC of alcohol; asking the right questions. *BMJ* 1981; 283:1458–1459. Discusses the value of the CAGE screening questions as well as other measures for identifying alcohol abuse.
7. Sibarte V, Shanahan F. Clinical examination of the gastrointestinal system in the 21st century—is the emphasis right? *Am J Gastroenterol* 2004; 99:1874–1875.
8. Walton S, Bennett JR. Skin and gullet. *Gut* 1991; 32:694–697. An excellent review of skin signs in gastroenterology.
9. Beitman RG, Rost SS, Roth JL. Oral manifestations of gastrointestinal disease. *Dig Dis Sci* 1981; 26:741–747. A detailed review.
10. Naylor CD. Physical examination of the liver. (The rational clinical examination.) *JAMA* 1994; 271:1859–1865. A valuable review of technique. Palpation is probably superior to percussion (in part because the midclavicular line is a 'wandering landmark'). Auscultation is usually of minimal value.
11. McGee S, *Evidence-based physical diagnosis*, 2nd edn. St Louis: Saunders, 2007.
12. Fink HA, Lederle FA et al. The accuracy of physical to detect abdominal aortic aneurysm. *Arch Intern Med* 2000;160:833–836.
13. Chervu A, Clagett GP, Valentine RJ, Myers SI, Rossi PJ. Role of physical examination in detection of abdominal aortic aneurysms. *Surgery* 1995; 117:454–457.
14. Thomson WH, Francis DM. Abdominal wall tenderness: a useful sign in the acute abdomen. *Lancet* 1977; 2:1053–1054. While abdominal wall

pain can be recognised when the patient tenses the abdominal wall muscles, intraperitoneal inflammation can cause a false-positive sign.

15. Srinivasan R, Greenbaum DS. Chronic abdominal wall pain: a frequently overlooked problem. Practical approach to diagnosis and management. *Am J Gastroenterol* 2002; 97:824–830.

16. Editorial. Abdominal wall tenderness test: could Carnett cut costs? *Lancet* 1991; 337:1134.

17. Williams JW Jr, Simel DL. Does this patient have ascites? How to divine fluid in the abdomen. (The rational clinical examination.) *JAMA* 1992; 267:2645–2648. This review provides information on the discriminant value of signs. Bulging flanks, shifting dullness and a fluid wave are each reasonably sensitive and specific. The presence of ascites is more easily predicted than its absence.

18. Muris JW, Starmans R, Wolfs GG, Pop P, Knottnerus JA. The diagnostic value of rectal examination. *Family Practice* 1993; 10:34–37. A useful procedure in patients with rectal or prostatic symptoms. Based on a literature review but studies in general practice are lacking.

19. Talley NJ. How to do and interpret a rectal examination in gastroenterology. *Am J Gastroenterol* 2008; 108:802–3.

20. Dobben AC, Terra MP, Deutekom M, et al. Anal inspection and digital rectal examination compared to anorectal physiology tests and endoanal ultrasonography in evaluating faecal incontinence. *Int J Colorectal Dis* 2007; 22:783–790.

21. Longstreth GF. Checking for *'the occult'* with a finger: a procedure of little value. *J Clin Gastroenterol* 1988; 10:133–134. A faecal occult blood test from the glove after rectal examination has too many false-positive and false-negative results to be of value.

22. Wagner JM, Mckinney WP, Carpenter JL. Does this patient have appendicitis? *JAMA* 1996; 276:1589–1594. A 'must read' that discusses the key symptoms and signs that help make the correct diagnosis.

23. Murtagh J. Acute abdominal pain: a diagnostic approach. *Aust Fam Phys* 1994; 23:358–361, 364–374.

Suggested reading

Browse NL. *An introduction to the symptoms and signs of surgical disease*, 4th edn. London: Arnold, 2005.

Ellis H, Calne RY, Watson CJE. *Lecture notes on general surgery*, 11th edn. Oxford: Blackwell, 2006.

Feldman M et al. *Sleisenger & Fordtran's gastrointestinal disease*, 9th edn. Philadelphia: Saunders, 2010.

Silen W. *Cope's early diagnosis of the acute abdomen*, 20th edn. New York: Oxford University Press, 2000.

Talley NJ, Martin CJ, eds. *Clinical gastroenterology. A practical problem-based approach*, 3rd edn. Sydney: Elsevier, 2010.

Yamada T, Alpers DH, Laine L, Owyang C, Powell DW. *Textbook of gastroenterology*, 5th edn. Oxford: Blackwell, 2008.

Chapter 7

The genitourinary system

You know my method. It is founded upon the observation of trifles.

Sherlock Holmes, created by Sir Arthur Conan Doyle (1859–1930)

Despite their very different functions the male and female genital and urinary symptoms are intimately associated anatomically and usually assessed together.

The genitourinary history
Presenting symptoms (Table 7.1)
These may include a change in the appearance of the urine, abnormalities of micturition, suprapubic or flank pain or the systemic symptoms of renal failure. Some patients have no symptoms but are found to be hypertensive or to have abnormalities on routine urinalysis or serum biochemistry. Others may feel unwell but not have localising symptoms (*Questions box 7.1*). The major renal syndromes are set out in Table 7.2.

Examination anatomy
Figure 7.1 shows an outline of the anatomy of the urinary tract. Figure 7.2 shows the arterial supply of the kidneys as demonstrated on a CT renal angiogram and Figure 7.3 shows the outline of the renal collecting system. Problems with function can arise in any part, from the arterial blood supply of the kidneys, the renal parenchyma, the ureters and bladder (including their innervation), to the urethra.

TABLE 7.1 Genitourinary history

Major symptoms

Change in appearance of urine, e.g. haematuria	Urethral discharge
Change in urine volume or stream	Symptoms suggestive of chronic renal failure (uraemia)
• Polyuria	• Oliguria, nocturia, polyuria
• Nocturia	• Anorexia, a metallic taste, vomiting, fatigue, hiccup, insomnia
• Anuria	• Itch, bruising, oedema
• Decrease in stream size	Menses
• Hesitancy	• Age of onset
• Dribbling	• Regularity
• Urine retention	• Last period (date)
• Strangury	• Dysmenorrhoea, menorrhagia
• Pis-en-deux—double-voiding (incomplete bladder emptying)	Erectile dysfunction
• Incontinence of urine	Loss of libido
Renal colic	Infertility
Dysuria (painful micturition)	Pregnancies: number and any complications
Frequency, urgency	Urethral or vaginal discharge
Fever, loin pain	Genital rash

Questions box 7.1

Questions to ask the patient with renal failure or suspected renal disease

! denotes symptoms for the possible diagnosis of an urgent or dangerous problem.

1 How did your kidney problems begin? Have you had tiredness, the need to pass urine at night (nocturia) or loss of appetite?

2 Was the kidney trouble thought to be brought on by any medications you were taking (e.g. non-steroidal anti-inflammatory drugs, ACE inhibitors/angiotensin receptor blockers, or contrast used for an X-ray procedure)?

3 Were you told there was inflammation of the kidneys (glomerulonephritis) or protein in the urine?

4 Have you had kidney infections recently or as a child?

5 Have you had kidney stones or urinary obstruction?

! 6 Have you passed blood in the urine?—Urinary tract malignancy

7 Have you had a biopsy of your kidney? Do you know the result?

8 Have you had diabetes or high blood pressure?

9 Have you had cardiovascular disease or peripheral vascular disease?

10 Have you had kidney surgery or removal of a kidney, or have you been told you have only one functioning kidney?

11 Is there a history in the family of enlarged kidneys and high blood pressure?—Polycystic kidneys

12 Have you had problems with rashes or arthritis?— Systemic lupus erythematosus, scleroderma

13 Have you had problems with swelling or shortness of breath?—Fluid retention

14 Have you been told how bad your kidney function is and whether you may need dialysis one day?

15 Are you taking medications to help the kidney function?

16 What tablets and medications (including over-the-counter products, herbal remedies, etc.) are you taking?

TABLE 7.2 The major renal syndromes

Name	Definition	Example
Nephrotic	Massive proteinuria	Minimal change disease
Nephritic	Haematuria, renal failure	Post-streptococcal glomerulonephritis
Tubulointerstitial nephropathy	Renal failure, mild proteinuria	Analgesic nephropathy
Acute renal failure*	Sudden fall in function, rise in creatinine	Acute tubular necrosis
Rapidly progressive renal failure	Fall in renal function, over weeks	Malignant hypertension or 'crescentic' glomerulonephritis
Asymptomatic urinary abnormality	Isolated haematuria, or mild proteinuria	Immunoglobulin A nephropathy

* Newly defined as acute kidney injury, AKI; Levin A, Warnock D, Mehta R, Kellum J, Shah S, Melitoris B, Ronco C. Improving outcome for AKI. *Am J Kidney Dis* 2007; 50(1):1–4.

Basic male and female reproductive anatomy is shown in Figures 7.9 (page 216) and 7.13 (page 218).

Change in appearance of the urine

Some patients present with discoloured urine. A red discoloration suggests haematuria (blood in the urine).[1] Urethral inflammation or trauma, or prostatic disease, can cause haematuria at the beginning of micturition which then clears, or haematuria only at the end of micturition (Table 7.3). Patients with porphyria can have urine that changes colour on standing. Consumption of certain drugs (e.g. rifampicin) or of large amounts of beetroot and, rarely, haemoglobinuria (due to destruction of red blood cells and release of free haemoglobin) can cause red discoloration of the urine (page 212). Patients with severe muscle trauma may have myoglobinuria as a result of muscle breakdown. This can also cause red discoloration. Foamy, tea-coloured or brown urine may be a presenting sign of nephrosis or kidney failure. It is worth noting that the colour of the urine is not a reliable guide to its concentration.

Urinary tract infection (UTI)

This condition includes both upper urinary tract (renal) infection and lower UTI (mostly the bladder—cystitis). Possibly as many as 50% of lower UTIs also involve the kidneys. Renal infection may be difficult to distinguish clinically from lower UTIs but is a more serious condition and more likely to involve systemic complications such as septicaemia.

Urinary tract infection is much more common in women than in men, but there are a number of risk factors for the disease (Table 7.4). It can be strongly suspected on the basis of the patient's symptoms.[2] These include: dysuria (pain or stinging during urination), frequency (need to pass small amounts of urine frequently), haematuria, and loin (more suggestive of upper UTI) or back pain. Physical examination may reveal fevers, rigors, lower abdominal discomfort and loin pain when the renal angle is balloted posteriorly. The latter findings are more suggestive of complicated UTI or pyelonephritis. The presence of a vaginal discharge is against the diagnosis. Elderly patients with a

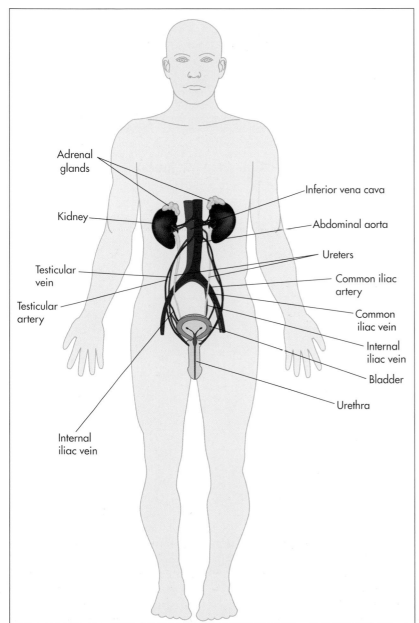

Adrenal glands

Kidney

Testicular vein

Testicular artery

Internal iliac vein

Inferior vena cava

Abdominal aorta

Ureters

Common iliac artery

Common iliac vein

Internal iliac vein

Bladder

Urethra

Figure 7.1 The anatomy of the kidneys and urinary tract

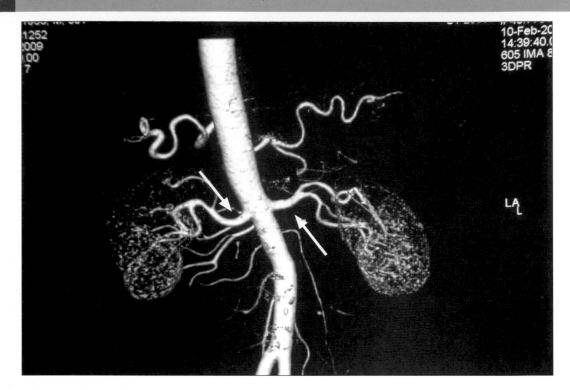

Figure 7.2 CT angiogram showing the origins and course of the renal arteries (large arrows) from the abdominal aorta; the left and right inferior phrenic arteries are visible arising superiorly

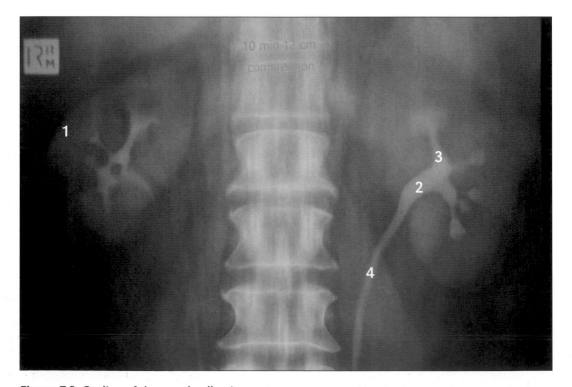

Figure 7.3 Outline of the renal collecting system
This intravenous pyelogram shows the outline of the kidneys (1), the renal pelves (2) and the calyces (3) and ureters (4).

TABLE 7.3 Haematuria
1 Favours urinary tract infection   Dysuria   Fever (prostatitis, pyelonephritis)   Suprapubic pain (cystitis)   Moderate flank or back pain (pyelonephritis)
2 Favours renal calculi   Severe loin pain
3 Favours source not glomerular   Clots in urine
4 Favours blood not in urine   Menstruation
5 Favours immunoglobulin A nephropathy   Multiple episodes over months
6 Favours trauma   Recent indwelling urinary catheter or procedure   Recent back or abdominal injury
7 Favours bleeding disorder   Use of anticoagulant drugs

TABLE 7.4 Risk factors for urinary tract infection (UTI)
Female sex
Coitus
Pregnancy
Diabetes
Indwelling urinary catheter
Previous UTI
Lower urinary tract symptoms of obstruction

urinary tract infection often present with confusion and few other symptoms or signs. A UTI in a male or frequent, relapsing or recurrent UTI in a female suggests an anatomical abnormality and requires urological evaluation.

Urinary obstruction

Urinary obstruction is a common symptom in elderly men and is most often due to prostatism (now called lower urinary tract symptoms— LUTS) or bladder outflow obstruction. The patient may have noticed hesitancy (difficulty starting micturition—urination), followed by a decrease in the size of the stream of urine and terminal dribbling of urine. Strangury (recurrently, a small volume of bloody urine is passed with a painful desire to urinate each time) and pis-en-deux/ double-voiding (the desire to urinate despite having just done so) may occur.[3] When obstruction is complete, overflow incontinence of urine can occur. Obstruction is associated with an increased risk of urinary infection.

Renal calculi can cause ureteric obstruction (Figure 7.4). The presenting symptom here, however, is usually severe colicky or constant loin or lower quadrant pain which may radiate down towards the symphysis pubis or perineum or testis (renal colic). Urinary obstruction can be a cause of acute renal failure (kidney injury) (Table 7.5).

Urinary incontinence

This is the inability to hold urine in the bladder voluntarily. It is not a consequence of normal ageing alone. The problem can occur transiently with urinary tract infections, delirium, excess urine output (e.g. from the use of diuretics), immobility (because patients are unable to reach the toilet), urethritis or vaginitis, or stool impaction.

Causes of established urinary incontinence include: (i) *stress incontinence* (instantaneous

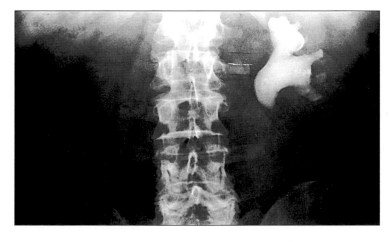

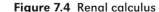

Figure 7.4 Renal calculus
Phleboliths (calcifications related to blood vessels) are rounded opacities seen in the pelvis below the level of the ischial spines, whereas ureteric calculi lie above this level, in the line of the ureters. The large staghorn calculus shown here is occupying the calyces of the left renal pelvis. This type of calculus is almost always radio-opaque. An abdominal ultrasound examination (IVPs are almost never performed in this context today) is necessary to check whether there is an obstruction at the pelviureteric junction. In general, 90% of renal calculi are radio-opaque and visible on plain X-ray films. A significant proportion of patients presenting with renal colic due to calcium calculi have hyperparathyroidism.

TABLE 7.5 Causes of acute renal failure (acute kidney injury, AKI*)

a. Onset over days

This is defined as a rapid deterioration in renal function severe enough to cause accumulation of waste products, especially nitrogenous wastes, in the body. Usually the urine flow rate is less than 20 mL/hour or 400 mL/day, but occasionally it is normal or increased (high-output renal failure).

Prerenal

Fluid loss: blood (haemorrhage), plasma or water and electrolytes (diarrhoea and vomiting, fluid volume depletion)

Hypotension: myocardial infarction, septicaemic shock, drugs

Renovascular disease: embolus, dissection or atheroma

Increased renal vascular resistance: hepatorenal syndrome

Renal

Acute-on-chronic renal failure (precipitated by infection, fluid volume depletion, obstruction or nephrotoxic drugs)—see Table 7.7

Acute renal disease:
- e.g. primary or secondary glomerulonephritis, connective tissue diseases

Acute tubular necrosis secondary to:
- ischaemia (hypovolaemia)
- toxins and drugs (such as aminoglycoside, antibiotics, radiocontrast material, heavy metals)
- rhabdomyolysis, haemoglobinuria

Tubulointerstitial disease:
- e.g. drugs (such as proton pump inhibitors, sulfonamides, cyclosporin A), urate or calcium deposits, phosphate, oxalate, crystal nephropathy

Vascular disease:
- e.g. vasculitis, scleroderma

Myeloma

Acute pyelonephritis (rare)

Postrenal (complete urinary tract obstruction)

Urethral obstruction:
- e.g. calculus or blood clot, sloughed papillae, trauma, phimosis or paraphimosis

At the bladder neck:
- e.g. calculus or blood clot, prostatic hypertrophy or cancer

Bilateral ureteric obstruction:
- intraureteric, e.g. blood clot, pyogenic debris, calculi
- extra-ureteric, e.g. retroperitoneal fibrosis (due to radiation, methysergide or idiopathic), retroperitoneal/pelvic tumour or surgery, uterine prolapse

b. Causes of rapidly progressive renal failure (onset over weeks to months)

Urinary tract obstruction

Rapidly progressive glomerulonephritis

Bilateral renal artery stenosis (may be precipitated by angiotensin-converting enzyme inhibitor or angiotensin receptor blocker use)

Multiple myeloma

Scleroderma renal crisis

Malignant hypertension

Haemolytic uraemic syndrome

Note: Anuria may be due to urinary obstruction, bilateral renal artery occlusion, rapidly progressive (crescentic) glomerulonephritis, renal cortical necrosis or a renal stone in a solitary kidney.

* Levin A, Warnock D, Mehta R, Kellum J, Shah S, Melitoris B, Ronco C. Improving outcome for AKI. *Am J Kidney Dis* 2007; 50(1):1–4.

leakage after the stress of coughing or after a sudden rise in intra-abdominal pressure of any cause)—this problem is more common in women due to vaginal deliveries or an atrophic vaginal wall postmenopause causing a hypermobile urethra; (ii) urge incontinence (*overactivity of the detrusor muscle*) which is characterised by an intense urge to urinate and then leakage of urine in the absence of cough or other stressors—this occurs in men and women; (iii) *detrusor underactivity*—this is rare and is characterised by urinary frequency, nocturia and the frequent leaking of small amounts of urine from neurological disease; (iv) overflow incontinence (*urethral obstruction*)—this occurs typically in men with disease of the prostate, and is characterised by dribbling incontinence after incomplete urination; and (v) a *vesico/urethral fistula*—a complication of obstructed labour.

Chronic renal failure (chronic kidney disease)

The clinical features of chronic renal failure can be deduced in part by considering the normal functions of the kidneys.

1 Failure of excretory function leads to accumulation of numerous 'uraemic' toxins, hence the widely used term 'uraemia'. This frequently leads to malaise, lethargy, anorexia, malnutrition and hiccups.

2 Urinary concentrating ability may be lost early, leading to the risk of dehydration; nocturia can be an early symptom.

3 Various factors such as the failure to excrete sodium may lead to hypertension.

4 Damage to the renal tubules may lead to sodium loss and hypotension.

5 Excretion of potassium depends in part on urine volume. Hyperkalaemia usually becomes a problem when a patient is oliguric (passes less than 400 mL urine/day) and may occur when taking potassium-sparing diuretics or agents that promote potassium retention (ACE inhibitors, angiotensin receptor blockers, non-steroidal anti-inflammatory drugs).

6 Failure of acid excretion leads to metabolic acidosis.

7 Disordered mineral and bone metabolism (abnormal levels of calcium, phosphorus, parathyroid hormone [PTH] and vitamin D) may lead to abnormalities in bone and vascular or soft-tissue calcification.[4]

8 Failure to secrete erythropoietin leads to normochromic normocytic anaemia.

9 Alterations in the metabolism of those medications which are excreted by the kidneys.

Adequacy of renal function is defined by the glomerular filtration rate (GFR). This is the volume of blood filtered by the kidneys per unit of time. The normal range is 90–120 mL/min. The GFR is estimated by calculating the clearance of creatinine (a normal breakdown product of muscle) from the blood. The serum creatinine and urea levels also provide a measure of accumulation of uraemic toxins and therefore of renal function. Most laboratories now provide an estimated GFR (eGFR) measurement calculated from the serum

TABLE 7.6 Classification of chronic kidney disease by glomerular filtration rate (GFR)

Stage	Description	GFR (mL/min/1.73 m³)
–	Increased risk for chronic kidney disease (e.g. diabetes, hypertension)	>90
1	Kidney damage but normal GFR	>90
2	Kidney damage and mild GFR reduction	60–89
3	Moderate reduction in GFR	30–59
4	Severe reduction in GFR	15–29
5	Kidney failure	<15

creatinine and the patient's age and sex.

A new definition and classification of chronic kidney disease (CKD) has been introduced. CKD is defined as kidney damage or GFR <60 mL/min/1.73 m² for 3 months or more, irrespective of cause.[5] Further kidney disease has been divided into 6 groups according to GFR (Table 7.6). These allow planning of investigations and treatment that might slow progression of the disease.

A uraemic patient may present with anuria (defined as failure to pass more than 50 mL urine daily), oliguria (less than 400 mL urine daily), nocturia (the need to get up during the night to pass urine) or polyuria (the passing of abnormally large volumes of urine) (page 297). Nocturia may be an indication of failure of the kidneys to concentrate urine normally, and polyuria may indicate complete inability to concentrate the urine.

The more general symptoms of renal failure include anorexia, vomiting, fatigue, hiccups and insomnia. Pruritus (a general itchiness of the skin), easy bruising and oedema due to fluid retention may also be present. Other symptoms indicating complications include bone pain, fractures because of renal bone disease, and the symptoms of hypercalcaemia (including anorexia, nausea, vomiting, constipation, increased urination, mental confusion) because of tertiary (or primary) hyperparathyroidism.[a] Patients may also present with the features of pericarditis, hypertension, cardiac failure, ischaemic heart disease, neuropathy or peptic ulceration.

---

[a]   In secondary hyperparathyroidism, serum calcium is low and phosphate is high. In tertiary hyperparathyroidism, where parathyroid function has become autonomous, serum calcium and phosphate levels are both high.

Questions box 7.2

Questions to ask the dialysis patient

! denotes symptoms for the possible diagnosis of an urgent or dangerous problem.

1 What fluid restriction have you been recommended?

2 Have phosphate-binding drugs been prescribed? When do you take these relative to meals?

3 Do you use haemodialysis or peritoneal dialysis? Do you do this at home? How many times a week?

! 4 Have you had abdominal pain or fever recently?—Peritonitis related to peritoneal dialysis

5 Have there been any problems with haemodialysis, such as low blood pressure, or with the fistula used for haemodialysis? Have there been any problems with peritonitis with peritoneal dialysis?

6 How much weight do you gain between each haemodialysis?

7 Do you still pass any urine? If so, how much?

8 Are you on a renal transplant list or have previously had a transplant?

9 Do you follow recommended dietary restrictions?

10 What other medications do you take?

11 Have you had heart or blood vessel problems?

12 Have you had overactive parathyroid glands or parathyroid surgery?

Find out whether the patient is undergoing dialysis and whether this is haemodialysis or peritoneal dialysis. There are a number of important questions that must be asked of dialysis patients (*Questions box 7.2*).

Ask about any complications that have occurred, including recurrent peritonitis with peritoneal dialysis or problems with vascular access for haemodialysis.

A common form of treatment for renal failure is renal transplantation. A patient may know how well the graft is functioning, and what the most recent renal function tests have shown. Find out whether the patient knows of rejection episodes, how these were treated, and if there has been more than one renal transplant. It is necessary to ascertain if there have been any problems with recurrent infection, urine leaks or side-effects of treatment. Long-term problems with immunosuppression may have

occurred, including the development of cancers, chronic nephrotoxicity (e.g. from cyclosporin or tacrolimus), obesity and hypertension from steroids, or recurrent infections. The patient should be aware of the need to avoid skin exposure to the sun and women should know that they need regular Papanicolaou[b] (Pap) smears for cancer surveillance.

Menstrual and sexual history

A menstrual history should always be obtained. The menarche or date of the first period is important (page 296). The regularity of the periods over the preceding months or years and the date of the last period are both relevant. The patient may complain of dysmenorrhoea (painful menstruation) or menorrhagia (an abnormally heavy period or series of periods).

Vaginal discharge can occur in patients with infections of the genital tract. Sometimes the type of discharge is an indication of the type of infection present. The history of the number of pregnancies and births is relevant: gravidity refers to the number of times a woman has conceived, while parity refers to the number of babies delivered (live births or stillbirths). One should also ask about any complications that occurred during pregnancy (e.g. hypertension).

The sexual history is also relevant.[6] Ask about contraceptive methods and the possibility of pregnancy.[7] Ask men about erectile dysfunction (impotence). Erectile dysfunction is defined as inability to achieve or maintain a satisfactory erection, for more than 3 months. Most causes are organic (neurogenic [e.g. diabetes] or vascular, or drug related [e.g. beta-blockers, thiazide diuretics]), with a slow onset and loss of morning erections in older men.

Treatment

A detailed drug history must be taken. Note all the drugs, including steroids and immunosuppressants, and their dosages. In patients with decreased renal function, the dosages of many drugs that are cleared by the kidneys must be adjusted. The patient with chronic renal failure should be well informed about the need for protein, phosphate, potassium, fluid or salt restriction. Patients with urinary tract infections may have had a number of courses of antibiotics. Treatment of hypertension should be documented. Certain drugs should be used with caution. For example, non-steroidal anti-

---

b Georgios N Papanicolaou (1884–1962). After studying at the University of Athens he worked in the pathology department at New York Hospital.

inflammatory drugs can worsen renal function or cause CKD.

Past history

Find out whether there have been previous or recurrent urinary tract infections or renal calculi. There may have been operations to remove urinary tract stones, or pelvic surgery may have been performed because of urinary incontinence in women or prostatism in men. The patient may know about the previous detection of proteinuria or microscopic haematuria at a routine examination. Glomerulonephritis will usually have been diagnosed by renal biopsy, a procedure that is often a memorable event. History of other urological disorders and results for prior urological evaluations are important. Histories of diabetes mellitus or gout are relevant, as these diseases may lead to renal complications. It is most important to find out about hypertension, because this may not only cause renal impairment but is also a common complication of renal disease. Similarly, a history of acute kidney failure episodes, history of cancer treated with chemotherapy or radiotherapy, severe allergic reactions, and exposures to nephrotoxic substances are all relevant. A history of childhood enuresis (bedwetting) beyond the age of three years may be relevant: it can be associated with vesicoureteric reflux and subsequent renal scarring.

Ask about previous myocardial infarction, congestive heart failure or valvular heart disease and about liver disease, especially hepatitis and about other systemic infections. Renovascular disease is more likely if there is a history of vascular disease elsewhere, such as myocardial ischaemia or cerebrovascular disease. In elderly patients, specific questions relating to ingestion of Bex or Vincent's powders may suggest a diagnosis of analgesic nephropathy. This is particularly important as these patients require surveillance for urothelial malignancy in addition to managing their renal impairment.

Social history

Occupational and travel exposure to toxins or infections, tobacco exposure, and excess consumption of alcohol are important.

Patients with chronic renal failure may have many social problems. There may be a need for access to equipment at home for dialysis. Whom does the patient contact if there is a problem with home dialysis? One must ask detailed questions to find out how the patient and his or her family is coping with the chronic illness and its complications. Has the patient been able to work? Find out how well-informed the patient is about the transplant, if this has been the treatment. Also find out what sort of support the patient has obtained from relatives and friends.

Family history

Some forms of renal disease are inherited. Polycystic kidney disease, for example, is an autosomal-dominant condition. Ask about diabetes and hypertension in the family. A family history of deafness and renal impairment suggests Alport's[c] syndrome, a hereditary form of nephritis. A family history of kidney disease of any type is a risk factor for development of CKD.

The genitourinary examination

A set examination of the genitourinary system is not routinely performed. However, if renal disease is suspected or known to be present then certain signs must be sought. These are mostly the signs of chronic renal failure (uraemia) and its causes (Table 7.7). On the other hand, examination of the male genitalia or female pelvis is part of the routine general examination.

General appearance

The general inspection remains crucial. Look for *hyperventilation*, which may indicate an underlying metabolic acidosis. *Hiccupping* may be present and can be an ominous sign of advanced uraemia. There may be the ammoniacal fish breath ('*uraemic fetor*') of kidney failure. This musty smell is not easy to describe but once detected is easily remembered. Patients with chronic renal failure commonly have a sallow complexion (a dirty brown appearance or '*uraemic tinge*'). This may be due to impaired excretion of urinary pigments (urochromes) combined with anaemia. The skin colour may be from slate grey to bronze, due to iron deposition in dialysis patients who have received multiple blood transfusions, but these signs are becoming less frequent with the use of exogenous erythropoietin. In terminal renal failure, patients become drowsy and finally sink into a coma due to nitrogen or toxin retention. Twitching due to myoclonic jerks, and tetany and epileptic seizures due to neuromuscular irritability or a low serum calcium level, occur late in renal failure. Over-vigorous correction of acidosis (e.g. with bicarbonate infusions) may also precipitate seizures and coma. There may be

---

c   Cecil Alport, 1880–1959, South African physician who worked in London and Egypt, described this syndrome in 1927 while working at St Mary's Hospital, London.

TABLE 7.7 Causes of chronic renal failure (chronic kidney disease, CKD*)

This is defined as a severe reduction in nephron mass over a variable period of time resulting in uraemia.[†]

1	Glomerulonephritis
2	Diabetes mellitus
3	Systemic vascular disease
4	Analgesic nephropathy
5	Reflux nephropathy
6	Hypertensive nephrosclerosis
7	Polycystic kidney disease
8	Obstructive nephropathy
9	Amyloidosis
10	Renovascular disease
11	Atheroembolic disease
12	Hypercalcaemia, hyperuricaemia, hyperoxaluria
13	Autoimmune diseases
14	Haematological diseases
15	Toxic nephropathies
16	Granulomatous diseases
17	Chronic tubulointerstitial nephritis

Clinical features suggesting that renal failure is chronic rather than acute

Small kidney size (except with polycystic kidneys, diabetes, amyloidosis and myeloma)

Renal bone disease

Anaemia (with normal red blood cell indices)

Peripheral neuropathy

* Levey A, Eckarrdt K, Tsukanoto Y, Levin A, Coresh J, Rossert J, Zeeuw W, Hostetter T, Lamiere N, Eknoyan G. Definition and classification of CKD: A position statement of KDIGO. *Kidney Int* 2005; 67:2089–2100.

[†] Note that this list is not all-inclusive.

typical skin nodules related to calcium phosphate deposition.

It is essential to assess the state of fluid balance in all patients with renal disease. Severe fluid-volume depletion can be a cause of acute renal failure and can cause precipitous decompensation in patients with chronic renal failure. Conversely, volume excess can result from intravenous infusions of fluid used in an attempt to correct acute renal failure, resulting in pulmonary oedema. Patients should be weighed regularly as an objective measure of their fluid status.

The distinctive ketone-like smell of a UTI may be apparent. There may be evidence of urinary incontinence on the patient's clothing.

The hands

The *nails* should be inspected: look for leuconychia; Muehrcke's nails[d] refer to paired white transverse lines near the end of the nails; these occur in hypoalbuminaemia (e.g. nephrotic syndrome).[8] A single transverse white band (Mees' lines,[e] Figure 7.5) may occur in arsenic poisoning, as well as in renal failure. Half-and-half nails (distal nail brown or red, proximal nail pink or white) are also seen in chronic renal failure. Non-pigmented indented transverse bands can occur with any cause of a catabolic state (Beau's lines[f]).

Anaemia is common and causes palmar crease pallor. There are a number of causes of anaemia in patients with chronic renal failure, including poor nutrition (especially folate deficiency), blood loss, erythropoietin deficiency, haemolysis, bone marrow depression and the chronic disease state.

Asterixis may be present in terminal chronic renal failure.

Inspect the wrist and forearms for scars and palpate for surgically created arteriovenous fistulae or shunts, used for haemodialysis access. There is a longitudinal swelling and a palpable continuous thrill present over the fistula. There may be scars from previous thrombosed shunts or carpal tunnel syndrome surgery present on either side. Look for signs of the carpal tunnel syndrome.

The arms

Bruising occurs because of nitrogen retention which causes impaired prothrombin consumption, a defect in platelet factor III, and abnormal platelet aggregation in chronic renal failure. *Skin pigmentation* is common, reflecting a failure to excrete urinary pigments. *Scratch marks and excoriations*, due to uraemic pruritus, often associated with hyperphosphataemia, may be present. This occurs commonly and can be extremely debilitating. *Uraemic frost* is a fine white powder present on the skin where very high concentrations of urea have precipitated out of the sweat in terminal chronic renal failure; it is very rare. Evidence of *vasculitis*, which can cause renal disease, should also be sought.

An arterio-venous fistula may be visible and

---

d   RC Meuhrcke reported this sign in the *British Medical Journal* in 1956.

e   RA Mees, Dutch physician, reported this sign in 1919. It had previously been reported (1901) in the *Lancet* by E Reynolds among drinkers of beer contaminated by arsenic in the north of England.

f   Joseph Honoré Simon Beau (1806–1865), Paris physician.

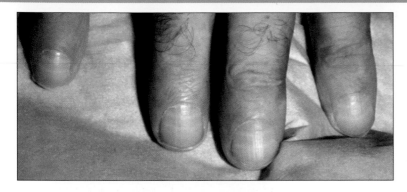

Figure 7.5 Mees' lines
(From McDonald FS, ed., *Mayo Clinic images in internal medicine*, with permission. © Mayo Clinic Scientific Press and CRC Press.)

or excessive replacement of calcium in patients with chronic renal failure.

The mouth should always be examined. A uraemic *fetor* may be present. This is an ammoniacal, musty odour due to breakdown of urea to ammonia in the saliva. Mucosal *ulcers* can occur as there is a decrease in saliva flow, and patients with chronic renal failure are prone to infection (e.g. thrush), due to decreased acute inflammatory responses as a result of nitrogen retention. Transplant patients treated with calcineurin inhibitors (cyclosporin and tacrolimus) frequently develop *gingival hyperplasia* (thickening of the gums).

The presence of a *rash* or skin tethering may indicate an underlying connective tissue disease such as systemic lupus erythematosus or systemic sclerosis.

The presence of hearing aids may be consistent with Alport's syndrome (hereditary nephritis often with sensorineural hearing loss and eye disease of the retina or cornea).

The neck

Carefully check the *jugular venous pressure* to help assess the intravascular volume status. Auscultate for *carotid artery bruits*; these provide a clue that there may be generalised atherosclerotic disease (which can cause renal artery stenosis or complicate chronic renal failure). Look for signs of previous *jugular vein puncture* due to previous vascular access insertion ('vascath') for haemodialysis. Surgical scars from previous *parathyroidectomy* performed for management of tertiary hyperparathyroidism may be present.

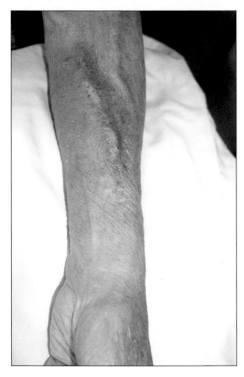

Figure 7.6 Arterio-venous fistula in the forearm of a haemodialysis patient

palpable in the forearm. A working fistula has a characteristic buzzing feel. This is used for vascular access for dialysis (Figure 7.6).

Look for signs of *peripheral neuropathy* in the limbs. Sensory impairment is more marked than motor impairment initially. Myopathy and bone tenderness can also occur.

The face

The eyes are important; look for signs of *anaemia* and, rarely, *jaundice* (retention of nitrogenous wastes can cause haemolysis). *Band keratopathy* is a calcium deposition beneath the corneal epithelium in line with the interpalpebral fissure—it is due to secondary or tertiary hyperparathyroidism,

The chest

Examine the heart and lungs. In chronic renal failure there may be *congestive cardiac failure* due to fluid retention, and *hypertension* as a result of sodium and water retention or excess vasoconstrictor activity or both. Signs of *pulmonary oedema* may also be present due to uraemic lung disease (a type of non-cardiogenic pulmonary oedema associated with typical 'bat's wing' pattern on chest X-ray; see Figure 4.61, page 99), volume overload or uraemic cardiomyopathy.

Pericarditis, which can be fibrinous or haemorrhagic in chronic renal failure, is secondary to retained metabolic toxins and can cause a pericardial effusion; there may be a pericardial rub or signs of cardiac tamponade. Lung infection is also common due to the immunosuppression present from the chronic renal failure itself or as a result of treatment.

The abdominal examination

Abdominal examination is performed as described on page 194. However, particular attention must be paid to the following.

Inspection

The presence of a Tenckhoff catheter (peritoneal dialysis catheter) should be noted. It is important to look for nephrectomy *scars* (see Figure 6.18, page 165). These are often more posterior than one might expect. It may be necessary to roll the patient over and look in the region of the loins. Renal transplant scars are usually found in the right or left iliac fossae. A *transplanted kidney* may be visible as a bulge under the scar, as it is placed in a relatively superficial plane. Peritoneal dialysis results in small scars from catheter placement in the peritoneal cavity; these are situated on the lower abdomen, at or near the midline.

The abdomen may be distended because of large polycystic kidneys or *ascites* (as a result of the nephrotic syndrome, or peritoneal dialysis fluid).

Inspect the scrotum for masses and genital oedema.

Palpation

Particular care is required here so that renal masses (Table 7.8) are not missed. Remember that an enlarged kidney usually bulges forwards, while perinephric abscesses or collections tend to bulge backwards. Transplanted kidneys in the right or left iliac fossa may be palpable as well. In polycystic kidney disease, hepatomegaly from hepatic cysts may be found (Table 7.9). Feel for the presence of an enlarged bladder. Also palpate for an abdominal aortic aneurysm. In the patient with abdominal pain, renal colic should be suspected if there is renal tenderness (positive LR 3.6) or loin tenderness (positive LR 27.7).[9]

Balloting

From the French word meaning *to shake about*, balloting is an examination technique for palpating

TABLE 7.8 Renal masses
1 Unilateral palpable kidney
Renal cell carcinoma
Hydronephrosis or pyonephrosis
Xanthogranulomatous pyelonephritis
Polycystic kidneys (with asymmetrical enlargement)
Normal right kidney or solitary kidney
Acute renal vein thrombosis (unilateral)
Acute pyelonephritis
Renal abscess
Compensatory hypertrophy of single functioning kidney
2 Bilateral palpable kidneys
Polycystic kidneys
Hydronephrosis or pyonephrosis bilaterally
Renal cell carcinoma bilaterally
Diabetic nephropathy (early)
Nephrotic syndrome (Table 7.12)
Infiltrative disease, e.g. amyloid, lymphoma
Acromegaly
Bilateral renal vein thrombosis

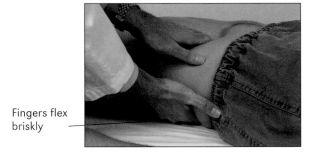

Fingers flex briskly

Figure 7.7 Balloting the kidneys

the kidney by attempting to flick it forward. One hand is placed under the renal angle and the examiner's fingers flick upwards while the other hand, placed anteriorly in the right or left upper quadrant, waits to feel the kidney move upwards and then float down again (Figure 7.7).

Percussion

This is necessary to confirm the presence of ascites by examining for shifting dullness. Also percuss for an enlarged bladder. Obesity and ascites make direct percussion of the bladder difficult. This is an opportunity to attempt *auscultatory percussion*.[10] The diaphragm of the stethoscope is placed just above the border of the symphysis pubis and direct percussion of the abdominal wall performed, starting at the subcostal margin in the middle line. There is a sudden increase in loudness when the

TABLE 7.9 Adult polycystic kidney disease

If you find polycystic kidneys, remember these very important points.

1 Take the blood pressure (75% have hypertension).

2 Examine the urine for haematuria (due to haemorrhage into a cyst) and proteinuria (usually less than 2 g/day).

3 Look for evidence of anaemia (due to chronic renal failure) or polycythaemia (due to high erythropoietin levels). Note that the haemoglobin level is higher than expected for the degree of renal failure.

4 Note the presence of hepatomegaly or splenomegaly (due to cysts). These may cause confusion when one is examining the abdomen.

5 Tenderness on palpation may indicate an infected cyst.

Note: Subarachnoid haemorrhage occurs in 3% of patients with polycystic kidney disease due to rupture of an associated intracranial aneurysm. As polycystic kidney disease is an autosomal-dominant condition, all family members should also be assessed.

upper border of the bladder is reached. It is even possible to estimate the volume of urine in the bladder by this method. An upper border less than 2 cm from the stethoscope suggests a fairly empty bladder, while an upper border more than 8 cm higher corresponds to a urine volume of between 750 mL and a litre.

Auscultation

The important sign here is the presence of a *renal bruit*. Renal bruits are best heard above the umbilicus, about 2 cm to the left or right of the midline. Listen with the diaphragm of the stethoscope over both these areas. Next ask the patient to sit up, and listen in both flanks. The presence of a systolic and diastolic bruit is important. A diastolic component makes the bruit more likely to be haemodynamically significant. Its presence suggests renal artery stenosis due to fibromuscular dysplasia or atherosclerosis. Approximately 50% of patients with renal artery stenosis will have a bruit. In a patient with hypertension that is difficult to control, the presence of a systolic/diastolic abdominal bruit has a positive LR for renal artery stenosis of over 40.[9] On the other hand, if only a soft systolic bruit is audible, at least half these patients do not have any significant renal artery stenosis. In such cases the aorta or splenic artery may be the source of the sound. The absence of hypertension makes the diagnosis of renal artery stenosis less likely. The occurrence of unexplained pulmonary oedema of sudden onset ('flash' pulmonary oedema) in a patient with renal impairment and hypertension makes a diagnosis of renal artery stenosis more likely.

Rectal and pelvic examination

Here the presence of prostatomegaly[11,12] in men and a frozen pelvis from cervical cancer in women is important, as this may be a cause of urinary tract obstruction and secondary renal failure.

The back

Strike the vertebral column gently with the base of the fist to elicit bony tenderness. This may be due to renal osteodystrophy from osteomalacia, secondary hyperparathyroidism or multiple myeloma. Back pain in the context of renal failure should always raise the possibility of an underlying paraproteinaemia.

Gentle use of the clenched fist to strike the patient in the renal angle is known as Murphy's kidney punch (Figure 7.8) and is designed to elicit renal tenderness in patients with renal infection. Similar information may be gained from more gentle balloting of the renal angle when the patient lies supine. Look also for sacral oedema in a patient confined to bed, particularly if the nephrotic syndrome or congestive cardiac failure is suspected. The presence of ulcerations of the toes suggests atheroembolic disease.

The legs

The important signs here are oedema, purpura (page 226), livedo reticularis (a red-blue reticular pattern from vasculitis or atheroembolic

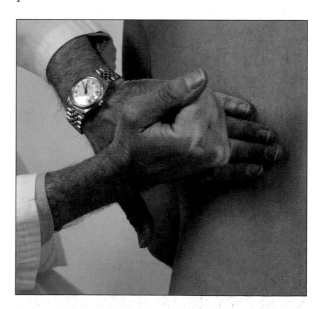

Figure 7.8 Murphy's kidney punch (not too hard)

disease), pigmentation, scratch marks and signs of peripheral vascular disease. Examination for peripheral neuropathy and myopathy is indicated, as in the arms. Gouty tophi or the presence of gouty arthropathy may very occasionally provide an explanation for the patient's renal failure (although secondary uric acid retention is common with chronic renal failure, it rarely causes clinical gout).

The blood pressure

It is of the utmost importance to take the blood pressure in every patient with renal disease. This is because hypertension can be the cause of renal disease or one of its complications. Test for postural hypotension, as hypovolaemia may precipitate acute renal failure.

The fundi

Examination of the fundi is important. Look especially for Keith-Wegerer hypertensive changes and diabetic changes. Diabetes can be a cause of chronic renal failure.

The urine

The ghosts of dead patients that haunt us do not ask why we did not employ the latest fad of clinical investigation; they ask why did you not test my urine?
Sir Robert Hutchison (1871–1960)

This valuable fluid must not be discarded in any patient in whom a renal, diabetic, gastrointestinal or other major system disease is suspected.

Colour

Look at the colour of the urine (Table 7.10).

Transparency

Phosphate or urate deposits can occur normally and produce white (phosphate) or pink (urate) cloudiness.

Fainter cloudiness may be due to bacteria. Pus, chyle or blood can cause a more turbid appearance.

Smell

A mild ammoniacal smell is normal. A urinary tract infection causes a fishy smell, and antibiotics can sometimes be smelt in the urine, as can asparagus.

Specific gravity

A urinometer, which is a weighted float with a scale, is used to measure specific gravity. The depth to which the float sinks in the urine indicates the

TABLE 7.10 Some causes of urine colour changes

Colour	Underlying causes
Very pale or colourless	Dilute urine (e.g. overhydration, recent excessive beer consumption, diabetes insipidus, post-obstructive diuresis)
Yellow-orange	Concentrated urine (e.g. dehydration)
	Bilirubin
	Tetracycline, anthracene, sulfasalazine, riboflavin, rifampin
Brown	Bilirubin
	Nitrofurantoin, phenothiazines; chloroquine, senna, rhubarb (yellow to brown or red)
Pink	Beetroot consumption
	Phenindione, phenolphthalein (laxatives), uric acid crystalluria (massive)
Red	Haematuria, haemoglobinuria, myoglobinuria (may also be pink, brown or black)
	Porphyrins, rifampicin, phenazopyridine, phenytoin, beetroot
Green	Methylene blue, triamterene
Black	Severe haemoglobinuria
	Methyldopa, metronidazole, unipenem
	Melanoma, ochronosis; porphryins, alkaptonuria (red to black on standing)
White/milky	Chlyuria

specific gravity, which is read off the scale on the side. The specific gravity can also be estimated by dipstick methods.

Water has a specific gravity of 1, and the presence of solutes (especially heavy solutes such as glucose or an iodine contrast medium) in urine increases the specific gravity. The normal range is 1.002 to 1.025. A consistently low specific gravity suggests chronic renal failure (as there is failure of the kidneys to concentrate the urine) or diabetes insipidus (where there is a deficiency of antidiuretic hormone resulting in passage of a large volume of dilute urine). A high specific gravity suggests fluid volume depletion, or diabetes mellitus with the presence of large amounts of glucose in the urine.

There is a rough correlation between the specific gravity of the urine and its osmolarity. For example, a specific gravity of 1.002 corresponds to an osmolarity of 100 mOsm/kg, while a specific gravity of 1.030 corresponds to 1200 mOsm/kg.

Chemical analysis

A chemical reagent colour strip allows simultaneous multiple analyses of pH, protein, glucose, ketones, blood, nitrite, specific gravity, presence of leucocytes, bile and urobilinogen. The strip is dipped in the urine and colour changes are measured after a set period. The colours are compared with a chart provided. It should be noted that specific gravity by dipstick is pH dependent and insensitive to non-ionised molecules, and therefore correlates poorly with urine osmolality.

pH

Normal urine is acid, except after meals when for a short time it becomes alkaline (the alkaline tide). Measuring the pH of urine is helpful in a number of critical circumstances. Sometimes the urine has to be made alkaline for therapeutic purposes, such as treating myoglobinuria or recurrent urinary calculi due to uric acid or cystine. Distal renal tubular acidosis should be suspected if the early morning urine is consistently alkaline and cannot be acidified. Urinary tract infections with urea-splitting organisms, such as *Proteus mirabilis*, can also cause an alkaline urine which, in turn, favours renal struvite stone formation.

Protein

The colours are compared with a chart provided. The strip tests give only a semi-quantitative measure of urinary protein (+ to ++++) and, if positive, must be confirmed by other tests. It is very important to note that the dipstick is sensitive to albumin but not to other proteins. A reading of + of proteinuria may be normal, as up to 150 mg of protein a day is lost in the urine. Causes of abnormal amounts of protein in the urine are listed in Tables 7.11 and 7.12. Chemical dipsticks do not detect the presence of Bence-Jones proteinuria[g] (immunoglobulin light chains).

If proteinuria is detected on dipstick testing, this should be quantified and careful urine (phase-contrast) microscopy should be carried out to look for evidence of active renal disease.

Glucose and ketones

A semi-quantitative measurement of glucose and ketones is available. Glycosuria usually indicates diabetes mellitus, but can occur with other diseases (Table 7.13). False-positive or false-negative results can occur with vitamin C (large doses), bacteria, oxidising detergents and hydrochloric acid,

tetracyclines or levodopa ingestion.

Ketones in the urine of patients with diabetes mellitus are an important indication of the

TABLE 7.11 Causes of proteinuria

Persistent proteinuria

1. Renal disease

Almost any renal disease may cause a trace of proteinuria. Moderate or large amounts tend to occur with glomerular disease (Table 7.12).

2. No renal disease (functional)

Exercise

Fever

Hypertension (severe)

Congestive cardiac failure

Burns

Blood transfusion

Postoperative

Acute alcohol abuse

Orthostatic proteinuria

Proteinuria that occurs when a patient is standing but not when recumbent is called orthostatic proteinuria. In the absence of abnormalities of the urine sediment, diabetes mellitus, hypertension or reduced renal function, this entity probably has a benign prognosis.

TABLE 7.12 Nephrotic syndrome

Definition

1 Proteinuria (>3.5 g per 24 hours) (*Note:* the other features can all be explained by loss of protein.)

2 Hypoalbuminaemia (serum albumin <30 g/L, due to proteinuria)

3 Oedema (due to hypoalbuminaemia)

4 Hyperlipidaemia (due to increased LDL and cholesterol, possibly from loss of plasma factors that regulate lipoprotein synthesis)

Causes

Primary renal pathology

1 Membranous glomerulonephritis

2 Minimal change glomerulonephritis

3 Focal and segmental glomerulosclerosis

Secondary renal pathology

1 Drugs: e.g. penicillamine, lithium, heroin, non-steroidal anti-inflammatory drugs

2 Systemic disease: e.g. SLE, diabetes mellitus, amyloidosis

3 Malignancy: e.g. carcinoma, lymphoma, multiple myeloma

4 Infections: e.g. hepatitis B, hepatitis C, infective endocarditis, malaria, HIV

LDL = low density lipoprotein.
SLE = systemic lupus erythematosus.
HIV = human immunodeficiency virus.

---

g   Henry Bence-Jones (1818–73), physician at St George's Hospital, London, described this in 1848.

presence of diabetic ketoacidosis (Table 7.13). The three ketone bodies are acetone, beta-hydroxybutyric acid and acetoacetic acid. Lack of glucose (starvation) or lack of glucose availability for the cells (diabetes mellitus) causes activation of carnitine acetyltransferase, which accelerates fatty-acid oxidation in the liver. However, the pathway for the conversion of fatty acids becomes saturated, leading to ketone body formation. The strip colour tests react only to acetoacetic acid. Ketonuria may also be seen associated with fasting, vomiting and strenuous exercise.

Blood

Blood in the urine (haematuria) is abnormal and can be seen with the naked eye if 0.5 mL is present per litre of urine (Table 7.14). Blood may be a contaminant of the urine when women are menstruating. A positive dipstick test is abnormal and suggests haematuria, haemoglobinuria (uncommon) or myoglobinuria (also uncommon). The presence of more than a trace of protein in the urine in addition suggests that the blood is of renal origin. False-positives may occur when there is a high concentration of certain bacteria and false-negative results can occur if vitamin C is being taken.

Nitrite

If positive, this usually indicates infection with bacteria that produce nitrite. More-specific dipstick tests for white cells are now available; a positive test has an LR of 4.2 for a urinary infection and a negative test has an LR of 0.3.[9]

The urine sediment

Every patient with suspected renal disease should have a midstream urine sample examined. Centrifuge 10 mL of the urine at 2000 rpm for 4 minutes. Remove the supernatant, leaving 0.5 mL; shake well to re-suspend, then place one drop on a slide with a coverslip. Look at the slide using a low-power microscope, and at specific formed elements under the high-power field (hpf) for identification. There is a significant false-negative rate when there are low numbers of formed elements in the urine.

Look for red blood cells, white blood cells and casts.

Red blood cells (RBCs)

These appear as small circular objects without a nucleus. Usually none are seen, although up to 5 RBCs/low-power field (lpf) may be normal in very concentrated urine. If their numbers are increased, try to determine whether the RBCs originate from

---

TABLE 7.13 Causes of glycosuria and ketonuria

Glycosuria

Diabetes mellitus

Other reducing substances (false-positives): metabolites of salicylates, ascorbic acid, galactose, fructose

Impaired renal tubular ability to absorb glucose (renal glycosuria)

- e.g. Fanconi* syndrome (proximal renal tubular disease)

Ketonuria

Diabetic ketoacidosis

Starvation

* Guido Fanconi (1892–1972), Zürich paediatrician. Considered a founder of modern paediatrics, he described this in 1936. It had previously been described by Guido De-Toni in 1933 and is sometimes called the De-Toni-Fanconi syndrome.

TABLE 7.14 Causes of positive dipstick test for blood in the urine

Haematuria

Renal

Glomerulonephritis

Polycystic kidney disease

Pyelonephritis

Renal cell carcinoma

Analgesic nephropathy

Malignant hypertension

Renal infarction, e.g. infective endocarditis, vasculitis

Bleeding disorders

Renal tract

Cystitis

Calculi

Bladder or ureteric tumour

Prostatic disease, e.g. cancer, benign prostatic hypertrophy

Urethritis

Haemoglobinuria

Intravascular haemolysis, e.g. microangiopathic haemolytic anaemia, march haemoglobulinuria, prosthetic heart valve, paroxysmal nocturnal haemoglobinuria, chronic cold agglutinin disease

Myoglobinuria

This is due to rhabdomyolysis (muscle destruction):

- Muscle infarction, e.g. trauma
- Excessive muscle contraction, e.g. convulsions, hyperthermia, marathon running
- Viral myositis, e.g. influenza, Legionnaires' disease
- Drugs or toxins, e.g. alcohol, snake venom, statins
- Idiopathic

the glomeruli (more than 80% of the RBCs are dysmorphic—irregular in size and shape) or the renal tract (the RBCs are typically uniform).

White blood cells (WBCs)

These cells have lobulated nuclei. Usually fewer than 6 WBCs/hpf are present, although up to 10 may be normal in very concentrated urine. Tubular epithelial cells have a compact nucleus and are larger. Pyuria indicates urinary tract inflammation. Bacteria may also be seen if there is infection, but bacterial contamination is more likely if squamous epithelial cells (which are larger and have single nuclei) are prominent. Sterile pyuria is characteristic of renal tuberculosis but may also occur in acute or chronic tubulo-interstitial disease. Multistix test strips will often test for the presence of WBCs.

Casts

Casts are cylindrical moulds formed in the lumen of the renal tubules or collecting ducts. They are signs of a damaged glomerular basement membrane or damaged tubules. The size of a cast is determined by the dimension of the lumen of the nephron in which it forms. The presence of casts is a very important abnormality and means renal disease.

Hyaline casts are long cylindrical structures. One or two RBCs or WBCs may be present in the cast. Normally there are fewer than 1 per lpf. They consist largely of Tamm-Horsfall mucoprotein secreted by the renal tubules.

Granular casts are abnormal cylindrical granular structures that arise from the tubules, usually in patients with proteinuria. They consist of hyaline material containing fragments of serum proteins.

Red cell casts are always abnormal and indicate primary glomerular disease (haematuria of glomerular origin or vasculitis). They contain 10 to 50 red cells, which are well defined.

With **white cell casts** many WBCs adhere to or inside the cast. These are abnormal, indicating bacterial pyelonephritis or, less commonly, glomerulonephritis, kidney infarction or vasculitis.

Fatty casts (i.e. the presence of fat in casts) are suggestive of the nephrotic syndrome.

Male genitalia

Inspect the genitals (Figures 7.9 and 7.10) for evidence of mucosal ulceration. This can occur in a number of systemic diseases, including Reiter's syndrome and the rare Behçet's syndrome. For aesthetic and protective reasons, it is essential to wear gloves for this examination. Retract the foreskin to expose the glans penis. This mucosal surface is prone to inflammation or ulceration in both infective and connective tissue diseases (Table 7.15). Look also for urethral discharge. If there is a history of discharge, attempt to express fluid by compressing or 'milking' the shaft. Any fluid obtained must be sent for microscopic examination and culture.

Inspect the scrotum with the patient standing. Usually the left testis hangs lower than the right. This is the only part of the body that consistently does not appear bilaterally symmetrical on inspection. Torsion of the testis may cause the involved testis to appear higher and to lie more transversely than normal. Inspect for oedema of the skin, sebaceous cysts, tinea cruris (an erythematous rash caused by a fungal infection of the moist skin of the groin) or scabies. Scrotal oedema is common in severe cardiac failure and may occur with the nephrotic syndrome and ascites.

Palpate each testis gently using the fingers and thumb of the right hand or cradle the testis between the middle and index fingers of the right hand and palpate it with the ipsilateral thumb.[13] The testes are normally equal in size, smooth and relatively firm. Absence of one or both testes may be due to previous excision, failure of the testis to descend, or a retractile testis. In children the testes may retract as examination of the scrotum begins because of a marked cremasteric reflex. A maldescended testis (one that lies permanently in the inguinal canal or higher) has a high chance of developing malignancy. An exquisitely tender, indurated testis suggests orchitis.[14] This is often due to mumps in postpubertal patients and occurs about 5 days after the parotitis. An undescended testis may be palpable in the inguinal canal, usually at or above the external inguinal ring. The presence of small firm testes suggests an endocrine disease (hypogonadism) or testicular atrophy due to

TABLE 7.15 Causes of genital lesions
Ulcerative
Herpes simplex (vesicles followed by ulcers: tender)
Syphilis (non-tender)
Malignancy (squamous cell carcinoma: non-tender)
Chancroid (*Haemophilus ducreyi* infection: tender)
Behçet's syndrome
Non-ulcerative
Balanitis, due to Reiter's syndrome or poor hygiene
Venereal warts
Primary skin disease, e.g. psoriasis
Note: Always consider HIV infection.

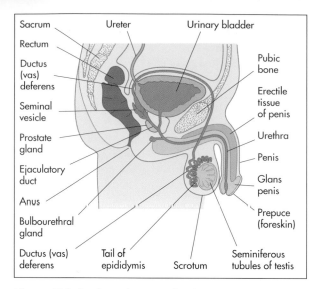

Figure 7.9 Basic male reproductive anatomy

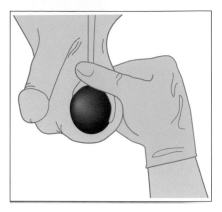

(a) To palpate the epididymis, feel along the posterior pole of the testis

alcohol or drug ingestion.

Feel posteriorly for the epididymis and then upwards for the vas deferens and the spermatic cord. It should be possible to differentiate the vas from the testis.

A varicocele feels like a bag of worms in the scrotum. The testis on the side of the varicocele often lies horizontally. It is unclear whether this is a cause or effect of the varicocele. A left varicocele is sometimes found when there is underlying left renal tumour or left renal vein thrombosis. The significance of the rarer right varicocele is disputed.[15]

Differential diagnosis of a scrotal mass
(Figure 7.11)

If a mass is palpable in the scrotum, decide first whether it is possible to get above it. Have the patient stand up. If no upper border is palpable, it must be descending down the inguinal canal from the abdomen and is therefore an inguino-scrotal hernia (page 178).

If it is possible to get above the mass, it is necessary to decide whether it is separate from or part of the testis, and to test for translucency. This is performed using a transilluminoscope (a torch) (Figure 7.12). With the patient in a darkened room, a small torch is applied to the side of the swelling by invaginating the scrotal wall. A cystic mass will light up while a solid mass remains dark.

A mass that is part of the testis and that is solid (non-translucent) is likely to be a tumour, or rarely a syphilitic gumma. The testes may be enlarged and hard in men with leukaemia. A

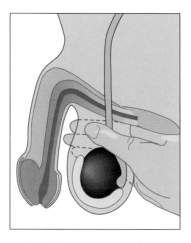

(b) Scrotal swelling—fingers can 'get above' mass

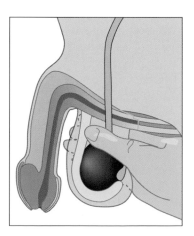

(c) Inguinal hernia with descent into the scrotum—fingers cannot 'get above' mass

Figure 7.10 Examination of scrotum
(From Douglas G, Nicol F and Robertson C, *Macleod's Clinical Examination*, 12th edn. Edinburgh: Churchill Livingstone, 2009, with permission)

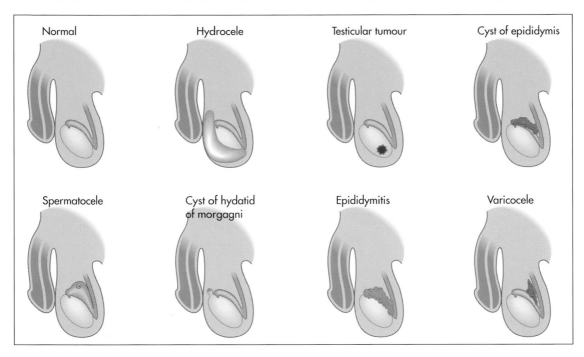

Figure 7.11 Differential diagnosis of a scrotal mass
(Adapted from Dunphy JE, Botsford TW. *Physical examination of the surgical patient. An introduction to clinical surgery*, 4th edn. Philadelphia: WB Saunders, 1975.)

mass that is cystic (translucent) with the testis within it is a hydrocele (a collection of fluid in the tunica vaginalis of the testis). A mass that appears separate from the testis and transilluminates is probably a cyst of the epididymis, while a similar mass that fails to transilluminate is probably the result of chronic epididymitis. By feeling along the testicular–epididymal groove it is usually possible to separate an epididymal mass from the testis itself.

Pelvic examination

The pelvic examination should be performed as the final part of any complete physical examination.[16] It is essential to obtain informed consent and for male students and doctors to have a chaperone. The patient's privacy must be promised and ensured. Gloves must be worn (Figure 7.13).

The patient should have first emptied her bladder. She should be on her back with her legs apart, ankles together and her knees bent (the frog-legged position). The left lateral position is used when the woman cannot assume the lithotomy position or when a view of the anterior vaginal wall is required: for example, when a urinary fistula is suspected.

The perineum should be brightly illuminated by a lamp. Put a glove on each hand. Inspect first

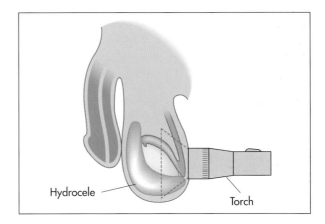

Figure 7.12 Transillumination of the scrotum

the external genitalia. Note any rash (e.g. sclerotic white areas of leucoplakia, or redness, swelling and excoriation from thrush or trichomoniasis), ulceration, warts, scars, sinus openings or other lesions. Separate the labia with the thumb and forefinger of the right hand. A Bartholin[h] cyst or abscess is palpated between the thumb and

---

h   Caspar Bartholin Secundus (1655–1738), professor of philosophy at Copenhagen at the age of 19, then professor of medicine, anatomy and physics. He described the glands in 1677.

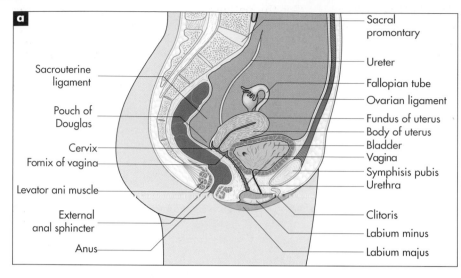

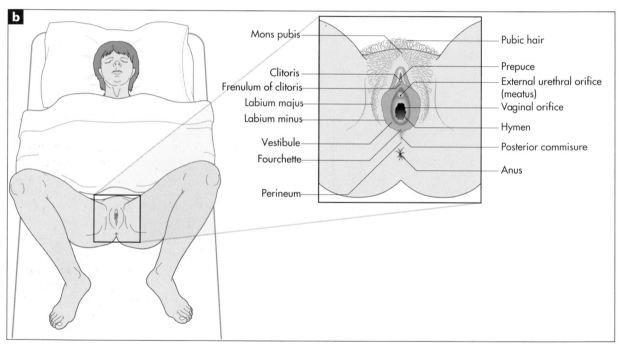

Figure 7.13 Basic female reproductive anatomy
(a) Lateral view, showing the relationship of the genitals to the rectum and bladder. (b) Position for examination. (From Douglas G, Nicol F and Robertson C, *Macleod's Clinical Examination*, 12th edn. Edinburgh: Churchill Livingstone, 2009, with permission)

index finger in the posterior part of the labia major; the normal gland is impalpable. Note the size and shape of the clitoris, and the presence or absence of a discharge from the urethral orifice and vaginal outlet. A bloody vaginal discharge suggests menstruation, a miscarriage, cancer or a cervical polyp or erosion. A purulent discharge suggests vaginitis, cervicitis or endometritis (e.g. gonorrhoea) or a retained tampon. *Trichomonas vaginalis* causes a frothy, watery, pale, yellow-white discharge, while thrush (*Candida albicans*) causes a thick cheesy discharge associated with excoriations and pruritus. Physiological discharge

may be present, this is almost colourless.

Ask the patient to bear down; a cystocele (descent of the bladder through the anterior vaginal wall) or rectocele (descent of the rectum through the posterior vaginal wall) or uterine prolapse may become apparent. Then ask the patient to cough; this may demonstrate stress incontinence. Note the presence of vaginal atrophy in older women.

Next insert the lubricated index and middle finger into the vagina. Locate the cervix first: it normally points towards the posterior vaginal wall. Note the position, size, shape, consistency, tenderness and mobility. Next palpate the anterior, posterior and lateral fornices. Usually the ovaries are not palpable. If a mass is palpable, its characteristics and location should be noted.

Bimanual palpation of the uterus is now performed; the fingers in the vagina are kept high up and rotated to face upwards while the left hand presses downwards and backwards above the pubic symphysis. Note whether the uterus is anterior (anteverted) or posterior (retroverted). Also note its size, shape and consistency and feel for tenderness and mobility. A large nodular mobile uterus suggests fibroids, while smooth enlargement of the uterus suggests pregnancy, adenomyosis or submucous fibroids.

A speculum examination of the vagina and cervix is made by introducing a well-lubricated warm bivalve speculum in an upwards direction and with the blades (bills) parallel to the labia and closed, while the other hand separates the labia. Lubricant may interfere with some cytology examinations and warm water can be used instead. The blades are opened under direct inspection once the speculum is fully introduced and rotated. The vagina and cervix are inspected. A smear for cervical cytology (Papanicolaou or 'Pap' smear) can be taken to detect cervical dysplasia or cancer. This is done using a spatula that is placed firmly against the cervical os and rotated through 360 degrees. The test is more accurate if some endocervical cells are also obtained. This can be done with a separate brush designed to fit into the os. A smear of vaginal wall cells for hormonal assessment can be taken with the other end of the spatula. The samples are smeared thinly on microscopic slides and placed immediately in fixative. Wet slides can also be prepared for *Trichomonas* or thrush, and cultures obtained for chlamydia and gonorrhoea if indicated.

Summary
Examination of a patient with chronic kidney disease: a suggested method
(Figure 7.14)
Lay the patient flat in bed while performing the usual **general inspection**. Note particularly the patient's mental state and the presence of a sallow complexion, whether the patient appears properly hydrated and whether there is any hyperventilation or hiccupping.

The detailed examination begins with the **hands** and the examination of the nails, which may reveal leuconychia, white transverse lines (Muehrcke's nails), a single white band (Mees' lines), or a distal brown arc (half-and-half nails). Examine the wrists and arms for a vascular access fistula.

Get the patient to hold out the hands and look for asterixis. Then inspect the **arms** for bruising, subcutaneous nodules (calcium phosphate deposits), pigmentation, scratch marks and gouty tophi.

Go on now to the **face** and begin by examining the eyes for anaemia, jaundice or band keratopathy. Examine the mouth for dryness, ulcers or fetor, and note the presence of any vasculitic rash on the face.

Check the **neck** for surgical scars, and listen for carotid bruits. Look at the jugular venous pressure with the patient at 45 degrees.

The patient should next be lying flat while the **abdomen** is examined for scars indicating peritoneal dialysis or operations, including renal transplants. Palpate for the kidneys, including transplanted kidneys, then examine the liver and spleen. Feel for an abdominal aortic aneurysm. Percuss over the bladder, determine if there is ascites, and listen for renal bruits. Rectal examination is indicated to detect prostatomegaly or bleeding.

Sit the patient up and palpate the **back** for tenderness and sacral oedema.

Examine the **heart** for signs of pericarditis or cardiac failure and the **lungs** for pulmonary oedema.

Lay the patient down again. Look at the **legs** for oedema (due to the nephrotic syndrome or cardiac failure), bruising, pigmentation, scratch marks or the presence of gout. Examine for peripheral neuropathy (decreased sensation, loss of the more distal reflexes).

Urinalysis is performed, testing for specific gravity, pH, glucose, blood, protein or leucocytes. Examination ends with measurement of the **blood pressure**, lying and standing (for orthostatic hypotension), and **fundoscopy** to look for hypertensive and diabetic changes.

References
1. Marazzi P, Gabriel R. The haematuria clinic. *BMJ* 1994; 308:356.
2. Bent S, Nallamothu BK, Simel DL et al. Does this woman have an acute uncomplicated urinary tract infection? *JAMA* 2002, 287; 20:2701–2710. Dysuria, frequency, haematuria, back pain and costovertebral tenderness increase the likelihood of urinary tract infection (positive LRs between 1.5 and 2.0). No vaginal discharge or irritation decreased the likelihood.
3. Dawson C, Whitfield H. Urological evaluation (ABC of urology). *BMJ* 1996; 312:695–698. This article provides useful definitions and interpretation of symptoms.
4. Moe S, Cunningham J, Goodman W, Martin K,

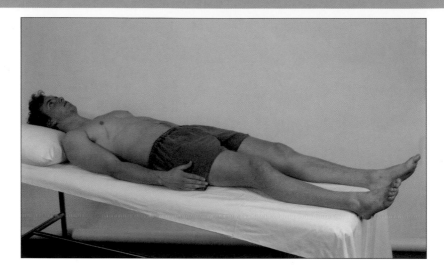

Figure 7.14 Chronic kidney disease examination

1. **General inspection**
   Mental state
   Hyperventilation (acidosis), hiccups
   Sallow complexion ('uraemic tinge')
   Hydration
   Subcutaneous nodules (calcium phosphate deposits)
2. **Hands**
   Nails—leuconychia; white lines; distal brown arc
   Arterio-venous fistulae
   Asterixis
   Neuropathy
3. **Arms**
   Bruising
   Pigmentation
   Scratch marks/excoriations
   Myopathy
4. **Face**
   Eyes—anaemia, jaundice, band keratopathy
   Mouth—dryness, ulcers, fetor, gingival hypertrophy
   Rash (lupus, vasculitis etc)
5. **Neck**
   Jugular venous pressure
   Carotid bruits
   Scars from previous vascath insertion
   Parathyroidectomy scars
6. **Abdomen**
   Tenckhoff catheter
   Scars—dialysis, operations
   Kidneys—transplant kidney
   Bladder

Liver
Lymph nodes
Ascites
Bruits
Rectal examination (prostatomegaly, frozen pelvis, bleeding)

7. **Back**
   Nephrectomy scar
   Tenderness
   Oedema
8. **Chest**
   Heart—heaving apex, pericarditis, failure
   Lungs—infection, pulmonary oedema
9. **Legs**
   Oedema—nephrotic syndrome, cardiac failure
   Bruising
   Pigmentation
   Scratch marks/excoriation
   Neuropathy
   Vascular access
10. **Urine analysis**
    Specific gravity, pH
    Glucose—diabetes mellitus
    Blood—'nephritis', infection, stone
    Protein—'nephritis' etc
11. **Other**
    Blood pressure—lying and standing
    Fundoscopy—hypertensive and diabetic changes etc
    Rash, livedo reticularis

Olgaard K, Ott S, Sprague S, Lamiere N, Eknoyan G. Definition, evaluation, and classification of renal osteodystrophy: A position statement of the Kidney Disease: Improving Global Outcomes (KDIGO). *Kidney Int* 2006; 69:1945–1953.

5. Levey A, Eckarrdt K, Tsukanoto Y, Levin A, Coresh J, Rossert J, Zeeuw W, Hostetter T, Lamiere N, Eknoyan G. Definition and classification of CKD: A position statement of KDIGO. *Kidney Int* 2005; 67:2089–2100.

6. Dean J. ABC of sexual health: examination of patient with sexual problems. *BMJ* 1998; 317:1641–1643.

7. Bastian LA, Pistcitelli JT. Is this patient pregnant? Can you reliably rule in or rule out early pregnancy by clinical examination? *JAMA* 1997; 278:586–591. Clinical features (amenorrhoea, morning sickness, tender breasts, enlarged uterus after 8 weeks with a soft cervix) cannot reliably diagnose early pregnancy—a pregnancy test, however, can.

8. Muehrcke RC. The fingernails in chronic hypoalbuminaemia: a new physical sign. *BMJ* 1956; 1:1327–1328. The classic description of this sign.

9. McGee S. *Evidence-based physical diagnosis*, 2nd edn. St Louis: Saunders, 2007.

10. Guarino JR. Auscultatory percussion of the urinary bladder. *Arch Intern Med* 1985; 145:1823–1825. This careful study makes a convincing case for the use of this technique, especially in obese patients or those with ascites.

11. Guinan P, Bush I, Ray V et al. The accuracy of the rectal examination in the diagnosis of prostate carcinoma. *N Engl J Med* 1980; 303:499–503. Suggests that rectal examination is an excellent technique for distinguishing benign prostatic hyperplasia and cancer, but this has subsequently been questioned.

12. Schroder FH. Detection of prostate cancer. *BMJ* 1995; 310:140–141.

13. Zornow DH, Landes RR. Scrotal palpation. *Am Fam Physician* 1981; 23:150–154. Describes standard examination techniques.

14. Rabinowitz R, Hulbert WC Jr. Acute scrotal swelling. *Urol Clin Nth Am* 1995; 22:101–105.

15. Roy CR, Wilson T, Raife M, Horne D. Varicocele as the presenting sign of an abdominal mass. *J Urol* 1989; 141:597–599. A sign of late-stage renal cell carcinoma, due to testicular vein compression, but can be on the left or right side!

16. Deneke M, Wheeler L, Wagner G, Ling FW, Buxton BH. An approach to relearning the pelvic examination. *J Fam Pract* 1982; 14:782–783. Provides some useful hints.

Suggested reading

Davison AM et al (ed). *Oxford textbook of clinical nephrology.* Oxford: Oxford University Press, 2005.

Chapter 8
The haematological system

[T]he blood is the generative part, the fountain of life, the first to live, the last to die and the primary seat to the soul.

William Harvey (1578–1657)

The haematological history
Presenting symptoms (Table 8.1)

TABLE 8.1 Haematological history

Major symptoms
Symptoms of anaemia: weakness, tiredness, dyspnoea, fatigue, postural dizziness
Bleeding (menstrual, gastrointestinal, after dental extractions)
Easy bruising, purpura, thrombotic tendency
Lymph gland enlargement
Bone pain
Infection, fever or jaundice
Enlargement of the tongue from amyloidosis
Paraesthesiae (e.g. B_{12} deficiency)
Skin rash
Weight loss

Patients with anaemia may present with weakness, tiredness, dyspnoea, fatigue or postural dizziness. Anaemia due to iron deficiency is often the result of gastrointestinal blood loss, or sometimes recurrent heavy menstrual blood loss, and so these symptoms should be sought. Disorders of platelet function or blood clotting may present with easy-bruising or bleeding problems. Recurrent infection may be the first symptom of a disorder of the immune system, including leukaemia or HIV infection. The patient may have noticed lymph node enlargement, which can occur with lymphoma or leukaemia. Not all lumps are lymph nodes; consider the differential diagnosis (Table 8.2). Ask about fever, its duration and pattern. Lymphomas can be a cause of chronic fever, and viral infections such as cytomegalovirus and infectious mononucleosis are associated with haematological abnormalities and fever.

TABLE 8.2 Differential diagnosis of lymphadenopathy

1	Lipoma—usually large and soft; may not be in lymph node area
2	Abscess—tender and erythematous, may be fluctuant
3	Sebaceous cyst—intradermal location
4	Thyroid nodule—forms part of thyroid gland
5	Secondary to recent immunisation

Treatment

Anaemia may have been treated with iron supplements or B_{12} injections. Anti-inflammatory drugs or anticoagulants may be the cause of bleeding. Treatment for leukaemia or lymphoma may have involved chemotherapy, radiotherapy, or both; or bone marrow transplant. There may have been blood transfusions in the past.

Past history

A history of gastric surgery or malabsorption may give a clue regarding the underlying cause of an anaemia. Anaemia in patients with systemic disease such as rheumatoid arthritis or uraemia can be multifactorial. Previous blood transfusions may have been required to treat the anaemia. On the other hand, patients with polycythaemia may have had many venesections (page 236).

TABLE 8.3 Causes of ecchymoses
Trauma
Thrombocytopenia or platelet dysfunction (Table 8.4)
Coagulation disorders
Acquired
Vitamin K deficiency (leading to factor II, VII, IX and X deficiency)
Liver disease (impaired synthesis of clotting factors)
Anticoagulants, e.g. heparin, warfarin, proteins with anticoagulant activity
Disseminated intravascular coagulation
Congenital (rarely cause ecchymoses and usually present with haemorrhage)
Haemophilia A (factor VIII deficiency)
Haemophilia B (factor IX deficiency, Christmas disease)
Von Willebrand's disease (an inherited abnormality of the von Willebrand protein, which is part of the factor VIII complex and causes a defect in platelet adhesion)
Senile ecchymoses (due to loss of skin elasticity)

Social history

A patient's racial origin is relevant. Thalassaemia is common in people of Mediterranean or southern Asian origin. Rarely, very strict vegetarian diets can result in vitamin B_{12} deficiency. Find out the patient's occupation and whether there has been work exposure to toxins such as benzene (risk of leukaemia). Has the patient had previous chemotherapy for a malignancy (drug-related development of leukaemia)? Does the patient drink alcohol?

Family history

There may be a history of thalassaemia or sickle cell anaemia in the family. Haemophilia is a sex-linked recessive disease while von Willebrand's disease[a] is autosomal dominant with incomplete penetrance (Table 8.3).

The haematological examination

Haematological assessment does not depend only on the microscopic examination of the blood constituents. Physical signs, followed by examination of the blood film, can give vital clues about underlying disease. Haematological disease can affect the red blood cells, the white cells, the platelets and other haemostatic mechanisms as well as the mononuclear-phagocyte (reticuloendothelial) system.

Examination anatomy

An important part of the examination involves assessment of all the palpable groups of lymph nodes. As each group is examined its usual drainage area must be kept in mind (Figure 8.1). It follows that whenever an abnormality is discovered anywhere that might be due to infection or malignancy its draining lymph nodes must be examined.

General appearance

Position the patient as for the gastrointestinal examination—lying on the bed with one pillow. Look for signs of wasting and for *pallor* (which may be an indication of anaemia—*Good signs guide 3.1*, page 26).[1-3] Note the patient's *racial* origin (e.g. thalassaemia). If there is any *bruising*, look at its distribution and extent. *Jaundice* may be present and can indicate haemolytic anaemia. *Scratch marks* (following pruritus, which sometimes occurs with lymphoma and myeloproliferative disease) should be noted.

The hands

The detailed examination begins in the usual way with assessment of the hands. Look at the nails for *koilonychia*—these are dry, brittle, ridged, spoon-shaped nails, which are rarely seen today. They can be due to severe iron deficiency anaemia, although the mechanism is unknown. Occasionally koilonychia may be due to fungal infection. They may also be seen in Raynaud's phenomenon. Digital infarction (Figure 8.2) may be a sign of abnormal globulins (e.g. cryoglobulinaemia). Pallor of the nail beds may occur in anaemia but is an unreliable sign. Pallor of the *palmar creases* suggests that the haemoglobin level is less than 70 g/L, but this is also a rather unreliable sign.[1]

Note any changes of rheumatoid or gouty *arthritis*, or connective tissue disease (Chapter 9). Rheumatoid arthritis, when associated with splenomegaly and neutropenia, is called Felty's syndrome[b]: the mechanism of the neutropenia is unknown, but it can result in severe infection. Felty's syndrome can also be associated with thrombocytopenia (Figure 8.3), haemolytic anaemia, skin pigmentation and leg ulceration. Gouty tophi and arthropathy may be present in the hands. Gout may be a manifestation of a myeloproliferative disease. Connective tissue diseases can cause anaemia because of the associated chronic inflammation.

Now take the *pulse*. A tachycardia may be

---

a   EA von Willebrand (1870–1949), Swedish physician, described this in 1926.

b   Augustus Roi Felty (1895–1963), physician, Hartford Hospital, Connecticut, described this in 1924.

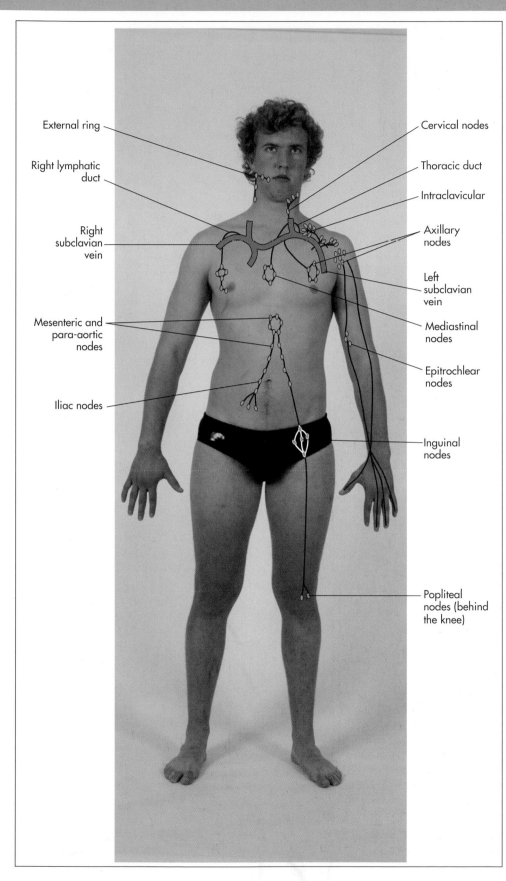

External ring

Right lymphatic duct

Right subclavian vein

Mesenteric and para-aortic nodes

Iliac nodes

Cervical nodes

Thoracic duct

Intraclavicular

Axillary nodes

Left subclavian vein

Mediastinal nodes

Epitrochlear nodes

Inguinal nodes

Popliteal nodes (behind the knee)

Figure 8.1 Usual drainage areas of lymph nodes (Adapted from Epstein O et al, *Clinical Examination*, 4th edn, Edinburgh: Mosby, 2008.)

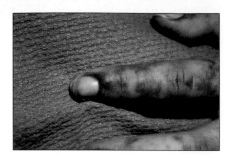

Figure 8.2 Digital infarction

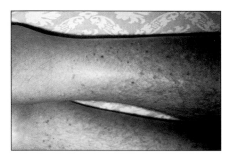

Figure 8.3 Thrombocytopenic purpura

present. Anaemic patients have an increased cardiac output and compensating tachycardia because of the reduced oxygen-carrying capacity of their blood.

Look for *purpura* (Figure 8.3), which is really any sort of bruising, due to haemorrhage into the skin. The lesions can vary in size from pinheads called *petechiae* (from Latin *petechia* 'a spot') (Table 8.4) to large bruises called *ecchymoses* (Table 8.3).

If the petechiae are raised (*palpable purpura*), this suggests an underlying systemic vasculitis, where the lesions are painful, or bacteraemia.

The forearms

If thrombocytopenia or capillary fragility is suspected, the Hess test[c] can be performed.[d]

---

[c] Alfred Hess (1875–1933), professor of paediatrics, New York, described this in 1914.
[d] This test is only of historical interest these days, as a platelet count can be obtained almost as quickly in most hospitals and clinics. A blood pressure cuff, placed over the upper arm, is inflated to a point 10 mmHg above the diastolic blood pressure. Wait for 5 minutes, then deflate the cuff and wait for another 5 minutes before inspecting the arm. Look for petechiae, which are usually most prominent in the cubital fossa and near the wrist, where the skin is most lax. Fewer than 5 petechiae per cm² is normal, while more than 20 is definitely abnormal, suggesting thrombocytopenia, abnormal platelet function or capillary fragility.

TABLE 8.4 Causes of petechiae

Thrombocytopenia
Platelet count <100 x 10⁹/L

Increased destruction
Immunological:
- immune thrombocytopenic purpura (ITP)
- systemic lupus erythematosus
- drugs, e.g. quinine, sulfonamides, methyldopa

Non-immunological:
- damage, e.g. prosthetic heart valve
- consumption, e.g. disseminated intravascular coagulation (DIC)
- loss, e.g. haemorrhage

Reduced production
Marrow aplasia, e.g. drugs, chemicals, radiation
Marrow invasion, e.g. carcinoma, myeloma, leukaemia, fibrosis

Sequestration
Hypersplenism

Platelet dysfunction
Congenital or familial
Acquired:
- myeloproliferative disease
- dysproteinaemia
- chronic renal failure, chronic liver disease
- drugs, e.g. aspirin

Bleeding due to small vessel disease
Infection:
- infective endocarditis
- septicaemia (e.g. meningococcal)
- viral exanthemata (e.g. measles)

Drugs, e.g. steroids
Scurvy (vitamin C deficiency)—classically perifollicular purpura on the lower limbs, which is almost diagnostic of this condition
Cushing's syndrome
Vasculitis:
- polyarteritis nodosa
- Henoch-Schönlein purpura*

Fat embolism
Dysproteinaemia

* Eduard Henoch (1820–1910), professor of paediatrics, Berlin, described this in 1865, and Johannes Schönlein (1793–1864), Berlin physician, described it in 1868.

Epitrochlear nodes

These must always be palpated. The best method is to flex the patient's elbow to 90 degrees, abduct the upper arm a little and then place the palm of the right hand under the patient's right elbow (Figure 8.4). The examiner's thumb can then be placed over the appropriate area, which is proximal and slightly anterior to the medial epicondyle.

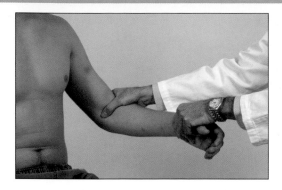

Figure 8.4 Feeling for the epitrochlear lymph node

This is repeated with the left hand for the other side. An enlarged epitrochlear node is usually pathological. It occurs with local infection, non-Hodgkin's lymphoma[e] or rarely syphilis. Note the features and different causes as listed in Tables 8.5 and 8.6. Certain symptoms and signs suggest that lymphadenopathy may be the result of a significant disease (*Good signs guide 8.1*).

Axillary nodes

To palpate these, the examiner raises the patient's arm and, using the left hand for the right side, pushes his or her fingers as high as possible into the axilla. The patient's arm is then brought down to rest on the examiner's forearm. The opposite is done for the other side (Figure 8.5).

There are five main groups of axillary nodes: (i) central; (ii) lateral (above and lateral); (iii) pectoral (medial); (iv) infraclavicular; and (v) subscapular (most inferior) (Figure 8.6). An effort should be made to feel for nodes in each of these areas of the axilla.

The face

The *eyes* should be examined for the presence of scleral jaundice, haemorrhage or injection (due to increased prominence of scleral blood vessels, as in polycythaemia). Conjunctival pallor suggests anaemia and is more reliable than examination of the nail beds or palmar creases.[3] In northern Europeans the combination of prematurely grey hair and blue eyes may indicate a predisposition to the autoimmune disease *pernicious anaemia*, where there is a vitamin B_{12} deficiency due to lack

TABLE 8.5 Characteristics of lymph nodes
During the palpation of lymph nodes the following features must be considered:
Site
Palpable nodes may be localised to one region (e.g. local infection, early lymphoma) or generalised (e.g. late lymphoma). The palpable lymph node areas are: • epitrochlear • axillary • cervical and occipital • supraclavicular • para-aortic (rarely palpable) • inguinal • popliteal
Size
Large nodes are usually abnormal (greater than 1 cm)
Consistency
Hard nodes suggest carcinoma deposits, soft nodes may be normal, and rubbery nodes may be due to lymphoma
Tenderness
This implies infection or acute inflammation
Fixation
Nodes that are fixed to underlying structures are more likely to be infiltrated by carcinoma than mobile nodes
Overlying skin
Inflammation of the overlying skin suggests infection, and tethering to the overlying skin suggests carcinoma

TABLE 8.6 Causes of localised lymphadenopathy
1 Inguinal nodes; infection of lower limb, sexually transmitted disease, abdominal or pelvic malignancy; immunisations
2 Axillary nodes; infections of the upper limb, carcinoma of the breast, disseminated malignancy; immunisations
3 Epitrochlear nodes; infection of the arm, lymphoma, sarcoidosis
4 Left supraclavicular nodes; metastatic malignancy from the chest, abdomen (especially stomach—Troiser's sign) or pelvis
5 Right supraclavicular nodes; malignancy from the chest or oesophagus

of intrinsic factor secretion by an atrophic gastric mucosa.

The *mouth* should be examined for hypertrophy of the gums, which may occur with infiltration by leukaemic cells, especially in acute monocytic leukaemia, or with swelling in scurvy. Gum bleeding

---

[e] Thomas Hodgkin (1798–1866), famous student at Guy's Hospital, London, described his disease in 1832. The first case he described was a patient of Richard Bright's. Hodgkin was one of the first to use the stethoscope in England. On failing to be appointed a physician, he gave up medicine and became a missionary.

GOOD SIGNS GUIDE 8.1 Factors suggesting lymphadenopathy is associated with significant disease

	LR if present	LR if absent
Age > 40	2.4	0.4
Weight loss	3.4	0.8
Fever	NS	NS
Head and neck but not supraclavicular	NS	NS
Supraclavicular	3.2	0.8
Axillary	0.0	NS
Inguinal	0.6	NS
Size:		
< 4 cm²	0.4	—
4–9 cm²	NS	—
> 9 cm²	8.4	—
Hard texture	3.3	NS
Tender	0.4	1.3
Fixed node	10.9	NS
3 or fewer nodes	0.04	—
5 or 6 nodes	5.1	—
7 or more nodes	21.9	—

From McGee S, *Evidence-based physical diagnosis*, 2nd edn. St Louis: Saunders, 2007.

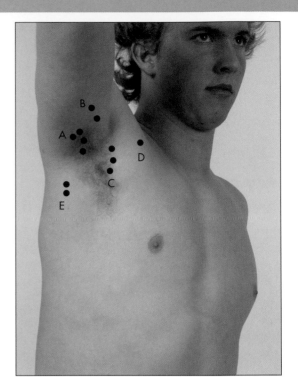

Figure 8.6 The main groups of axillary lymph nodes A = central; B = lateral; C = pectoral; D = infraclavicular; E = subscapular.

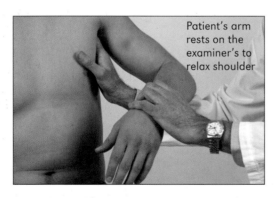

Patient's arm rests on the examiner's to relax shoulder

Figure 8.5 Feeling for the axillary lymph nodes

must also be looked for, and ulceration, infection and haemorrhage of the buccal and pharyngeal mucosa noted. Atrophic glossitis occurs with megaloblastic anaemia or iron deficiency anaemia. Multiple telangiectasiae may appear around the mouth or in the mouth in patients with *hereditary haemorrhagic telangiectasia*. Look to see if the tonsils are enlarged. *Waldeyer's ring*[f] is a circle

of lymphatic tissue in the posterior part of the oropharynx and nasopharynx, and includes the tonsils and adenoids. Sometimes non-Hodgkin's lymphoma will involve Waldeyer's tonsillar ring, but Hodgkin's disease rarely does.

Cervical and supraclavicular nodes

Sit the patient up and examine the cervical nodes from behind. There are eight groups. Attempt to identify each of the groups of nodes with your fingers (Figure 8.7). First palpate the submental node, which lies directly under the chin, and then the submandibular nodes, which are below the angle of the jaw. Next palpate the jugular chain, which lies anterior to the sternomastoid muscle, and then the posterior triangle nodes, which are posterior to the sternomastoid muscle. Palpate the occipital region for occipital nodes and then move to the postauricular node behind the ear and the preauricular node in front of the ear. Finally from the front, with the patient's shoulders slightly shrugged, feel in the supraclavicular fossa and at the base of the sternocleidomastoid muscle for the

---

f   Heinrich Wilhelm Gottfried von Waldeyer-Hartz (1836–1921), Berlin anatomist.

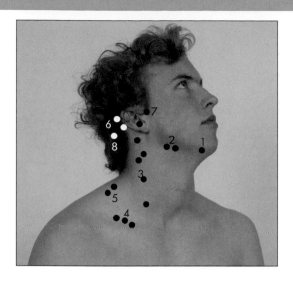

Figure 8.7 Cervical and supraclavicular lymph nodes
1 = submental; 2 = submandibular; 3 = jugular chain;
4 = supraclavicular; 5 = posterior triangle;
6 = postauricular; 7 = preauricular; 8 = occipital.

TABLE 8.7 Causes of lymphadenopathy

Generalised lymphadenopathy

Lymphoma (rubbery and firm)

Leukaemia (e.g. chronic lymphocytic leukaemia, acute lymphocytic leukaemia)

Infections: viral (e.g. infectious mononucleosis, cytomegalovirus, HIV), bacterial (e.g. tuberculosis, brucellosis, syphilis), protozoal (e.g. toxoplasmosis)

Connective tissue diseases: e.g. rheumatoid arthritis, systemic lupus erythematosus

Infiltration: e.g. sarcoid

Drugs: e.g. phenytoin (pseudolymphoma)

Localised lymphadenopathy

Local acute or chronic infection

Metastases from carcinoma or other solid tumour

Lymphoma, especially Hodgkin's disease

---

supraclavicular nodes. Causes of lymphadenopathy, localised and generalised, are given in Table 8.7. Note that small cervical nodes are often palpable in normal young people.[4,5]

The detection of lymphadenopathy should lead to a search of the area drained by the enlarged nodes. This may reveal the likely cause (see Table 8.6).

Bone tenderness

While the patient is sitting up, tap over the spine with the fist for bony tenderness. This may be caused by an enlarging marrow due to infiltration by myeloma, lymphoma or carcinoma, or due to malignant disease of the bony skeleton. Also gently press the sternum and both clavicles with the heel of the hand and then test both shoulders by pushing them towards each other with your hands.

The abdominal examination

Lay the patient flat again. Examine the abdomen carefully, especially for splenomegaly[6] (Table 8.8, *Good signs guide 8.2*), hepatomegaly, para-aortic nodes (rarely palpable), inguinal nodes and testicular masses. Remember that a central deep abdominal mass may occasionally be due to enlarged para-aortic nodes. Para-aortic adenopathy strongly suggests lymphoma or lymphatic leukaemia. The rectal examination may reveal evidence of bleeding or a carcinoma.

Assessment of the patient with suspected malignancy is presented in Table 8.9.[7]

Inguinal nodes

There are two groups—one along the inguinal ligament and the other along the femoral vessels. Small, firm mobile nodes are commonly found in otherwise normal subjects (Figure 8.8).

The legs

Inspect for any bruising, pigmentation or scratch marks. Palpable purpura over the buttocks and legs are present in Henoch-Schönlein purpura[g] (Figure 8.9). Leg ulcers may occur above the medial or lateral malleolus in association with haemolytic anaemia (including sickle cell anaemia and hereditary spherocytosis), probably as a result of tissue infarction due to abnormal blood viscosity. Leg ulcers can also occur with thalassaemia, macroglobulinaemia, thrombotic thrombocytopenic purpura and polycythaemia, as well as in Felty's syndrome. Chronic use of hydroxyurea for myeloproliferative disorders can cause malar ulcers.

Very occasionally, popliteal nodes may be felt in the popliteal fossa.

The legs should also be examined for evidence of the neurological abnormalities caused by vitamin B_{12} deficiency: peripheral neuropathy and subacute combined degeneration of the spinal cord. Vitamin B_{12} is an essential cofactor in the conversion of homocysteine to methionine; in B_{12} deficiency, the lack of methionine impairs methylation of myelin basic protein. Deficiency of vitamin B_{12} can

---

g   Henoch-Schönlein purpura is also characterised by glomerulonephritis (manifested by haematuria and proteinuria), arthralgias and abdominal pain.

TABLE 8.8 Causes of splenomegaly

Massive
Common
Chronic myeloid leukaemia
Myelofibrosis

Rare
Malaria
Kala azar
Primary lymphoma of spleen

Moderate
The above causes
Portal hypertension
Lymphoma
Leukaemia (acute or chronic)
Thalassaemia
Storage diseases, e.g. Gaucher's disease*

Small
The above causes
Other myeloproliferative disorders:
• polycythaemia rubra vera
• essential thrombocythaemia
Haemolytic anaemia
Megaloblastic anaemia (rarely)
Infection:
• viral (e.g. infectious mononucleosis, hepatitis)
• bacterial (e.g. infective endocarditis)
• protozoal (e.g. malaria)
Connective tissue diseases:
• rheumatoid arthritis
• systemic lupus erythematosus
• polyarteritis nodosa
Infiltrations:
• e.g. amyloid, sarcoid
Splenomegaly may be found in 3%–12% of the normal population.

Note: Secondary carcinomatosis is a very *rare* cause of splenomegaly.
* Phillipe Charles Ernest Gaucher (1854–1918), who described this in 1882, was physician and dermatologist at the Hôpital St-Louis, Paris.

GOOD SIGNS GUIDE 8.2 Splenomegaly

Finding	Positive LR	Negative LR
Spleen palpable	8.5	0.5
Spleen percussion positive	1.7	0.7

From McGee S, *Evidence-based physical diagnosis*, 2nd edn. St Louis: Saunders, 2007.

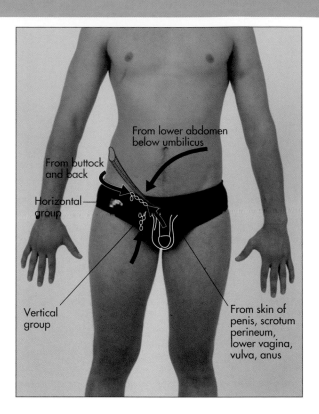

Figure 8.8 The groups of inguinal lymph nodes, their drainage areas and the position of the spleen
(Adapted from Epstein O et al, *Clinical Examination*, 4th edn, Edinburgh: Mosby, 2008.)

TABLE 8.9 Assessing the patient with suspected malignancy

1 Palpate all draining lymph nodes

2 Examine all remaining lymph node groups

3 Examine the abdomen, particularly for hepatomegaly and ascites

4 Feel the testes

5 Perform a rectal examination and pelvic examination

6 Examine the lungs

7 Examine the breasts

8 Examine all the skin and nails for melanoma

The fundi

Examine the fundi. An increase in blood viscosity, which occurs in diseases such as macroglobulinaemia, myeloproliferative disease or chronic granulocytic leukaemia, can cause engorged retinal vessels and later papilloedema. Haemorrhages may occur because of a haemostatic disorder. Retinal lesions (multiple yellow-white patches) may be present in toxoplasmosis (see Figure 16.5) and cytomegalovirus infections (see Figure 16.6).

also result in optic atrophy and mental changes. Lead poisoning causes anaemia and foot (or wrist) drop.

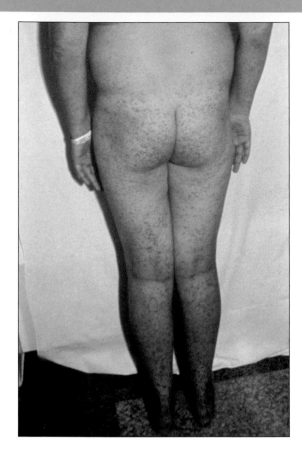

Figure 8.9 Henoch-Schönlein purpura
(From McDonald FS, ed., *Mayo Clinic images in internal medicine*, with permission. © Mayo Clinic Scientific Press and CRC Press.)

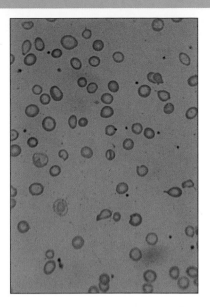

Figure 8.10 Iron-deficiency anaemia
Red cells show varying shape and size and are generally hypochromic.

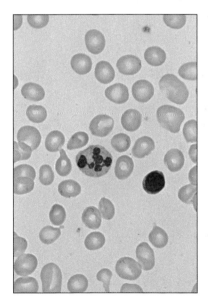

Figure 8.11 Megaloblastic anaemia
Red cells are macrocytic with many oval forms and the neutrophil is hypersegmented.

Examination of the peripheral blood film

This is a simple and useful clinical investigation.

A properly made peripheral blood film is one of the simplest, least invasive and most readily accessible forms of 'tissue biopsy', and can be a very useful diagnostic tool in clinical medicine. An examination of the patient's blood film can (i) assess whether the morphology of red cells, white cells and platelets is normal; (ii) help to characterise the type of anaemia; (iii) detect the presence of abnormal cells and provide clues about quantitative changes in plasma proteins—e.g. paraproteinaemia; and (iv) help to make the diagnosis of an underlying infection, malignant infiltration of the bone marrow or primary proliferative haematological disorder. The following pages present illustrated examples of some clinical problems diagnosed by examination of the blood film (Figures 8.10 to 8.22).

Correlation of physical signs and haematological disease
Anaemia

Anaemia is a reduction in the concentration of haemoglobin below 135 g/L in an adult man and 115 g/L in an adult woman. Anaemia is not a disease itself but results from an underlying pathological process (Table 8.10, page 235). It can be classified according to the blood film. Red blood cells with

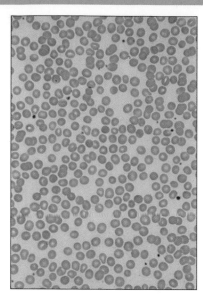

Figure 8.12 Spherocytic anaemia
Hereditary spherocytosis or autoimmune haemolytic anaemia. The numerous red blood cells which are small, round and lack central pallor are spherocytes (the big red blood cells are probably reticulocytes).

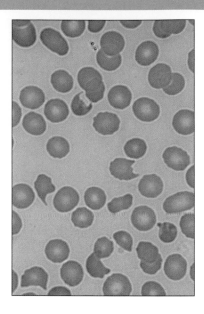

Figure 8.14 Microangiopathic haemolysis (e.g. disseminated intravascular coagulation)
Frequent fragmented (bitten) red cells.

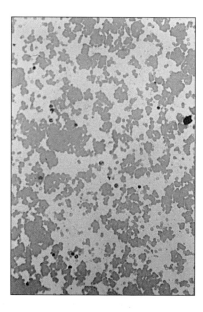

Figure 8.13 Autoagglutination
Cold haemagglutinin disease. Film shows clumping of red cells (low power).

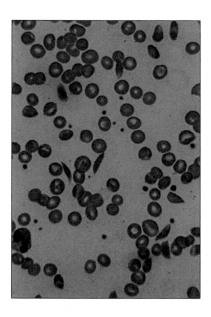

Figure 8.15 Sickle cell anaemia
Film shows several sickle-shaped cells with target cells probably secondary to the 'autosplenectomy' that occurs in this disease.

a low mean cell volume (MCV) appear small (microcytic) and pale (hypochromic). Those with a high MCV appear large and round or oval-shaped (macrocytic). Alternatively, the red blood cells may be normal in shape and size (normochromic, normocytic) but reduced in number.

Signs of a severe anaemia of any cause include pallor, tachycardia, wide pulse pressure, systolic ejection murmurs due to a compensatory rise in cardiac output, and cardiac failure if myocardial reserve is reduced. There may be signs of the underlying cause.

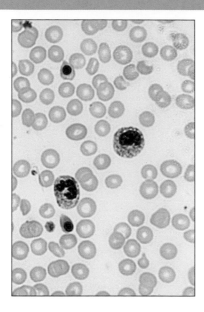

Figure 8.16 Leucoerythroblastic film
Film indicative of bone marrow infiltration. Shows circulating nucleated red blood cells and immature white cells.

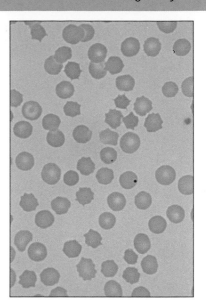

Figure 8.18 Postsplenectomy picture
Film shows several Howell-Jolly bodies, target cells and crenated cells.

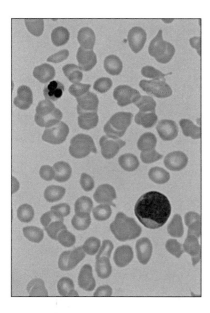

Figure 8.17 Myelofibrosis
Film shows a dysplastic nucleated red blood cell, frequent tear-drop poikilocytes and a primitive granulocyte.

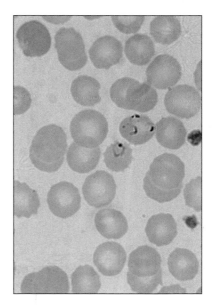

Figure 8.19 Malaria
The two red cells in the centre show the trophozoite.

Pancytopenia

Signs

There may be clinical evidence of anaemia, leucopenia (reduced numbers of white blood cells resulting in susceptibility to infection) and thrombocytopenia (petechiae and bleeding)—a deficiency in all three bone marrow cell lines. If confirmed on a blood count, this condition is called pancytopenia.

Causes

- **Aplastic anaemia:** severe hypoplasia of the

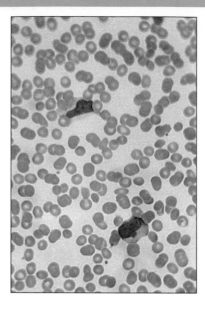

Figure 8.20 Viral illness (e.g. infectious mononucleosis)
Film shows two atypical or 'switched-on' lymphocytes.

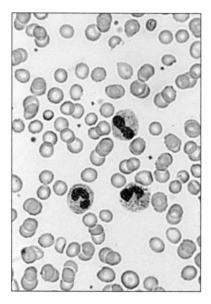

Figure 8.21 Bacterial infection (e.g. pneumonia, infective endocarditis)
The white cell in the centre is a band form with prominent 'toxic' granules.

erythroid, myeloid and platelet precursor cell lines in the bone marrow, resulting in a bone marrow that is fatty and empty of cells. The causes are listed in Table 8.10; 50% have no cause identified.
- **Marrow infiltration** by leukaemia, lymphoma, carcinoma, myeloma, myelofibrosis or granulomata.

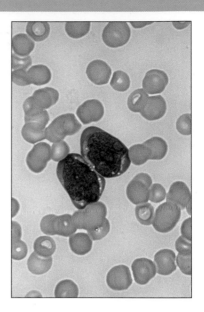

Figure 8.22 Acute leukaemia
The film shows two very primitive white cells with prominent nucleoli.

- **Other:** acute leukaemia (subleukaemic phase), pernicious anaemia, hypersplenism, systemic lupus erythematosus, folate deficiency, paroxysmal nocturnal haemoglobinuria (PNH).

Acute leukaemia

Leukaemia is a neoplastic proliferation of one of the blood-forming cells. Acute leukaemia presents with marrow failure from progressive infiltration of the marrow with immature cells. The course is rapidly fatal without treatment. Acute leukaemias can be divided into two main types: acute lymphoblastic leukaemia and acute myeloid leukaemia.

General signs of acute leukaemia

Pallor (anaemia), fever (which usually indicates infection secondary to neutropenia) and petechiae (thrombocytopenia) are all due to bone marrow failure. Weight loss, muscle wasting (hypercatabolic state) and localised infections (e.g. of the tonsils or perirectal region, due to leucopenia) also occur.

Signs of infiltration of the haemopoietic system

These include: (i) bony tenderness, due to infiltration or infarction; (ii) lymphadenopathy (slight to moderate, especially in acute lymphoblastic leukaemia); (iii) splenomegaly (slight to moderate, occurs especially in acute lymphoblastic leukaemia; the spleen may be tender due to splenic infarction); and (iv) hepatomegaly (slight to moderate).

TABLE 8.10 Causes of anaemia

Microcytic anaemia

Iron-deficiency anaemia (iron is essential for haem production)

- chronic bleeding (commonest cause, usually from gastrointestinal or menstrual loss)
- malabsorption, e.g. gastrectomy, coeliac disease
- hookworm (blood loss)
- pregnancy (increased demand)
   Note: Dietary inadequacy alone is rarely the sole cause.

Thalassaemia minor (an abnormal haemoglobin)

Sideroblastic anaemia (iron incorporation into haem is abnormal)

Long-standing anaemia of chronic disease

Macrocytic anaemia

Megaloblastic bone marrow (oval macrocytes on the blood film)

- vitamin B_{12} deficiency due to:
   pernicious anaemia
   gastrectomy
   tropical sprue or bacterial overgrowth
   ileal disease, e.g. Crohn's disease, ileal resection (>60 cm)
   fish tapeworm (*Diphyllobothrium latum*) in Scandinavia especially
   poor diet (vegans, very rare)
- folate deficiency due to:
   dietary deficiency, especially alcoholics
   malabsorption, especially coeliac disease
   increased cell turnover, e.g. pregnancy, leukaemia, chronic haemolysis, chronic inflammation
   antifolate drugs, e.g. phenytoin, methotrexate, sulfasalazine

Non-megaloblastic bone marrow (round macrocytes on the blood film)

- alcohol
- cirrhosis of the liver
- reticulocytosis, e.g. haemolysis, haemorrhage
- hypothyroidism
- marrow infiltration
- myelodysplastic syndrome
- myeloproliferative disease

Normocytic anaemia

Bone marrow failure:

- aplastic anaemia (bone marrow fatty or empty), e.g. drugs (such as chloramphenicol, indomethacin, phenytoin, gold, sulfonamides, antineoplastics), radiation, systemic lupus erythematosus, viral hepatitis, pregnancy, Fanconi syndrome, idiopathic
- ineffective haematopoiesis (normal or increased bone marrow cellularity), e.g. myelodysplastic syndrome, paroxysmal nocturnal haemoglobinuria (PNH)
- infiltration, e.g. leukaemia, lymphoma, myeloma, granuloma, myelofibrosis

Anaemia of chronic disease:

- chronic inflammation, e.g. infection (abscess, tuberculosis), connective tissue disease
- malignancy
- endocrine deficiencies, e.g. hypothyroidism, hypopituitarism, Addison's disease
- liver disease
- chronic renal failure
- malnutrition

Haemolytic anaemia:

- intracorpuscular defects, e.g. hereditary spherocytosis, elliptocytosis; haemoglobinopathies—sickle cell anaemia, thalassaemia; paroxysmal nocturnal haemoglobinuria (PNH)
- extracorpuscular defects: e.g. immune—autoimmune (warm or cold antibody) incompatible blood transfusion; hypersplenism; trauma (marathon runners, prosthetic heart valves); microangiopathic—disseminated intravascular coagulation); toxic—malaria

Signs of infiltration of other areas

There may be: (i) tonsillar enlargement (especially in acute lymphoblastic leukaemia); (ii) swelling or bleeding of the gums, especially in monocytic leukaemia; (iii) pleural effusions; (iv) nerve palsies, involving the spinal nerve roots or the cranial nerves; or (v) meningism due to infiltration of the meninges, especially in acute lymphoblastic leukaemia.

Chronic leukaemia

This is a haematological malignancy in which the leukaemic cell is at first well differentiated. These have a better prognosis untreated than acute leukaemia. There are two main types: chronic myeloid leukaemia and chronic lymphocytic leukaemia.

Signs of chronic myeloid leukaemia

This is one of the myeloproliferative disorders. There is an expanded granulocytic mass in the bone marrow, liver and spleen.

General signs may include pallor (anaemia due to bone marrow infiltration) and secondary gout (common).

Haemopoietic system signs include massive splenomegaly and moderate hepatomegaly. (*Note:* Lymphadenopathy is usually a sign of blast transformation.)

Signs of chronic lymphocytic leukaemia

There may be tiredness and pallor. Recurrent acute infections occur.

Haemopoietic system signs include marked or moderate lymphadenopathy and moderate hepatosplenomegaly.

Other abnormalities may include a Coombs'[h] test—positive haemolytic anaemia, herpes zoster skin infections and nodular infiltrates. Patients may note a hypersensitivity to insect bites before the diagnosis is made.

Myeloproliferative disease

This is a group of disorders of the haematopoietic stem cell. These include polycythaemia rubra vera, primary myelofibrosis, chronic myeloid leukaemia and essential thrombocythaemia. Overlapping clinical and pathological features occur in these disorders. Therefore, patients may have signs of one or more of the conditions. Any of them may progress to acute myeloid leukaemia.

[h] Robin Coombs (b. 1921), Quick professor of biology, Cambridge.

TABLE 8.11 Polycythaemia

Signs of polycythaemia rubra vera

Plethoric appearance including engorged conjunctival and retinal vessels (not specific)

Scratch marks (generalised pruritus)

Splenomegaly (80%)

Bleeding tendency (platelet dysfunction)

Peripheral vascular and ischaemic heart disease (thrombosis, slow circulation)

Gout

Mild hypertension

Causes of polycythaemia

Absolute polycythaemia (increased red cell mass)

Idiopathic: polycythaemia rubra vera

Secondary polycythaemia

• Increased erythropoietin:

    renal disease—polycystic disease, hydronephrosis, tumour; after renal transplantation

    hepatocellular carcinoma

    cerebellar haemangioblastoma

    uterine fibroma

    virilising syndromes

    Cushing's syndrome

    phaeochromocytoma

• Hypoxic states (erythropoietin secondarily increased):

    chronic lung disease

    sleep apnoea

    living at high altitude

    cyanotic congenital heart disease

    abnormal haemoglobins

    carbon monoxide poisoning

Relative polycythaemia (decreased plasma volume)

Dehydration

Stress polycythaemia: Gaisböck's* disease

* Felix Gaisböck (1868–1955), German physician, described this in 1905.

Polycythaemia

This is an elevated haemoglobin concentration and can result from an increased red blood cell mass or a decreased plasma volume. Polycythaemia rubra vera results from an autonomous increase in the red blood cell production. Patients with polycythaemia often have a striking ruddy, plethoric appearance. To examine a patient with suspected polycythaemia, assess for both the manifestations of polycythaemia rubra vera and for other possible underlying causes of polycythaemia (Table 8.11).

Look at the patient and estimate the state of hydration (dehydration alone can cause an elevated haemoglobin due to haemoconcentration). Note if there is a Cushingoid (page 309) or virilised (page 315) appearance. Cyanosis may be present because of an underlying condition such as cyanotic congenital heart disease or chronic lung disease. Look for nicotine staining (smoking). All these diseases can result in secondary polycythaemia.

The arms should be inspected for scratch marks; post-bathing pruritus occurs in polycythaemia rubra vera, possibly due to basophil histamine release. Take the blood pressure: very rarely a phaeochromocytoma will cause secondary polycythaemia and hypertension.

Examine the eyes. Look for injected conjunctivae. Fundal hyperviscosity changes, including engorged, dilated retinal veins and haemorrhages, may be present. Inspect the tongue for central cyanosis.

Examine the cardiovascular system for signs of cyanotic congenital heart disease and the respiratory system for signs of chronic lung disease. The abdomen must be carefully assessed for splenomegaly, which occurs in 80% of cases of polycythaemia rubra vera but does not usually occur with the other causes of polycythaemia. There may be evidence of chronic liver disease or hepatocellular carcinoma, which may cause secondary polycythaemia. Palpate for the kidneys and perform a urinalysis. In women palpate the uterus. Polycystic kidney disease, hydronephrosis, renal carcinoma and uterine fibromata can all rarely cause secondary polycythaemia.

The legs must be inspected for scratch marks, gouty tophi (Figure 9.57, page 282) and arthropathy, as well as for signs of peripheral vascular disease. In polycythaemia rubra vera, secondary gout occurs due to the increased cellular turnover resulting in hyperuricaemia. Peripheral vascular disease occurs in polycythaemia rubra vera because of thrombosis (as there is increased platelet adhesiveness and accelerated atherosclerosis) and slowed circulation due to hyperviscosity.

Look for cerebellar signs, which may be due to the presence of a cerebellar haemangioblastoma, a very rare cause of secondary polycythaemia. Examine the central nervous system for signs of a stroke due to thrombosis.

Primary myelofibrosis

This is a clonal haemopoietic stem cell disorder with fibrosis as a secondary phenomenon. Gradual replacement of the marrow by fibrosis and progressive splenomegaly characterise the disease.

- **General signs** include pallor (anaemia occurs in most patients eventually) and petechiae (in 20% of patients, due to thrombocytopenia).
- **Haemopoietic system signs** include splenomegaly (in almost all cases, and often to a massive degree—there may also be a splenic

rub due to splenic infarction), hepatomegaly (occurs in 50% of patients and can be massive) and lymphadenopathy (very uncommon).
- **Other signs** are bony tenderness (uncommon) and gout (occurs in 5% of patients).

Chronic myeloid leukaemia
(See page 236.)

Essential thrombocythaemia

This is a sustained elevation of the platelet count above normal without any primary cause.
- **General signs** include spontaneous bleeding and thrombosis.
- **Haemopoietic system signs** include splenomegaly.
- **Causes of thrombocytosis** (platelet count more than 450×10^9/L) include: (i) following haemorrhage or surgery; (ii) postsplenectomy; (iii) iron deficiency; (iv) chronic inflammatory disease; (v) malignancy.
- **Causes of thrombocytosis** (platelet count more than 800×10^9/L) include: (i) myeloproliferative disease; (ii) secondary to recent splenectomy, malignancy, or marked inflammation occasionally.

Lymphoma (Figure 8.23)

This is a malignant disease of the lymphoid system. There are two main clinicopathological types: Hodgkin's disease (with the characteristic Reed-Sternberg cell[i]) and non-Hodgkin's lymphoma. Signs of lymphoma depend on the stages of the disease (Table 8.12).

Hodgkin's disease often presents in stage I or II, while non-Hodgkin's lymphoma usually presents in stage III or IV.

Signs of Hodgkin's disease

1 Lymph node enlargement: discrete, rubbery, painless, large and superficial nodes, often confined to one side and one lymph node group.
2 Weight loss and fever with or without infection (reduced cell-mediated immunity) suggest a poor prognosis.
3 Splenomegaly and hepatomegaly. Splenomegaly does not always indicate extensive disease.
4 Organ infiltration occurs with late disease. Look especially for signs of: (i) lung disease, such as a pleural effusion; (ii) bone pain or pathological fractures (rare); (iii) spinal cord or

---

[i] Dorothy Reed (1874–1964), pathologist at Johns Hopkins Hospital, Baltimore, described these cells in 1906 and Karl Sternberg (1872–1935), pathologist, described giant cells in 1898.

TABLE 8.12 Staging of lymphoma: Ann Arbor classification

Stage I
Disease confined to a single lymph node region or a single extralymphatic site (IE)

Stage II
Disease confined to two or more lymph node regions on one side of the diaphragm

Stage III
Disease confined to lymph nodes on both sides of the diaphragm with or without localised involvement of the spleen (IIIS), other extralymphatic organ or site (IIIE), or both (IIIES)

Stage IV
Diffuse disease of one or more extralymphatic organs (with or without lymph node disease)

For any stage: a = no symptoms; b = fever, weight loss greater than 10% in 6 months, night sweats.
E involves direct invasion from lymph node into surrounding tissue.

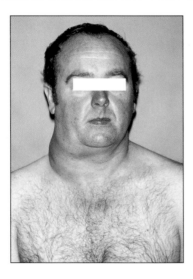

Figure 8.23 Cervical lymph node enlargement in a patient with lymphoma
(From Mir MA, *Atlas of Clinical Diagnosis*, 2nd edn. Edinburgh: Saunders, 2003, with permission.)

nerve compression (rare); and (iv) nodular skin infiltrates (rare).

Signs of non-Hodgkin's lymphoma

1 Lymph node enlargement: often more than one site is involved and Waldeyer's ring is more commonly affected.
2 Hepatosplenomegaly is common.
3 Systemic signs (for example weight loss or fever) are less common.
4 Signs of extranodal spread are more common.

5 The disease may sometimes arise at an extranodal site (e.g. the gastrointestinal tract).

Multiple myeloma
This is a disseminated malignant disease of plasma cells.

General signs
There may be signs of anaemia (due to bone marrow infiltration or as a result of renal failure), purpura (due to bone marrow infiltration and thrombocytopenia) or infection (particularly pneumonia).

Bony tenderness and pathological fractures may be present. Weight loss may be a feature.

Skin changes include hypertrichosis, erythema annulare, yellow skin and secondary amyloid deposits.

There may be signs of spinal cord compression, or mental changes (due to hypercalcaemia).

Look for signs of chronic renal failure (which may be due to tubular damage from filtered light chains, uric acid nephropathy, hypercalcaemia, urinary tract infection, secondary amyloidosis or plasma cell infiltration).

Summary
The haematological examination: a suggested method (Figure 8.24)
This will be a targeted examination during follow-up consultations but should be completed in full for the first visit.

Position the patient as for a gastrointestinal examination. Make sure he or she is fully undressed, in stages and with a gown for women. Look for bruising, pigmentation, cyanosis, jaundice and scratch marks (due to myeloproliferative disease or lymphoma). Also note the presence of frontal bossing and the racial origin of the patient.

Pick up the patient's **hands**. Look at the nails for koilonychia (spoon-shaped nails, which are rarely seen today and indicate iron deficiency) and the changes of vasculitis. Pale palmar creases may indicate anaemia (typically the haemoglobin level has to be lower than 70 g/L). Evidence of arthropathy may be important (e.g. rheumatoid arthritis and Felty's syndrome, recurrent haemarthroses in bleeding disorders, secondary gout in myeloproliferative disorders).

Examine the **epitrochlear nodes**. Note any bruising. Remember, petechiae are pinhead haemorrhages, while ecchymoses are larger bruises.

Go to the **axillae** and palpate the axillary nodes. There are five main areas: central, lateral (above and

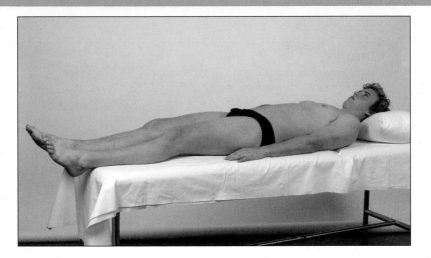

Figure 8.24 Haematological system examination

Lying flat (1 pillow)

1. **General inspection**
   Weight (normal, reduced, increased)
   Bruising (thrombocytopenia, scurvy etc)
   • Petechiae (pinhead bleeding)
   • Ecchymoses (large bruises)
   Pigmentation (lymphoma)
   Rashes and infiltrative lesions (lymphoma)
   Ulceration (neutropenia)
   Cyanosis (polycythaemia)
   Plethora (polycythaemia)
   Jaundice (haemolysis)
   Scratch marks (myeloproliferative diseases, lymphoma)
   Racial origin
2. **Hands**
   Nails—koilonychia, pallor
   Palmar crease pallor (anaemia)
   Arthropathy (haemophilia, secondary gout, drug treatment etc)
   Pulse
3. **Epitrochlear and axillary nodes**
4. **Face**
   Sclera—jaundice, pallor, conjunctival suffusion (polycythaemia)
   Mouth—gum hypertrophy (monocytic leukaemia etc.), ulceration, infection, haemorrhage (marrow aplasia etc.); atrophic glossitis, angular stomatitis (iron, vitamin deficiencies)
   Tongue—amyloidosis
5. **Cervical nodes (sitting up)**
   Palpate from behind
6. **Bony tenderness**
   Spine
   Sternum
   Clavicles
   Shoulders
7. **Abdomen (lying flat) and genitalia**
   Inguinal nodes
   Detailed examination
8. **Legs**
   Vasculitis (Henoch-Schönlein purpura—buttocks, thighs)
   Bruising
   Pigmentation
   Ulceration (e.g. haemoglobinopathies)
   Neurological signs (subacute combined degeneration, peripheral neuropathy)
9. **Other**
   Fundi (haemorrhages, infection etc)
   Temperature chart (infection)
   Urine analysis (haematuria, bile etc)
   Rectal and pelvic examination (blood loss)

lateral), pectoral (most medial), infraclavicular and subscapular (most inferior).

Look at the **face**. Inspecting the eyes, note jaundice, pallor or haemorrhage of the sclerae, and the injected sclerae of polycythaemia. Examine the mouth. Look for peri-oral telangiectasiae. Note gum hypertrophy (e.g. from acute monocytic leukaemia or scurvy), ulceration, infection, haemorrhage, atrophic glossitis (e.g. from iron deficiency, or vitamin B_{12} or folate deficiency) and angular stomatitis. Look for tonsillar and adenoid enlargement (Waldeyer's ring).

Sit the patient up. Examine the **cervical nodes** from behind. There are eight groups: submental, submandibular, jugular chain, supraclavicular, posterior triangle, postauricular, preauricular and occipital. Then feel the supraclavicular area from the front. Tap the spine with your fist for **bony tenderness** (caused by an enlarging marrow—e.g. in myeloma or carcinoma). Also gently press the sternum, clavicles and shoulders for bony tenderness.

Lay the patient flat again. Examine the **abdomen**. Focus on the liver and spleen. Feel for para-aortic nodes. Don't forget to feel the testes, and to perform a rectal and pelvic examination (for tumour or bleeding). Spring the hips for pelvic tenderness. Palpate the inguinal nodes. There are two groups—along the inguinal ligament and along the femoral vessels.

Examine the **legs**. Note particularly leg ulcers. Examine the legs from a neurological aspect, for evidence of vitamin B_{12} deficiency or peripheral neuropathy from other causes. Remember, hypothyroidism can cause anaemia and neurological disease.

Finally, examine the **fundi**, look at the **temperature** chart, and test the **urine**.

References

1. Strobach RS, Anderson SK, Doll DC, Ringenberg QS. The value of the physical examination in the diagnosis of anaemia: correlation of the physical findings and the haemoglobin concentrations. *Arch Intern Med* 1988; 148:831–832. Palmar crease pallor can occur above a haemoglobin of 70 g/L.

2. Nardone DA, Roth KM, Mazur DJ, McAfee JH. Usefulness of physical examination in detecting the presence or absence of anemia. *Arch Intern Med* 1990; 150:201–204.

3. Sheth TN, Choudray NK, Bowes M, Detsky AS. The relation of conjunctival pallor to the presence of anemia. *J Gen Intern Med* 1997; 12:102–106. The presence of conjunctival pallor is a useful indicator of anaemia, but its absence is unhelpful. It is also a reliable sign.

4. Linet OI, Metzler C. Practical ENT: incidence of palpable cervical nodes in adults. *Postgrad Med* 1977; 62:210–211, 213. In young adults without chronic disease, palpable cervical lymph nodes are often detected but are not clinically important. Remember, posterior cervical nodes are almost never normal.

5. Robertson TI. Clinical diagnosis in patients with lymphadenopathy. *Med J Aust* 1979; 2:73–76.

6. Grover SA, Barkun AN, Sackett DL. Does this patient have splenomegaly? *JAMA* 1993; 270:2218–2221. A valuable guide to assessment of splenomegaly, although the recommendations are controversial. A combination of percussion and palpation may best identify splenomegaly, but in contrast to hepatomegaly, percussion may be modestly more sensitive, according to the few available studies. Our conclusion is that this needs to be better established; in practice splenomegaly is often missed by percussion alone.

7. Anonymous. Cancer detection in adults by physical examination. US Public Health Service. *Am Fam Phys* 1995; 51:871–874, 877–880, 883–885.

Suggested reading

Hoffbrand AV, Moss P, Pettit JE. *Essential haematology*, 5th edn. London: Blackwell, 2006.

Provan D, ed. *ABC of clinical haematology*, 3rd edn. London: BMJ Publishing Group, 2007.

Chapter 9

The rheumatological system

The rheumatism is a common name for many aches and pains which have yet got no peculiar appellation, though owing to very different causes.

William Heberden (1710–1801)

Rheumatology is 'the study of the Rheumatic Diseases including arthritis, rheumatic fever, fibrositis, neuralgia, myositis, bursitis, gout and other conditions producing somatic pain, stiffness and soreness' (Oxford English Dictionary, 2nd edn, 1989). The rheumatological system therefore includes diseases of the joints, tendons and muscles.

The rheumatological history
Presenting symptoms (Table 9.1)
Peripheral joints

Pain and swelling. The underlying aetiology of joint pain can often be determined by establishing the distribution and duration of joint involvement. Remember, *arthralgia* is the presence of joint pain without swelling, while with *arthritis* there is usually pain and swelling. Determine whether one or many joints are involved.

It is often useful to ask the patient to point to the painful place or area. For example, pain said to affect the knee may be in the popliteal fossa, the knee joint itself, or in the supra- or infra-patellar bursa. Remember also that pain in the knee or lower thigh may be referred from the hip (Figure 9.1).

Find out if the symptoms are of an acute or chronic nature and whether they are getting better or worse. The effect of rest and exercise on the joint pain should be determined. Patients with rheumatoid arthritis have joint symptoms which are worse after rest, while those with osteoarthritis have pain which is worse after exercise. Ask

TABLE 9.1 Rheumatological history—major symptoms

Joints
Pain
Swelling
Morning stiffness
Stiffness after inactivity
Loss of motion
Loss of function
Deformity
Weakness
Instability
Changes in sensation

Eyes
Dry eyes and mouth
Red eyes

Systemic
Raynaud's phenomenon
Rash, fever, fatigue, weight loss, diarrhoea, mucosal ulcers

about the sequence of onset of joint involvement. Precipitating factors such as trauma should be noted. The causes of monoarthritis (single joint) and polyarthritis (more than one joint), and the patterns of polyarthritis in various diseases, are presented in Tables 9.2, 9.3 and 9.4.

Morning stiffness. Ask about the presence of early-morning stiffness and the length of time that this stiffness lasts. Morning stiffness classically occurs in rheumatoid arthritis and other inflammatory arthropathies, and the duration of stiffness is a guide to its severity. Stiffness after inactivity, such as sitting, is characteristic of osteoarthritis of the hip or knee.

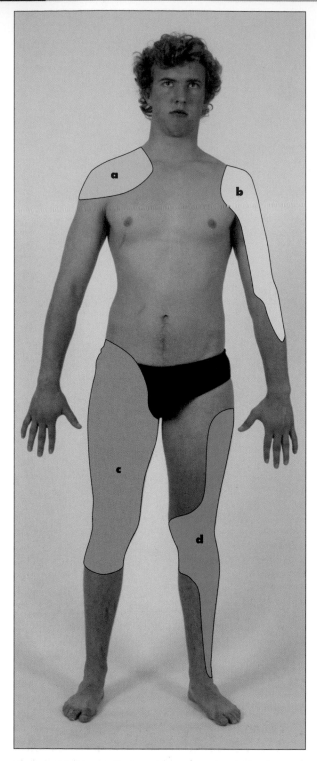

Figure 9.1 Map of referral patterns for different joints
(a) Acromioclavicular and sternoclavicular joints.
(b) Scapulohumeral joint. (c) Hip. (d) Knee.
(Adapted from Epstein O et al, *Clinical Examination*, 4th edn. Edinburgh: Mosby, 2008.)

TABLE 9.2 Causes of monoarthritis

A single hot red swollen joint (acute monoarthritis)
Septic arthritis
- Haematogenous—e.g. staphylococcal or gonococcal (latter may be polyarticular)
- Secondary to penetrating injury

Traumatic
Gout, pseudogout, or hydroxyapatite arthropathy
Haemarthrosis—e.g. haemophilia (Figure 9.2)
Seronegative spondyloarthritis (occasionally)

A single chronic inflamed joint (chronic monoarthritis)
Chronic infection—e.g. atypical mycobacterial infection
Seronegative spondyloarthritis
Pigmented villonodular synovitis
Synovial (osteo)chondromatosis

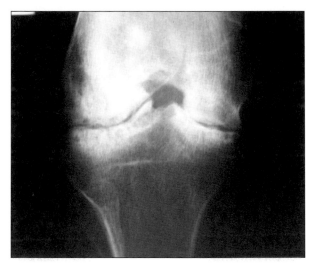

Figure 9.2 Haemophilia
X-ray of the knee showing loss of joint space and some deformity of the adjacent bone. Although the tibia and femur are sclerotic adjacent to the destructive change, the bones are generally osteopenic with mild overgrowth of the epiphysis.
(Courtesy Canberra Hospital X-ray library.)

Deformity. The patient may have noticed deformity of a joint or bone. If there has been progressive change in the shape of the area this is more likely to be significant.

Instability. Joint instability may be described by the patient as a 'giving way', or occasionally 'coming out', of the joint in certain conditions. This may be due to true dislocation (for example, with the shoulder or the patella) or alternatively to muscle weakness or ligamentous problems.

TABLE 9.3 Causes of polyarthritis
Acute polyarthritis
Infection—viral, bacterial
Onset of chronic polyarthritis
Chronic polyarthritis
Rheumatoid arthritis
Seronegative spondyloarthritis
Primary osteoarthritis
Gout, pseudogout, or hydroxyapatite arthropathy
Connective tissue disease, e.g. systemic lupus erythematosus
Infection, e.g. spirochaetal infection (rare)

TABLE 9.4 Patterns of polyarthropathy
Rheumatoid arthritis
This is usually a symmetrical polyarthritis.
Hands: proximal interphalangeal, metacarpophalangeal and wrist joints
Elbows
Small joints of the upper cervical spine
Knees
Ankles
Feet: tarsal and metatarsophalangeal joints
Cervical spine and temporomandibular joints may also be affected
Seronegative spondyloarthritis
Ankylosing spondylitis
Sacroiliac joints and spine
Hips, knees and shoulders
Psoriatic arthritis
Asymmetric oligoarthritis
Sausage digits
Terminal interphalangeal joints
Sacroiliac joints
Rheumatoid pattern
Reiter's syndrome
Sacroiliac joints and spine
Hips
Knees
Ankles and joints of the feet
Primary osteoarthritis
This is usually symmetrical and can affect many joints.
Fingers: distal (Heberden's nodes) and proximal (Bouchard's nodes) interphalangeal joints, and metacarpophalangeal joints of the thumbs
Acromioclavicular joints
Small joints of the spine (lower cervical and lumbar)
Knees
Metatarsophalangeal joints of the great toes
Secondary osteoarthritis
This is:
1 asymmetrical and affects previously injured, inflamed or infected weightbearing joints, particularly hip and knee
2 a result of metabolic conditions, e.g. haemochromatosis; symptoms and findings are generalised

Change in sensation. Change in sensation may occur as a result of nerve entrapment or injury, and sometimes as a result of ischaemia. Ask about numbness or paraesthesiae (pins and needles). The distribution of the change of sensation should help to distinguish nerve damage or entrapment (a specific distribution) from ischaemia.

Back pain

This is a very common symptom. It is most often a consequence of local musculoskeletal disease.

Ask where the pain is situated, whether it began suddenly or gradually, whether it is localised or diffuse, whether it radiates to the limbs or elsewhere, and whether the pain is aggravated by movement, coughing or straining. Musculoskeletal pain is characteristically well localised and is aggravated by movement. If there is a spinal nerve root irritation there may be pain that occurs in a dermatomal distribution. This helps to localise the level of the lesion. Diseases such as osteoporosis (with crush fractures), infiltration of carcinoma, leukaemia or myeloma may cause progressive and unremitting back pain, which is often worse at night (Table 9.6). The pain may be of sudden onset but is usually self-limiting if it results from the crush fracture of a vertebral body. In ankylosing spondylitis the pain is usually situated over the sacroiliac joints and lumbar spine, it is also worse at night and is associated with morning stiffness. The pain of ankylosing spondylitis is typically better with activity which helps distinguish it from mechanical back pain.[1,2] Pain from diseases of the abdomen and chest (e.g. dissecting abdominal or thoracic aortic aneurysm) can also be referred to the back.

Limb pain

This can occur from disease of the musculoskeletal system, the skin, the vascular system or the nervous system.

Musculoskeletal pain may be due to trauma or inflammation. Muscle disease such as *polymyositis* can present with an aching pain in the proximal muscles around the shoulders and hips, associated with weakness. Pain and stiffness in the shoulders and hips in patients over the age of 50 years may be due to *polymyalgia rheumatica*. The acute or subacute onset of symptoms in multiple locations suggests an inflammatory process. Bone disease

TABLE 9.5 Functional assessment in rheumatoid arthritis

Class	Assessment
Class 1	Normal functional ability
Class 2	Ability to carry out normal activities, despite discomfort or limited mobility of one or more joints
Class 3	Ability to perform only a few of the tasks of the normal occupation or of self-care
Class 4	Complete or almost complete incapacity with the patient confined to wheelchair or to bed

TABLE 9.6 Alarm features for back pain

Age > 50 years
Cancer history
Weight loss (unexplained)
Pain on waking from sleep
Pain for longer than one month and unresponsive to simple analgesics
Fever
History of drug use by injection
Bowel or bladder dysfunction

such as osteomyelitis, osteomalacia, osteoporosis or tumours can cause limb pain. Inflammation of tendons (*tenosynovitis*) can produce local pain over the affected area.

Vascular disease may also produce pain in the limbs. Acute arterial occlusion causes severe pain of sudden onset, often with coolness or pallor. Chronic peripheral vascular disease can result in calf pain on exercise that is relieved by rest. This is called intermittent claudication. Venous thrombosis can also cause diffuse aching pain in the legs associated with swelling.

Spinal stenosis can cause pseudo-claudication—pain on walking but relieved by leaning forward.

Nerve entrapment and *neuropathy* can both cause limb pain which is often associated with paraesthesiae or weakness. The usual cause is synovial thickening or joint subluxation—especially for patients with rheumatoid arthritis. The vasculitis associated with the inflammatory arthropathies can also cause neuropathy leading to diffuse peripheral neuropathy or mononeuritis multiplex. Patients with chronic rheumatoid arthritis often develop subluxation of the cervical spine at the atlanto-axial joint. This is caused by erosion of the transverse ligament around the posterior aspect of the odontoid process (dens). The patient may describe shooting paraesthesiae down the arms and an occipital headache. Neck flexion leads to indentation of the cord by the dens and can cause tetraplegia or sudden death. The abnormality may be obvious on lateral X-rays of the cervical spine (Figure 9.3). Injury to peripheral nerves can result in vasomotor changes and severe limb pain. This is called *causalgia*. Even following amputation of a limb, phantom limb pain may develop and persist as a chronic problem.

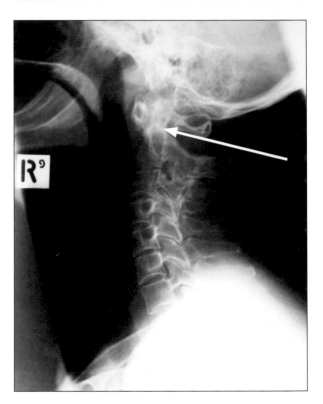

Figure 9.3 Rheumatoid arthritis
Lateral X-ray of the cervical spine showing anterior subluxation of the anterior arch of the dens of the axis (C2, arrow).
(Courtesy Canberra Hospital X-ray library.)

Raynaud's phenomenon

Raynaud's phenomenon[a] is an abnormal response of the fingers and toes to cold. Classically, the fingers first turn white, then blue and finally red after exposure to cold. It is during the red phase that the pain may be most severe, but pain during the white stage may also be severe, as a result of

a   Maurice Raynaud (1834–1881) described this in his first work, published in Paris in 1862.

TABLE 9.7 Causes of Raynaud's phenomenon (white-blue-red fingers and toes in response to cold)

Reflex
Raynaud's disease (idiopathic)
Vibrating machinery injury
Cervical spondylosis

Connective tissue disease
Scleroderma, diffuse or limited type
Mixed connective tissue disease
Systemic lupus erythematosus
Polyarteritis nodosa
Rheumatoid arthritis
Polymyositis
Vasculitis

Arterial disease
Embolism or thrombosis
Buerger's disease (thromboangiitis obliterans)—smokers
Trauma

Haematological
Polycythaemia
Leukaemia
Dysproteinaemia
Cold agglutinin disease

Poisons
Drugs: beta-blockers, ergotamine
Vinyl chloride

TABLE 9.8 Clinical features of Sjögren's syndrome

In this syndrome mucus-secreting glands are infiltrated by lymphocytes and plasma cells, which cause atrophy and fibrosis of glandular tissue.

1 Dry eyes: conjunctivitis, keratitis, corneal ulcers (rarely vascularisation of the cornea)

2 Dry mouth

3 Chest: infection secondary to reduced mucus secretion or interstitial pneumonitis

4 Kidneys: renal tubular acidosis or nephrogenic diabetes insipidus

5 Genital tract: atrophic vaginitis

6 Pseudolymphoma: lymphadenopathy and splenomegaly, which may rarely progress to a true (usually non-Hodgkin's) lymphoma

Note: This syndrome occurs in rheumatoid arthritis and with the connective tissue diseases.

ischaemia. Patients with Raynaud's disease have Raynaud's phenomenon without an obvious underlying cause. The disease tends to be familial and females are more likely to be affected. In connective tissue diseases, especially scleroderma, Raynaud's phenomenon can occur and may lead to the formation of digital ulcers (Table 9.7).

Dry eyes and mouth
Dry eyes and dry mouth are characteristic of Sjögren's syndrome (Table 9.8). This syndrome may occur in isolation (primary Sjögren's) and is very common in association with rheumatoid arthritis and other connective tissue disease. Mucus-secreting glands become infiltrated with lymphocytes and plasma cells, which cause atrophy and fibrosis. The dry eyes can result in conjunctivitis, keratitis and corneal ulcers. Sjögren's syndrome can also have an effect on other organs such as the lungs or kidneys.

Red eyes
The seronegative spondyloarthropathies and Behçet's[b] syndrome but not rheumatoid arthritis may be complicated by iritis (eye pain with central scleral injection—a 'red eye'—radiating out from the pupil) (see Figure 9.51, page 279). In other diseases, such as Sjögren's, red eyes may be due to dryness, episcleritis or scleritis.

Systemic symptoms
A number of other symptoms may occur with specific rheumatological diseases. *Fatigue* is common with connective tissue disease. *Weight loss* and *diarrhoea* may occur with scleroderma, because of small-bowel bacterial overgrowth. Mucosal ulcers are common in some connective tissue diseases such as systemic lupus erythematosus (SLE). Specific rashes can also occur. *Generalised stiffness* can be due to rheumatoid arthritis or scleroderma, but other causes include systemic infection (e.g. influenza), excessive exercise, polymyalgia rheumatica, neuromuscular disease (e.g. extrapyramidal disease, tetanus, myotonia, dermatomyositis) and hypothyroidism. Finally, on occasion *fever* may be associated with the connective tissue diseases, especially SLE, but infection should always be excluded.

Treatment history
Document current and previous anti-arthritic medications (e.g. aspirin, other non-steroidal anti-inflammatory drugs, gold, methotrexate, penicillamine, chloroquine, steroids, anti-tumour

b   Halushi Behçet (1889–1948), Turkish dermatologist.

necrosis factor α therapy, or other biological agents). Any side-effects of these drugs (e.g. gastric ulceration or haemorrhage, from aspirin) also need to be identified. Ask about physiotherapy and joint or tendon surgery in the past.

Past history

It is important to inquire about any history of trauma or surgery in the past. Similarly, a history of recent infection, including hepatitis, streptococcal pharyngitis, rubella, dysentery, gonorrhoea and tuberculosis, may be relevant to the onset of arthralgia or arthritis. A history of tick bite may indicate that the patient has Lyme disease. Inflammatory bowel disease can be associated with arthritis, as described on page 191. A history of psoriasis may indicate that the arthritis is due to psoriatic arthropathy. It is also important to inquire about any history of arthritis in childhood. The smoking history is important: rheumatoid arthritis is more common in smokers, and smoking adds to their already increased risk of cardiovascular disease.

Social history

Determine the patient's domestic set-up and occupation. This is particularly relevant if a chronic disabling arthritis has developed. Any history of sexually transmitted disease in the past is important, but non-specific urethritis and gonorrhoea are especially relevant.

Family history

Some diseases associated with chronic arthritis run in families. These include rheumatoid arthritis, gout and primary osteoarthritis, haemochromatosis, the seronegative spondyloarthropathies and inflammatory bowel disease. A family history of bleeding disorder may explain an acutely swollen tender joint in a boy (haemophilia).

Examination anatomy

Joint structures (Figure 9.4)

Inflammatory arthritis affects first the joint synovium. Thickening of this may be palpable and is called *pannus*. Later, destruction of surrounding structures including tendons, articular cartilages and the bone itself occur.

Joint pain may be well localised if there is inflammation close to the skin, but deeper joint abnormalities may cause pain to be referred. The areas where joint pain is felt correspond to the innervation of the muscle attached to that joint—the myotome. For example, the glenohumeral joint of the shoulder and the posterior scapular muscles are supplied from C5 and C6, so pain over the shoulder or scapula may arise from any structure supplied from these nerve roots—including the shoulder muscles and joints but also the C5 and C6 segments of the spine. Figure 9.1 shows a map of approximate referral patterns for important joints.

The extra-articular structures that surround a joint—the ligaments, tendons and nerves—may also be the source of joint pain. Disease of the joint itself tends to limit movement of the joint in all directions, both active movement (moved by the patient) and passive movement (moved by the examiner). Extra-articular disease causes variable limitation of movement in different directions, and tends to cause more limitation of active than of passive movement.

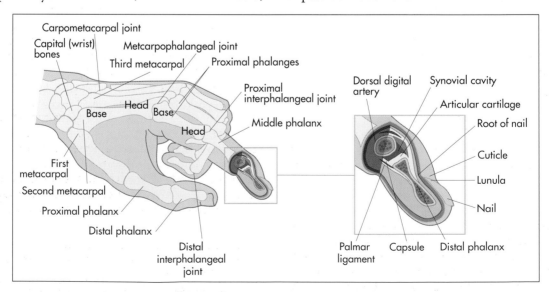

Figure 9.4 Hand bones and finger joint—a typical synovial joint

The rheumatological examination

There are certain established ways of examining the joints and related structures[3] and it is important to be aware of the numerous systemic complications of rheumatological diseases. The actual system of examination depends on the patient's history and sometimes on the examiner noticing an abnormality on general inspection. Formal examination of all the joints is rarely part of the routine physical examination, but students should learn how to handle each joint properly and a formal examination is an important part of the evaluation of patients who present with joint symptoms or who have an established diagnosis and active symptoms. Diseases of the extra-articular soft tissues are particularly common.

General inspection

This is important for two reasons: first, it gives an indication of the patient's functional disability, which is essential in all rheumatological assessments; and second, certain conditions can be diagnosed by careful inspection. Look at the patient as he or she walks into the room. Does walking appear to be painful and difficult? What posture is taken? Does the patient require assistance such as a stick or walking frame? Is there obvious deformity, and what joints does it involve? Note the pattern of joint involvement, which gives a clue about the likely underlying disease (Tables 9.2 to 9.4).

For a more detailed examination the patient should be undressed as far as practical, usually to the underclothes. Depending on the patient's condition and the parts of the body to be examined, the examination may best be begun with the patient in bed, or sitting over the side of the bed or in a chair, or standing. The opportunity of watching the patient remove the clothes should not be lost because arthritis can interfere with this essential daily task.

Principles of joint examination

Certain general rules apply to the examination of all the joints and they can be summarised as: *look, feel, move, measure,* and *compare with the opposite side.*

Look

The first principle is always to compare right with left. Remember that joints are three-dimensional structures and need to be inspected from the front, the back and the sides. The skin is inspected for *erythema* indicating underlying inflammation and suggesting active, intense arthritis or infection, *atrophy* suggesting chronic underlying disease, *scars* indicating previous operations such as tendon repairs or joint replacements, and *rashes.* For example, psoriasis is associated with a rash and polyarthritis (inflammation of more than one joint). The psoriatic rash consists of scaling erythematous plaques on extensor surfaces. The nails are often also affected (page 252). Also look for a vasculitic skin rash (inflammation of the blood vessels of the skin), which can range in appearance from palpable purpura or livedo reticularis (bluish-purple streaks in a net-like pattern) to skin necrosis.

A small, firm, painless swelling over the back (dorsal surface) of the wrist is usually a synovial cyst—a ganglion.[c] A larger, localised, soft area of swelling of the dorsum of the wrist generally indicates tenosynovitis.

Note any *swelling* over the joint. There are a number of possible causes: these include effusion into the joint space, hypertrophy and inflammation of the synovium (e.g. rheumatoid arthritis), or bony overgrowths at the joint margins (e.g. osteoarthritis). It may also occur when tissues around the joints become involved, as with the tendinitis or bursitis of rheumatoid arthritis. Swelling of the lower legs may be due to fluid retention, which is painless and can occur in association with inflammation anywhere in the leg. Painful swelling may result from inflammation of the ankle joints or tendons, or of the fascia, or from inflammatory oedema of the skin and subcutaneous tissue.

Deformity is the sign of a chronic, usually destructive, arthritis, and ranges from mild ulnar deviation of the metacarpophalangeal joints in early rheumatoid arthritis to the gross destruction and disorganisation of a denervated (Charcot's[d]) joint (Figure 10.20, page 319). Deviation of the part of the body away from the midline is called *valgus* deformity, and towards the midline, *varus* deformity. For example, *genu valgum* means knock-kneed and *genu varum*, bow-legged.

Look for abnormal bone alignment. *Subluxation* is said to be present when displaced parts of the joint surfaces remain partly in contact. *Dislocation* is used to describe displacement where there is loss of contact between the joint surfaces.

Muscle wasting results from a combination of disuse of the joint, inflammation of the surrounding tissues and sometimes nerve entrapment. It tends

---

c   The traditional treatment, striking the lesion very hard with the family Bible, is not effective.

d   Jean Martin Charcot (1825–1893), Parisian physician and neurologist. He became professor of nervous diseases, holding the first Chair of Neurology in the world. His pupils included Babinski, Marie and Freud.

to affect muscle groups adjacent to the diseased joint (e.g. quadriceps wasting with active arthritis of the knee) and is a sign of chronicity.

Feel

Palpate for skin *warmth*. This is done traditionally with the backs of the fingers where temperature appreciation is said to be better. A cool joint is unlikely to be involved in an acute inflammatory process. A swollen and warm joint may be affected by active synovitis (see below), infection (e.g. *Staphylococcus*) or crystal arthritis (e.g. gout).

Tenderness is a guide to the acuteness of the inflammation, but may be present over the muscles of patients with fibromyalgia. The patient must be told to let the examiner know if the examination is becoming uncomfortable. Tenderness can be graded as follows:

Grade I—patient complains of pain
Grade II—patient complains of pain and winces
Grade III—patient complains of pain, winces and withdraws the joint
Grade IV—patient does not allow palpation.

This may result from joint inflammation or from lesions outside the joints (periarticular tissues), including inflamed tendons, bursae, or attachments (entheses). Infected joints are extremely tender and patients will often not let the examiner move the joint at all. Palpation of a joint or area for tenderness must be performed gently, and the patient's face rather than the joint itself should be watched for signs that the examination is uncomfortable.

Palpate the joint deliberately now, if possible, for evidence of *synovitis*, which is a soft and spongy (boggy) swelling. This must be distinguished from an *effusion*, which tends to affect large joints but can occur in any joint. Here the swelling is fluctuant and can be made to shift within the joint. *Bony swelling* feels hard and immobile, and suggests osteophyte formation or subchondral bone thickening.

Move

Much information about certain joints is gained by testing the range of *passive* movement. (Passive movement is obviously contraindicated in cases of recent injury to the limb or joint, such as a suspected fracture.) The patient is asked to relax and let the examiner move the joint. This must be attempted gently and will be limited if the joint is painful (secondary to muscle spasm), if a tense effusion is present, if there is capsular contraction or if there is a fixed deformity. The joints may have limited extension (called fixed flexion deformity) or limited flexion (fixed extension deformity). Passive movement of the spine is not a practical manoeuvre (unless the examiner is very strong), and active movement is tested here. *Active* movement is more helpful in assessing integrated joint function. Hand function and gait are usually applied as tests of *function*. *Pain on motion* indicates a joint or periarticular problem.

Stability of the joint is important and depends largely on the surrounding ligaments. This is tested by attempting to move the joint gently in abnormal directions to its usual limits, set by ligaments and muscular tone.

Joint crepitus, which is a grating sensation or noise from the joint, indicates irregularity of the articular surfaces. Its presence suggests chronicity.

Measure

Accurate measurement of the range of movement of a joint is possible with a goniometer, which is a hinged rod with a protractor in the centre. The jaws are opened and lined up with the joint. Measurement of joint movements is performed from the zero starting position. For most joints this is the anatomical position in extension—e.g. the straightened knee. Movement is then recorded as the number of degrees of flexion from this position. A knee with a fixed flexion deformity may be recorded as '30 to 60 degrees', which indicates that there is 30 degrees of fixed flexion deformity and that flexion is limited to 60 degrees. At some joints both flexion and extension from the anatomical position can be measured, as at the wrists. The goniometer is not routinely used by non-rheumatologists and there is a wide range of normal values for joint movement. Most clinicians estimate the approximate joint angles.

A tape measure is useful for measuring and following serially the quadriceps muscle bulk and in examination of spinal movements.

Assessment of individual joints

The hands and wrists (Figures 9.5 to 9.9)

Examination anatomy. The articulations between the phalanges are synovial hinge joints. The eight bones of the wrist (carpal bones) form gliding joints which allow wrist movements—flexion/extension and abduction/adduction as they slide over each other.

History. *Pain* may be present in some or all of the joints. It is more likely to be vague or diffuse if it has radiated from the shoulder or neck or is due to carpal tunnel syndrome, and to be localised if it is due to arthritis. *Stiffness* is typically worse in

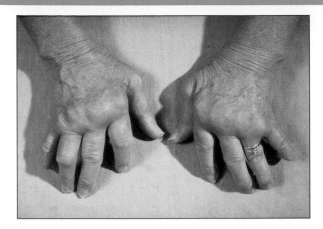

Figure 9.5 Examination of the hands and wrists

Sitting up (hands on a pillow)

1. **General inspection**
   Cushingoid
   Weight
   Iritis, scleritis, etc
   Obvious other joint disease
2. **Look**
   Dorsal aspect
   - Wrists
     Skin—scars, redness, atrophy, rash
     Swelling—distribution
     Deformity
     Muscle wasting
   - Metacarpophalangeal joints
     Skin
     Swelling—distribution
     Deformity—ulnar deviation, volar subluxation etc

- Proximal and distal interphalangeal joints
  Skin
  Swelling—distribution
  Deformity—swan necking, boutonnière, Z, etc
- Nails
  Psoriatic changes—pitting, ridging, onycholysis, hyperkeratosis, discoloration
3. **Feel and move passively**
   Wrists
   - Synovitis
   - Effusions
   - Range of movement
   - Crepitus
   - Ulnar styloid tenderness
   Metacarpophalangeal joints
   - Synovitis
   - Effusions
   - Range of movement
   - Crepitus
   - Subluxation
   Proximal and distal interphalangeal joints
   - As above
   Palmar tendon crepitus
   Carpal tunnel syndrome tests
   Palmar aspect
   - Skin—scars, palmar erythema, palmar creases (anaemia)
   - Muscle wasting
4. **Hand function**
   Grip strength
   Key grip
   Opposition strength
   Practical ability
5. **Other**
   Elbows—subcutaneous nodules—psoriatic rash
   Other joints
   Signs of systemic disease

the mornings in rheumatoid arthritis. *Swelling* of the wrist may indicate arthritis or tendon sheath inflammation. Swelling of individual joints suggests arthritis. *Deformity* of the fingers and hand due to rheumatoid arthritis or of the fingers as a result of arthritis or gouty tophi may be the presenting complaint. The sudden onset of deformity suggests tendon rupture. *Locking or snapping* of a finger (trigger finger) is typical of inflammation of a flexor tendon sheath (tenovaginitis). *Loss of function* is a serious problem when it involves the numerous functions of the hand and wrist. The history should include an assessment of the difficulties the patient has in using the hands and wrists. *Neurological symptoms* as a result of nerve compression may cause paraesthesiae or limitation of strength or of complicated hand functions.

Figure 9.6 (right) X-ray of normal hand
(Courtesy M Thomson, National Capital Diagnostic Imaging, Canberra.)

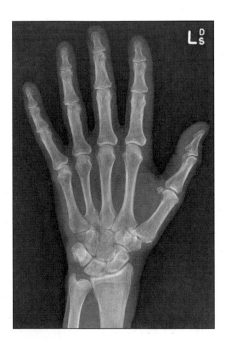

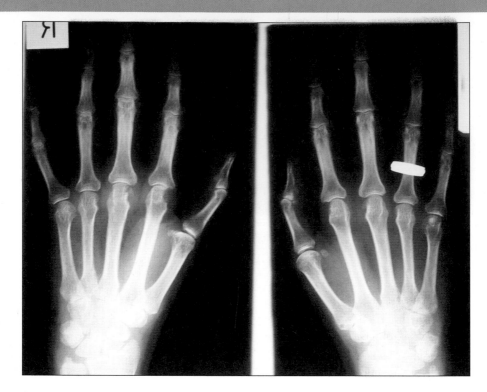

Figure 9.7 Rheumatoid arthritis, early findings
X-ray of the hands of a patient with early rheumatoid arthritis. Note erosions of the heads of the metacarpophalangeal joints and of the ulnar styloid, and reduced amounts of cartilage in the joint spaces. (Courtesy Canberra Hospital X-ray library.)

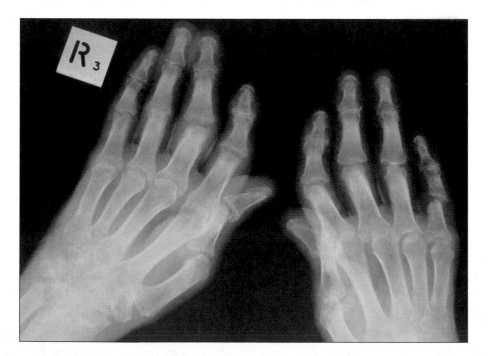

Figure 9.8 Rheumatoid arthritis, late findings
X-ray of the hands of a patient with advanced rheumatoid arthritis. Note loss of joint space and destruction of the right carpal joints, subluxation of metacarpophalangeal and poximal interphalangeal (PIP) joints, and Z deformity of the thumb. There are erosions of the PIP joints, a sign of active disease. (Courtesy Canberra Hospital X-ray library.)

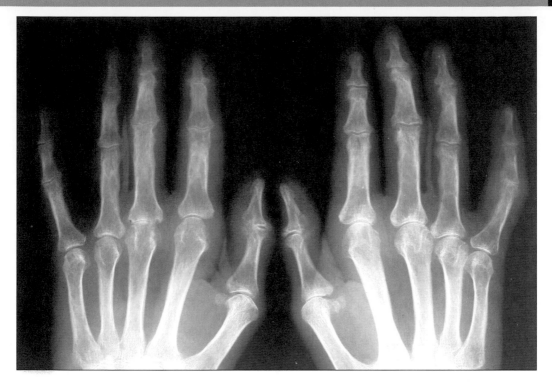

Figure 9.9 Osteoarthritis arthritis
X-ray of the hands showing the typical findings of osteoarthritis with joint-space narrowing and proliferative changes in the distal joints. Also note erosive and destructive changes at multiple proximal interphalangeal joints. (Courtesy Canberra Hospital X-ray library.)

Examination. First sit the patient over the side of the bed and place the hands on the pillow with palms down. Often examination of the hands alone will give enough information for the examiner to make a diagnosis. As a result this is quite a popular test in viva voce examinations.

Look. Start the examination at the *wrists and forearms*. Inspect the skin for erythema, atrophy, scars and rashes. Look for swelling and its distribution. Next look at the wrist for swelling, deformity, ulnar and hyloid prominence. Then look for muscle wasting of the intrinsic muscles of the hand. This results in the appearance of hollow ridges between the metacarpal bones. It is especially obvious on the dorsum of the hand.

Go on to the *metacarpophalangeal joints*. Again note any skin abnormalities, swelling or deformity. Look especially for ulnar deviation and volar (palmar) subluxation of the fingers. Ulnar deviation is deviation of the phalanges at the metacarpophalangeal joints towards the medial (ulnar) side of the hand. It is usually associated with anterior (Volar) subluxation of the fingers (Figure 9.10). These deformities are characteristic but not pathognomonic of rheumatoid arthritis (Table 9.9).

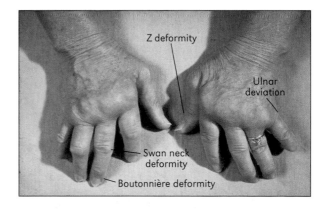

Figure 9.10 The hands in rheumatoid arthritis

Next inspect the *proximal interphalangeal* and *distal interphalangeal* joints. Again note any skin changes and joint swelling. Look for the characteristic deformities of *rheumatoid arthritis*. These include *swan neck* and *boutonnière* deformity of the fingers and Z *deformity* of the thumb (Figure 9.10). They are due to joint destruction and tendon dysfunction. The swan neck deformity is hyperextension at the proximal interphalangeal joint and fixed flexion deformity at the distal

TABLE 9.9 Differential diagnosis of a deforming polyarthropathy

Rheumatoid arthritis
Seronegative spondyloarthropathy, particularly psoriatic arthritis, ankylosing spondylitis or Reiter's disease
Chronic tophaceous gout (rarely symmetrical)
Primary generalised osteoarthritis
Erosive or inflammatory osteoarthritis

interphalangeal joint. It is due to subluxation at the proximal interphalangeal joint and tendon shortening at the distal interphalangeal joint. The boutonnière (buttonhole) deformity consists of fixed flexion of the proximal interphalangeal joint and extension of the distal interphalangeal joints. This is due to protrusion of the proximal interphalangeal joint through its ruptured extensor tendon. The Z deformity of the thumb consists of hyperextension of the interphalangeal joint and fixed flexion and subluxation of the metacarpophalangeal joint.

Now look for the characteristic changes of *osteoarthritis* (Figure 9.11). Here the distal interphalangeal and first carpometacarpal joints are usually involved. *Heberden's nodes*[e] are a common deformity caused by marginal osteophytes that lie at the base of the distal phalanx. Less commonly, the proximal interphalangeal joints may be involved and osteophytes here are called *Bouchard's*[f] nodes.

Look also to see if the phalanges appear *sausage-shaped*. This is characteristic of psoriatic arthropathy, but can also occur in patients with Reiter's disease. It is due to interphalangeal arthritis and flexor tendon sheath oedema. Finger shortening due to severe destructive arthritis also occurs in psoriatic disease and is called *arthritis mutilans*. The hand may take up a *main en lorgnette* ('hand holding long-handled opera glasses') appearance due to a combination of shortening and telescoping of the digits.

Now examine the *nails*. Characteristic *psoriatic* nail changes may be visible: these include pitting (small depressions in the nail), onycholysis (Figure 9.12) and, less commonly, hyperkeratosis (thickening of the nail), ridging and discoloration. The presence of *vasculitic* changes around the nailfolds implies active disease. These consist of black to brown 1–2 mm lesions due to skin infarction and occur typically in rheumatoid

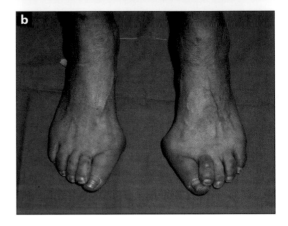

Figure 9.11 The hands (a) and the feet (b) of a patient with osteoarthritis
Showing Heberden's nodes (distal interphalangeal joints), Bouchard's nodes (proximal interphalangeal joints) and bunions.

arthritis (Figure 9.13). Splinter haemorrhages may be present in patients with systemic lupus erythematosus (and infective endocarditis) and are due to vasculitis. Unlike nailfold infarcts they are located under the nails in the nail beds. Periungual telangiectasiae occur in systemic lupus erythematosus, scleroderma or dermatomyositis.

The hands should now be turned over and the *palmar surfaces* revealed. Look at the palms for scars (from tendon repairs or transfers), palmar erythema, and muscle wasting of the thenar or hypothenar eminences (due to disuse, vasculitis or peripheral nerve entrapment). Telangiectasia here would support the diagnosis of scleroderma.

Feel and move. Turn the hands back again to the palm-down position. Palpate the *wrists* with both thumbs placed on the dorsal surface by the wrists, supported underneath by the index fingers (Figure 9.14). Feel gently for synovitis (boggy swelling) and effusions. The wrist should be gently dorsiflexed (normally possible to 75 degrees) and palmar flexed (also possible to 75 degrees) with the examiner's thumbs. Then radial and ulnar

---

e   William Heberden (1710–1801), London physician, and doctor to George III and Samuel Johnson, described these in 1802. He was the first person to describe angina.
f   Charles Jacques Bouchard (1837–1915), Parisian physician.

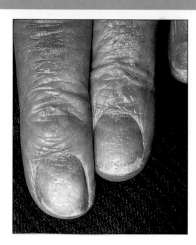

Figure 9.12 Psoriatic nails
Showing onycholysis and discoloration, with typical pitting and ridging.

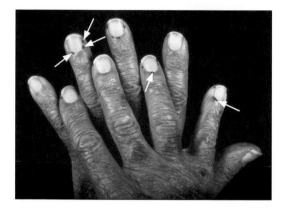

Figure 9.13 Rheumatoid vasculitis (arrows)

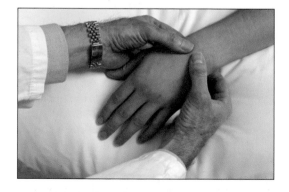

Figure 9.14 Palpating the wrist joint—approved method

deviation (20 degrees) is tested (Figure 9.15). Note any tenderness or limitation of movement or joint crepitus. Palpate the ulnar styloid for tenderness, which can occur in rheumatoid arthritis.

Test for tenderness at the tip of the radial styloid. This suggests de Quervain's[g] tenosynovitis.

Feel for tenderness in the anatomical snuff box if scaphoid injury is suspected (Figure 9.15). Test for tenderness distal to the head of the ulna for extensor carpi ulnaris tendinitis.

Go on now to the *metacarpophalangeal joints*, which are palpated in a similar way with the two thumbs. Again passive movement is tested. Volar subluxation can be demonstrated by flexing the metacarpophalangeal joint with the proximal phalanx held between the thumb and forefinger. The metacarpophalangeal joint is then rocked backwards and forwards (Figure 9.16). Very little movement occurs with this manoeuvre at a normal joint. Considerable movement may be present when ligamentous laxity or subluxation is present.

Palpate the *proximal* and *distal interphalangeal* joints for tenderness, swelling and osteophytes.

Next test for *palmar tendon crepitus*. The palmar aspects of the examiner's fingers are placed against the palm of the patient's hand while he or she flexes and extends the metacarpophalangeal joints. Inflamed palmar tendons can be felt creaking in their thickened sheaths and nodules can be palpated. This indicates tenosynovitis.

A *trigger finger* may also be detected by this manoeuvre. Here the thickening of a section of digital flexor tendon is such that it tends to jam when passing through a narrowed part of its tendon sheath. Rheumatoid arthritis is an important cause. Typically, flexion of the finger occurs freely up to a certain point where it sticks and cannot be extended (as flexors are more powerful than extensors). The application of greater force overcomes the resistance with a snap.

If the carpal tunnel syndrome is suspected, ask the patient to flex both wrists for 30 seconds—paraesthesiae will often be precipitated in the affected hand if the syndrome is present (*Phalen's*[h] *wrist flexion test*). The paraesthesiae (pins and needles) are in the distribution of the median nerve (page 363), when thickening of the flexor retinaculum has entrapped the nerve in the carpal tunnel (Table 9.10). This test is more reliable than *Tinel's sign*,[i] in which tapping over the flexor retinaculum (which lies at the proximal part of the palm) may cause similar paraesthesiae.[4]

Now test active movements. First assess *wrist flexion and extension* as shown in Figure 9.17. Compare the two sides. Now go on to *thumb*

g   Fritz de Quervain (1868–1940), professor of surgery in Berne, Switzerland.
h   George Phalen, orthopaedic surgeon, the Cleveland Clinic.
i   Jules Tinel (1879–1952), physician and neurologist in Paris. In 1915 he described tingling in the distribution of a nerve that had been severed and was regrowing when it was percussed.

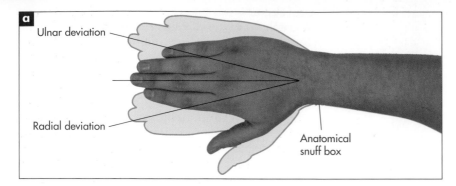

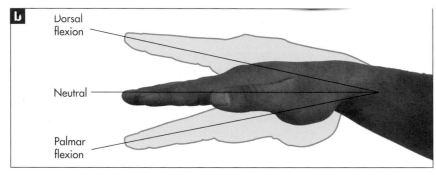

Figure 9.15 Movements of the wrist
(a) Ulnar and radial deviation. (b) Dorsal and palmar flexion.

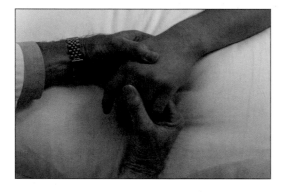

Figure 9.16 Examination for volar subluxation at the metacarpophalangeal joints

TABLE 9.10 Causes of carpal tunnel syndrome	
Occupation-related: working with wrists and hands flexed	Pregnancy
	Gout
Rheumatoid arthritis	Obesity
Hypothyroidism	Amyloidosis
Acromegaly	Diabetes mellitus
	Idiopathic
	Carpal bone osteomyelitis

movements (Figure 9.18). The patient holds the hand flat, palm upwards, and the examiner's hand holds the patient's fingers. Test *extension* by asking the patient to stretch the thumb outwards, *abduction* by asking for the thumb to be pointed straight upwards, *adduction* by asking him or her to squeeze the examiner's finger, and *opposition* by getting the patient to touch the little finger with the thumb. Look for limitation of these movements and discomfort caused by them. Next test *metacarpophalangeal and interphalangeal movements*. As a screening test, ask the patient to make a fist then to straighten out the fingers (Figure 9.19). Then test the fingers

individually. If active flexion of one or more fingers is reduced, test the superficial and profundus flexor tendons (Figure 9.20). Hold the proximal finger joint extended and instruct the patient to bend it; the distal fingertip will flex if the flexor profundus is intact. Then hold the other fingers extended (to inactivate the profundus) and check finger flexion (inability indicates the superficialis is unable to work). The most common tendon ruptures are of the extensors of the fourth and fifth fingers.

Function. It is important to test the function of the hand. *Grip strength* is tested by getting the patient to squeeze two of the examiner's fingers. Even an angry patient will rarely cause pain if given only two fingers. Serial measurements of

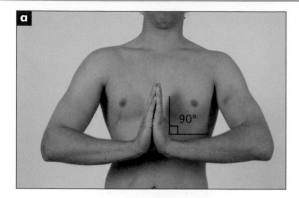

grip strength can be made by asking the patient to squeeze a partly inflated sphygmomanometer cuff and noting the pressure reached. *Key grip* (Figure 9.21) is the grip with which a key is held between the pulps of the thumb and forefinger. Ask the patient to hold this grip tightly and try to open up his or her fingers. *Opposition strength* (Figure 9.22) is where the patient opposes the thumb and individual fingers. The difficulty with which these can be forced apart is assessed. Finally, *a practical test*, such as asking the patient to undo a button or write with a pen, should be performed.

Tests of hand function should be completed by formally assessing for neurological changes (page 362).

Examination of the hands is not complete without feeling for the *subcutaneous nodules* of rheumatoid arthritis near the elbows (Figure 9.23). These are 0.5–3 cm firm, shotty, non-tender lumps which occur typically over the olecranon. They may be attached to bone. They are found in rheumatoid-factor-positive rheumatoid arthritis. Rheumatoid nodules are areas of fibrinoid necrosis with a characteristic histological appearance and are probably initiated by a small vessel vasculitis. They are localised by trauma but can occur elsewhere, especially attached to tendons, over pressure areas

Figure 9.17 (a) Active wrist extension and (b) active wrist flexion

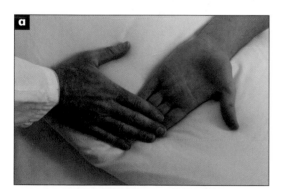
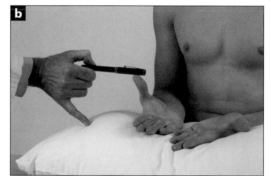
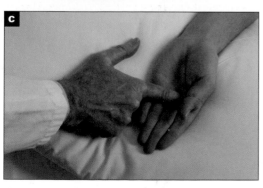
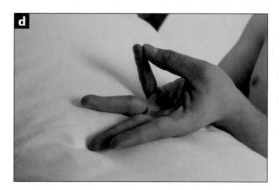

Figure 9.18 Thumb movements
(a) Extension. (b) Abduction. (c) Adduction. (d) Opposition.

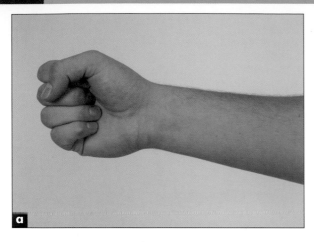
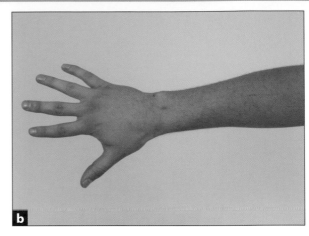

Figure 9.19 Screening metacarpophalangeal and interphalangeal movements
(a) Flexion. (b) Extension.

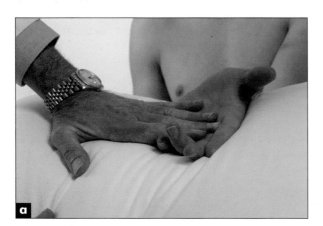
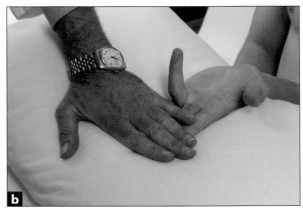

Figure 9.20 Testing the superficial and profundus flexor tendons
(a) Flexor profundus. (b) Flexor superficialis.

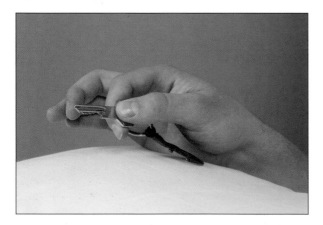
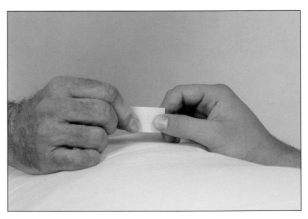
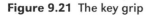

Figure 9.21 The key grip

Figure 9.22 Testing opposition strength

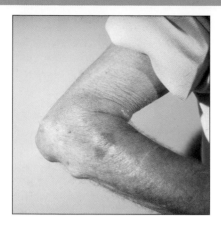

Figure 9.23 Subcutaneous nodules in rheumatoid arthritis

TABLE 9.11 Causes of arthritis plus nodules*

Rheumatoid arthritis
Systemic lupus erythematosus (rare)
Rheumatic fever (Jaccoud's[†] arthritis) (very rare)
Granulomas—e.g. sarcoidosis (very rare)

* Gouty tophi and xanthomata from hyperlipidaemia may cause confusion.
† François Jaccoud (1830–1913), professor of medicine, Geneva.

in the hands or feet, in the lung, pleura, myocardium or vocal cords. The combination of arthritis and nodules suggests the diagnostic possibilities listed in Table 9.11.

The elbows

Examination anatomy (Figure 9.24). The humerus, radius and ulna meet at the elbow, which is a hinge and a pivot joint. Pivoting occurs between the radius and ulna, and the articulation between all three bones forms a hinge joint.

History. *Pain* from the elbow is usually diffuse and may radiate down the forearm. It may occur over the lateral or medial epicondyle if the patient has tendinitis (tennis or golfer's elbow). The patient may have noticed some swelling as a result of inflammation. *Swelling* over the back suggests olecranon bursitis. *Stiffness* may interfere with elbow movements and the patient may complain of difficulty combing the hair. When supination and pronation are affected the patient may complain of difficulty with carrying and holding. If the patient is aware of the elbow moving abnormally this suggests *instability* of the joint and may be a result of rheumatoid arthritis or trauma. Ulnar nerve trauma at the elbow may lead to a complaint of *numbness* or *paraesthesiae* in the distribution of that nerve.

Examination. Watch as the patient undresses, for difficulty disentangling the arms from clothing. The upper arms should be exposed completely. Note any deformity or difference in the normal 5–10 degree valgus position (carrying angle) as the patient stands with the palms facing forward.

Look for a joint effusion, which appears as a swelling on either side of the olecranon. Discrete swellings over the olecranon or over the proximal subcutaneous border of the ulna may be due to rheumatoid nodules, gouty tophi, an enlarged olecranon bursa or, rarely, to other types of nodules (Table 9.11).

Feel for tenderness, particularly over the lateral and medial epicondyles which may indicate tennis or golfer's elbow, respectively. Palpate any discrete swellings. Rheumatoid nodules are quite hard, may be tender and are attached to underlying structures. Gouty tophi have a firm feeling and often appear yellow under the skin, but are sometimes difficult to distinguish from rheumatoid nodules. A fluid collection in the olecranon bursa is softly fluctuant and may be tender if inflammation is present. These collections are associated with rheumatoid arthritis and gout, but often occur independently of these diseases.

Small amounts of fluid or synovitis of the elbow joint may be detected by the examiner, facing the patient, placing the thumb of the opposite hand along the edge of the ulnar shaft just distal to the olecranon where the synovium is closest to the surface. Full extension of the elbow joint will cause a palpable bulge in this area if fluid is present.

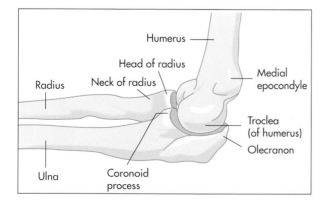

Figure 9.24 Anatomy of the elbows

Move the elbow joints passively. The elbow is a hinge joint. The zero position is when the arm is fully extended (0 degrees). Normal flexion is possible to 150 degrees. Limitation of extension is an early sign of synovitis.

If lateral epicondylitis is suspected, ask the patient to extend the wrist actively against resistance (see Figure 9.70, page 291). Test the range of active movements by standing in front of the patient and demonstrating. If there is any deformity or complaint of numbness, a neurological examination of the hand and arm are indicated for ulnar nerve entrapment.

The shoulders

Examination anatomy (Figure 9.25). The shoulder joint includes the clavicle, scapula and humerus. The acromioclavicular joint is formed by the acromion of the scapula and the clavicle. Movements of the shoulder are a result of a combination of ball-and-socket articulation at the glenohumeral joint (between the glenoid cavity of the scapula and the ball-shaped end of the humerus) and motion between the scapula and the thorax. It is the most mobile joint in the body.

The joint is encased in a capsule and is lined with synovium.

This complicated joint is frequently affected by a number of non-arthritic conditions involving its bursa, capsule and surrounding tendons— e.g. 'frozen (stiff) shoulder' (adhesive capsulitis), tendinitis, bursitis. All of these disorders affect movement of the shoulder.

History. *Pain* is the most common symptom of a patient with shoulder problems.[5] Typically it is felt over the front and lateral part of the joint. It may radiate to the insertion of the deltoid or even further. Pain felt over the top of the shoulder is more likely to come from the acromioclavicular joint or from the neck. *Deformity* has to be severe before it becomes obvious. *Pain and stiffness* may severely limit shoulder movement. *Instability* may cause the alarming feeling that the shoulder is jumping out of its socket. This is most likely to occur during abduction and external rotation (e.g. while attempting to serve a tennis ball). *Loss of function* may result in difficulty using the arms at above shoulder height or reaching around to the back.

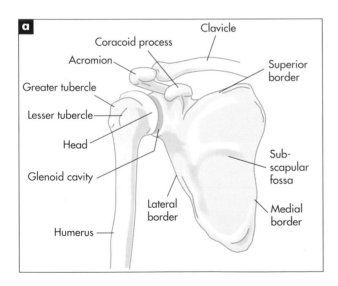
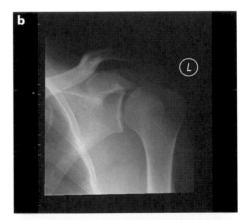
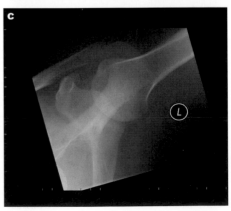

Figure 9.25 Examination of the shoulders
(a) Anatomy of the shoulder. (b) X-ray of left shoulder in the neutral position; the relative positions of the humeral head, clavicle and scapulae can be seen. (c) X-ray of left shoulder in abduction. Abduction of the arm rotates the head of the humerus and the clavicle moves upwards.
(X-rays courtesy M Thomson, National Capital Diagnostic Imaging, Canberra.)

Examination. Watch the patient undressing and note forward, backward and upward movements of the shoulders and whether these seem limited or cause the patient pain. Stand back and compare the two sides. The arms should be held at the same level and the outlines of the acromioclavicular joints should be the same. There may be wasting of one of the deltoid muscles that will not be obvious unless the two are compared.

Look at the joint. A swelling may be visible anteriorly, but unless effusions are large and the patient is thin these are difficult to detect. Look for asymmetry and for scars as a result of injury or previous surgery.

Feel for tenderness and swelling. Stand beside the patient, rest one hand on the shoulder and move the arm into different positions (see below). As the shoulder moves, feel the acromioclavicular joint and then move the hand along the clavicle to the sternoclavicular joint.

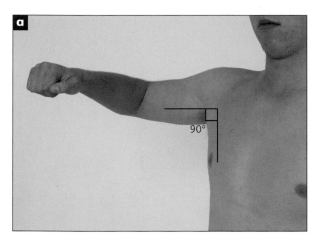

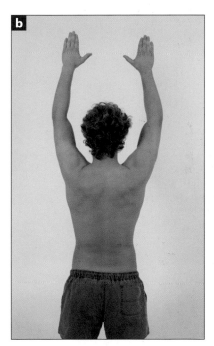

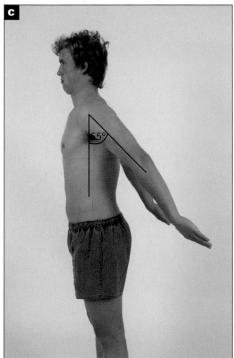

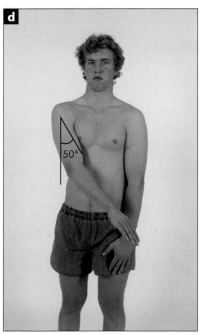

Figure 9.26 Movements of the shoulder joint
(a) Abduction using the glenohumeral joint. (b) Abduction using the glenohumeral joint and the scapula. (c) Extension. (d) Adduction.

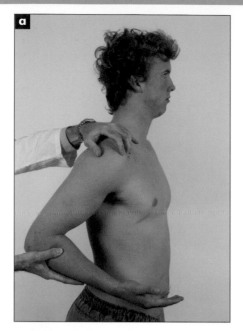

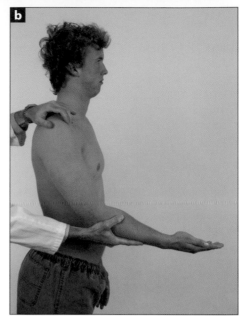

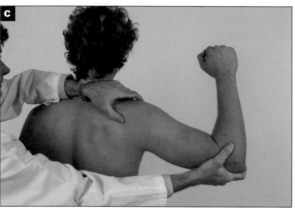

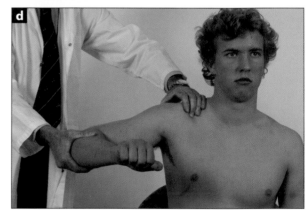

Figure 9.27 Examining the shoulder joint
(a) Extension. (b) Flexion. (c) Apprehension test. (d) Internal rotation and abduction.

Move the joint (Figures 9.26 and 9.27). The zero position is with the arm hanging by the side of the body so that the palm faces forwards. *Abduction* tests glenohumeral abduction, which is normally possible to 90 degrees. For the right shoulder the examiner stands behind the patient resting the left hand on the patient's shoulder, while the right hand abducts the elbow from the shoulder. *Elevation* is usually possible to 180 degrees when it is performed actively, as movement of the scapula is then included. *Adduction* is possible to 50 degrees. The arm is carried forwards across the front of the chest. *External rotation* is possible to 65 degrees. With the elbow bent to 90 degrees the arm is turned laterally as far as possible. *Internal rotation* is usually possible to 90 degrees. It is tested actively by asking

the patient to place his or her hand behind the back and then to try to scratch the back as high up as possible with the thumb. Patients with rotator cuff problems complain of pain when they perform this manoeuvre. *Flexion* is possible to 180 degrees, of which the glenohumeral joint contributes about 90 degrees. *Extension* is possible to 65 degrees. The arm is swung backwards as in marching. During all these manoeuvres, limitation with or without pain and joint crepitus are assessed.

Rapid assessment of shoulder movement is possible using the three-step 'Apley[j] scratch test' (Figure 9.28). Stand behind and ask the patient to scratch an imaginary itch over the opposite scapula, first by reaching over the opposite shoulder, next by reaching behind the neck and finally by reaching behind the back.

j   Alan Apley, orthopaedic surgeon, St Thomas's Hospital, London.

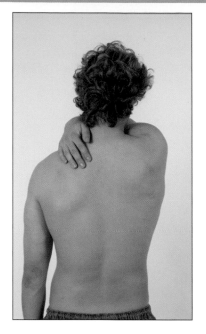
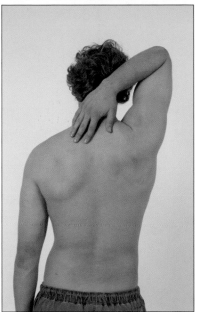
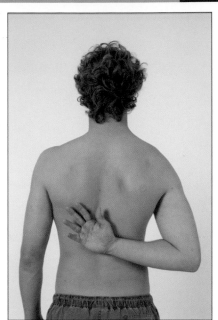

Figure 9.28 Apley scratch test to assess shoulder movements

The anterior stability of the shoulder joint is best assessed by the 'apprehension' test. Stand behind the patient, abduct, extend and externally rotate the shoulder (Figure 9.27c) while pushing the head of the humerus forwards with the thumb. The patient will strongly resist this manoeuvre if there is impending dislocation. There will be a similar response if the arm is adducted and internally rotated and posterior dislocation is about to occur.

This is also the time to test biceps function. The patient flexes the elbow against resistance. A ruptured biceps tendon causes the biceps muscle to roll up into a ball.

As a general rule, intra-articular disease produces *painful* limitation of movement in *all* directions, while tendinitis produces painful limitation of movement in *one* plane only, and tendon rupture or neurological lesions produce *painless* weakness. For example, if the abnormal sign is limited shoulder abduction in the middle range (45–135 degrees), this suggests 'rotator cuff' problems (i.e. the supraspinatus, infraspinatus, subscapularis and teres minor muscles) rather than arthritis.

In bicipital tendinitis there is localised tenderness on palpating over the groove. The supraspinatus tendon is a little higher, just under the anterior surface of the acromion. Supraspinatus tendinitis is common. Testing for it involves placing a finger over the head of the tendon while the shoulder is in extension. As this pushes the tendon forwards against the examiner's finger, the movement is painful. When the shoulder is then flexed the tendon moves away and the pain disappears.

Don't forget that arthritis affecting the acromio-clavicular joint can be confused with glenohumeral disorders. Also remember to examine the neck and axillae in patients with shoulder pain.

The temporomandibular joints

History. The usual symptoms of temporomandibular joint dysfunction include clicking and pain on opening the mouth. The jaw may sometimes lock in the open position.

Examination. Look in front of the ear for swelling. **Feel** by placing a finger just in front of the ear while the patient opens and shuts the mouth (Figure 9.29). The head of the mandible is palpable as it slides forwards when the jaw is opened. Clicking and grating may be felt. This is sometimes associated with tenderness if the joint is involved in an inflammatory arthritis. Rheumatoid arthritis may affect the temporomandibular joint.

The neck

Examination anatomy—the spine. The spinal column (Figure 9.30) is like a tower of bones that protects the spinal cord and houses its blood supply and efferent and afferent nerves. It provides mechanical support for the body and is flexible enough to allow bending and twisting movements. There are diarthrodial joints between the articular processes of the vertebral bodies, and the vertebral

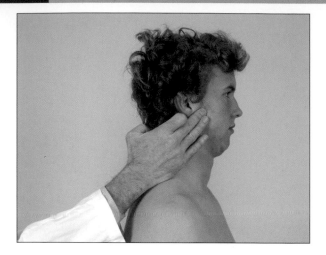

Figure 9.29 Examining the temporomandibular joints

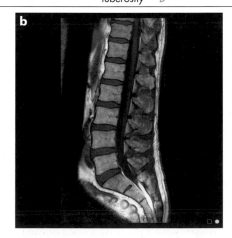

a

Tip of Dens of axis

Posterior arch of atlas (C1)

Transverse process of third cervical vertebra C3

Spinous process of axis (C2)

Vertebra prominens (spinous process of C7)

Facet for head of first rib

Transverse process of first thoracic vertebra T1

Demi-facet for second rib on T2

Pedicle of T4

Intervertebral disc T3–4

Articular surface for tubercle of sixth rib

Intervertebral foramen

Inferior vertebral notch of T9

Transverse process of T7

Superior vertebral notch of T10

Spinous process of T9

Transverse process of first lumbar vertebra (L1)

Spinous process of L1

Superior articular process of L3

Inferior articular process of L3

L5 Vertebra

Superior articular process of sacrum

Sacral promontory

Median sacral crest

Auricular surface of sacrum

Sacral tuberosity

Coccyx

b

Figure 9.30 (a) Structure of the spine (b) MRI scan of the lumbar spine showing the anatomical features seen in (a)
(MRI scan courtesy M Thomson, National Capital Diagnostic Imaging, Canberra.)

bodies are separated by the vertebral discs. These pads of cartilage are flexible enough to allow movement between the vertebrae. In the cervical spine from C3 to C7, the uncovertebral joints of Luschka[k] are present. These are formed between a lateral bony extension (uncinate process) from the margin of the more inferior vertebral body with the one above. Osteoarthritic hypertrophy of these joints may result in pain or nerve root irritation.

History. *Pain* is the most common neck symptom. Musculoskeletal neck pain usually arises in the structures at the back of the neck: the cervical spine, the splenius, semispinalis and trapezius muscles, or in the cervical nerves or nerve roots. Pain in the front of the neck may come from the oesophagus, trachea, thyroid gland or anterior neck muscles e.g. the sternocleidomastoid and platysma. Pain may be referred to the front of the neck from the heart.

There may be a history of trauma from direct injury or a sudden deceleration causing hyperextension of the neck; 'whiplash' injury. Injury can also be caused by attempted therapeutic neck manipulations by physiotherapists or chiropractors. The possibility of spinal cord injury must be considered in these patients. Ask about weakness or altered sensation in the arms and legs and any problem with bowel or bladder function.

The pain may have begun suddenly, suggesting a disc prolapse, or more gradually due to disc degeneration.

---

k   Hubert von Luschka (1820–75), professor of anatomy in Tübingen.

Postural tendon and muscle strains are common causes of temporary neck pain. These are often related to overuse. Ask for the patient's occupation and whether work or recreational activities involve repeated and prolonged extension of the neck, e.g. painters and bicyclists. These patients often describe neck stiffness, and pain and muscle spasm are often present. The repeated holding of a telephone between the shoulder and the ear can cause nerve root problems. Neck movement may cause *radicular symptoms* such as paraesthesiae in the distribution of a cervical nerve after a hyperextension injury or cervical spine arthritis. Ask about paraesthesiae and weakness in the arms and hands.

Deformity may occur as a result of muscle spasm or sometimes following disc prolapse. *Torticollis* is a chronic and uncontrollable twisting of the neck to one side as a result of a muscle dystonia or cervical nerve root problem.

Examination. The patient should be undressed so as to expose the neck, shoulders and arms.

Look at the cervical spine while the patient is sitting up, and note particularly his or her posture (Figure 9.31). **Movement** should be tested actively. Flexion is tested by asking the patient to try to touch his or her chest with the chin (normal flexion is possible to 45 degrees). Extension (Figure 9.32a) is tested by asking the patient to look up and back (normally possible to 45 degrees). Lateral bending (Figure 9.32b) is tested by getting the patient to touch his or her shoulder with the ear; lateral bending is normally possible to 45 degrees. Rotation is tested by getting the patient to look over the shoulder to the right and then to the left. This is normally possible to 70 degrees.

Feel the posterior spinous processes. This is often easiest to do when the patient lies prone with the chest supported by a pillow and the neck slightly flexed. The examiner should feel for tenderness and uneven spacing of the spinous processes. Tenderness of the facet joints will be elicited by feeling a finger's breadth lateral to the middle line on each side (Figure 9.33).

Neurological examination of the upper limbs, including testing of shoulder abduction (C5, C6) and the serratus anterior muscle (C5, C6, C7), is part of the assessment of the neck.

The thoracolumbar spine and sacroiliac joints

History. Lower back pain is a very common symptom (Table 9.12). The discomfort is usually worst in the lumbosacral area. Ask whether the onset was sudden and associated with lifting or

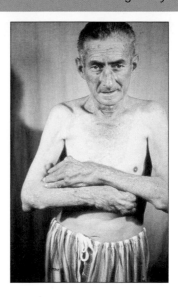

Figure 9.31 Rheumatoid arthritis
Note the head tilt due to right atlanto-axial subluxation, the rheumatoid hands and the subcutaneous rheumatoid nodules.

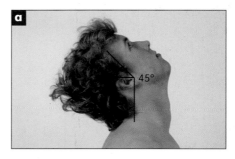

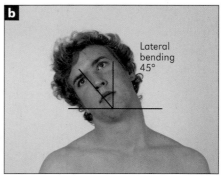

Figure 9.32 Movements of the neck
(a) Extension—'Look up and back'. (b) Lateral bending—'Now touch your right ear onto your shoulder' (45 degrees); rotation—'Now look over your shoulder to the right and then to the left' (70 degrees).

straining or whether it was gradual.[1,2] Stiffness and pain in the lower back that is worse in the morning is characteristic of an inflammatory spondyloarthropathy. Pain that shoots from the

TABLE 9.12 Differential diagnoses for back pain

Remember that serious causes of back pain are rare in otherwise well patients (<1%).

❗ denotes symptoms for the possible diagnosis of an urgent or dangerous problem.

Suggests non-specific or musculoskeletal cause
(although often said to be due to disc herniation, there is little correlation between MRI-scan-detected disc herniation and pain—it is found in 30% of asymptomatic people)

Gradual onset

No neurological symptoms or signs

Recent minor injury

Suggests ankylosing spondylitis

Systemic symptoms

Pain at rest

❗ **Suggests malignant pain**

Worse at rest, keeps patient awake

Present for more than 4 weeks

Weight loss

Known malignancy

❗ **Suggests abscess**

Worse at rest

Fever

Immunosuppression

❗ **Suggests cauda equina syndrome** (compression of sacral nerve roots usually due to large midline herniation of a disc, but can be caused by infection or malignancy that causes narrowing of the spinal canal)

Severe pain

Urinary retention or incontinence

Faecal incontinence

Saddle anaesthesia

Leg weakness

Suggests fracture of vertebral body

Sudden onset of severe pain

Known osteoporosis

Steroid use

Trauma

Tenderness over vertebral body

Suggests sciatica (irritation or compression of L4–S1 nerve roots)

Pain radiates down the leg beyond the knee

Suggests spinal canal stenosis

Pain worse with walking

Improved by sitting forward

Suggests referred pain

Abdominal pain (diverticular abscess, pyelonephritis)

Nausea and vomiting, dysuria (pyelonephritis)

Sudden-onset tearing pain, hypotension, shock (ruptured abdominal aortic aneurysm)

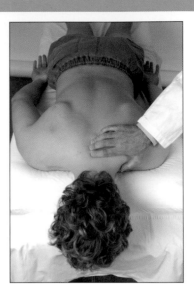

Figure 9.33 Examining the spinous processes

back into the buttock and thigh along the sciatic nerve distribution is called '*sciatica*'. In sciatic nerve compression at a lumbosacral nerve root, the pain is often aggravated by coughing or straining. 'Lumbago' however is often due to referred pain (e.g. from the vertebral joints). There may be other *neurological symptoms* in the legs due to nerve compression or irritation. The distribution of the paraesthesiae or weakness may indicate the level of spinal cord or nerve root abnormality. One should also ask about urinary incontinence and retention as well as numbness in the 'saddle region', erectile dysfunction and bowel incontinence, which can be a result of cauda equina involvement.

Examination. To start the examination, have the patient standing and clothed only in underpants. **Look** for deformity, inspecting from both the back and side. Note especially loss of the normal thoracic kyphosis and lumbar lordosis, which is typical of ankylosing spondylitis. Also note any evidence of scoliosis, a lateral curvature of the spine which may be simple ('C' shaped) or compound ('S' shaped) and which can result from trauma, developmental abnormalities, vertebral body disease (e.g. rickets, tuberculosis) or muscle abnormality (e.g. polio).

Feel each vertebral body for tenderness and palpate for muscle spasm.[1]

Movement is assessed actively. Bending movements largely take place at the lumbar spine, while rotational movements occur at the thoracic spine. Range of movement is tested by observation (Figure 9.34) and the use of Schober's test (see below) (Figure 9.35).

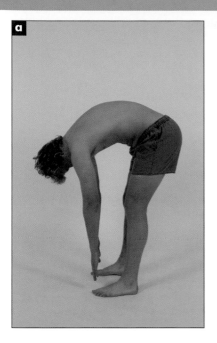

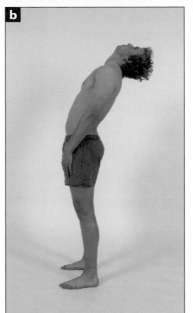

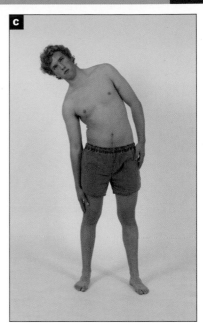

Figure 9.34 Movements of the thoracolumbar spine
(a) Flexion. (b) Extension. (c) Lateral bending. (d) Rotation.

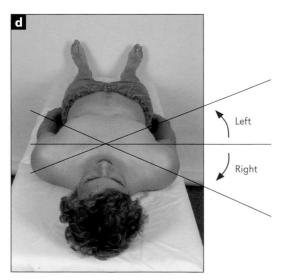

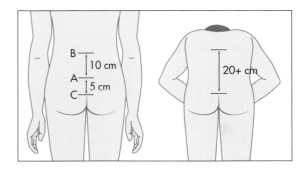

Figure 9.35 Schober's test
(From Douglas G, Nicol F and Robertson C, *Macleod's Clinical Examination*, 12th edn. Edinburgh: Churchill Livingstone, 2009, with permission.)

Flexion is tested by asking the patient to touch the toes with the knees straight. The normal range of flexion is very wide. Many people can reach only halfway down the shins when the knees are kept straight. As the patient bends, look at the spine: there is normally a gentle curve along the back from the shoulders to the pelvis. Patients with advanced ankylosing spondylitis have a flat ankylosed spine and all the bending occurs at the hips. Test *extension* by asking the patient to lean backwards. Patients with back pain usually find this less uncomfortable than bending forwards. *Lateral bending* is assessed by getting the patient to slide the right hand down the right leg as far as possible without bending forwards, and then the

same for the left side. This movement tends to be restricted early in ankylosing spondylitis. *Rotation* is tested with the patient sitting on a stool (to fix the pelvis) and asking him or her to rotate the head and shoulders as far as possible to each side. This is best viewed from above.

Measure the lumbar flexion with *Schober's test* (Figure 9.35). A mark is made at the level of the posterior iliac spine on the vertebral column (approximately at L5). One finger is placed 5 cm below and another 10 cm above this mark. The patient is then asked to touch the toes. An increase of less than 5 cm in the distance between the two fingers indicates limitation of lumbar flexion. The finger-to-floor distance at full flexion can be measured serially to give an objective indication of disease progression.

Assess *straight leg raising* (Lasègue's[l] test includes passive ankle dorsiflexion). With the patient lying down, lift the straightened leg if sciatica is suspected (normally to 80–90 degrees). This will be limited by pain in lumbar disc prolapse (less than 60 degrees).

Press directly on the anterior superior iliac spines and apply lateral pressure so as to attempt to separate them. This will cause pain in the sacroiliac joints when patients have sacroiliitis.

Now get the patient to lie in bed on the stomach. Look for gluteal wasting. The sacroiliac joints lie deep to the dimples of Venus.[m] By tradition, firm palpation with both palms overlying each other is used to elicit tenderness in patients with sacroiliitis. Test each side separately.

Now ask the patient to lie on one side. Apply firm pressure to the upper pelvic rim. This will also elicit pain in the sacroiliac joints.

The complete examination of the back also requires neurological assessment of the lower limbs.[6]

The hips

Examination anatomy (Figure 9.36). The hip is a ball-and-socket synovial joint. The socket is formed by three bones: the ilium, ischium and pubis. The ball is the head of the femur. Surrounding tendons and nerves may cause symptoms that need to be distinguished from hip abnormalities.

History (Table 9.13). The word 'hip' is used variably by patients to indicate a number of sites including the buttocks, low back, or trochanteric region. Ask the patient to point to the site of pain. The patient with true hip joint problems will often have *pain* that is felt anteriorly in the groin or may radiate to the knee. Athletes with 'groin strain' often have adductor tendinitis or osteitis pubis caused by trauma or overuse. Find out what sport the patient plays. The condition is common in sports involving running. Typically the pain is present at the start of exercise and improves as the athlete 'warms up', only to recur later at rest. Take a detailed work history. Overuse syndromes related to work may be worst on Fridays and improve over the weekend. Jumping down off trucks or platforms may cause repeated trauma to the joint.

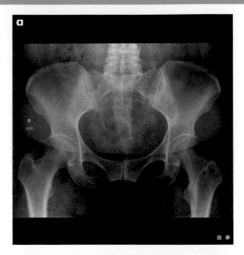

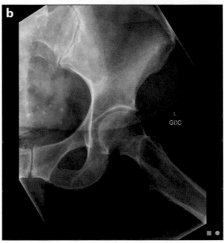

Figure 9.36 X-rays of (a) pelvis and hip joints; (b) hip in abduction
(Courtesy M Thomson, National Capital Diagnostic Imaging, Canberra.)

A *limp* may be noticed by the patient. When associated with pain it is a compensating mechanism but, when painless, may be due to differing limb length or instability of the joint. Patients are sometimes aware of *clicking* or *snapping* coming from the region of the hip. This may be due to a psoas bursitis or to slipping of the tendon of the gluteus maximus over the edge of the greater trochanter. *Functional impairment* usually results in difficulty walking and climbing stairs. Sitting down and standing up can become progressively more uncomfortable because of stiffness and pain.

A history of a fall and inability to walk or bear weight on the leg suggests a fracture of the neck of the femur. A history of rheumatoid arthritis and pain which is present at rest suggests rheumatoid arthritis of the hip. Osteoarthritis is more likely to

---

l   Charles E Lasègue (1816–83), Professor of Medicine in Paris and pupil of Trousseau.
m   Roman goddess of love—her ancient Greek equivalent was Aphrodite.

TABLE 9.13 Differential diagnosis of hip and thigh pain

Favours fractured neck of femur
Known osteoporosis
History of a fall
Severe sudden pain
Inability to bear weight

Favours osteoarthritis
Advanced age
Obesity
Gradual onset
Pain when walking
Work involves jumping off trucks or platforms

Favours rheumatoid arthritis
Pain at rest
Pain worst in the morning
Other typical joint involvement
Walking may be severely limited

Favours septic arthritis
Fever
Malaise

Favours aseptic necrosis of the femoral head
Sudden onset of pain
Inability to bear weight on leg
Steroid use
Known fracture
Diabetes mellitus
Sickle cell anaemia

Favours meralgia paraesthetica (lateral cutaneous nerve of the thigh entrapment)
Anterior thigh pain with paraesthesiae
Occupation involves long periods of sitting
Use of a constricting lumbar support belt

Favours trochanteric bursitis
Pain involves lateral thigh
Worse when climbing stairs

evolve gradually in older people and is associated with obesity and with recurrent trauma.

Ask about systemic symptoms such as fever and weight loss which might be a sign of septic arthritis.

Pain which is associated with paraesthesiae and radiates in the distribution of the lateral cutaneous nerve of the thigh suggests an entrapment syndrome (meralgia paraesthetica).

Examination. Watch the patient walking into the room and note the use of a walking stick, a slow and obviously uncomfortable gait, or a limp.

Get the patient to lie down, first on the back.

Looking at the hip joint itself is not possible because so much muscle overlies it. However, the examiner must inspect for scars and deformity. The patient may adopt a position with one leg rotated because of pain.

Feel just distal to the midpoint of the inguinal ligament for joint tenderness. This point lies over the only part of the femoral head that is not intra-acetabular. Now feel for the positions of the greater trochanters. The examiner's thumbs are placed on the anterior superior iliac spines on each side while the fore and middle fingers move posteriorly to find the tips of the greater trochanters. These should be at the same level. If one side is higher than the other, the higher side is likely to be the abnormal one.

Move the hip joint passively (Figure 9.37). *Flexion* is tested by flexing the patient's knee and moving the thigh towards the chest. The examiner keeps the pelvis on the bed by holding the other leg down. A fixed flexion deformity (inability to extend a joint normally) may be masked by the patient's arching the back and tilting the pelvis forward and increasing lumbar lordosis unless *Thomas's test*[n] is applied. The legs are fully flexed to straighten the pelvis. One leg is then extended. A fixed flexion deformity (e.g. as result of osteoarthritis) will prevent straightening. *Rotation* is tested with the knee and hip flexed. One hand holds the knee, the other the foot. The foot is then moved medially (*external rotation of the hip*, normally possible to 45 degrees), then laterally (*internal rotation of the hip*, normal to 45 degrees). *Abduction* is tested by standing on the same side of the bed as the leg to be tested. The right hand grasps the heel of the right leg while the left hand is placed over the anterior superior iliac spine to steady the pelvis. The leg is then moved outwards as far as possible. This is normally possible to 50 degrees. *Adduction* is the opposite. The leg is carried immediately in front of the other limb and this is normally possible to 45 degrees.

Ask the patient to roll over onto the stomach. *Extension* is then tested by placing one hand over the sacroiliac joint while the other elevates each leg. This is normally possible to about 30 degrees. Ask the patient to stand now and perform the Trendelenburg[o] test. The patient stands first on one leg and then on the other. Normally the non-weightbearing hip rises, but with proximal myopathy

---

n   Hugh Thomas (1834–91), 'the father of orthopaedic surgery', worked in Liverpool as a bone-setter but did not have a hospital appointment.
o   Friedrich Trendelenburg (1844–1924), professor of surgery at Rostock, Bonn and Leipzig.

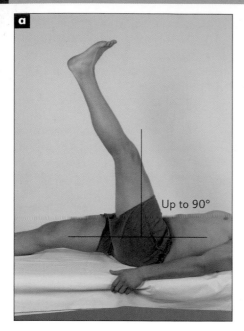

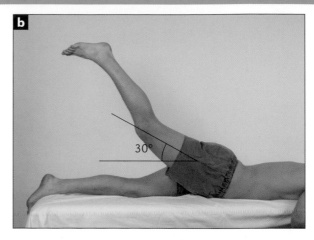

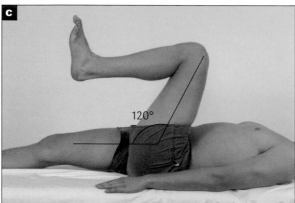

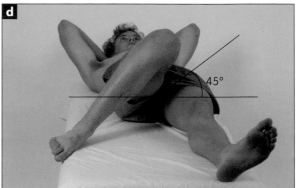

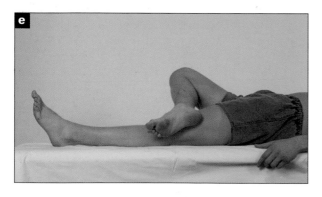

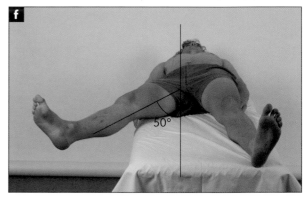

Figure 9.37 Movements of the hip
(a) Flexion. (b) Extension. (c) Flexion, knee bent. (d) Internal rotation. (e) External rotation. (f) Abduction.

or hip joint disease the non-weightbearing side sags.

Finally, the true *leg length* (from the anterior superior iliac spine to the medial malleolus) and apparent leg length (from the umbilicus to the same lower point) for each leg should be measured. A difference in true leg length indicates hip disease on the shorter side, while apparent leg length differences are due to tilting of the pelvis.

In patients with osteoarthritis of the joint, internal rotation, abduction and extension are usually restricted.[7] Osteoarthritic joints (Figure 9.38) show loss of joint space, sclerosis (thickening and increased radiodensity) at the joint margins and osteophyte (bony outgrowth) formation on plain X-ray films.

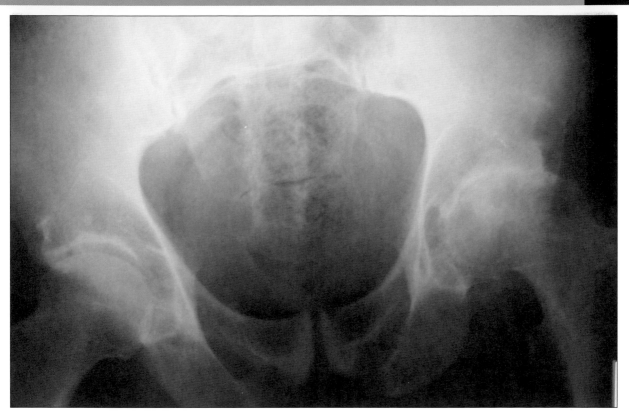

Figure 9.38 Osteoarthritis arthritis
Anteroposterior X-ray of the hip showing the features of osteoarthritis. The left side is more severely affected than the right; note sclerosis, osteophyte formation and asymmetrical joint space narrowing. (Courtesy Canberra Hospital X-ray library.)

The knees
Examination anatomy (Figure 9.39). The knee is a complex hinge joint formed by the distal femur, the patella and the proximal end of the tibia. The bones are enclosed in a joint capsule with an extensive synovial membrane. Lateral stability is provided by the lateral collateral ligaments and antero-posterior movement is restricted by the cruciate ligaments. There is extensive articular cartilage which acts as a shock absorber and allows smooth gliding movements between the ends of the bones.

History (Table 9.14). *Pain* is a common knee problem. If there has been an injury or it is due to a mechanical abnormality, it is often localised. Inflammatory diseases more often cause diffuse pain. Ask the patient to point to the place where the pain is most severe. *Stiffness* is usually of gradual onset and is typical of osteoarthritis. It tends to be worse after inactivity. *Locking* of the knee usually means there is a sudden inability to reach full extension. The knee is often stuck at about 45 degrees of flexion. Unlocking may occur just as suddenly, sometimes following some

form of manipulation by the patient. The cause is mechanical: a loose body or torn meniscus has become wedged between the articular surfaces of the joint. *Swelling* may occur suddenly after an injury, suggesting it is due to haemarthrosis from a fracture or ligamentous tear; if swelling occurs after a few hours a torn meniscus is more likely to be the cause. Arthritis and synovitis cause a chronic swelling. Patients sometimes notice *deformity*, which in later life is usually due to arthritis. Sometimes the patient may complain that the knee is *unstable* or *gives way*. Patellar instability and ruptured ligaments may present this way. One should always ask about *loss of function*. There is often a reduced ability to walk distances, climb stairs and get into and out of chairs.

Osteoarthritis of the knee is very common. Older age, previous injury and stiffness lasting less than half an hour are in favour of this diagnosis as the cause of knee pain. *Good signs guide 9.1* outlines the symptoms and signs of this condition. Physically active adolescents may present with pain and swelling below the knee at the point of attachment of the patellar tendon to the tibial tuberosity—tibial

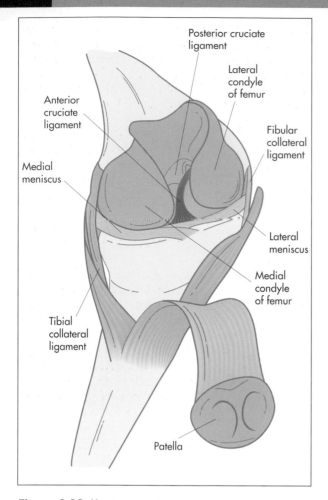

Figure 9.39 Knee anatomy

Labels in figure:
- Posterior cruciate ligament
- Lateral condyle of femur
- Anterior cruciate ligament
- Fibular collateral ligament
- Medial meniscus
- Lateral meniscus
- Medial condyle of femur
- Tibial collateral ligament
- Patella

TABLE 9.14 Differential diagnosis of knee pain	
Area of pain	**Associated features**
Lateral aspect of knee	
Tear of lateral meniscus	History of trauma
	Locking or clicking
	Swelling delayed after injury
Tear of lateral collateral ligament	Knee gives way
Biceps femoris strain	Overuse or injury
Medial aspect of knee	
Tear of medial meniscus	History of trauma
	Locking or clicking
	Swelling delayed after injury
Tear or strain of medial collateral ligament	Knee gives way
Hamstring strain	Overuse or injury
Patellofemoral syndrome	Overuse
	Chronic symptoms
Back of the knee	
Baker's cyst	Sudden pain
	Localised swelling and tenderness
Bursitis, e.g. popliteal, semimembranosus	Overuse pattern
	Chronic pain
Hamstring strain	Injury or overuse
Deep venous thrombosis	
Front of the knee	
Patellar fracture	Injury
	Sudden pain and tenderness
	Swelling
	Separation of fractured segments, visible or palpable
Patellar tendinitis	Overuse
Osteoarthritis	Chronic pain
	Worse with walking
	History of old injuries
Prepatellar bursitis (housemaid's knee*)	Occupation
Infrapatellar bursitis (clergyman's knee)	Occupation

* Described by Henry Hamilton Bailey (1894–1961) as 'the most elementary diagnosis in surgery'.

apophysitis or Osgood Schlatter's disease.[p] This is the most common *traction apophysitis*.

Ask if there has been previous knee surgery or arthroscopy.

Take an occupational and sporting history. Injury and overuse syndromes are often related to exercise (particularly competitive sport) and occupations associated with repetitive minor injuries to the knees.

Examination. This is performed with the patient in a number of positions and, of course, walking.[8,9] Even more than with the other joints, it is important to examine the more normal or uninjured knee first. This will help with the interpretation of changes in

p   Robert Osgood (1873–1956). He worked in France during the First World War and then at the Massachusetts General Hospital where he founded the X-ray department and subsequently developed several radiation-induced skin tumours.
     Carl Schlatter (1864–1934), professor of surgery in Zurich. He pioneered a total gastrectomy operation in 1897.

GOOD SIGNS GUIDE 9.1 Osteoarthritis as the cause of chronic knee pain

Symptom or sign	LR positive	LR negative
Stiffness < 30 mins	3.0	0.2
Crepitus on passive movement	2.1	0.2
Bony enlargement	11.8	0.5
Palpable increase in temperature	0.3	1.6
Valgus deformity	1.4	0.9
Varus deformity	3.4	0.8
At least 3 of the above	3.1	0.1

From McGee S, *Evidence-based physical diagnosis*, 2nd edn. St Louis: Saunders, 2007.

the other knee and give the patient more confidence that the examination will not be painful.

Look first with the patient lying down on the back with both knees and thighs fully exposed. The affected knee will often be flexed, the most comfortable position. Note any quadriceps wasting. This begins quite soon after knee abnormalities lead to disuse of the muscle. Examine the knees themselves for skin changes, scars (including those from previous surgery or arthroscopy), swelling and deformity. Compare each side with the other. Localised swellings may move about as the knee flexes and extends. They are often cartilaginous loose bodies. Fixed lumps in the line of the joint may be meniscal cysts.

Swelling of the synovium or a knee effusion is usually seen medial to the patella and in the joint's suprapatellar extension. Loss of the peripatellar grooves may be an early sign of an effusion. Assess fixed flexion deformity by squatting down and looking at each knee from the side. A space under the knee will be visible if there is permanent flexion deformity arthritis.

Varus and valgus deformity may be obvious here but are more easily seen when the patient stands. Varus deformity is often related to osteoarthritis and valgus deformity to rheumatoid arthritis.

Now watch as the patient flexes and straightens each knee in turn. As the knee extends the patella glides upwards and remains centred over the femoral condyles. If there is patellar subluxation it will slip laterally during knee flexion and return to the midline during knee extension.

Feel the quadriceps for wasting. Palpate over the knees for warmth and synovial swelling.

Test carefully for a joint effusion. The *patellar tap* is used to confirm the presence of large effusions

(Figure 9.40). One hand rests over the lower part of the quadriceps muscle and compresses the suprapatellar extension of the joint space. The other hand pushes the patella downwards. The sign is positive if the patella is felt to sink and then comes to rest with a tap as it touches the underlying femur. The *bulge sign* is used to detect small effusions. Here the left hand compresses the suprapatellar pouch while the fingers of the right hand are run along the groove beside the patella on one side and then the other. A bulging along the groove due to a fluid wave, on the side not being compressed, is a sign of a small effusion.

Examine for patellofemoral lesions by sliding the patella sideways across the underlying femoral condyles.

Move the joint passively. Test *flexion* (normally possible to 135 degrees) and *extension* (normal to 5 degrees) by resting one hand on the knee cap while the other moves the leg up and down (Figure 9.41a). The range of movements and the presence of crepitus are noted. While holding the knee flexed, feel for and attempt to localise tenderness. Feel gently for tenderness along the joint line at the patellar ligament and at the sites of attachment of the collateral ligaments.

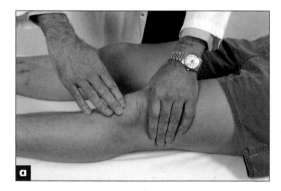

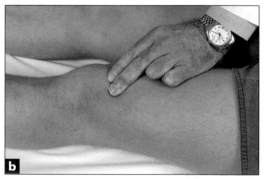

Figure 9.40 Testing for patellar effusion
(a) The patellar tap. (b) The bulge sign: compressing the suprapatellar pouch.

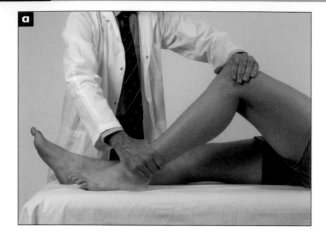

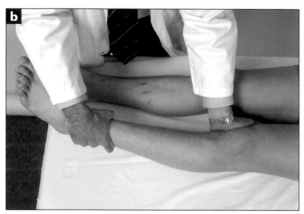

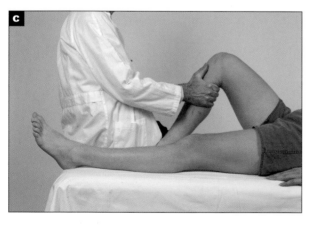

Figure 9.41 Knee examination
(a) Testing knee flexion. (b) Testing the collateral ligaments.
(c) Testing the cruciate ligaments.

Test the *ligaments* next. The lateral and medial *collateral ligaments* are assessed by having the knee slightly flexed while holding the leg, with the examiner's forearm resting along the length of the tibia; lateral and medial movements of the leg on the knee joint are tested (Figure 9.41b). Meanwhile the thigh is steadied with the other hand. Movements of more than 5–10 degrees are

abnormal. The *cruciate ligaments* (Figure 9.41c) are tested next. The examiner steadies the patient's foot with an elbow or by sitting on it. The patient's knee is flexed to 90 degrees. The examiner's hands grasp the tibia and attempt anterior and posterior movements of the leg on the knee joint. Movement may be detected by the examiner's thumbs positioned at the joint margins. Again, movement of more than 5–10 degrees is abnormal. Increased anterior movement suggests anterior cruciate ligamentous laxity, and increased posterior movement suggests posterior cruciate ligamentous laxity. The Lachman test may be more accurate (positive LR 42.0, negative LR 0.1).[8] Here the knee is flexed 20–30 degrees while the patient is lying supine. Grasp the femur (place your hand above the knee) to steady it, then grab the lower leg below the knee and give it a quick forward tug. It is abnormal when there is exaggerated anterior tibial movement or the knee fails to stop with a thud.

When recurrent dislocation or subluxation of the patella is suspected, the *patellar apprehension test* should be performed. Push the patella firmly in a lateral direction while slowly flexing the knee. The patient's face should be studied for the anxious look that suggests impending dislocation (it is then time to suspend the test).

Ask the patient to roll into the prone position. Look and feel in the popliteal fossa for a Baker's cyst.[q] This is a pressure diverticulum of the synovial membrane that occurs through a hiatus in the knee capsule (Figure 9.42). It is best seen with the knee extended. Rupture of this into the calf muscle produces signs that may mimic a deep venous thrombosis. Rupture is often associated with the 'crescent sign'— ecchymoses below the malleoli of the ankle. A Baker's cyst must be distinguished from an aneurysm of the popliteal artery, which will be pulsatile, and a bony tumour (very hard).

This is also the position in which Apley's *grinding test* may be performed (Figure 9.43). This is a test of meniscal damage. The patient's leg is flexed to 90 degrees, the examiner stabilises the thigh by kneeling lightly on it and while pressing on the foot rotates the leg backwards and forwards. Pain or clicking make the test positive. The *distraction test* is the opposite. Here the patient's leg is pulled upwards so as to take the strain off the menisci and stretch the ligaments. If the patient finds the test painful, a ligamentous abnormality may be the cause.

---

q   William Baker (1839–96), surgeon at St Bartholomew's Hospital, London, described this in 1877.

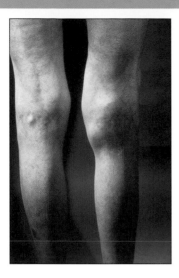

Figure 9.42 Baker's cyst of the right knee, viewed from behind

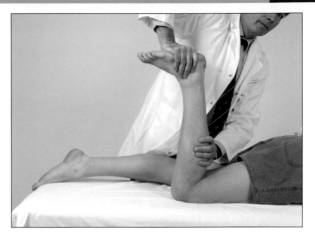

Figure 9.43 Apley's grinding test (push hard)

McMurray's[r] test (Figure 9.44) is another way of detecting a meniscal tear. The patient lies on the back, the examiner stands on the side to be tested and holds the ankle. The examiner's other hand sits on the medial side of the knee and pushes to apply valgus force. The patient's leg is then extended from the flexed position while being internally and then externally rotated. The test is positive if there is a popping sensation, which may be followed by inability to extend the knee.

Stand the patient up. Look particularly for varus (bow-leg) and valgus (knock-knee) deformity.

Finish with a test of function. Get the patient to walk to and fro. Study the gait and the movement of the knees, particularly for a sideways wobble.

The ankles and feet

Examination anatomy (Figure 9.45). The ankle is a synovial hinge joint formed between the distal ends of the tibia and the fibula, and the talus bone. Protrusions from the ends of the tibia and fibula, which are called malleoli, form a socket that in combination with lateral ligaments stabilises the joint. The proximal part of the foot is called the *tarsus* and contains the seven tarsal bones (talus, calcaneus [heel] navicular, cuboid and the three cuneiform bones) with their supporting ligaments and joint capsules. The joints and ligaments around these bones allow the movements of the foot: inversion and eversion, dorsi- (upward) and plantar (downward) flexion.

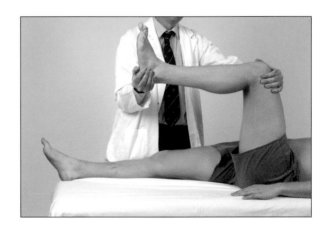

Figure 9.44 McMurray's test of the knee

History. The usual symptom is pain. If this is present only when the patient wears shoes, the shoes rather than the feet may be the problem. There may be a specific area that is painful and the patient should be asked to point to this. There may be a history of injury or of intensive or unusual exercise. Ankle injuries are common in certain sports that involve twisting of the foot on the leg (e.g. netball, football) (Table 9.15). Rupture of the Achilles tendon occurs in squash and tennis players in patients over 50 and following forced dorsiflexion of the foot.

Patients with foot (Table 9.16) or ankle pain may have a history of rheumatoid arthritis. This can cause pain and deformity and affect the ankle subtalar, midtarsal and metatarsophalangeal joints.

Very severe pain involving the first metatarso-phalangeal joint is usually due to gout. Pain right over one of the metatarsals that comes on after unusually vigorous exercise may be due to a stress fracture.

r   Thomas McMurray (1888–1949), the first professor of orthopaedic surgery in Liverpool.

GOOD SIGNS GUIDE 9.2 Ligament and meniscal injuries

Finding[+]	Sensitivity (%)	Specificity (%)	Positive LR	Negative LR
Detecting anterior cruciate ligament tear*				
Anterior drawer sign	27–88	91–99	11.5	0.5
Lachman's sign	48–96	90–99	17.0	0.2
Pivot shift sign	6–32	96–99	8.0	NS
Detecting meniscal injury*				
McMurray sign	17–29	96–98	8.2	0.8
Joint line tenderness	58–85	30–53	NS	NS
Block to full extension	44	86	3.2	0.7

NS = not significant.

* Diagnostic standard: for anterior cruciate tear, tear demonstrated by MRI imaging, arthroscopy, or surgery; for meniscal tear, arthroscopy.

[+] Definition of findings: see text.

From McGee S, *Evidence-based physical diagnosis*, 2nd edn. St Louis: Saunders, 2007.

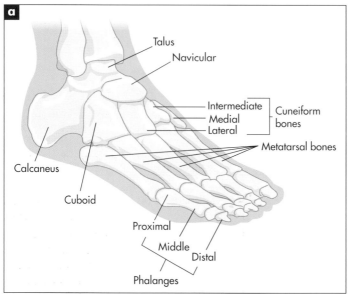

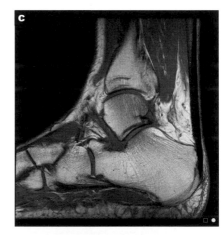

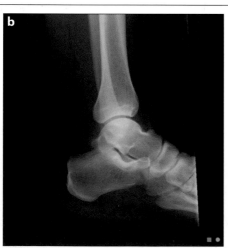

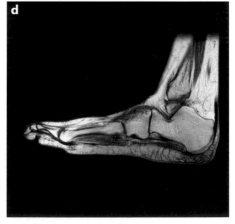

Figure 9.45 The ankles and feet
(a) Anatomy of the ankle and foot. (b) X-ray of the ankle.
(c) MRI scan of the ankle. (d) MRI scan of the left foot.
(X-ray and MRI scans courtesy M Thomson, National Capital Diagnostic Imaging, Canberra.)

TABLE 9.15 Differential diagnoses of ankle pain
Chronic or persistent pain suggests
Osteoarthritis (worse with walking)
Inflammatory arthritis (often painful at rest)
Pain behind the ankle suggests
Achilles tendinitis (tender lump behind foot, associated with rheumatoid arthritis)
Achilles tendon rupture (pain sudden and severe)
Pain over lateral aspect of ankle suggests
Lateral ligament injury—sprain (history of forced inversion of the ankle)
Lateral malleolus fracture (severe pain, history of trauma)
Pain over medial aspect of ankle suggests
Deltoid ligament injury—sprain (history of forced eversion of the ankle)
Posterior tibial tendinitis
Tarsal tunnel syndrome (posterior tibial nerve entrapment)
Fracture of medial malleolus (severe pain, history of trauma)

TABLE 9.16 Differential diagnoses of foot pain
Hind foot or midfoot pain suggests
Osteoarthritis
Rheumatoid arthritis
Plantar fibromas
Plantar fasciitis (heel pain)
Forefoot pain suggests
Metatarsalgia
Metatarsal fracture
Interdigital neuroma (interdigital nerve entrapment neuropathy)
Gout (severe pain and swelling, usually of first metatarsophalangeal joint)
Toe problems (bunions, ingrown toenail, claw toes, hammer toes)

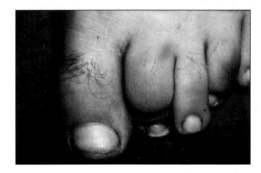

Figure 9.46 Sausage-shaped first and second toes in psoriatic arthritis

There may be deformity involving the ankle or toes. Patients find this especially troublesome if it makes it difficult to put on shoes. The patient may have noticed swelling; ask if this is painful or not and whether it involves one or both feet. Bilateral swelling is more likely due to inflammation. Swelling over the medial aspect of the first metatarsal head (a bunion) occurs commonly as people get older, but may be associated with rheumatoid arthritis.

Paraesthesiae in the feet may have been noticed. Try to find out the distribution of the abnormal sensation, which may be a result of peripheral nerve injury or peripheral neuropathy. Coldness of the feet is very common but cyanosis and ulceration are more worrying problems. Chronic foot ulcers mean diabetes must be excluded.

Examination. This examination includes the ankles, feet and toes.

Look at the skin. Note any swelling, scars, deformity or muscle wasting. Deformities affecting the forefoot include hallux valgus (fixed lateral deviation of the main axis of the big toe), clawing (fixed flexion deformity) and crowding of the toes, as occurs in rheumatoid arthritis. Sausage deformities of the toes occur with psoriatic arthropathy or Reiter's[s] disease (Figure 9.46).

Look for the nail changes that suggest psoriasis. Inspect the transverse arch of the foot, which runs underneath the metatarsophalangeal joints, and the longitudinal arch, which runs from the first metatarsophalangeal joint to the heel. These arches, which bear the weight of the body, may be flattened in arthritic conditions of the foot like rheumatoid arthritis. Calluses over the metatarsal heads on the plantar surface of the foot occur with subluxation of these joints (Figure 9.47).

Feel, starting with the ankle, for swelling around the lateral and medial malleoli. This should not be confused with pitting oedema. If an ankle fracture is suspected because of a history of injury, tenderness over the posterior medial malleolus is a reliable sign (positive LR 4.8).[10]

Move the *talar (ankle) joint*, grasping the midfoot with one hand. *Dorsiflexion* is tested by raising the foot towards the knee—normally possible to 20 degrees—and *plantar flexion* by performing the opposite manoeuvre, which is normally possible to 50 degrees.

With the subtalar joint, only *inversion* and

---

s Hans Reiter (1881–1969), professor of hygiene in Berlin, described the syndrome in 1916. This was well before he became an enthusiastic Nazi.

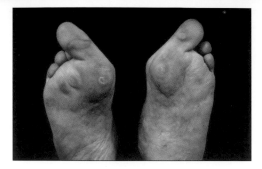

Figure 9.47 Rheumatoid feet showing bilateral hallux valgus and calluses over the metatarsal heads

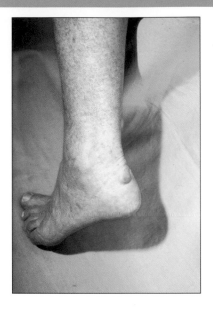

Figure 9.48 Rheumatoid nodule of the Achilles tendon

eversion of the foot on the ankle are tested. Pain on movement is more important than range at this joint. The midtarsal (midfoot) joint allows rotation of the forefoot when the hindfoot is fixed. This is done by steadying the ankle with one hand and rotating (twisting) the forefoot. Again, pain on motion rather than loss of range of movement is noted.

Squeeze the *metatarsophalangeal joints* by compressing the first and fifth metatarsals between your thumb and forefinger. Tenderness suggests inflammation, common in early rheumatoid arthritis. Press upwards from the sole of the foot just proximal to the metatarsophalangeal joints of the third and fourth toes. Pain here suggests *Morton's*[t] neuroma. This is due to entrapment and swelling of the digital nerve between the toes. It is associated with pain and numbness of the sides of these toes.

Each *individual interphalangeal joint* is then assessed by feeling and moving. These are typically affected in the seronegative spondyloarthropathies. Extremely tender involvement of the first metatarsophalangeal joint is characteristic of acute gout. In this case the joint also looks red and swollen.

Palpate the *Achilles tendon* for rheumatoid nodules (Figure 9.48) and tenderness due to Achilles tendinitis. An old Achilles tendon rupture may be detected by squeezing the calf: normally the foot plantar flexes unless the tendon has previously ruptured (Simmonds'[u] test). Also palpate the inferior aspect of the *heel* for tenderness; this may indicate plantar fasciitis, which occurs in the seronegative spondyloarthropathies and sometimes for no apparent reason.

Correlation of physical signs and rheumatological disease

Rheumatoid arthritis (Figures 9.30 and 9.49)

This is a chronic systemic inflammatory disease of unknown aetiology which characteristically involves the joints. In the majority of cases, patients with rheumatoid arthritis have rheumatoid factor present in the serum (seropositive disease). These are heterogeneous antibodies directed against the Fc portion of immunoglobulin G (IgG), but are not specific for rheumatoid arthritis.

To examine the patient with suspected rheumatoid arthritis, sit him or her up in bed or on a chair.

General inspection

Look to see whether the patient has a Cushingoid appearance due to steroid treatment (page 309), or whether there are signs of weight loss that may indicate active disease.

The hands

Put the hands on a pillow. Look especially for symmetrical small joint synovitis (the distal interphalangeal joints are usually spared). The other common abnormalities are ulnar deviation, volar subluxation of the metacarpophalangeal joints,

---

t   Thomas Morton (1835–1903), general and eye surgeon, Philadelphia Hospital, performed one of the first appendicectomies.

u   Franklin Simmonds, orthopaedic surgeon, Rowley Bristow Hospital, Surrey, UK; he is now retired.

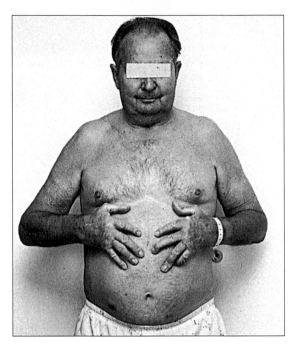

Figure 9.49 Rheumatoid arthritis

1. **General inspection**
   Cushingoid appearance
   Weight
2. **Hands**
3. **Arms**
   Entrapment neuropathy (e.g. carpal tunnel)

   Subcutaneous nodules
   Elbow joint
   Shoulder joint
   Axillary nodes
4. **Face**
   Eyes—dry eyes (Sjögren's), scleritis, episcleritis, scleromalacia perforans, anaemia, cataracts (steroids, chloroquine)
   Fundi—hyperviscosity
   Face—parotids (Sjögren's)
   Mouth—dryness, ulcers, dental caries
   Temporomandibular joint (crepitus)
5. **Neck**
   Cervical spine
   Cervical nodes
6. **Chest**
   Heart—pericarditis, valve lesions
   Lungs—effusion, fibrosis, infarction, infection, nodules (and Caplan's syndrome)
7. **Abdomen**
   Splenomegaly (e.g. Felty's syndrome)
   Inguinal nodes
8. **Hips**
9. **Knees**
10. **Lower limbs**
    Ulceration (vasculitis)
    Calf swelling (ruptured synovial cyst)
    Peripheral neuropathy
    Mononeuritis multiplex
    Cord compression
11. **Feet**
12. **Other**
    Urine: protein, blood (drugs, vasculitis, amyloidosis)
    Rectal examination (blood)

and Z deformity of the thumb with swan neck and boutonnière deformity of the fingers. Examine the fingernails and periungual areas for splinter-like vasculitic changes and look for wasting of the small muscles of the hand. Look at the palms for palmar erythema. Feel the palms for palmar tendon crepitus while the patient extends and flexes the fingers. Look for signs of an ulnar nerve palsy (from ulnar nerve entrapment at the elbow) and a median nerve palsy (carpal tunnel).

The wrists

Look for synovial thickening and perform Phalen's sign (carpal tunnel).

The elbows

Look around the elbows for rheumatoid nodules, which suggest seropositive disease, and examine the elbow joint. Flexion contractures are common.

The shoulders and axillae

Here examine for tenderness and limitation of movement. Also palpate the axillary nodes because enlarged nodes may indicate active disease of joints in the area that they drain.

The eyes

Look at the eyes for redness which may indicate the dryness of Sjögren's syndrome (Table 9.8), which occurs in 10%–15% of cases. Note also nodular scleritis (an elevated white or purple-red lesion, which is pathologically a rheumatoid nodule and usually appears surrounded by the intense redness of the injected sclera) (Figure 9.50). These nodules occur especially in the superior parts of the sclera and are often bilateral, but affect only 1% of patients. Iritis does *not* occur.

With severe scleritis, scleral thinning may occur, exposing the underlying choroid. This is called *scleromalacia*. Look for cataracts due to steroid treatment. Conjunctival pallor may be present, indicating anaemia due to iron deficiency. This can be a result of blood loss from non-steroidal anti-inflammatory drug use, folate deficiency from a poor diet, hypersplenism or chronic inflammation, or some combination of these.

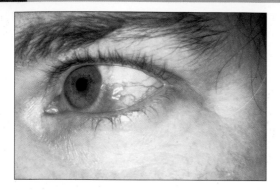

Figure 9.50 Nodular scleritis involving the sclera lateral to the iris

The parotids

Look for enlargement of the parotid glands, as occurs with Sjögren's syndrome.

The mouth

Look for dryness of the mouth and dental caries (Sjögren's syndrome), and ulcers related to drug treatment (e.g. methotrexate).

The temporomandibular joints

Feel the temporomandibular joints for crepitus as the patient opens and shuts the mouth.

The neck

Go on to examine the cervical spine for tenderness, muscle spasm and reduction of rotational movement. Examine for cervical lymphadenopathy.

The chest

Now examine the lungs for signs of pleural effusions or pulmonary fibrosis. Caplan's syndrome[v] is the presence of rheumatoid lung nodules in combination with pneumoconiosis.

The heart

Listen to the heart for a pericardial rub (relatively common) and for murmurs indicating valvular regurgitation (especially the aortic valve), which may occur due to nodular involvement of a heart valve.

The abdomen

Feel the abdomen for splenomegaly (this occurs in up to 10% of patients and suggests the possibility of Felty's syndrome, page 229) and hepatomegaly. Feel the inguinal lymph nodes.

---

v   Anthony Caplan, Welsh physician, described this in 1953.

The lower limbs

Examine the hips for limitation of joint movement. The knees, however, are more often affected and here one must note any quadriceps wasting, synovial effusions and flexion contractures. Valgus deformity and ligamentous instability may occur as late complications. Look in the popliteal fossae for Baker's cysts. Go on to look at the lower parts of the legs for ulceration; this can occur as a vasculitic complication of Felty's syndrome. Examine for a stocking distribution peripheral neuropathy and for mononeuritis multiplex of the nerves of the lower limbs. There may also be signs of spinal cord compression due to anterior dislocation of the first cervical vertebra or vertical subluxation of the odontoid process.

The ankles and feet (Figures 9.47 and 9.48)

Now look for foot drop (peroneal nerve entrapment or vasculitis) and examine the ankle joint for limitation of movement. Look at the metatarsophalangeal joints for swelling and subluxation. There may also be lateral deviation and clawing of the toes. Remember that the interphalangeal joints are very rarely involved. Finally, feel the Achilles tendon for nodules—a sign of seropositive disease.

Seronegative spondyloarthropathies

Four conditions are generally accepted as belonging to this group: ankylosing spondylitis, psoriatic arthritis, Reiter's disease (reactive arthritis) and enteropathic arthritis. These are called the seronegative spondyloarthropathies because they were originally distinguished from rheumatoid arthritis by the absence of rheumatoid factor in the serum. However, up to 30% of patients with otherwise classical rheumatoid arthritis are rheumatoid factor negative. The seronegative spondyloarthropathies overlap clinically and pathologically, and have an association with HLA-B27.

Ankylosing spondylitis

The following areas should be examined.

The back and sacroiliac joints: may show loss of lumbar lordosis and thoracic kyphosis; severe flexion deformity of the lumbar spine (rare); tenderness of the lumbar vertebrae; reduction of movement of the lumbar spine in all directions; and tenderness of the sacroiliac joints.

The legs: Achilles tendinitis; plantar fasciitis; signs of cauda equina compression (rare)—lower limb weakness, loss of sphincter control, saddle sensory loss.

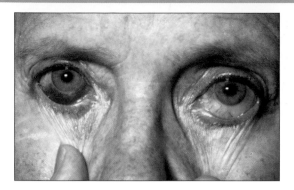

Figure 9.51 Iritis of the right eye

The lungs: decreased chest expansion (less than 5 cm); signs of apical fibrosis.

The heart: signs of aortic regurgitation.

The eyes: acute iritis (tends to recur)—painful red eye (10%–15%) (Figure 9.51).

Rectal and stool examination: signs of inflammatory bowel disease (either ulcerative colitis or Crohn's disease). *Note:* signs of secondary amyloidosis—for example, hepatosplenomegaly, renal enlargement, proteinuria—may be present, although this is a very rare complication.

X-rays of the spine and sacroiliac joints (Figure 9.52): may show ankylosis (fusion) of the sacroiliac joints and 'squaring' of the vertebral bodies as a result of loss of their anterior corners and periostitis of their waists. 'Bridging syndesmophytes'[w] occur as a result of ossification of the fibres of the joint annulus. Severe disease causes the changes called *bamboo spine* visible on X-ray.

Reiter's syndrome (reactive arthritis)

Classically this disease follows urethritis or diarrhoea, with conjunctivitis and arthritis (usually asymmetrical) of the large weightbearing joints such as the hip, knee or ankle. The following areas should be examined.

The genital region: urethral discharge; circinate balanitis—scaly, superficial reddened erosions with well-demarcated borders on the glans penis (Figure 9.53).

The prostate: prostatitis.

The eyes: conjunctivitis; iritis (rare).

The mouth: painless smooth mucosal lesions, especially of the tongue.

The back: sacroiliac joints (may be unilaterally involved).

The lower limbs (more commonly affected):

w   A syndesmosis is a joint where the bones are joined by fibrous ligaments or sheets.

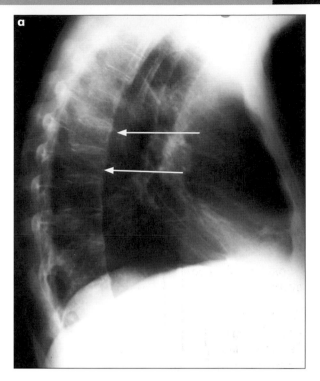

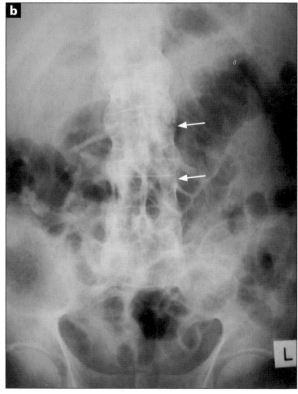

Figure 9.52 Ankylosing spondylitis
Anteroposterior (a) and lateral (b) X-rays of the thoracic spine showing ankylosis of the sacroiliac joints, extensive syndesmophyte formation (short arrows) and squaring of the vertebral bodies (long arrows).
(Courtesy Canberra Hospital X-ray library.)

knees, ankles; metatarsophalangeal joints and toes ('sausage toes'); plantar fasciitis, Achilles tendinitis; keratoderma blennorrhagica on the sole (non-tender reddish-brown macules, which become scaling papules; Figure 9.54)—this is indistinguishable from pustular psoriasis; nails thickened, opaque and brittle.

The hands (less commonly involved): wrists; metacarpophalangeal joints, proximal interphalangeal joints, distal interphalangeal joints; keratoderma blennorrhagica on the palms; nail changes.

Cardiovascular system: aortic regurgitation (rare).

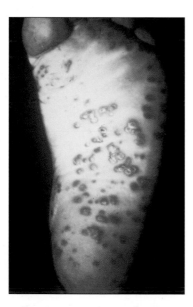

Figure 9.53 Circinate balanitis

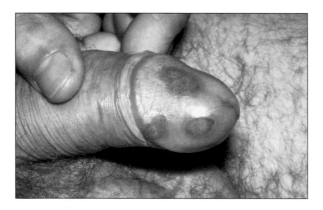

Figure 9.54 Reiter's syndrome with keratoderma blennorrhagica
(From FS McDonald, ed., *Mayo Clinic images in internal medicine*, with permission. © Mayo Clinic Scientific Press and CRC Press.)

X-ray findings: the first attack of arthritis is associated with soft-tissue changes and subsequent attacks may lead to joint-space narrowing and proliferative erosions at the joint margins. Changes in the sacroiliac joints and spine resemble those of ankylosing spondylitis except that the sacroiliac joint changes and spinal syndesmophytes tend to be asymmetrical. Calcaneal spurs (Figure 9.55)—a result of plantar fasciitis—are characteristic.

Psoriatic arthritis

Ten per cent of patients with psoriasis (page 446) have arthritis.

Examine as for rheumatoid arthritis, but include the spine and sacroiliac joints. There are five distinct groups of psoriatic arthritis, but overlap is common.

1 Monoarticular and asymmetrical oligoarticular arthritis of the hands and feet and other joints (note sausage-shaped digits in Figure 9.46). Most psoriatic arthritis is of this type.
2 Symmetrical polyarthritis, similar to rheumatoid arthritis (but seronegative).
3 Distal interphalangeal joint involvement with psoriatic nail changes (Figure 9.12).

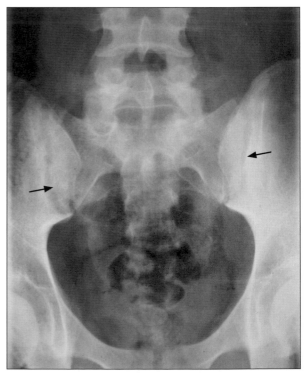

Figure 9.55 Reiter's syndrome
X-ray of the pelvis of a patient with Reiter's syndrome, showing loss of joint space in the sacroiliac joints (arrows). (Courtesy Canberra Hospital X-ray library.)

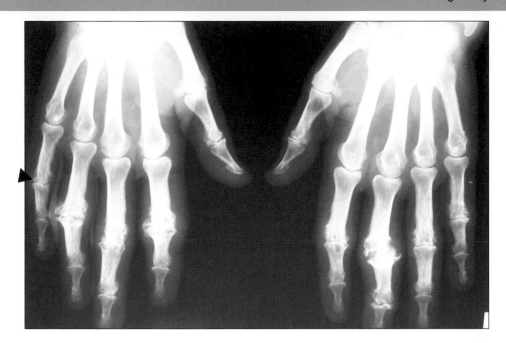

Figure 9.56 Psoriatic arthritis
X-ray of the wrist of a patient with psoriatic arthritis; note the 'pencil in cup' deformity (tapered proximal osseous surface and expanded base) of the distal bone of the fingers, early ankylosis [arrowhead] of the proximal interphalangeal joint of the right little finger and erosions with proliferative change of the little finger). Note also the lack of osteoporosis.
(Courtesy Canberra Hospital X-ray library.)

4 Arthritis mutilans (destructive polyarthritis).
5 Sacroiliitis with or without peripheral joint involvement.

X-ray findings (Figure 9.56): in mild cases X-rays are normal or show only joint-space narrowing and erosive changes. Unlike the X-rays of rheumatoid joints the bone density is maintained and there may be sclerotic changes in the small bones. Ankylosis of peripheral joints and *arthritis mutilans* can occur in either condition. The involvement of the spine and sacroiliac joints is asymmetrical, as in Reiter's syndrome.

Enteropathic arthritis

There are two patterns of involvement of the joints with ulcerative colitis and Crohn's disease.
1 **Peripheral joint disease.** This is an asymmetrical oligoarthropathy, usually affecting the lower limbs, especially the knees and ankles. It rarely causes deformity.
2 **Sacroiliitis.** This is indistinguishable clinically from ankylosing spondylitis.

Gouty arthritis

Begin with the feet, as acute gouty arthritis affects the metatarsophalangeal joint of the great toe in 75% of cases. Next examine the ankles and knees, which tend to be involved after recurrent attacks. The fingers, wrists and elbows are affected late (Figure 9.57). Inspect and palpate for gouty tophi (these are urate deposits with inflammatory cells surrounding them) (Latin *tophus,* 'chalk stone'). The presence of tophi indicates chronic recurrent gout. They tend to occur over the joint synovia, the olecranon bursa, the extensor surface of the forearm, the helix of the ear (Figure 9.58), and in the infrapatellar and Achilles tendons.

Finally, examine for signs of the causes of secondary gout: increased purine turnover due to myeloproliferative disease (page 236), lymphoma (page 237) or leukaemia; and decreased renal urate excretion due to renal disease or hypothyroidism. Hypertension, diabetes mellitus and ischaemic heart disease are more common among sufferers of gout.

X-rays (Figure 9.59) show multiple juxta-articular erosions which may obliterate the joint space.

Calcium pyrophosphate arthropathy (pseudogout)

This may present a similar picture to that described above for true gout, but usually large joints (especially the knees) and wrists are involved. In a

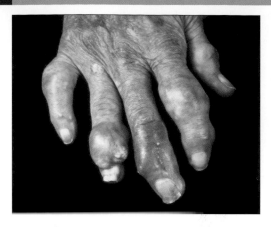

Figure 9.57 Gouty tophi of the fingers

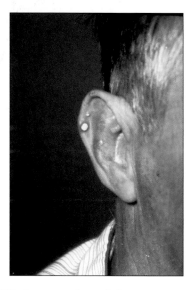

Figure 9.58 Gouty tophus of the ear

minority of patients there will be signs of hyperpara-thyroidism, haemochromatosis or true gout.

X-rays show joint-space narrowing, cyst form-ation under the cartilage and calcification of the joint cartilage (chondrocalcinosis). Chondrocalcinosis on X-ray is typical of pseudogout but is not always present.

Calcium hydroxyapatite arthropathy
This causes large-joint arthritis (especially knee and shoulder) and is more common in elderly patients.

Systemic lupus erythematosus (SLE)
This is a multisystemic chronic inflammatory disease of unknown origin, named because the erosive nature of the condition was likened to the damage caused by a hungry wolf (Latin *lupus*[x] 'wolf') (Figure 9.60).

General inspection
Look for weight loss (due to chronic inflammation) or a Cushingoid appearance (steroid treatment). While taking the history note any abnormal mental state—psychosis may occur due to the lupus itself or to steroid therapy.

Hands
Note any vasculitic-appearing lesions around the nail bed, or telangiectasia and erythema of the skin of the nail base. A rash may occur—photosensitivity is common. The hand rash of lupus tends to occur over the phalanges, as opposed to that of dermatomyositis which affects the knuckles.

Raynaud's phenomenon may occur if the weather is cold (Table 9.7).

Examine for arthropathy: synovitis of the proximal and metacarpophalangeal joints. The arthritis of SLE is not erosive, but if severe may lead to reducible deformities due to damage to supporting structures.

Forearms
Livedo reticularis may occur here; in Latin this describes skin discoloration in the form of a small net. This is formed by connected bluish-purple streaks without discrete borders. They occur usually on the limbs and are associated with various connective tissue diseases.[11] Look for purpura (due to vasculitis[12] or autoimmune thrombocytopenia). Examine for a proximal myopathy (due to the disease itself or to steroid treatment). Subcutaneous nodules very rarely occur in SLE. The axillary nodes may be enlarged but will not be tender.

The head and neck
Alopecia (hair loss) is an important diagnostic clue that occurs in about two-thirds of patients and may be associated with scarring. Look especially for lupus hairs, which are short, broken hairs above the forehead. The hair as a whole may be coarse and dry, as in hypothyroidism.

Examine the eyes for scleritis and episcleritis (see Figure 9.50). The eyes may be red and dry (Sjögren's syndrome). Pallor of the conjunctivae occurs with anaemia, usually due to chronic disease. Occasionally jaundice due to autoimmune haemolytic anaemia may be found. Perform a fundoscopy for cytoid bodies, which are hard exudates (white spots) due to aggregates of swollen nerve fibres and are secondary to vasculitis.

x   Lupus has been used as a name for any erosive disease of the skin; for
    example, lupus vulgaris is tuberculosis of the skin.

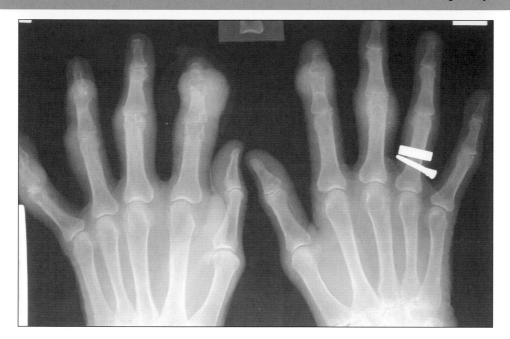

Figure 9.59 Gout
X-ray of the hands of a patient with severe gouty arthritis. Note multiple juxta-articular erosions with relative preservation of the joint space, and erosions with overhanging edges. There are large soft-tissue swellings over the distal interphalangeal joints of the index fingers. (Courtesy Canberra Hospital X-ray library.)

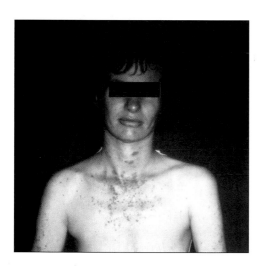

Figure 9.60 Systemic lupus erythematosus

1. **General inspection**
   Cushingoid appearance
   Weight
   Mental state
2. **Hands**
   Vasculitis
   Rash
   Arthropathy
3. **Arms**
   Livedo reticularis
   Purpura
   Proximal myopathy (active disease or steroids)
4. **Head**
   Alopecia, with or without scarring, lupus hairs
   Eyes—scleritis, cytoid lesions, etc.
   Mouth—ulcers, infection
   Rash—butterfly
   Cranial nerve lesions
   Cervical adenopathy
5. **Chest**
   Cardiovascular system—pericarditis
   Respiratory system—pleural effusion, pleurisy, pulmonary fibrosis, collapse or infection
6. **Abdomen**
   Hepatosplenomegaly
   Tenderness
7. **Hips**
   Aseptic necrosis
8. **Legs**
   Feet—red soles, small-joint synovitis
   Rash
   Ulcers over the malleoli, e.g. antiphospholipid syndrome
   Proximal myopathy
   Neuropathy
   Mononeuritis multiplex
   Cerebellar ataxia
   Hemiplegia
9. **Other**
   Urine analysis (proteinuria)
   Blood pressure (hypertension)
   Temperature chart

A facial rash may be diagnostic (Figure 9.61). The classical rash is an erythematous 'butterfly rash' over the cheeks and bridge of the nose and must be distinguished from rosacea. Mouth ulcers on the soft or hard palate may occur and the mouth may be dry (Sjögren's syndrome).

The *rash of discoid lupus* may be found in the same area or affect different parts of the body. Lesions begin as spreading red plaques which have a central area of hyperkeratosis and follicular plugging. An active lesion has an oedematous edge. The appearance may suggest psoriasis. A healed lesion may have marginal hyperpigmentation with central atrophy and depigmentation. The scalp, external ear and face are most commonly affected, but in some patients lesions may occur all over the arms and chest. Extensive annular or psoriaform lesions may indicate the presence of subacute cutaneous lupus.

After examining the face, feel for cervical lymphadenopathy, which is usually non-tender.

The chest

Signs of a pericardial rub (from pericarditis) may be found. In the respiratory examination a pleural rub (pleuritis) or signs suggesting the presence of a pleural effusion, pulmonary fibrosis, pulmonary collapse or pulmonary hypertension may be detected. Chest disease is probably most often secondary to an interstitial pneumonitis rather than to vasculitis of the lungs.

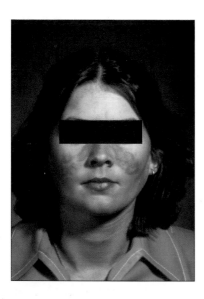

Figure 9.61 Butterfly rash of systemic lupus erythematosus

The abdomen

Splenomegaly, usually mild, can be detected in 10% of cases. Hepatomegaly (mild) may occur in uncomplicated cases. Chronic liver disease due to chronic hepatitis ('lupoid hepatitis') is a separate autoimmune disease rather than a variant of SLE.

The hips

Examine the hip joint movements: in aseptic (avascular) necrosis there is pain on movement, with preservation of hip extension but loss of the other movements. This is due to ischaemia of the femoral head and may be related to steroid use or to the SLE itself.

The legs

Examine for proximal myopathy and peripheral neuropathy (mainly sensory).

Rarely there may be signs of hemiplegia, cerebellar ataxia or chorea.

Leg ulceration over the malleoli, due to vasculitis or the antiphospholipid syndrome,[11] is important. Very occasionally the toes may be gangrenous. There may be ankle oedema from the nephrotic syndrome or fluid retention from steroids. Livedo reticularis may be present on the legs.

Urine and blood pressure

Perform a urine analysis (for proteinuria and haematuria) and take the blood pressure (for hypertension). Renal disease is a common complication of SLE.

Temperature

Take the temperature, as fever is common in SLE, either from secondary infection or from the disease per se.

Scleroderma (progressive systemic sclerosis)

This is a disorder of connective tissue with variable cutaneous fibrosis and with abnormalities of the microvasculature of the fingers, gut, lungs, heart and kidneys. In diffuse cutaneous scleroderma there is more prominent skin sclerosis and these patients may have pulmonary fibrosis. In limited cutaneous scleroderma (CREST syndrome—*Calcinosis*, *Raynaud's* phenomenon, *oEsophageal* motility disturbance, *Sclerodactyly* and *Telangiectasia*), diffuse skin sclerosis and interstitial lung disease do not occur but patients are at risk of developing pulmonary hypertension.

General inspection (Figure 9.62)

Look for cachexia due to dysphagia (from an

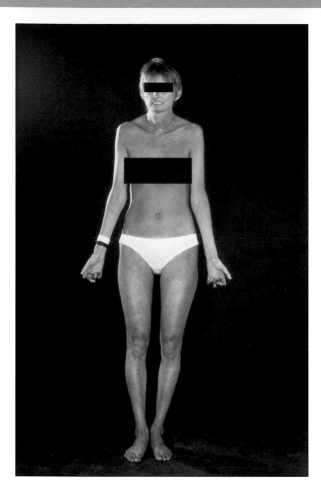

Figure 9.62 Scleroderma

1. **General appearance**
   'Bird-like' facies
   Weight-loss (malabsorption)
2. **Hands**
   CRST—calcinosis, atrophy distal tissue pulp
       (Raynaud's), sclerodactyly, telangiectasia
   Dilated capillary loops (nailfolds)
   Small-joint arthropathy and tendon crepitus
   Fixed flexion deformity
   Hand function
3. **Arms**
   Oedema (early), or skin thickening and tightening
   Pigmentation
   Vitiligo
   Hair loss
   Proximal myopathy
4. **Head**
   Alopecia
   Eyes—loss of eyebrows, anaemia, difficulty with
       closing
   Mouth—puckered, difficulty with opening
   Pigmentation
   Telangiectasia
   Neck muscles—wasting and weakness
5. **Dysphagia**
6. **Chest**
   Tight skin ('Roman breastplate')
   Heart—cor pulmonale, pericarditis, failure
   Lungs—fibrosis, reflux pneumonitis, chest infections
7. **Legs**
   Skin lesions
   Vasculitis
8. **Other**
   Blood pressure (hypertension with renal involvement)
   Urine analysis (proteinuria)
   Temperature chart (infection)
   Stool examination (steatorrhoea)

oesophageal motility disturbance) or malabsorption (due to bacterial overgrowth).

Skin changes in scleroderma vary. There may be an early oedematous phase with non-tender pitting oedema of the hands which appear tightly swollen. In patients with progressive disease the oedematous skin is replaced by indurated skin which appears thickened, hard and tight. This phase usually begins in the fingers (Table 9.17).

The hands

Examine the hands. Note particularly *calcinosis* (palpable nodules due to calcific deposits in the subcutaneous tissue of the fingers), *Raynaud's phenomenon* sometimes causing atrophy of the finger pulps (due to ischaemia) (Figure 9.63), *sclerodactyly* (tightening of the skin of the fingers leading to tapering), and multiple large *telangiectasia* on the fingers (Figure 9.64).

Look for *contraction deformity of the fingers*, which is relatively common (Figure 9.65), and for synovitis, although this is uncommon. The nails can

be affected by Raynaud's. It can be useful to inspect the nailfolds using a hand-held magnifying glass: in scleroderma you may see dilated capillary loops but this is not diagnostic. These are best viewed on the fourth digit. Assessing hand function is important in this disease.

The arms

Determine the extent of skin tethering in the arms. If the skin thickening extends above the wrists to the arms, legs or trunk, the diagnosis is *diffuse scleroderma* rather than *CREST*. If the skin thickening extends only to the elbows and face this is called *limited scleroderma*. Assess for proximal myopathy due to myositis.

The face

The skin of the face is involved in progressive disease. There is loss of normal wrinkles and skinfolds as well as of the eyebrows. The face appears pinched and expressionless ('bird-like'

TABLE 9.17 Differential diagnosis of thickened tethered skin

Systemic sclerosis (scleroderma), diffuse type; milder changes in limited cutaneous scleroderma

Mixed connective tissue disease (a distinct disorder with features of scleroderma, systemic lupus erythematosus, rheumatoid arthritis and myositis)

Eosinophilic fasciitis—widespread skin thickening due to inflammation of the fascia often following excessive muscle exercise; occurs in association with eosinophilia and hypergammaglobulinaemia

Localised morphea—heterogeneous group of disorders where there are small areas of sclerosis: most common type is morphea, which begins with large plaques of red or purple skin that evolve into sclerotic areas and may regress spontaneously over years

Chemically induced: vinyl chloride, pentazocine, bleomycin

Pseudoscleroderma: porphyria cutanea tarda, acromegaly, carcinoid syndrome

Scleroedema: thickened skin over the shoulders and upper back in diabetes mellitus

Graft versus host disease

Silicosis

Eosinophilic myalgia syndrome (L-tryptophan)

Toxic oil syndrome

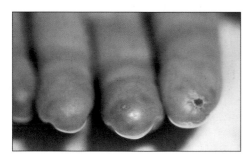

Figure 9.63 Digital infarcts

facies). Inspect for malar telangiectasia and look for salt-and-pepper pigmentation. Ask the patient to close the eyes—skin tethering may make this incomplete. The eyes may be dry (Sjögren's syndrome), though this is uncommon, and the conjunctivae pale (there are a number of reasons for anaemia, including the presence of chronic disease, bleeding from oesophagitis, watermelon stomach and microangiopathic haemolytic anaemia).

Ask the patient to open the mouth fully. It may appear puckered and narrow. Inability to open the mouth so that there is more than 3 cm of

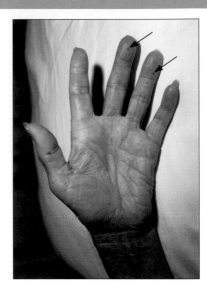

Figure 9.64 Telangiectasia of the hands in the CREST syndrome

clearance between the incisors indicates abnormal restriction.

The chest

Inspect the skin of the chest wall, which may have acquired a tight, thickened appearance, like ancient Roman breastplate armour.

Examine the lungs for pulmonary fibrosis, evidence of reflux pneumonitis, or (rarely) a pleural effusion or alveolar cell carcinoma.

Examine the heart for cor pulmonale secondary to pulmonary fibrosis or for pericarditis. Left ventricular failure may also occur due to myocardial involvement.

The legs

Look for signs of vasculitis, ulceration and skin involvement. Peripheral neuropathy is rare.

Urinalysis and blood pressure

These are very important because renal involvement is common in scleroderma and is often associated with severe hypertension. Renal disease is one of the most common causes of death.

The stool

Look for evidence of steatorrhoea (due to malabsorption from bacterial overgrowth). A summary of the physical signs that can be found in scleroderma is presented in Figure 9.62.

Rheumatic fever

This is an inflammatory disease which is a delayed sequel to infection with group A beta-haemolytic

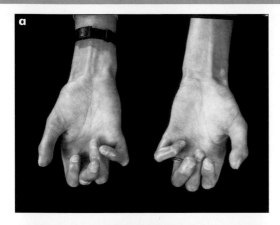

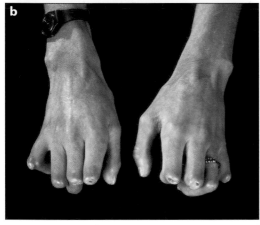

Figure 9.65 Systemic sclerosis: signs in the hands
Sclerodactyly, tethered smooth skin, calcinosis and
ulceration, atrophy of finger pulps due to Raynaud's
phenomenon, and fixed flexion deformities of the fingers.

Streptococcus; it is uncommon in Western nations today. It is diagnosed by finding two major or one major and two minor criteria, plus evidence of recent streptococcal infection.

Major criteria: (i) carditis (causing tachycardia, murmurs, cardiac failure, pericarditis); (ii) polyarthritis; (iii) chorea (page 399); (iv) erythema marginatum (see below); (v) subcutaneous nodules (painless mobile swellings).

Minor criteria: (i) fever; (ii) arthralgia; (iii) previous rheumatic fever; (iv) acute phase proteins; (v) prolonged PR interval on the ECG.

Examining the patient with suspected rheumatic fever

First examine the large joints of the limbs for effusions and synovitis. Two or more joints must be involved (classically there is a transient migratory polyarthritis). Feel for subcutaneous nodules over bony prominences. Look for a rash. Erythema marginatum is a slightly raised pink or red rash that blanches with pressure. The red rings have a clear centre and round margins, and occur on the trunk and proximal limbs; the rash is not found on the face. Look for choreiform movements. Their onset is usually delayed until about 3 months after the throat infection.

Now examine the cardiovascular system for any signs of pancarditis: (i) a pericardial rub due to pericarditis; (ii) congestive cardiac failure due to myocarditis; (iii) mitral or aortic regurgitation due to acute endocarditis.

Finally, take the temperature.

The vasculitides

This is a heterogeneous group of disorders characterised by inflammation and damage to blood vessels.[12] The clinical features and major vessels involved are shown in Table 9.18.

Soft-tissue rheumatism

This includes a number of common, painful conditions that arise in soft tissue, often around a joint. The problem may be general—for example, fibromyalgia; or restricted to a single anatomical region—for example, tendon, tenosynovium, enthesis or bursa. There are a large number of these conditions; the more common ones are described here.

Fibromyalgia syndrome

This syndrome is a common, frequently overlooked condition that mostly affects women in their 40s and 50s. It presents with a variable group of symptoms including widespread musculoskeletal aches and pains, and usually with symptoms of chronic fatigue. The musculoskeletal pain is mostly axial (neck and back) and diffuse. It is made worse by stress or cold. Pain may be felt 'all over' and is unresponsive to anti-inflammatory drug treatment. The combination of pain and fatigue may cause the patient severe disability. There is usually a poor sleep pattern. The patient wakes up not feeling refreshed, and more tired in the morning than later in the day. Note that no abnormal pathology has been found in the joints, muscles or tendons of these patients.

Examination. Test for the characteristic multiple hyperalgesic tender points (Figure 9.66). These areas may be tender to finger pressure in normal people but in affected patients there is marked tenderness and a definite withdrawal response. This response should be obtained in at least 11 of 18 sites in the upper and lower limbs and on both sides (i.e. it is widespread and symmetrical). Next

TABLE 9.18 The vasculitides

Name	Vessels	Characteristics
Small vessel vasculitis		
Wegener's* granulomatosis	Small to medium-sized capillaries, venules, arterioles, small arteries	Granulomatous inflammation affecting the respiratory tract, often with necrotising glomerulonephritis Saddle-nose deformity
Churg-Strauss syndrome	Small	Asthma, eosinophilia, skin nodules, mononeuritis multiplex, pulmonary infiltrates
Henoch-Schonlein purpura	Small	Children affected; purpura over buttocks, abdominal pain, arthritis of knee and ankle, nephritis (40%)
Microscopic polyangiitis	Small	Glomerulonephritis, alveolar haemorrhage, neuropathy, pleural effusions
Mixed essential cryoglobulinaemia	Small	Arthritis, palpable purpura of extremities, Raynaud's disease, neuropathy Hepatitis C common
Medium-sized vessel vasculitis		
Polyarteritis nodosa	Medium-sized to small	Myalgia, arthralgia, fever, palpable purpura, skin ulceration or infarction, weight loss, testicular tenderness, neuropathy (involvement of vasa nervorum), hypertension, renal infarction Hepatitis B associated
Kawasaki's disease	Medium-sized (coronary artery involvement)	Children affected; desquamating rash over extremities, strawberry tongue
Large vessel vasculitis		
Giant cell arteritis (temporal arteritis)	Medium to large (temporal and ophthalmic arteries and their branches)	Localised headache, systemic symptoms, tenderness temporal artery, jaw pain, visual loss—posterior ciliary artery (age ≥50 years)
Takayasu's disease[†]	Large (aorta, brachial, carotid, ulnar and axillary arteries)	Systemic symptoms, claudication, loss of pulses (typically Asian race ≤40 years)

GIT = gastrointestinal tract. SLE = systemic lupus erythematosus. PAN = polyarteritis nodosa. CNS = central nervous system.
* Frederich Wegener, German pathologist, described this in 1936.
[†] Mikito Takayasu (1860–1938), Japanese professor of ophthalmology.

examine for hyperalgesia at control sites such as the forehead or distal forearm, where it should be absent.

The diagnosis is based on the presence of typical symptoms and multiple hyperalgesic tender sites (with negative control sites). Inflammatory and endocrine disease must be excluded.

Shoulder syndromes

Soft-tissue disorders of the shoulder are common and have certain particular clinical features.

Rotator cuff syndrome

Supraspinatus tendinitis is the commonest form of rotator cuff syndrome. It is associated with degeneration and subsequent inflammation in the supraspinatus tendon as it is compressed between the acromion and humeral head when the arm is raised. It mostly affects 40- to 50-year-olds. Symptoms may begin following unaccustomed physical activities such as gardening.

Examination. Examine the shoulder joint. Note pain on abduction of the arm (Figure 9.67), with a painful arc of movement between 60 and 120 degrees of abduction. Involvement of other rotator cuff tendons causes similar painful movement. Biceps tendinitis is present in the majority of patients with a rotator cuff syndrome. Yergason's[y] sign for biceps tendinitis is helpful (positive LR

---

y Robert Mosley Yergason, American surgeon born in 1885, described this sign in 1931.

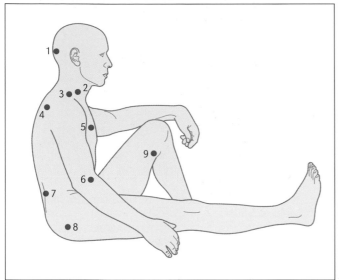

Figure 9.66 Frequent sites of localised tenderness in fibromyalgia
18 tender point sites (test bilaterally) are:
1   Insertion of suboccipital muscle
2   Under lower sternocleidomastoid muscle
3   Insertion of supraspinatus muscle
4   Trapezius muscle (mid upper)
5   Near second costochondral junction
6   2 cm distal to lateral epicondyle
7   At prominence of greater trochanter
8   Upper outer quadrant of buttock
9   At medial fat pad of knee

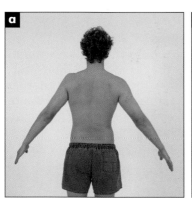
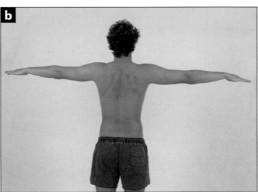
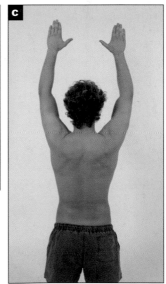

Figure 9.67 Inflammation of the rotator cuff tendons may cause a 'painful arc' during abduction of the arm
The initial movement (a) is painless but the next 90 degrees of movement (b) causes pain. When the arm reaches full abduction (c) the pain eases as the pressure is taken off the rotator cuff apparatus.

2.8).[10] The patient flexes the elbow to 90 degrees and pronates the wrist. The examiner holds the wrists and attempts to prevent the patient's attempts to supinate the forearm. Inflammation of the head of the biceps causes pain in the shoulder since this muscle is the main supinator of the forearm.

Frozen shoulder

Capsulitis of the shoulder, or frozen shoulder, is associated with limitation of active and passive arm movements in all directions. It may follow immobilisation of the arm after a stroke. There is typically a sudden onset of shoulder pain, which is worse at night and radiates to the base of the neck and down the arm. Pain is made worse by shoulder movement and may be bilateral. Pain and stiffness usually subside over a period of months. Complete movement may not be regained.

Examination. Examine the shoulders. There is global restriction of both active and passive movement of the shoulder—that is, it is frozen.

Elbow epicondylitis (tennis and golfer's elbow)

Many contact and non-contact sports can cause physical injury, although serious injuries are rather

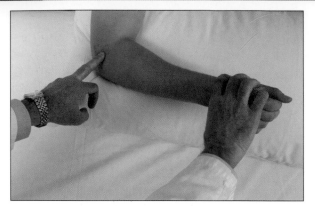

Figure 9.68 Examination of the elbow
Looking for signs of lateral epicondylitis. Palpation over the forearm extensor muscle origin elicits pain. Straining the muscles by resisted extension of the wrist exacerbates the symptoms.

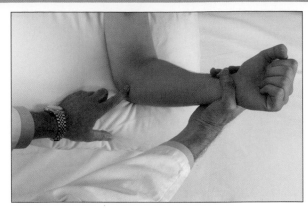

Figure 9.69 Examination to elicit signs of medial epicondylitis
Local pressure over the medial epicondyle elicits pain. Symptoms are exacerbated by resisted flexion of the wrist and fingers.

uncommon with certain sports (e.g. synchronised swimming). There may be pain over the epicondyles of the elbow. The *lateral epicondyle* is the most often affected and is called 'tennis elbow'. Pain arises from the site of insertion of the extensor muscle tendons into the lateral epicondyle (enthesis). Involvement of the medial epicondyle at the site of insertion of the flexor tendons of the forearm causes medial epicondylitis—'golfer's elbow'. These conditions are also common in manual workers such as painters.

Examination. Examine for local tenderness over the lateral (Figure 9.68) or medial epicondyle (Figure 9.69). Ask the patient to extend the fingers against resistance (Figure 9.70). This will make the pain of lateral epicondylitis worse. Ask the patient to flex the fingers against resistance. This will exacerbate the pain of medial epicondylitis.

Tenosynovitis of the wrist

Inflammation of the synovial tubes in which tendons run can occur in patients with rheumatoid arthritis but also in otherwise healthy people. The cause is often unaccustomed repetitive movement. A common site for tenosynovitis is at the wrist, where it involves the long extensor and abductor tendons of the thumb (de Quervain's tenosynovitis; Figure 9.71).

Examination. This reveals tenderness and swelling on the radial side of the wrist (radial styloid). There is pain on active or passive movement of the thumb. Confirm the diagnosis by performing Finkelstein's test.[z] Hold the patient's hand with the thumb tucked

into the palm and then quickly turn the wrist into full ulnar deviation (Figure 9.72). An alternative approach that is reported to produce fewer false-positives involves gripping the patient's thumb rather than tucking the thumb into the palm.[13] Sharp pain will occur in the tendon sheath when the test is positive. Examine also the other common sites of tendon involvement—the flexor tendons of the fingers and the Achilles tendon.

Bursitis

Bursae are found in areas exposed to mechanical strain or trauma, either at the site where muscle or tendon glides over bone or muscle, or superficially where bony prominences are exposed to mechanical stress. Bursitis usually occurs as a local soft-tissue inflammatory reaction to unusual mechanical pressure. It may be associated with rheumatoid arthritis, gout or sepsis. Common sites include the prepatellar area (housemaid's knee) (Figure 9.73), over the olecranon (olecranon bursitis) and over the greater trochanter (trochanteric bursitis).

Nerve entrapment syndromes

These are caused by compression of peripheral nerves at vulnerable sites and are associated with pain, paraesthesiae and numbness in a particular nerve distribution.

Carpal tunnel syndrome

Compression of the median nerve at the wrist is the most frequent form. This seems hardly

---

z   Harry Finkelstein (1865–1939), surgeon, Hospital for Joint Diseases, New York.

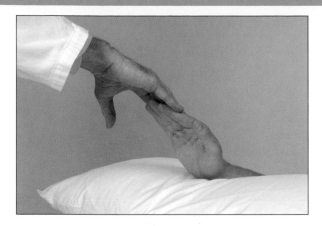

Figure 9.70 Testing for lateral epicondylitis

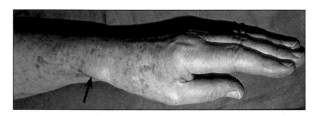

Figure 9.71 A patient with de Quervain's tenosynovitis
There is characteristic swelling of the tendon sheath of the abductor pollicis brevis over the styloid process of the radius.

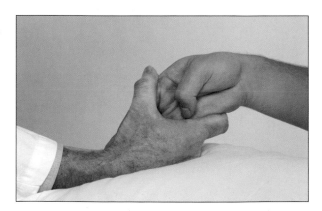

Figure 9.72 Finkelstein's test

wake patients from sleep and may radiate up the forearm (one-third of cases). The commonest cause is an overuse tenosynovitis of the flexor tendon sheaths at the wrist. Fluid retention during pregnancy or from use of the oral contraceptive pill can also produce carpal tunnel symptoms. In addition, median nerve compression can occur in rheumatoid arthritis, hypothyroidism, acromegaly and amyloidosis.

Examination. Symptoms can be reproduced by gentle percussion over the carpal tunnel while the wrist is held in extension (Tinel's sign). This sign is negative in up to 30% of patients with electrophysiologically proven median nerve compression. Prolonged (60 seconds) passive wrist flexion (Phalen's test) has a lower false-negative rate (positive LR 1.3, negative LR 0.7).[10] Look for wasting in the median nerve distribution, and loss of motor (thenar muscle strength: weak thumb abduction) and sensory function. These signs occur only in advanced cases.

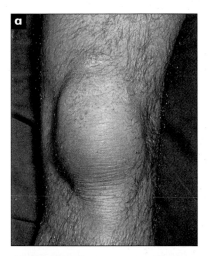

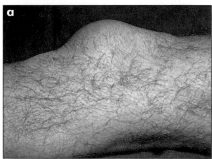

Figure 9.73 A red, swollen and painful prepatellar bursa
(a) Anterior view. (b) Lateral view.

surprising when one remembers that the carpal tunnel, sandwiched between the carpal bones and the carpal ligament, contains 9 flexor tendons as well as the median nerve. These patients complain of numbness and paraesthesiae in the median nerve distribution (the 3 radial fingers and the radial side of the ring finger). Symptoms often

Meralgia[aa] paraesthetica

Compression of the lateral cutaneous nerve of the thigh causes paraesthesiae and sensory loss over the lateral side of the thigh (page 375). This entirely sensory nerve passes through the lateral part of the inguinal ligament only just medial to the anterior superior iliac spine. Here it is subject to compression in patients who are obese, wear tight or heavy belts or spend long periods sitting. Diabetes, pregnancy and trauma can also be causes of problems with the nerve.

Tarsal tunnel syndrome

This may be caused by compression of the posterior tibial nerve in its fibro-osseous canal formed by the flexor retinaculum and the tarsal bones. Symptoms include burning pain and paraesthesiae in toe, sole and heel. Patients are often woken with pain at night and, as with the carpal tunnel syndrome, this may radiate upwards. Walking may improve the symptoms. Causes include diabetes, synovitis from rheumatoid arthritis, bony deformity and flexor tenosynovitis. Hypertrophy of the abductor hallucis muscle, which occurs in intemperate runners, is an occasional cause.

Examination. There is usually tenderness over the nerve posterior to the medial malleolus. There may be a positive Tinel's sign over the tarsal tunnel. Motor findings include weakness of toe flexion and of the intrinsic muscles of the foot.

Morton's 'neuroma'

This is caused by compression of one or more of the interdigital plantar nerves by the transverse metatarsal ligament. Patients complain of a burning pain or ache that extends distally from the affected web space to the toes (most often the third and fourth).

Metatarsalgia is a non-localised ache that spreads across the forefoot involving the area of some or all of the metatarsal heads. It can occur in normal feet after prolonged standing but also occurs in a number of other foot conditions (Table 9.19), and is often associated with poor-fitting shoes. *Morton's metatarsalgia* is interdigital nerve entrapment (usually between the third and fourth metatarsal bones. Patients describe burning pain between the metatarsal bones and may have numbness on the adjacent toes. They get relief by removing their shoes and massaging the foot.

TABLE 9.19 Causes of metatarsalgia

Tight or pointed shoes
Atrophy of metatarsal fat pad in elderly people
Plantar calluses
Metatarsophalangeal joint arthritis
Flat or cavus foot deformity
Overlapping toes
Interdigital entrapment
Hemiplegia
Peripheral vascular disease

Examination. There is often tenderness between the involved metatarsal heads, and a painful nodule may be palpable.

References

1. Van den Hoogen HMM, Koes BW, Van Eijk JTM, Bouter LM. On the accuracy of history, physical, and the erythrocyte sedimentation rate in diagnosing low back pain in general practice: a criteria based review of the literature. *Spine* 1995; 20:318–327. Unfortunately, distinguishing mechanical from non-mechanical causes of low back pain such as ankylosing spondylitis is clinically difficult. However, tenderness to pressure over the anterior superior iliac spines and over the lower sacrum may, based on other studies, be somewhat helpful for the positive diagnosis of ankylosing spondylitis.

2. Deyo RA, Rainville J, Kent DL. What can the history and physical examination tell us about low back pain? *JAMA* 1992; 268:760–765.

3. Fuchs HA. Joint counts and physical measures. *Rheum Dis Clin Nth Am* 1995; 21:429–444. Describes useful quantitative methods to evaluate tenderness, pain on motion, swelling, deformity and limitation of movement.

4. Katz JN, Larson ME, Sabra A et al. The carpal syndrome: diagnostic utility of the history and physical examination findings. *Ann Intern Med* 1990; 112:321–327. This study compares the neurophysiological assessment of the carpal tunnel syndrome with the information obtained by examination and history. No single symptom or sign is sufficiently predictive.

5. Glockner SM. Shoulder pain: a diagnostic dilemma. *Am Fam Phys* 1995; 51:1677–1687, 1690–1692. Reviews the utility of symptoms and signs in differential diagnosis.

6. Katz JN, Dalgas M, Stucki G et al. Degenerative lumbar spinal stenosis. Diagnostic value of the history and physical examination. *Arth Rheum* 1995; 38:1236–1241. Describes symptoms (severe lower limb pain which is absent when the patient is seated) and signs (including a wide-based gait,

---

[aa] The Greek word *meros* means thigh and *algia* means painful.

positive Romberg's sign, thigh pain with lumbar extension) that help predict this rare condition in older patients.

7. Murtagh J. Diagnosis of early osteoarthritis of the hip joint: the four-step stress test. *Aust Fam Phys* 1990; 19:389. Discusses the diagnosis of osteoarthritis of the hip in a systematic way, suggesting a four-step approach.

8. Solomon DH, Simel DL, Bates DW et al. Does this patient have a torn meniscus or ligament of the knee? *JAMA* 2001; 286: 1610–1620.

9. Scholten RJ, Opstetten W, vander Plas CG et al. Accuracy of physical diagnostic tests for assessing ruptures of the anterior cruciate ligament: a meta-analysis. *J Fam Pract* 2003; 52:689–694.

10. McGee S. *Evidence-based clinical diagnosis*, 2nd edn. Phildelphia: Saunders, 2007.

11. Grob JJ, Bonerandi JJ. Cutaneous manifestations associated with the presence of the lupus-anticoagulant. *J Am Acad Dermatol* 1986; 15:211–219. Antiphospholipid antibody syndrome can be associated with leg ulcers (that resemble pyoderma gangrenosum), livedo reticularis and fingertip ischaemia.

12. Stevens GL, Adelman HM, Wallach PM. Palpable purpura: an algorithmic approach. *Am Fam Phys* 1995; 52:1355–1362.

13. Elliott BG. Finkelstein's test: a descriptive error that can produce a false-positive. *J Hand Surg Br* 1992; 17:481–482. Careful explanation of the performance of this test (which is often misunderstood) appears in this article. Movement with the thumb folded into the hand can produce a false-positive result.

Suggested reading

Hochberg M, Silman AJ, Smolen JS, Weinblatt ME, Weisman MH. *Rheumatology*, 4th edn. St Louis: Mosby, 2008.

Snaith ML. *ABC of rheumatology*, 3rd edn. London: BMJ Publishing Group, 2004.

Solomon L, Nayagam D, Warwiak D. *Apley's system of orthopaedics and fractures*, 9th edn. London: Butterworth-Heineman, 2009.

Chapter 10

The endocrine system

A physician is obligated to consider more than a diseased organ, more even than the whole man—he must view the man in his world.

Harvey Cushing (1869–1939)

The endocrine history

Presenting symptoms (Table 10.1)

Hormones control so many aspects of body function that the manifestations of endocrine disease are protean. Symptoms can include changes in body weight, appetite, bowel habit, hair distribution, pigmentation, sweating, height and menstruation, galactorrhoea (unexpected breast-milk production—in men and women), as well as polydipsia, polyuria, lethargy, headaches and loss of libido and erectile dysfunction. Many of these symptoms have other causes as well and must be carefully evaluated. On the other hand, the patient may know which endocrine organ or group of endocrine organs has been causing a problem. In particular, there may be a history of a thyroid condition or diabetes mellitus. A list of common symptoms associated with various endocrine diseases is presented in Table 10.1. In this section some of the important symptoms associated with endocrine disease will be discussed.

Changes in appetite and weight

An increased appetite associated with weight loss classically occurs in thyrotoxicosis or uncontrolled diabetes mellitus. An increased appetite with weight gain may occur in Cushing's syndrome, hypoglycaemia or in hypothalamic disease. A loss of appetite with weight loss can occur with adrenal insufficiency but is also seen in anorexia nervosa and with gastrointestinal disease (particularly malignancy). A loss of appetite with weight gain can occur in hypothyroidism.

Changes in bowel habit

Diarrhoea and an increase in the frequency of bowel movements are associated with hyperthyroidism and adrenal insufficiency, while constipation may occur in hypothyroidism and hypercalcaemia.

Changes in sweating

Increased sweating is characteristic of hyperthyroidism, phaeochromocytoma, hypoglycaemia and acromegaly, but may also occur in anxiety states and at the menopause (page 411).

Changes in hair distribution

Hirsutism refers to an increased growth of body hair in women. The clinical evaluation and differential diagnosis are presented on page 315. The absence of facial hair in a man suggests hypogonadism, while temporal recession of the scalp hair in women occurs with androgen excess. The decrease in adrenal androgen production that occurs as a result of hypogonadism, hypopituitarism or adrenal insufficiency can cause loss of axillary and pubic hair in both sexes.

Lethargy

This common symptom can be due to a number of different diseases. Patients with hypothyroidism, Addison's disease and diabetes mellitus can present with this problem. Anaemia, connective tissue diseases, chronic infection (e.g. HIV, infective endocarditis), drugs (e.g. sedatives, diuretics causing electrolyte disturbances), chronic liver disease, renal failure and occult malignancy may also result in lethargy. Importantly, depression is a common cause of this symptom (page 411).

TABLE 10.1 Endocrine history

Major symptoms
Appetite and weight changes
Disturbed defecation
Sweating
Hair distribution
Lethargy
Skin changes
Pigmentation
Stature
Loss of libido, erectile dysfunction
Menstruation
Polyuria
Lump in the neck (goitre)

Endocrine abnormalities and typical symptoms and signs

Thyrotoxicosis: preference for cooler weather, weight loss, increased appetite (polyphagia), palpitations, increased sweating, nervousness, irritability, diarrhoea, amenorrhoea, muscle weakness, exertional dyspnoea

Hypothyroidism (myxoedema): preference for warmer weather, lethargy, swelling of eyelids (oedema), hoarse voice, constipation, coarse skin, hypercarotenaemia

Diabetes mellitus: polyuria, polydipsia, thirst, blurred vision, weakness, infections, groin itch, rash (pruritus vulvae, balanitis), weight loss, tiredness, lethargy, disturbance of conscious state

Hypoglycaemia: morning headaches, weight gain, seizures, sweating

Primary adrenal insufficiency: pigmentation, tiredness, loss of weight, anorexia, nausea, diarrhoea, nocturia, mental changes, seizures (hypotension, hypoglycaemia)

Acromegaly: fatigue, weakness, increased sweating, heat intolerance, weight gain, enlarging hands and feet, enlarged and coarsened facial features, headaches, decreased vision, voice change, decreased libido, erectile dysfunction (impotence)

Cushing's syndrome: truncal obesity, purple striae, moon-like facies, buffalo hump, myopathy, bruises

Changes in the skin and nails

The skin becomes coarse, pale and dry in hypothyroidism, and dry and scaly in hypoparathyroidism. Flushing of the skin of the face and neck occurs in the carcinoid syndrome (due to the release of vasoactive peptides from the tumour). Soft-tissue overgrowth occurs in acromegaly and skin tags may appear in the axillae. These are called molluscum fibrinosum. Acanthosis nigricans can also occur in acromegaly and in insulin-resistant states including Cushing's syndrome and polycystic ovarian syndrome. Xanthelasma can be present in patients with diabetes or hypothyroidism.

Onycholysis occurs in Graves' disease and

Cushing's syndrome is associated with spontaneous ecchymoses, thin skin and purple striae.

Changes in pigmentation

Increased pigmentation may be reported in primary adrenal insufficiency, Cushing's syndrome or acromegaly. Decreased pigmentation occurs in hypopituitarism. Localised depigmentation is characteristic of vitiligo, which may be associated with certain endocrine diseases such as Hashimoto's[a] disease with hypothyroidism and Addison's disease with adrenal insufficiency as well as other auto-immune conditions.

Changes in stature

Tallness may occur in children for constitutional reasons (tall parents) or, rarely, may reflect growth hormone excess (leading to gigantism), gonadotrophin deficiency, Klinefelter's syndrome[b], Marfan's syndrome or generalised lipodystrophy. Short stature can also result from endocrine disease, as discussed on page 313.

Erectile dysfunction (impotence)

A persistent inability to attain or sustain penile erections may occasionally be due to primary hypogonadism or to secondary hypogonadism due to hyperprolactinaemia or hypopituitarism. More often, it is related to emotional disorders. Vascular disease, autonomic neuropathy (e.g. in diabetes mellitus or alcoholism), spinal cord disease or testicular atrophy can also cause this problem.

Galactorrhoea

Hyperprolactinaemia (usually the result of pituitary adenoma) can cause galactorrhoea in up to 80% of women and 30% of men. Galactorrhoea in men occurs from a normal-appearing male breast.

Menstruation

Failure to menstruate is termed *amenorrhoea*.

Primary amenorrhoea is defined as a failure to start menstruating by 17 years of age. True primary amenorrhoea may result from ovarian failure (e.g. X chromosomal abnormalities such as Turner's syndrome) or from pituitary or hypothalamic disease (e.g. tumour, trauma or idiopathic disease). Excess androgen production or systemic disease (e.g. malabsorption, chronic renal failure, obesity) can also result in primary amenorrhoea.

Apparent primary amenorrhoea can also occur

a   Hakaru Hashimoto (1881–1934), Japanese surgeon.
b   Harry Fitch Klinefelter (b. 1912), Baltimore physician, described the condition when he was a medical student.

if menstrual flow cannot escape: for example, if there is an imperforate hymen.

Secondary amenorrhoea is defined as the cessation of menstruation for 6 months or more. Pregnancy and menopause are common causes. The polycystic ovarian syndrome, hyperprolactinaemia, virilising syndromes or hypothalamic or pituitary disease can also result in this problem, as can use of the contraceptive pill or psychiatric disease.

Polyuria

Polyuria is defined as a urine volume of more than 3 litres/day. Patients who report urinary frequency may find it difficult to tell if large volumes of urine are being passed. Causes include diabetes mellitus (due to excessive filtration of glucose, a poorly resorbed solute); diabetes insipidus (due to inadequate renal water conservation from a central deficiency of antidiuretic hormone, or a lack of renal responsiveness to this hormone); primary polydipsia, where a patient drinks excessive water (due to psychogenic or hypothalamic disease or drugs such as chlorpromazine or thioridazine); hypercalcaemia; and tubulointerstitial or cystic renal disease.

Past history

A previous history of any endocrine condition must be uncovered. This includes surgery on the neck for a goitre. A partial thyroidectomy or radio-iodine (^{131}I) treatment in the past can lead to eventual hypothyroidism. The same may apply to radiation of the thyroid for carcinoma. A woman may have been diagnosed with diabetes mellitus after the birth of a large baby. There may be a past history of hypertension, which is occasionally due to an endocrine condition (e.g. phaeochromocytoma, Cushing's syndrome or Conn's syndrome). Previous thyroid surgery can be associated with hypoparathyroidism because of surgical damage to the parathyroid glands.

Previous treatment of a patient's thyroid problems may have included the use of antithyroid drugs, thyroid hormone or radioactive iodine. Surgery on the adrenals or pituitary may have been performed and this may leave the patient with decreased adrenal or pituitary function.

Patients with diabetes mellitus have an important chronic condition (*Questions box 10.7*, page 316). Treatment may be with diet, insulin or oral hypoglycaemic agents. One must determine how well the patient understands the condition, and whether he or she understands the principles of the diabetic diet and adheres to it. Find out how the blood sugar levels are monitored and whether

or not the patient adjusts the insulin dose. Most patients should now be able to monitor their own blood sugar levels at home using a glucometer. There is now good evidence that tight control of blood sugar levels reduces the incidence of diabetic complications. Patients should have records of home blood sugar measurements, and may know the results of tests such as the haemoglobin A1c (a measure of average blood sugar levels) and of tests of renal function and for protein in the urine.

The patient should be aware of the need for care of the feet and eyes to help prevent complications. Most diabetics have regular ophthalmological review, often using retinal photography. There may be a history of laser treatment for proliferative diabetic retinopathy.

Patients with hypopituitarism or hypoadrenalism may be on glucocorticoid (steroid) replacement; the latter also require mineralocorticoid replacement. Details of the patient's dosage schedule should be obtained.

Social history

Many of these conditions are chronic and their complications serious. How well the patient copes with various problems and the conditions at home and work will have an important effect on the success of treatment.

Family history

There may be a history in the family of thyroid conditions or diabetes mellitus. Occasionally a family history of a multiple endocrine neoplasia (MEN) syndrome may be obtained. These are rare autosomal-dominant conditions. They include pituitary tumours, medullary carcinoma of the thyroid, hyperparathyroidism, phaeochromocytoma and pancreatic islet cell tumours.

The endocrine examination

A formal examination of the whole endocrine system is set out on page 322. Usually there will be some clue from the history and general inspection to indicate what specific endocrine diseases should be pursued.

The thyroid
The thyroid gland[c]

Examination anatomy. Even when it is not enlarged, the thyroid (Figure 10.2) is the largest

---

c   The first person to distinguish an enlarged thyroid from cervical lymphadenopathy was the Roman medical writer Aulus Aurelius Cornelius Celsus (53 BC–7 AD). He is more famous for describing the four cardinal signs of inflammation: redness, swelling, heat and tenderness.

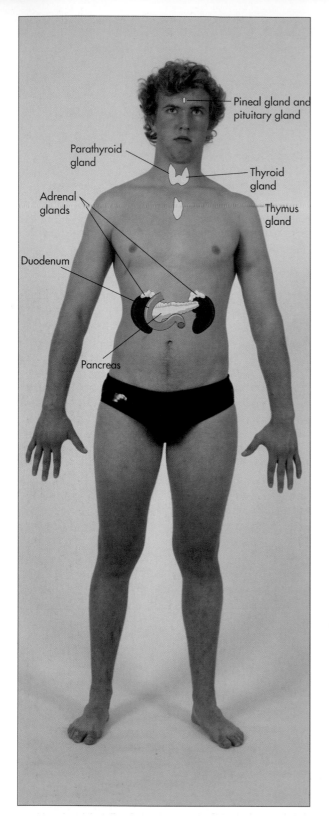

Figure 10.1 The endocrine glands

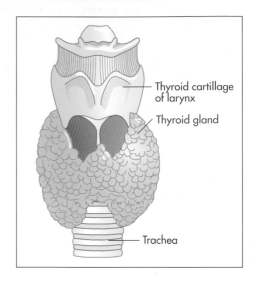

Figure 10.2 The anatomy of the thyroid

endocrine gland. Enlargement is common, occurring in 10% of women and 2% of men and more commonly in iodine-deficient parts of the world. The normal gland lies anterior to the larynx and trachea and below the laryngeal prominence of the thyroid cartilage. It consists of a narrow isthmus in the middle line (anterior to the second to fourth tracheal rings and 1.5 cm in size), and two larger lateral lobes each about 4 cm long. Although the position of the larynx varies, the thyroid gland is almost always about 4 cm below the larynx.

Inspection. The normal thyroid may be just visible below the cricoid cartilage in a thin young person (Table 10.2).[1,2]. Usually only the isthmus is visible as a diffuse central swelling. Enlargement of the gland, called a goitre (Latin *guttur*, 'throat'), should be apparent on inspection (see *Good signs guide 10.1*), especially if the patient extends the neck. Look at the front and sides of the neck and decide whether there is localised or general swelling of the gland. In normal people the line between the cricoid cartilage and the suprasternal notch should be straight. An outward bulge suggests the presence of a goitre (Figure 10.3). Remember that 80% of people with a goitre are biochemically euthyroid, 10% are hypothyroid and 10% are hyperthyroid.

The temptation to begin touching a swelling as soon as it has been detected should be resisted until a glass of water has been procured. The patient takes sips from this repeatedly so that swallowing is possible without discomfort. Ask the patient to swallow, and watch the neck swelling carefully.

TABLE 10.2 Causes of neck swellings

Midline

Goitre (moves up on swallowing)

Thyroglossal cyst (moves on poking out the tongue with the jaw stationary)

Submental lymph nodes

Lateral

Lymph nodes*

Salivary glands (e.g. stone, tumour)
- Submandibular gland
- Parotid gland (lower pole)

Skin: sebaceous cyst or lipoma

Lymphatics: cystic hygroma (translucent)

Carotid artery: aneurysm or rarely tumour (pulsatile)

Pharynx: pharyngeal pouch, or brachial arch remnant (brachial cyst)

Parathyroid gland (very rare)

* Aulus Celsus (page 297), the Roman medical writer who was active early in the 1st century AD, was the first to publish work distinguishing a goitre from cervical lymphadenopathy.

GOOD SIGNS GUIDE 10.1 Detection of a goitre (compared with ultrasound findings)

Sign	Positive LR	Negative LR*
No goitre on inspection or palpation	0.4	—
Goitre palpated and visible only on neck extension	NS	—
Goitre palpated and visible with neck in normal position	26.3	—

NS = not significant.

* No values available.

From McGee S, *Evidence-based physical diagnosis*, 2nd edn. St Louis: Saunders, 2007.

Only a goitre or a thyroglossal cyst, because of attachment to the larynx, will rise during swallowing. The thyroid and trachea rise about 2 cm as the patient swallows; they pause for half a second and then descend. Some non-thyroid masses may rise slightly during swallowing but move up less than the trachea and fall again without pausing. A thyroid gland fixed by neoplastic infiltration may not rise on swallowing, but this is rare. Swallowing also allows the shape of the gland to be seen better.

It should be noted whether an inferior border is visible as the gland rises. The thyroglossal cyst is a midline mass that can present at any age. It is an embryological remnant of the thyroglossal duct. Characteristically it rises when the patient protrudes the tongue.

Inspect the skin of the neck for scars. A thyroidectomy scar forms a ring around the base of the neck in the position of a high necklace. Also look for prominent veins. Dilated veins over the upper part of the chest wall, often accompanied by filling of the external jugular vein, suggest retrosternal extension of the goitre (thoracic inlet obstruction). Rarely, redness of the skin over the gland occurs in cases of suppurative thyroiditis.

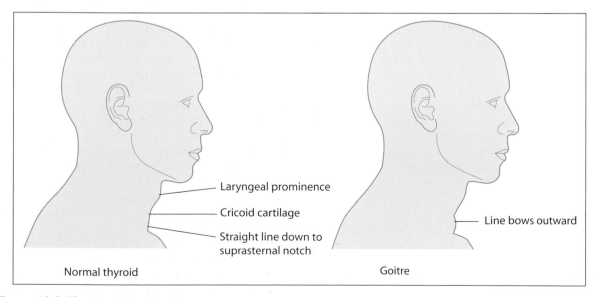

Normal thyroid — Laryngeal prominence / Cricoid cartilage / Straight line down to suprasternal notch

Goitre — Line bows outward

Figure 10.3 The thyroid and goitre

(Adapted from McGee S, *Evidence-based physical diagnosis*, 2nd edition, St Louis, Saunders, 2007.)

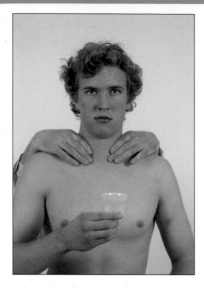

Figure 10.4 Palpating the thyroid from behind while the patient swallows sips of water

TABLE 10.3 Differential diagnosis of thyroid nodules
1 Carcinoma (5% of palpable nodules)—fixed to surrounding tissues, palpable lymph nodes, vocal cord paralysis, hard, larger than 4 cm (most are, however, smaller than this)
2 Adenoma—mobile, no local associated features
3 Big nodule in a multinodular goitre—palpable multinodular goitre

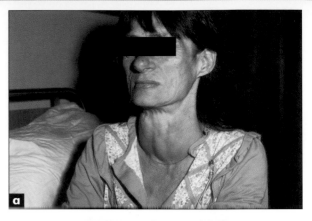

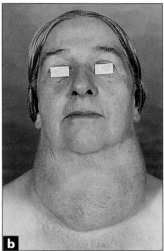

Figure 10.5 Goitre: (a) large; (b) massive

Palpation. Palpation is best begun from *behind* (Figure 10.4) but warn the patient. Both hands are placed with the pulps of the fingers over the gland. The patient's neck should be slightly flexed so as to relax the sternomastoid muscles. Feel systematically both lobes of the gland and its isthmus.

Consider the following:

- **Size:** only an approximate estimation is possible (Figure 10.5). Feel particularly carefully for a lower border, because its absence suggests retrosternal extension.
- **Shape:** note whether the gland is uniformly enlarged or irregular and whether the isthmus is affected. If a *nodule* that feels distinct from the remaining thyroid tissue is palpable, determine its location, size, consistency, tenderness and mobility. Also decide whether the whole gland feels nodular (multinodular goitre).
- **Consistency:** may vary in different parts of the gland. Soft is normal; the gland is often firm in simple goitre and typically rubbery hard in Hashimoto's thyroiditis. A stony, hard node suggests carcinoma (Table 10.3), calcification in a cyst, fibrosis or Riedel's thyroiditis.
- **Tenderness:** a feature of thyroiditis (subacute or rarely suppurative), or less often of a bleed into a cyst or carcinoma.
- **Mobility:** carcinoma may tether the gland.

Repeat the assessment while the patient swallows.

Decide if a thrill is palpable over the gland, as occurs when the gland is unusually metabolically active as in thyrotoxicosis.

Palpate the cervical lymph nodes (page 228). These may be involved in carcinoma of the thyroid.

Move to the *front*. Palpate again. Localised swellings may be more easily defined here. Note the position of the trachea, which may be displaced by a retrosternal gland.

TABLE 10.4 Goitre

Causes of a diffuse goitre (patient often euthyroid)

Idiopathic (majority)

Puberty or pregnancy

Thyroiditis
- Hashimoto's
- Subacute (gland usually tender)

Simple goitre (iodine deficiency)

Goitrogens—iodine excess, drugs (e.g. lithium)

Inborn errors of thyroid hormone synthesis—e.g. Pendred's* syndrome (an autosomal-recessive condition associated with nerve deafness)

Causes of a solitary thyroid nodule

Benign:
- Dominant nodule in a multinodular goitre
- Degeneration or haemorrhage into a colloid cyst or nodule
- Follicular adenoma
- Simple cyst (rare)

Malignant:
- Carcinoma—primary or secondary (rare)
- Lymphoma (rare)

*   Vaughan Pendred (b. 1869), London physician.

Percussion. The upper part of the manubrium can be percussed from one side to the other. A change from resonant to dull indicates a possible retrosternal goitre, but this is not a very reliable sign.

Auscultation. Listen over each lobe for a bruit (a swishing sound coinciding with systole). This is a sign of increased blood supply which may occur in hyperthyroidism, or occasionally from the use of antithyroid drugs. The differential diagnosis also includes a carotid bruit (louder over the carotid itself) or a venous hum (obliterated by gentle pressure over the base of the neck). If there is a goitre, apply mild compression to the lateral lobes and listen again for stridor.

Pemberton's sign. Ask the patient to lift both arms as high as possible. Wait a few moments, then search the face eagerly for signs of congestion (plethora) and cyanosis. Associated respiratory distress and inspiratory stridor may occur. Look at the neck veins for distension (venous congestion). Ask the patient to take a deep breath in through the mouth and listen for stridor. This is a test for thoracic inlet obstruction due to a retrosternal goitre or any retrosternal mass.[3] (Lifting the arms up pulls the thoracic inlet upward so that the goitre occupies more of this inflexible bony opening.)

Examination of the thyroid should be part of every routine physical examination. Causes of a goitre are listed in Table 10.4.

Hyperthyroidism (thyrotoxicosis)

This is a disease caused by excessive concentrations of thyroid hormones. The cause is usually over-production by the gland but may sometimes be due to accidental or deliberate use of thyroid hormone (thyroxine) tablets; *thyrotoxicosis factitia*. Thyroxine is sometimes taken by patients as a way of losing weight. The cause may be apparent in these cases if a careful history is taken (*Questions box 10.1*). The anti-arrhythmic drug *amiodarone* which contains large quantities of iodine can cause thyrotoxicosis in up to 12% of patients in low-iodine-intake areas.

Many of the clinical features of thyrotoxicosis

Questions box 10.1

Questions to ask the patient with suspected hyperthyroidism

! **denotes symptoms for the possible diagnosis of an urgent or dangerous problem.**

1   Have you any history of thyroid problems?

2   Have you a family history of thyrotoxicosis?—There is a familial incidence of Graves disease and associated auto-immune conditions such as vitiligo, Addison's disease, pernicious anaemia, type 1 diabetes, myasthenia gravis and premature ovarian failure

3   Have you taken amiodarone or thyroxine?

4   Have you had recent exposure to iodine?—Iodinated X-ray contrast materials can precipitate thyrotoxicosis (usually in patients with an existing multinodular goitre)

!   5   Have you had palpitations?—Thyrotoxicosis can present with atrial fibrillation which may precipitate heart failure

6   Have you noticed insomnia, irritability or hyperactivity?

7   Have you had loss of weight, diarrhoea or increased stool frequency, increased sweating or heat intolerance?

8   Have you had muscle weakness?—Proximal muscle weakness is common and the patient may have noticed difficulty getting out of a chair

9   Have you had eye problems such as double vision, grittiness, redness or pain behind the eyes?

GOOD SIGNS GUIDE 10.2 Thyrotoxicosis

Sign	Positive LR	Negative LR
Pulse		
≥90/min	4.4	0.2
Skin		
Moist and warm	6.7	0.7
Thyroid		
Enlarged	2.3	0.1
Eyes		
Eyelid retraction	31.5	0.7
Lid lag	17.6	0.8
Neurological		
Fine tremor	11.4	0.3

From McGee S, *Evidence-based physical diagnosis,* 2nd edn. St Louis: Saunders, 2007.

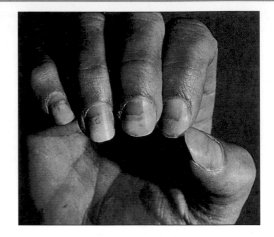

Figure 10.6 Onycholysis (Plummer's nails)

are characterised by signs of sympathetic nervous system overactivity such as tremor, tachycardia and sweating. The explanation is not entirely clear. Catecholamine secretion is usually normal in hyperthyroidism; however, thyroid hormone potentiates the effects of catecholamines, possibly by increasing the number of adrenergic receptors in the tissues.

The commonest cause of thyrotoxicosis in young people is Graves' disease,[d] an autoimmune disease where circulating immunoglobulins stimulate thyroid stimulating hormone (TSH) receptors on the surface of the thyroid follicular cells.

Examine a suspected case of thyrotoxicosis as follows (see *Good signs guide 10.2*).

General inspection. Look for signs of weight loss, anxiety and the frightened facies of thyrotoxicosis.

The hands. Ask the patient to put out his or her arms and look for a fine tremor (due to sympathetic overactivity). Laying a sheet of paper over the patient's fingers may more clearly demonstrate this tremor, to the amazement of less-experienced colleagues.

Look at the nails for *onycholysis* (Plummer's[e] nails) (Figure 10.6). Onycholysis (where there is separation of the nail from its bed) is said to occur particularly on the ring finger, but can occur on all the fingernails, and is apparently due to sympathetic

overactivity. Inspect now for thyroid acropathy (acropathy is another term for clubbing), seen rarely in Graves' disease but not with other causes of thyrotoxicosis.

Inspect for palmar erythema and feel the palms for warmth and sweatiness (sympathetic overactivity).

Take the pulse. Note the presence of sinus tachycardia (sympathetic overdrive) or atrial fibrillation (due to a shortened refractory period of atrial cells related to sympathetic drive and hormone-induced changes). The pulse may also have a collapsing character due to a high cardiac output.

Test for proximal myopathy and tap the arm reflexes for abnormal briskness, especially in the relaxation phase.

The eyes. Examine the eyes for exophthalmos, which is protrusion of the eyeball from the orbit (Figure 10.7, Table 10.5). This may be very obvious,

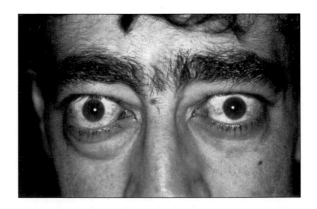

Figure 10.7 Thyrotoxicosis: thyroid stare and exophthalmos

---

d   Robert Graves (1796–1853), Dublin physician.
e   Henry Plummer (1874–1936), physician at the Mayo Clinic, USA.

TABLE 10.5 Causes of exophthalmos

Bilateral
Graves' disease
Unilateral
Tumours of the orbit: e.g. dermoid, optic nerve glioma, neurofibroma, granuloma
Cavernous sinus thrombosis
Graves' disease
Pseudotumours of the orbit

but if not, look carefully at the sclerae, which in exophthalmos are not covered by the lower eyelid. Next look from behind over the patient's forehead for exophthalmos, where the eye will be visible anterior to the superior orbital margin. Now examine for the complications of proptosis, which include: (i) chemosis (oedema of the conjunctiva and injection of the sclera, particularly over the insertion of the lateral rectus); (ii) conjunctivitis; (iii) corneal ulceration (due to inability to close the eyelids); (iv) optic atrophy (rare and possibly due to optic nerve stretching); and (v) ophthalmoplegia (the inferior rectus muscle power tends to be lost first, and later convergence is weakened).

The mechanism of exophthalmos is uncertain. It occurs only in Graves' disease. It may precede the onset of thyrotoxicosis, or may persist after the patient has become euthyroid. It is characterised by an inflammatory infiltrate of the orbital contents, but not of the globe itself. The orbital muscles are particularly affected, and an increase in their size accounts for most of the increased volume of the orbital contents and therefore for protrusion of the globe. It is probably due to an autoimmune abnormality.

Next examine for the components of thyroid ophthalmopathy, which are related to sympathetic overactivity and are not specific for Graves' disease. Look for the thyroid stare (a frightened expression) and lid retraction (Dalrymple's sign[f]), where there is sclera visible above the iris. Test for lid lag (von Graefe's sign[g]) by asking the patient to follow your finger as it descends at a moderate rate from the upper to the lower part of the visual field. Descent of the upper lid lags behind descent of the eyeball.

If ptosis is present, one should rule out myasthenia gravis, which can be associated with autoimmune disease.

The neck. Examine for thyroid enlargement, which is usually detectable (60%–90% of patients). In Graves' disease the gland is classically diffusely enlarged and is smooth and firm. An associated thrill is usually present but this finding is not specific for thyrotoxicosis caused by Graves' disease. Absence of thyroid enlargement makes Graves' disease unlikely, but does not exclude it. Possible thyroid abnormalities in patients who are thyrotoxic but do not have Graves' disease include a toxic multinodular goitre, a solitary nodule (toxic adenoma), and painless, postpartum or subacute (de Quervain's[h]) thyroiditis. In de Quervain's thyroiditis there is typically a moderately enlarged firm and tender gland. Thyrotoxicosis may occur without any goitre, particularly in elderly patients. Alternatively, in hyperthyroidism due to a rare abnormality of trophoblastic tissue (a hydatidiform mole or choriocarcinoma of the testis or uterus), or excessive thyroid hormone replacement, the thyroid gland will not usually be palpable.

If a thyroidectomy scar is present, assess for hypoparathyroidism (Chvostek's[i] or Trousseau's[j] signs; page 311). These signs are most often present in the first few days after operation.

The arms. Ask the patient to raise the arms above the head and so test for proximal myopathy.

The chest. Gynaecomastia (page 315) occurs occasionally. Examine the heart for systolic flow murmurs (due to increased cardiac output) and signs of congestive cardiac failure, which may be precipitated by thyrotoxicosis in older people.

The legs. Look first for pretibial myxoedema. This takes the form of bilateral firm, elevated dermal nodules and plaques, which can be pink, brown or skin-coloured. They are caused by mucopolysaccharide accumulation. Despite the name, this occurs only in Graves' disease and not in hypothyroidism. Test now for proximal myopathy and hyperreflexia in the legs which is present in only about a quarter of cases.

---

f   John Dalrymple (1803–52), British ophthalmic surgeon.
g   Friedrich von Graefe (1828–70), professor of ophthalmology in Berlin, described this in 1864. He was one of the most famous ophthalmologists of the 19th century; Horner was one of his pupils. He died of tuberculosis at the age of 42.

h   Fritz de Quervain (1868–1940), professor of surgery, Berne, Switzerland.
i   Franz Chvostek (1835–84), Viennese physician.
j   Armand Trousseau (1801–1867), Parisian physician.

TABLE 10.6 Thyrotoxicosis and hypothyroidism

Causes of thyrotoxicosis

Primary

Graves' disease

Toxic multinodular goitre

Toxic uninodular goitre: usually a toxic adenoma

Hashimoto's thyroiditis (early in its course; later it produces hypothyroidism)

Subacute thyroiditis (transient)

Postpartum thyroiditis (non-tender)

Iodine-induced ('Jod-Basedow phenomenon'*—iodine given after a previously deficient diet)

Secondary

Pituitary (very rare): TSH hypersecretion

Hydatidiform moles or choriocarcinomas: HCG secretion (rare)

Struma ovarii (rare)

Drugs, e.g. excess thyroid hormone ingestion, amiodarone

Causes of hypothyroidism

Primary

Without a goitre (decreased or absent thyroid tissue):
- Idiopathic atrophy
- Treatment of thyrotoxicosis—e.g. [131]I, surgery
- Agenesis or a lingual thyroid
- Unresponsiveness to TSH

With a goitre (decreased thyroid hormone synthesis):
- Chronic autoimmune diseases—e.g. Hashimoto's thyroiditis
- Drugs, e.g. lithium, amiodarone
- Inborn errors (enzyme deficiency)
- Endemic iodine deficiency or iodine-induced hypothyroidism

Secondary

Pituitary lesions (Table 10.8)

Tertiary

Hypothalamic lesions

Transient

Thyroid hormone treatment withdrawn

Subacute thyroiditis

Postpartum thyroiditis

---

* Carl von Basedow (1799–1854), German general practitioner, described this in 1840 (Jod = iodine in German).

TSH = thyroid stimulating hormone. HCG = human chorionic gonadotrophin.

Hypothyroidism (myxoedema)

Hypothyroidism (deficiency of thyroid hormone) is due to primary disease of the thyroid or, less commonly, is secondary to pituitary or hypothalamic failure (Table 10.6). Myxoedema implies a more severe form of hypothyroidism. In

Questions box 10.2

Questions to ask the patient with suspected hypothyroidism

1 Have you found cold weather more difficult to cope with recently?

2 Have you had problems with constipation?

3 Have you gained weight?

4 Have you noticed that your skin has become dry?

5 Do you think your memory is not as good as it was? Have you felt depressed?

6 Do you think your voice has become hoarse?—Hypothyroid speech (characteristically slow and nasal) occurs in one-third of patients

7 Have you noticed swelling of your legs?

GOOD SIGNS GUIDE 10.3 Hypothyroidism

Sign	Positive LR	Negative LR
Skin		
Coarse	5.6	0.7
Cool and dry	4.7	0.9
Cold palms	NS	NS
Dry palms	NS	NS
Periorbital puffiness	2.8	0.6
Puffiness of wrists	2.9	0.7
Loss of eyebrow hair	1.9	NS
Speech		
Hypothyroid speech	5.4	0.7
Thyroid gland		
Goitre	2.8	0.6
Pulse		
<70/min	4.1	0.8

NS = not significant.

From McGee S, *Evidence-based physical diagnosis*, 2nd edn. St Louis: Saunders, 2007.

---

myxoedema, for unknown reasons, hydrophilic mucopolysaccharides accumulate in the ground substance of tissues including the skin. This results in excessive interstitial fluid, which is relatively immobile, causing skin thickening and a doughy induration.

The symptoms of hypothyroidism are insidious but patients or their relatives may have noticed cold intolerance, muscle pains, oedema, constipation, a hoarse voice, dry skin, memory loss, depression or weight gain (*Questions box 10.2*).

Examine the patient with suspected hypothyroidism as follows (see *Good signs guide 10.3*).

General inspection. Look for signs of obvious mental and physical sluggishness, or evidence of the very rare 'myxoedema madness'. Hypothyroid speech is a feature in about a third of patients. This is characteristically slow, nasal and deep in pitch. Obesity is no more common than in euthyroid people.

The hands. Note peripheral cyanosis (due to reduced cardiac output) and swelling of the skin, which may appear cool and dry. The yellow discoloration of hypercarotenaemia (there is slowing down of hepatic metabolism of carotene) may be seen on the palms. Look for palmar crease pallor—anaemia may be due to: (i) chronic disease; (ii) folate deficiency secondary to bacterial overgrowth, or vitamin B_{12} deficiency due to associated pernicious anaemia; or (iii) iron deficiency due to menorrhagia.

Take the pulse, which may be of small volume and slow. Test for sensory loss, as the carpal tunnel is thickened in myxoedema.

The arms. Test for proximal myopathy (rare) and a 'hung-up' biceps or Achilles tendon reflex (see below).

The face. Inspect the face (Figure 10.8). The skin, but not the sclerae, may appear yellow due to hypercarotenaemia. The skin may be generally thickened, and alopecia may be present, as may

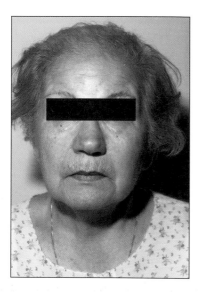

Figure 10.8 Myxoedema

vitiligo (an associated autoimmune disease).

Inspect the eyes for periorbital oedema. Loss or thinning of the outer third of the eyebrows can occur in myxoedema but is also common in healthy persons. Look for xanthelasma (due to associated hypercholesterolaemia). Palpate for coolness and dryness of the skin and hair. There may be thinning of the scalp hair.

Look at the tongue for swelling. Ask the patient to speak, and listen for coarse, croaking, slow speech. Bilateral nerve deafness may occur with endemic or congenital hypothyroidism.

The thyroid gland. A primary decrease in thyroid hormone results in a compensatory oversecretion of TSH. A goitre will result if there is viable thyroid tissue.

Many cases of hypothyroidism are not associated with an enlarged gland as there is little thyroid tissue. The exceptions include severe iodine deficiency, enzyme deficiency (inborn errors of metabolism), late Hashimoto's disease or treated (with radioactive iodine) thyrotoxicosis (Table 10.6).

The chest. Examine the heart for a pericardial effusion and the lungs for pleural effusions.

The legs. There may be non-pitting oedema. Ask the patient to kneel on a chair with the ankles exposed. Tap the Achilles tendon with a reflex hammer. There is apparently normal (in fact slightly slowed) contraction followed by delayed relaxation of the foot in hypothyroidism (the 'hung-up' reflex). Examine for signs of peripheral neuropathy and for other uncommon neurological abnormalities associated with hypothyroidism (Table 10.7).

The pituitary

Pituitary tumours can present in two ways: as a result of (i) local effects such as headaches, visual field loss and loss of acuity; and (ii) changes in pituitary hormone secretion. These changes include: (i) excess growth hormone, causing acromegaly; (ii) excess adrenocorticotrophic hormone (ACTH), causing Cushing's syndrome; (iii) excess prolactin, causing galactorrhoea, secondary amenorrhoea or male infertility or deficiency (hypopituitarism), and (iv) excess thyroid stimulating hormone (TSH), causing hyperthyroidism.

Panhypopituitarism (all pituitary hormones are deficient)

This is a deficiency of most or all of the pituitary hormones and is usually due to a space-occupying

TABLE 10.7 Neurological associations of hypothyroidism

Common
Entrapment: carpal tunnel, tarsal tunnel
Delayed ankle jerks
Muscle cramps

Uncommon
Peripheral neuropathy
Proximal myopathy
Hypokalaemic periodic paralysis
Cerebellar syndrome
Psychosis
Coma
Unmasking of myasthenia gravis
Cerebrovascular disease
High cerebrovascular fluid protein
Nerve deafness

Questions box 10.3

Questions to ask the patient with suspected pan-hypopituitarism

1 Have you had problems with lethargy, weakness and fatigue, or weight loss or poor appetite?—Adrenocorticoid deficiency

2 Have you gained weight, found cold weather more intolerable or had constipation?—Thyroid stimulating hormone deficiency

3 (Men) Have you noticed reduced sexual interest (libido), reduced muscle strength, erectile dysfunction or had problems with infertility?—Follicle stimulating hormone (FSH) deficiency

4 (Women) Have you had less bleeding during menstruation?—Oligomenorrhoea due to FSH deficiency

5 Have you noticed reduced exercise ability and energy?—Growth hormone deficiency in adults

6 Have you had headaches or visual disturbance?—Pituitary enlargement

lesion or destruction of the pituitary gland (Table 10.8). Hormone production is often lost in the following order: (i) growth hormone (dwarfism in children, insulin sensitivity in adults); (ii) prolactin (failure of lactation after delivery); (iii) gonadotrophins (loss of secondary sexual characteristics, secondary amenorrhoea in women, loss of libido and infertility in men); (iv) TSH (hypothyroidism); and (v) ACTH (hypoadrenalism, with loss of secondary sexual hair due to decreased adrenal androgen production).

However, isolated single hormonal deficiencies or multiple deficiencies may occur in any combination.

TABLE 10.8 Causes of hypopituitarism

Space-occupying lesion
• Pituitary tumour (non-secretory or secretory)
• Other tumours: craniopharyngioma, metastatic carcinoma, sarcoma
• Granulomata: e.g. sarcoid, tuberculosis

Iatrogenic: e.g. surgery or irradiation

Head injury

Sheehan's syndrome* (postpartum pituitary haemorrhage resulting in necrosis of the gland)

Empty sella syndrome (often an incidental MRI scan finding and not always associated with pituitary insufficiency)

Infarction or pituitary apoplexy

Idiopathic

* Harold Sheehan (b. 1900), professor of pathology, Liverpool, England, described the syndrome in 1937.

General inspection. The patient may be of short stature (failure of growth hormone secretion before growth is complete). Look for pallor of the skin (due to anaemia or occasionally ACTH deficiency because of the loss of its melanocyte-stimulating activity), fine-wrinkled skin and lack of body hair (due to gonadotrophin deficiency). There may be complete absence of the secondary sexual characteristics (Table 10.9) if gonadotrophin failure occurred before puberty.

The face. Look at the face more closely. Multiple skin wrinkles around the eyes are characteristic of gonadotrophin deficiency. Inspect the forehead carefully for hypophysectomy scars—transfrontal scars will be apparent (Figure 10.9) but not transsphenoidal ones, as this operation is performed through the base of the nose, via an incision under the upper lip.

Examine the eyes (Chapter 13). The visual fields must be assessed for any defects, especially bitemporal hemianopia (an enlarging pituitary tumour may compress the optic chiasm), and the fundi examined for optic atrophy (optic nerve compression from a pituitary tumour). Assess the third, fourth, sixth and first divisions of the fifth cranial nerves, as these may be affected by extrapituitary tumour expansion into the cavernous sinus (Figure 10.10).

Feel the facial hair over the bearded area in

TABLE 10.9 Secondary sexual development (Tanner stages)

This occurs at puberty in response to pituitary gonadotrophins

Males

1 Preadolescent
2 Enlargement of testes and scrotum
3 Lengthening of penis
4 Increase in penis breadth, glans development and scrotal darkening
5 Adult: above, plus public hair spread to medial surface of the thighs

Females

Breasts	Pubic hair
1 Preadolescent	1 No pubic hair
2 Breast bud (elevation of breasts and papilla)	2 Sparse growth, mainly over the labia
3 Enlargement of breast and areola (no separation of contours)	3 Darker, coarser, more curled hairs but sparse over the junction of the pubes
4 Areola and papilla project above breast level (secondary mound)	4 Adult type but no hair spread to medial surface of thighs
5 Adult: areola is recessed and papilla projects	5 Adult: horizontal pattern and hair spread to medial thighs

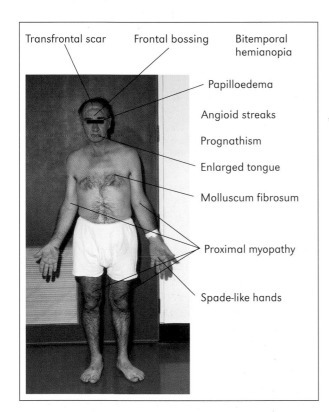

Transfrontal scar Frontal bossing Bitemporal hemianopia

Papilloedema

Angioid streaks

Prognathism

Enlarged tongue

Molluscum fibrosum

Proximal myopathy

Spade-like hands

Figure 10.9 Acromegaly

men for normal beard growth (which is lost with gonadotrophin deficiency).

The chest. Go on to the chest. Look for skin pallor and for a decrease in nipple pigmentation. In men,

decreased body hair (axillary and chest) may be present. In women, secondary breast atrophy may be found.

The genital region. Loss of pubic hair occurs in both sexes. In men, testicular atrophy may be present. Atrophied testes are characteristically small and firm. The normal-sized testis is about 15–25 mL in volume.

The ankle reflexes. Test for 'hung-up' jerks (Figure 10.11). These are an important sign of pituitary hypothyroidism. Occasionally, pituitary hypothyroid patients may be slightly overweight, but the classical myxoedematous appearance is usually absent.

Acromegaly[k]

This is excessive secretion of growth hormone, typically due to an eosinophilic pituitary adenoma.[l] Growth hormone stimulates the liver and other tissues to produce somatomedins which in turn promote growth. Growth hormone is also a protein anabolic hormone exerting its effects at the ribosomal level, and it is diabetogenic as it exerts an anti-insulin effect in muscle and increases hepatic glucose release. The disease has a very gradual onset and patients may not have noticed symptoms. Most patients, however, have headache

---

k The acral parts are the hands and feet.
l Acromegaly was first described by Pierre Marie in 1886 and was first called hyperpituitarism by Harvey Cushing in 1909.

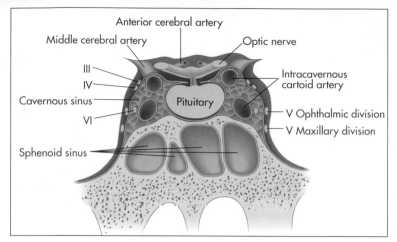

Figure 10.10 The cavernous sinus and its relationship with the cranial nerves and pituitary gland

caused by stretching of the dura by the enlarging pituitary tumour.

Gigantism is the result of growth hormone hypersecretion occurring before puberty and fusion of the epiphyses. It results in massive skeletal as well as soft-tissue growth. Acromegaly occurs when the growth plates have fused, so that only soft-tissue and flat-bone enlargement are possible.

General inspection. The face and body habitus[m] may be characteristic (Figure 10.9).

The hands. Sit the patient on the side of the bed or in a chair and look at the hands. Notice a wide spade-like shape (due to soft tissue and bony enlargement). Increased sweating and warmth of the palms may be noted. This is due to an increased metabolic rate. The skin may appear thickened. Changes of osteoarthritis in the hands are common and are due to skeletal overgrowth. Examine for median nerve entrapment, which can occur because of soft-tissue overgrowth in the carpal tunnel area.

The arms. Proximal myopathy may be present (page 391). Palpate behind the medial epicondyle (the 'funny bone') for ulnar nerve thickening.

The axillae. Carefully inspect the axillae for skin tags (called molluscum fibrosum, which are non-tender skin-coloured protrusions). Summon up courage and feel for greasy skin. Look for acanthosis nigricans.

The face. Look for a large supraorbital ridge, which causes frontal bossing (this may also

---

m From the Latin—*habitus* = the state or condition of a thing.

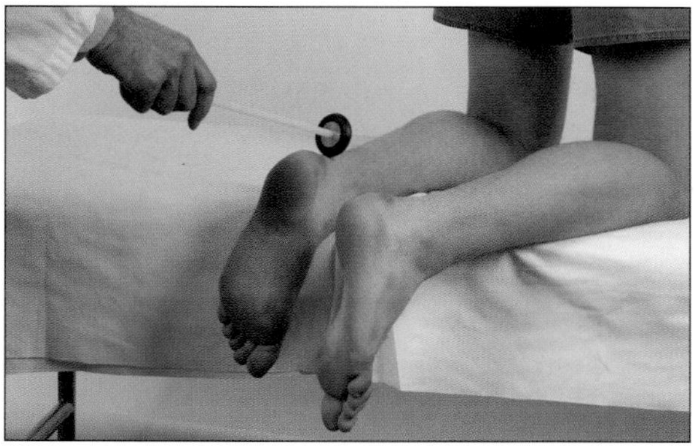

Figure 10.11 Testing ankle jerks (second method—see also page 372)
This method best demonstrates the 'hung-up' reflexes of hypothyroidism. Look for rapid dorsiflexion followed by slow plantar flexion after the tendon is tapped.

occur occasionally in Paget's disease, rickets, achondroplasia or hydrocephalus). The lips may be thickened.

Examine the eyes for visual field defects; classically there may be bitemporal hemianopia if the pituitary tumour is large. Look in the fundi for optic atrophy (due to nerve compression) and papilloedema (due to raised intracranial pressure with an extensive tumour). The presence of angioid streaks (red, brown or grey streaks that are three to five times the diameter of a retinal vein and appear to emanate from the optic disc) should also be sought: these are due to degeneration and fibrosis of Bruch's membrane. One should also note hypertensive changes or diabetic changes in the fundus. Ocular palsies may occur with an extensive pituitary tumour.

Look in the mouth for an enlarged tongue that may not fit neatly between the teeth. The teeth themselves may be splayed and separated, with malocclusion as the jaw enlarges. The lower jaw may look square and firm (as it does on some American actors). When the jaw protrudes it is called prognathism (Greek *pro* 'forwards', *gnathos* 'jaw').

The neck. The thyroid may be diffusely enlarged or multinodular (all the internal organs may enlarge under the influence of growth hormone). Listen to the voice for hoarseness.

The chest. Look for coarse body hair and gynaecomastia. Examine the heart for signs of arrhythmias, cardiomegaly and congestive cardiac failure, which may be due to ischaemic heart disease, hypertension or cardiomyopathy (all more common in acromegaly).

The back. Inspect for kyphosis.

The abdomen. Examine for hepatic, splenic and renal enlargement, and go on to look for testicular atrophy (the latter indicating gonadotrophin deficiency secondary to an enlarging pituitary tumour). Acromegaly can be associated with a mixed pituitary tumour and resultant hyperprolactinaemia can also cause testicular atrophy.

The lower limbs. Look for signs of osteoarthritis in the hips especially, and knees (page 269), and for pseudogout. Foot drop may be present because of common peroneal nerve entrapment (page 376).

The urine and blood pressure. Test the urine for glucose, as excess growth hormone is diabetogenic in 25% of cases. Take the blood pressure to test for hypertension.

Finally, decide if the disease is active or not. Signs of active disease include: (i) large numbers of skin tags (skin tags can occur commonly in normal people); (ii) excessive sweating; (iii) presence of glycosuria; (iv) increasing visual field loss; (v) enlarging goitre; and (vi) hypertension. *Note:* Headache also suggests disease activity.

Other pituitary syndromes

Cushing's syndrome can occur as a result of excess pituitary ACTH secretion. Hyperthyroidism can occur as a result of excess pituitary TSH production. Prolactinomas of the pituitary can cause galactorrhoea (production of milk) in both women and men.

The adrenals
Cushing's syndrome

This is due to a chronic excess of glucocorticoids. Steroids have multiple effects on the body, due to stimulation of the DNA-dependent synthesis of select messenger ribonucleic acids (RNAs). This leads to the formation of enzymes, which alter cell function and result in increased protein catabolism and gluconeogenesis. Remember that Cushing's disease is specifically pituitary ACTH overproduction, while Cushing's syndrome is due to excessive steroid hormone production from any cause (Table 10.10; see *Good signs guide 10.4*, *Questions box 10.4*).

The hands. Skinfold thickness is best assessed on the backs of the hands and may be reliable only as a sign of Cushing's in young women. The skinfold should be thicker than 1.8 mm.

Standing. Have the patient undress to the underpants and, if possible, stand up (Figure 10.12). Look from the front, back and sides. Note *moon-like facies* and *central obesity*. The limbs appear thin despite sometimes very gross truncal (mostly intra-abdominal rather than subcutaneous fat) obesity.[n] This is the characteristic fat distribution that occurs with steroid excess. *Bruising* may be present (due to loss of perivascular supporting tissue–protein catabolism). Look for excessive *pigmentation* on the extensor surfaces (because

---

[n] The enthusiastic student can calculate the central obesity index. This is the sum of three truncal circumferences (neck, chest and waist) divided by six peripheral ones (arms, thighs and legs on both sides). A normal index is less than 1.

TABLE 10.10 Causes of Cushing's syndrome
Exogenous administration of excess steroids or ACTH (most common)
Adrenal hyperplasia
• Secondary to pituitary ACTH production (Cushing's disease)
Microadenoma
Macroadenoma
Pituitary-hypothalamic dysfunction
• Secondary to ACTH-producing tumours— e.g. small cell lung carcinoma
Adrenal neoplasia
• Adenoma
• Carcinoma (rare)
ACTH = adrenocorticotrophic hormone.

GOOD SIGNS GUIDE 10.4 Cushing's syndrome

Sign	Positive LR	Negative LR
Vital signs		
Hypertension	2.3	0.8
Body habitus		
Moon face	1.6	0.1
Central obesity	3.0	0.2
General obesity	0.1	2.5
Skin findings		
Thin skinfold (women)	115.6	0.2
Plethora	2.7	0.3
Hirsutism (women)	1.7	0.7
Ecchymoses	4.5	0.5
Red or purple striae	1.9	0.7
Acne	2.2	0.6
Extremities		
Proximal muscle weakness	NS	0.4
Oedema	1.8	0.7

NS = not significant.

From McGee S, *Evidence-based physical diagnosis*, 2nd edn. St Louis: Saunders, 2007

Questions box 10.4

Questions to ask the patient with suspected Cushing's syndrome

❗ denotes symptoms for the possible diagnosis of an urgent or dangerous problem.

1 Have you gained a lot of weight recently? How much?
2 Do you bruise easily?
3 Has your skin become thin?
4 Have you had problems with acne?
❗ 5 Have you felt agitated and been unable to sleep?
6 Have you had problems with weakness of your muscles or difficulty getting up out of chairs?—Proximal myopathy
7 Have you had problems maintaining erections (men) or had amenorrhoea (women)?
8 Have you been diagnosed with diabetes?

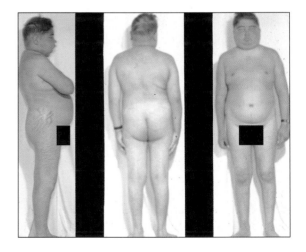

Figure 10.12 Buffalo hump and central obesity in Cushing's syndrome
(From McDonald FS, ed., *Mayo Clinic images in internal medicine*, with permission. © Mayo Clinic Scientific Press and CRC Press.)

of melanocyte-stimulating-hormone [MSH]-like activity in the ACTH molecule). Ask the patient to squat at this point to test for *proximal myopathy*, due to mobilisation of muscle tissue or excessive urinary potassium loss. Look at the back for the '*buffalo hump*', which is due to fat deposition over the interscapular area. Palpate for bony *tenderness* of the vertebral bodies due to crush fractures from osteoporosis (a steroid anti-vitamin-D effect and increased urinary calcium excretion may be responsible in part for disruption of the bone matrix).

Sitting. Ask the patient to sit on the side of the bed, but remember that he or she may be suffering from steroid psychosis and refuse to do anything you ask.

The face and neck. Look for plethora (this occurs in the absence of polycythaemia which, however, may also be present). The face may have a typical moon shape due to fat deposition in the upper part. Inspect for acne and hirsutism (if adrenal androgen secretion is also increased). Telangiectasiae may also be present.

Examine the visual fields for signs of a pituitary tumour, and the fundi for optic atrophy, papilloedema and hypertensive or diabetic changes. Look for supraclavicular fat pads.

The abdomen. Lay the patient in bed on one pillow. Examine the abdomen for purple striae, which are due to weakening and disruption of collagen fibres in the dermis, leading to exposure of vascular subcutaneous tissues. In patients with Cushing's syndrome these are wider (1 cm) than those seen in people who have gained weight rapidly for other reasons. They may also be present near the axillae on the upper arms or on the inside of the thighs. Palpate for adrenal masses (rarely a large adrenal carcinoma will be palpable over the renal area). Palpate for hepatomegaly due to fat deposition or rarely to adrenal carcinoma deposits.

The legs. Palpate for oedema (due to salt and water retention). Look for bruising and poor wound healing.

The urinalysis and blood pressure. Test the urine for sugar (as steroids are diabetogenic; this is due to an increase in hepatic gluconeogenesis and an anti-insulin effect on peripheral tissues). Hypertension is common due to salt and water retention (an aldosterone effect) and possibly to increased angiotensin secretion or a direct effect on blood vessels.

Synthesis of signs. Certain signs are of some aetiological value in Cushing's syndrome.

* **Signs which suggest that adrenal carcinoma may be the underlying cause:** (i) a palpable abdominal mass; (ii) signs of virilisation in the female; (iii) gynaecomastia in the male.
* **Signs which suggest that ectopic ACTH production may be the cause:** (i) absence of the Cushingoid body habitus unless the responsible tumour has been slow growing and allowed time for Cushingoid features to develop; (ii) more prominent oedema and hypertension; (iii) marked muscle weakness. *Note:* When Cushing's is due to ectopic ACTH production from a small cell carcinoma, the patient is much more likely to be male (positive LR 13)[4] and the history to be of more rapid onset of the symptoms and signs (18 months: positive LR 15).[4]
* **Significance of hyperpigmentation:** this suggests an extra-adrenal tumour, or enlargement of an ACTH-secreting pituitary adenoma following adrenalectomy (Nelson's[o] syndrome).

Addison's disease[p]

This is adrenocortical hypofunction with reduction in the secretion of glucocorticoids and mineral-

TABLE 10.11 Causes of Addison's disease

Chronic

Primary
Autoimmune adrenal disease
Infection (tuberculosis, HIV)
Granuloma
Following heparin therapy
Malignant infiltration
Haemochromatosis
Adrenoleucodystrophy

Secondary
Pituitary or hypothalamic disease

Acute
Septicaemia: meningococcal
Adrenalectomy
Any stress in a patient with chronic hypoadrenalism or abrupt cessation of prolonged high-dose steroid therapy

ocorticoids. It is most often due to autoimmune disease of the adrenal glands. Other causes are listed in Table 10.11.

If this disease is suspected, look for cachexia. Then, with the patient undressed, look for pigmentation in the palmar creases (Figure 10.13), elbows, gums and buccal mucosa, genital areas and in scars. This occurs because of compensatory ACTH hypersecretion in primary hypoadrenalism (when there is adrenal disease), as ACTH has melanocyte-stimulating activity. Also inspect for vitiligo (localised hypomelanosis), an autoimmune disease that is commonly associated with autoimmune adrenal failure.

Take the blood pressure and test for postural hypotension. Remember that the rest of the autoimmune disease cluster may be associated with autoimmune adrenal failure (Table 10.12).

Calcium metabolism
Primary hyperparathyroidism

This is due to excess parathyroid hormone (Table 10.13), which results in an increased serum calcium level, increased renal phosphate excretion and increased formation of 1,25-dihydroxycholecalciferol by activation of adenyl cyclase in the bone and kidneys. Primary hyperparathyroidism causes problems with 'stones' (renal stones), 'bones' (osteopenia and pseudogout), 'abdominal groans' (constipation, peptic ulcer and pancreatitis) and 'psychological moans' (confusion) (*Questions box 10.5*).

Other causes of hypercalcaemia are listed in Table 10.14.

---

[o] Warren Nelson (1906–64), American endocrinologist.
[p] Thomas Addison (1793–1860) described the disease in 1849. Addison, Bright and Hodgkin made up the famous trio of physicians at Guy's Hospital, London.

TABLE 10.12 A classification of conditions found in various combinations in autoimmune polyglandular syndromes

Type I (rare autosomal recessive)	Type II (more common, HLA DRB1, DQA1, DQB1)
1 Chronic mucocutaneous candidiasis	1 Insulin-requiring diabetes (type 1)
2 Hypoparathyroidism	2 Autoimmune thyroid disease
3 Addison's disease	3 Addison's disease
	4 Myasthenia gravis
	5 Pernicious anaemia
	6 Primary gonadal failure

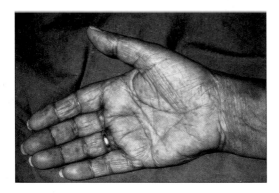

Figure 10.13 Palmar crease pigmentation in Addison's disease

TABLE 10.13 Types of hyperparathyroidism

Primary
Adenoma (80%)
Hyperplasia
Carcinoma (rare)
Secondary
Hyperplasia following chronic renal failure
Tertiary (autonomous)
The appearance of autonomous hyperparathyroidism is a complication of secondary hyperparathyroidism

General inspection. Note the mental state of the patient. Severe hypercalcaemia may cause coma or convulsions. Assess hydration (polyuria from hypercalcaemia may cause dehydration).

The face. Look in the eyes for band keratopathy, which is rare (page 209).

The body and lower limbs. Palpate the shoulders, sternum, ribs, spine and hips for bony tenderness, deformity or evidence of previous fractures. Test for proximal muscle weakness. Look for pseudogout. Take the blood pressure, as hypertension may occur.

Urinalysis. Test for blood in the urine (renal stones).

The MEN syndromes

The multiple endocrine neoplasias (MENs), types I and II, are autosomal dominant conditions. Hyperparathyroidism can be associated with both. MEN type I (due to a mutation on chromosome 11) is associated with tumours of the parathyroid, pituitary and pancreatic islet cells. MEN type IIA (due to a mutation on chromosome 10 involving the c-*ret* proto-oncogene) is associated with medullary

---

Questions box 10.5

Questions to ask the patient with suspected hyperparathyroidism

! denotes symptoms for the possible diagnosis of an urgent or dangerous problem.

1 Have you had kidney stones?

2 Have you had any fractures?

3 Have you been troubled by abdominal pain? Have you had constipation?

4 Have you been depressed or had hallucinations?—Psychiatric disorders

! 5 Have you had episodes of confusion, irritability, extreme tiredness or even unconsciousness?—Neurological symptoms

---

carcinoma of the thyroid, hyperparathyroidism and phaeochromocytoma. MEN type IIB is characterised by mucosal neuromas (often on the lips and tongue) and medullary carcinoma of the thyroid plus phaeochromocytoma.

Hypoparathyroidism

This results in hypocalcaemia with neuromuscular consequences (tetany) (*Questions Box 10.6*).

It is usually a postoperative complication after thyroidectomy, but can be idiopathic.

TABLE 10.14 Important causes of hypercalcaemia

Primary hyperparathyroidism
Carcinoma (from bone metastases or humoral mediators)
Thiazide diuretics
Vitamin D excess
Excessive production of vitamin D metabolites: e.g. sarcoidosis, certain T cell lymphomas
Thyrotoxicosis
Associated with renal failure (e.g. severe secondary hyperparathyroidism)
Multiple myeloma
Familial hypocalciuric hypercalcaemia
Prolonged immobilisation or space flight

Questions box 10.6

Questions to ask the patient with suspected hypocalcaemia

! denotes symptoms for the possible diagnosis of an urgent or dangerous problem.

1 Have you recently had surgery to remove the parathyroid glands?

2 Have you had tingling around the mouth or in the fingers?

3 Have you had muscle cramps?

! 4 Have you had fits or seizures?

TABLE 10.15 Causes of hypocalcaemia

Hypoparathyroidism: after thyroidectomy, idiopathic
Malabsorption
Deficiency of vitamin D
Chronic renal failure
Acute pancreatitis
Pseudohypoparathyroidism
Magnesium deficiency
Hypocalcaemia of malignant disease

Hypocalcaemia can also result from end-organ resistance to parathyroid hormone (pseudohypoparathyroidism) (Table 10.15).

Look first for Trousseau's and Chvostek's signs. *Trousseau's sign* is elicited with a blood pressure cuff placed on the arm with the pressure raised above the patient's systolic pressure. Typical contraction of the hand occurs within 2 minutes when hypocalcaemia has caused neuromuscular irritability. The thumb becomes strongly adducted, and the fingers are extended, except at the metacarpophalangeal joints. The appearance is that of an obstetrician about to remove the placenta manually and is called the *main d'accoucheur.*

Chvostek's sign is performed by tapping gently over the facial (seventh) cranial nerve under the ear. The nerve is hyperexcitable in hypocalcaemia and a brisk muscular twitch occurs on the same side of the face.

Next test for hyperreflexia, again due to neuromuscular irritability.

Look at the nails for fragility and monilial infection. Note any dryness of the skin. Go to the face and look for deformity of the teeth. Examine the eyes for cataracts or papilloedema. These signs may all occur in idiopathic hypoparathyroidism, an autoimmune disease. Cataracts may also follow surgically induced hypoparathyroidism.

Pseudohypoparathyroidism. In this disease the patients have tetany (due to hypocalcaemia) as well as typical skeletal abnormalities. These include short stature, a round face, a short neck, thin stocky build and very characteristically short fourth or fifth fingers or toes (due to metacarpal or metatarsal shortening; this can be unilateral or bilateral) (Figure 10.14). Ask the patient to make a fist to demonstrate the characteristic clinical signs.

Pseudopseudohypoparathyroidism. This amusing name is given to a disease where there is no tetany (calcium concentration in the blood is normal), but the characteristic skeletal deformities are present.

Syndromes associated with short stature

These conditions begin in childhood.

General inspection

First measure the height of the patient; in children this should be compared with percentile charts for age and sex. Look for the classical appearance of Turner's syndrome, Down syndrome, achondroplasia or rickets (Figure 10.15), which may explain the short stature. The height of parents and siblings should be checked as well.

Note any evidence of weight loss, including loose skinfolds, which may suggest a nutritional cause (starvation, malabsorption or protein loss). Look for signs of hypopituitarism or hypothyroidism,

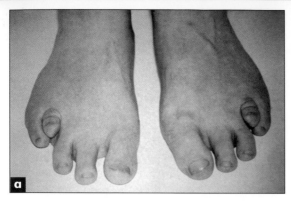

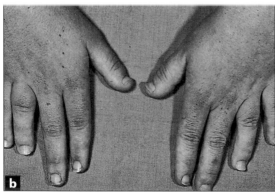

Figure 10.14 Pseudohypoparathyroidism: (a) feet; (b) hands
(From McDonald FS, ed., *Mayo Clinic images in internal medicine*, with permission. © Mayo Clinic Scientific Press and CRC Press.)

or steroid excess. Sexual precocity (early onset of secondary sexual characteristics) causes relative tallness at first but short stature later.

The chest
Examine for evidence of cyanotic congenital heart disease and pulmonary disease, such as cystic fibrosis.

The abdomen
Look for evidence of hepatic failure or renal failure (a cause of growth retardation when it occurs in children).

Turner's syndrome (45XO)
Sexual infantilism (failure of development of secondary sexual characteristics)—female genitalia.

Upper limbs. Lymphoedema of the hands; short fourth metacarpal bones; hyperplastic nails; increased carrying angle; hypertension.

Facies. Micrognathia (small chin); epicanthic folds ptosis; fish-like mouth; deformed or low-set ears; hearing loss.

Neck. Webbing of the neck; low hairline; redundant skinfolds on the back of the neck.

Chest. Widely spaced nipples (a shield-like chest); coarctation of the aorta.

Other. Pigmented naevi; keloid formation; lymphoedema of the legs.

Down syndrome (Trisomy 21)
Facies. Oblique orbital fissures; conjunctivitis; Brushfield spots on the iris; small simple ears; flat nasal bridge; mouth hanging open; protruding tongue; narrow high-arched palate.

Hands. Short broad hands; incurving fifth finger; single palmar crease; hyperflexible joints.

Chest. Congenital heart disease; especially endocardial cushion defects.

Other. Straight pubic hair; gaps between the first and second toes; mental deficiency usually present.

Rickets (Figure 10.15)
Defective mineralisation of the *growing* skeleton, due to lack of vitamin D (e.g. nutritional or chronic renal failure) or hypophosphataemia (e.g. renal tubular disorders).

Upper limbs. Tetany; hypotonia, proximal myopathy; bowing of the radius and ulna.

Facies. Frontal bossing; parietal flattening.

Chest. 'Rickety rosary'—thickening of costochondral junctions; Harrison's groove—indentation of lower ribs at the diaphragmatic attachment.

Lower limbs. Bowing of femur and tibia; hypotonia, proximal myopathy; fractures.

Achondroplasia (dwarfism)
This is an autosomal-dominant disease of cartilage caused by mutation of the fibroblast growth factor receptor gene.

Short stature, short limbs, normal trunk, relatively large head, saddle-shaped nose, exaggerated lumbar lordosis and occasionally spinal cord compression are features.

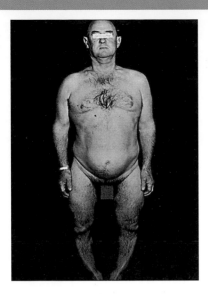

Figure 10.15 **Rickets (postrachitic patient)**
Look for frontal bossing, proximal myopathy of arms and thighs, and bowing of the ulna, femur and tibia.

TABLE 10.16 Causes of hirsutism
Polycystic ovary syndrome (commonest cause)
Idiopathic
Adrenal: androgen-secreting tumours e.g. Cushing's syndrome, congenital adrenal hyperplasia, virilising tumour (more often a carcinoma than an adenoma)
Ovarian: androgen-secreting tumour
Drugs: phenytoin, diazoxide, streptomycin, minoxidil, anabolic steroids e.g. testosterone
Other: acromegaly, porphyria cutanea tarda

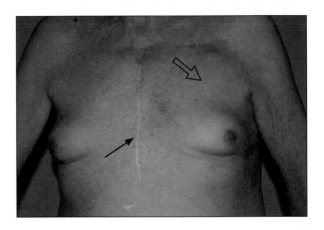

Figure 10.16 Gynaecomastia
This patient takes spironolactone for heart failure. Note median sternotomy scar (arrow) and defibrillator box (open arrow).

Hirsutism

This is excessive hairiness in a woman beyond what is considered normal for her race (Table 10.16). It is caused by androgen (including testosterone) excess. In the examination of such a patient, it is important to decide whether virilisation is also present. Virilisation is the appearance of male secondary sexual characteristics (clitoromegaly, frontal hair recession, male body habitus and deepening of the voice) and indicates that excessive androgen is present.

General inspection

Ask the patient to undress to her underwear. Note the hair distribution over the face and in the midline, front and back. In general, an obvious male balding pattern (a receding hairline), hair over the beard area or on the back and chest, and hair in the escutcheon (umbilicus to groin in the midline) is usually abnormal. Look for obvious acromegaly or Cushing's syndrome and for the skin changes of porphyria cutanea tarda.

Ask the patient to remove her underclothing and lie flat. Look for signs of virilism. These include breast atrophy and increased muscle bulk of the arms and legs, male pattern of pubic hair, and enlargement of the clitoris. Look in the axillae; the patient with polycystic ovarian syndrome may have acanthosis nigricans (and associated insulin resistance).

The abdomen

Palpate for adrenal masses, polycystic ovaries or an ovarian tumour (these are rarely palpable).

The blood pressure

Hypertension occurs in the rare C11-hydroxylase deficiency, which is a virilising condition.

Gynaecomastia (Figure 10.16)

This is 'true' enlargement of the male breasts.[5] Careful examination will detect up to 4 cm of palpable breast tissue in 30% of normal young men; this percentage increases with age. These men are unaware of any breast abnormality. Gynaecomastia occurs in up to 50% of adolescent boys, and also in elderly men in whom it is due to falling testosterone levels. Fat deposition ('false' enlargement) in obese men can be confused with gynaecomastia.

Examine the breasts (page 435) for evidence of localised disease (e.g. malignancy, which is rare), tenderness, which indicates rapid growth, and any discharge from the nipple. Detection of breast

TABLE 10.17 Differential diagnosis (causes) of pathological gynaecomastia

Increased oestrogen production

Leydig cell tumour (oestrogen)

Adrenal carcinoma (oestrogen)

Bronchial carcinoma (human chorionic gonadotrophin)

Liver disease (increased conversion of oestrogen from androgens)

Thyrotoxicosis (increased conversion of oestrogen from androgens)

Starvation

Decreased androgen production (hypogonadal states)

Klinefelter's syndrome

Secondary testicular failure: orchitis, castration, trauma

Testicular feminisation syndrome

Drugs

Oestrogen receptor binders: oestrogen, digoxin, marijuana

Anti-androgens: spironolactone, cimetidine

TABLE 10.18 Causes of diabetes mellitus

Criteria for diagnosis of diabetes mellitus: fasting plasma venous blood sugar level of 7.0 mmol/L or more (≥126 mg/dL), or a 2-hour postprandial blood sugar level of 11.1 mmol/L or more (≥200 mg/dL), on more than one occasion.

I. Type 1
- Type 1A (autoimmune destruction of beta cells in the pancreas)
- Adult-onset type 1 (islet cell antibodies)

II. Type 2 (insulin deficiency and resistance)

III. Other types of diabetes
- A. Mutations leading to abnormalities of β cell function
- B. Inherited defects of insulin action: e.g. lipoatrophic diabetes (characterised by generalised lipoatrophy, hepatomegaly, hirsutism, acanthosis nigricans, hyperpigmentation and hyperlipidaemia)
- C. Diseases of the exocrine pancreas: e.g. chronic pancreatitis, carcinoma, haemochromatosis
- D. Endocrine abnormalities: e.g. acromegaly, Cushing's syndrome, phaeochromocytoma, glucagonoma, somatostatinoma
- E. Drug-induced: e.g. steroids, the contraceptive pill, streptozotocin, diazoxide, phenytoin, thiazide diuretics
- F. Infections: e.g. cytomegalovirus, coxsackie, congenital rubella
- G. Rare forms of immune-mediated diabetes: e.g. anti-insulin receptor antibodies
- H. Genetic abnormalities associates with diabetes: e.g. Down's syndrome, Klinefelter's syndrome, Turner's syndrome
- J. Stiff person syndrome (progressive muscle stiffness of axial muscles)

IV. Gestational diabetes mellitus

tissue in men is best performed with the patient sitting up. Squeeze the breast behind the patient's nipple between the thumb and forefinger. Try to detect an edge between subcutaneous fat and true breast tissue.

Examine the genitalia now for sexual ambiguity and the testes for absence or a reduced size. Note any loss of secondary sexual characteristics.

Look especially for signs of *Klinefelter's syndrome* (47,XXY). These patients are tall, have decreased body hair and characteristically small, firm testes.

Look also for signs of panhypopituitarism or chronic liver disease. Thyrotoxicosis can occasionally be a cause.

Finally, examine the visual fields and fundi for evidence of a pituitary tumour.

Causes of pathological gynaecomastia are summarised in Table 10.17.

Diabetes mellitus[q]

Diabetes mellitus is characterised by hyperglycaemia due to an absolute or relative deficiency of insulin. The causes of diabetes are listed in Table 10.18. The disease can present with asymptomatic glycosuria detected on routine physical examination or with symptoms of diabetes (Table 10.1), ranging from polyuria to coma as a result of diabetic ketoacidosis (*Questions box 10.7*).

---

q   This disease was called diabetes by ancient Greek and Roman physicians because the word diabetes means a siphon, referring to the large urine volume. Rather courageously, they distinguished diabetes mellitus from diabetes insipidus by the sweet taste of the urine: *mellitus*, 'sweet'; *insipidus*, 'tasteless'.

General inspection (Figure 10.17)

Assess for evidence of dehydration because the osmotic diuresis caused by a glucose load in the urine can cause massive fluid loss. Note obesity (non-insulin-dependent diabetics are usually obese) or signs of recent weight loss (this can be evidence of uncontrolled glycosuria).

Look for one of the abnormal endocrine facies (e.g. Cushing's syndrome or acromegaly) and for pigmentation (e.g. haemochromatosis—bronze diabetes) as these may cause secondary diabetes.

The patient may be comatose due to dehydration, acidosis or plasma hyperosmolality. Kussmaul's breathing ('air hunger') is present in diabetic ketoacidosis due to the acidosis (this occurs because fat metabolism is increased to compensate for the lack of availability of glucose; excess acetyl-

Questions box 10.7

Questions to ask the diabetic patient

! denotes symptoms for the possible diagnosis of an urgent or dangerous problem.

1 What was your age at the time the diabetes was diagnosed?

2 Did you require insulin from the start?

! 3 What was the problem that led to the diagnosis?—**Polyuria**, **thirst**, weight loss, recurrent skin infections, screening assessment

4 What previous and current drug treatment are you taking for diabetes?

5 What diet has been prescribed? What do you understand about your diabetic diet?

6 What blood sugar testing do you do? What are the usual results?

! 7 Have you had any problems with hypoglycaemia (treatment-induced low blood sugar)? Have you had episodes of sweating, confusion, malaise or unconsciousness?

8 Do you know what action should be taken if these acute symptoms (of hypo- or hyperglycaemia) occur?—Check sugar level, take glucose tablet, go to hospital

9 Have you had keto-acidosis (very high blood sugars associated with acidosis) and needed admission to hospital?—Polyuria, dehydration, confusion, unconsciousness

10 Have you had complications of diabetes— eyes, nerves, blood vessels, kidneys?

11 What regular testing has been performed for these problems?

12 How do you and your family cope with this chronic condition?

13 Have you been able to work?

coenzyme A is produced, which is converted in the liver to ketone bodies, and two of these are organic acids).

The lower limbs

Unlike most other systematic examinations, assessment of the diabetic can profitably begin with the legs, as many of the major physical signs are found to be here. In particular, vascular and neurological abnormalities in the feet must not be missed.[6]

Inspection. Look at the skin. The *skin* of the feet and lower legs may be hairless and atrophied due to small-vessel vascular disease and resultant ischaemia (the mechanism is uncertain, but may be related to lipoprotein alterations in the vessel walls).

Note any leg *ulcers*, particularly on the toes or any area of the feet exposed to pressure (Figure 10.18). These ulcers are due to a combination of ischaemia and peripheral neuropathy (the cause of the neuropathy is unknown, but may be related to small vessel ischaemia and glycosylation of neural proteins).

Look for superficial skin *infection*, such as boils, cellulitis and fungal infections. These are more common in diabetics because of a combination of high tissue glucose levels and ischaemia, which provides a favourable environment for the growth of organisms.

Note any *pigmented scars* (late diabetic dermopathy). There may be small rounded plaques with raised borders lying in a linear fashion over the shins (diabetic dermopathy).

Necrobiosis lipoidica diabeticorum is a reasonably specific skin manifestation of diabetes mellitus, but is rare (fewer than 1% of diabetics) (Figure 10.19). It is found over the shins, where a central yellow scarred area is surrounded by a red margin when the condition is active. These plaques may ulcerate.

Look now at the thighs for insulin injection sites. These may be associated with localised *fat atrophy* and *fat hypertrophy*, and may be related to impure insulin use which causes a localised immune reaction (modern genetically engineered insulins have made these rare). Note any *quadriceps muscle wasting* due to femoral nerve mononeuropathy, which is called (inaccurately) diabetic amyotrophy.

Inspect the knees for the very rare Charcot's joints (grossly deformed disorganised joints, due to loss of proprioception or pain, or both; this leads to recurrent and unnoticed injury to the joint) (Figure 10.20).

Palpation. Palpate any injection sites for fat atrophy or hypertrophy. Feel all the peripheral pulses and the temperature of the feet, and test the capillary return. Absent peripheral pulses, cold extremities and reduced capillary return are all evidence of peripheral vascular disease.

Neurological examination. Assess formally for peripheral neuropathy, including dorsal column loss (diabetic pseudotabes), and tap the reflexes. Test proximal muscle power (diabetic amyotrophy).

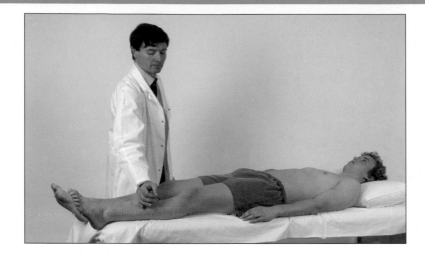

Figure 10.17 Diabetes mellitus

Lying

1. **General inspection**
   Weight—obesity
   Hydration
   Endocrine facies
   Pigmentation—haemochromatosis, etc
2. **Legs**
   Inspect
   • Skin—necrobiosis, hair loss, infection, pigmented scars, atrophy, ulceration, injection sites
   • Muscle wasting
   Palpate
   • Temperature of feet (cold, blue due to 'small' or 'large' vessel disease)
   • Peripheral pulses
   Femoral (auscultate)
   Popliteal
   Posterior tibial
   Dorsalis pedis
3. **Arms**
   Inspect
   • Injection sites
   • Skin lesions

   Pulse
4. **Eyes**
   Fundi—cataracts, rubeosis, retinal disease
   III nerve palsy, etc
5. **Mouth**
   Monilia
   Infection
6. **Neck**
   Carotid arteries—palpate, auscultate
7. **Chest**
   Signs of infection
8. **Abdomen**
   Liver—fat infiltration; rarely haemochromatosis
   Neurological assessment
   • Femoral nerve mononeuritis
   • Peripheral neuropathy
9. **Other**
   Urine analysis—glycosuria, ketones, proteinuria
   Blood pressure—lying and standing
   Oedema

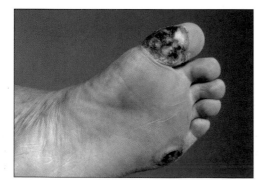

Figure 10.18 Diabetic (neuropathic) ulcer
(From McDonald FS, ed., *Mayo Clinic images in internal medicine*, with permission. © Mayo Clinic Scientific Press and CRC Press.)

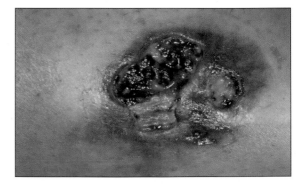

Figure 10.19 Necrobiosis lipoidica diabeticorum
(From McDonald FS, ed., *Mayo Clinic images in internal medicine*, with permission. © Mayo Clinic Scientific Press and CRC Press.)

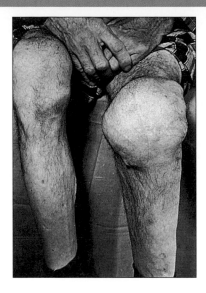

Figure 10.20 Charcot's joint of left knee

The upper limbs

Look at the nails for signs of *Candida* infection. Take the blood pressure lying and standing, as diabetic autonomic neuropathy can cause postural hypotension.

The face

The eyes. Test visual acuity. This may be permanently impaired because of retinal disease or temporarily disturbed because of changes in the shape of the lens associated with hyperglycaemia and water retention. Look for Argyll Robertson pupils[r], which are a rare complication of diabetes.

Using the ophthalmoscope, begin by examining for rubeosis (new blood vessel formation over the iris, which can cause glaucoma) (Figure 10.21). Then note any cataracts, which are related to sorbitol deposition in the lens (when glucose is present in high concentrations in the tissues it is converted to sorbitol by aldose reductase).

Now examine the retina, where many exciting changes may await the fundoscopist. There are two main types of retinal change in diabetes: non-proliferative and proliferative.

Non-proliferative changes (Figure 10.22) are directly related to ischaemia of blood vessels and include: (i) two types of haemorrhages—*dot haemorrhages,* which occur in the inner retinal layers, and *blot haemorrhages,* which are larger and

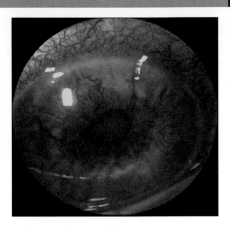

Figure 10.21 Rubeosis iridis
Shows new vessels on the anterior surface of the iris. These are secondary to ischaemia (often due to diabetes).

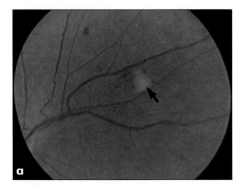

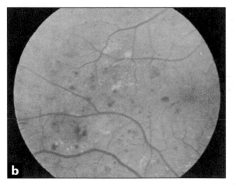

Figure 10.22 Diabetic retinopathy
(a) Soft exudate (arrow) and small haemorrhages.
(b) Microaneurysms (dots), retinal haemorrhages (blots) and hard yellow exudates.

which occur more superficially in the nerve fibre layer; (ii) *microaneurysms,* which are due to vessel wall damage; and (iii) two types of exudates— *hard exudates,* which have straight edges, and *soft exudates* (cottonwool spots), which have a fluffy appearance.

Proliferative changes (Figure 10.23) are changes in blood vessels in response to ischaemia of the

---

[r]   Douglas Argyll Robertson (1837–1909), a Scottish ophthalmic surgeon and President of the Royal College of Surgeons, described these in 1869. The pupils are small, irregular and unequal, and react briskly to accommodation but not to light. Tertiary syphilis is another cause.

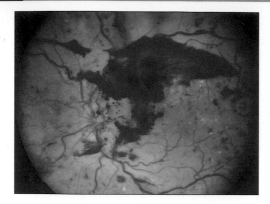

Figure 10.23 Proliferative diabetic retinopathy

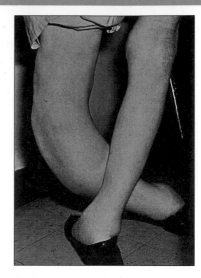

Figure 10.24 Paget's disease, showing bowing of the tibia

retina. They are characterised by new vessel formation, which can lead to vitreal haemorrhage, scar formation and eventually retinal detachment. The *detached retina* appears as an opalescent sheet that balloons forward into the vitreous. The underlying choroid is visible through the detached retina as a bright red-coloured sheet. Look also for *laser scars* (small brown or yellow spots), which are secondary to photocoagulation of new vessels by laser therapy.

Assess the third, fourth and sixth cranial nerves. In particular examine for a diabetic third nerve palsy from ischaemia, which usually spares the pupil (as infarction of the third nerve affects the inner pupillary fibres more than the outer fibres; in this way it differs from compressive lesions, which have the opposite effect).

Other cranial nerves may be affected sometimes because of cerebrovascular accidents (large vessel atheroma). *Rhinocerebral mucormycosis* may rarely develop in very poorly controlled diabetic patients, causing periorbital and perinasal swelling and cranial nerve palsies.

The ears. Look in the ears for evidence of infection. The rare *malignant otitis externa*, usually due to *Pseudomonas aeruginosa*, causes a mound of granulation tissue in the external canal, and facial nerve palsy in 50% of cases.

The mouth. Look for evidence of *Candida* infection.

The neck and shoulders

Examine the carotid arteries for evidence of vascular disease.

Rarely there may be thickening of the skin of the upper back and shoulders (scleroedema diabeticorum—this diffuse cutaneous infiltration has a very different distribution from scleroderma, with which it is sometimes confused). Look for acanthosis nigricans—associated with insulin resistance.

The abdomen

Palpate for hepatomegaly (fatty infiltration, or due to haemochromatosis).

Urinalysis

Test for glucose and protein. Diabetic nephropathy (from glomerulonephritis, renal arterial disease or pyelonephritis) can cause proteinuria. The presence of nitrite and/or blood is of value as asymptomatic urinary tract infections can occur. In advanced disease there may be signs of renal failure.

Paget's[s] disease (osteitis deformans)

This disease is characterised by excessive reabsorption of bone by osteoclasts and compensatory disorganised deposition of new bone. It is possibly a disease of viral origin.

General inspection

Note short stature (due to bending of the long bones of the limbs) and any obvious deformity of the head and lower limbs.

Head and face

Inspect the scalp for enlargement in the frontal and parietal areas and measure the head circumference

---

[s]   Sir James Paget (1814–99), a surgeon at St Bartholomew's Hospital, London, was also Queen Victoria's doctor.

(greater than 55 cm is usually abnormal). There may be prominent skull veins. Palpate for increased bony warmth and auscultate over the skull for systolic bruits. Both of these are due to increased vascularity of the skull vault. Oddly enough, bronchial breath sounds may be audible over the pagetic skull through the stethoscope. These are due to increased bone conduction of air. An area of very localised bony swelling and warmth may indicate development of a bony sarcoma (1% of cases of Paget's disease may develop this complication).

Examine the eyes. Assess visual acuity and visual fields, and look in the fundi for angioid streaks and optic atrophy. Retinitis pigmentosa occurs rather more rarely. Test for hearing loss (due to bony ossicle involvement or eighth nerve compression by bony enlargement).

Examine the remaining cranial nerves; all may be involved because of bony overgrowth of the foramina or be caused by basilar invagination (platybasia; where the posterior fossa becomes flat and the basal angle increased).

The neck

Patients with basilar invagination have a short neck and low hairline. The head is held in extension and neck movements are decreased. Assess the jugular venous pressure, as a high output cardiac failure may be present, particularly if there is coexistent ischaemic heart disease.

The heart

Examine for signs of cardiac failure.

The back

Inspect for kyphosis (due to vertebral involvement causing collapse of the vertebral bodies). Tap for

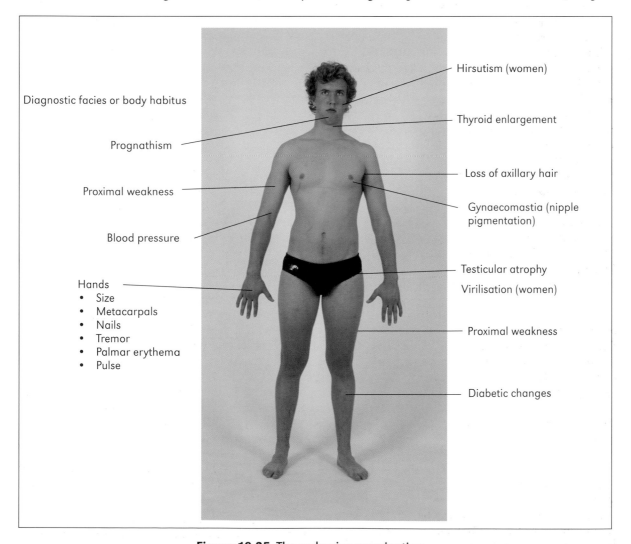

Figure 10.25 The endocrine examination

localised tenderness, feel for warmth and auscultate for systolic bruits over the vertebral bodies.

The legs

Inspect for anterior bowing of the tibia and lateral bowing of the femur (Figure 10.24). Feel for bony warmth and tenderness. Note any changes of osteoarthritis in the hips and knees, which often coexist with Paget's disease. Note any localised warm swelling, which may indicate sarcoma.

Examine for evidence of paraplegia, which is uncommon but can occur due to cord compression by bone or vascular shunting in the spinal cord Cerebellar signs may rarely be present due to platybasia.

Urinalysis

Check for blood (there is an increased incidence of renal stones in Paget's disease).

Summary

The endocrine system: a suggested method of examination (Figure 10.25)

Inspect the patient for one of the diagnostic facies or body habituses. If the diagnosis is obvious, proceed with the specific examination outlined previously. If not, examine as follows.

Pick up the **hands**. Look at the overall size (acromegaly), length of the metacarpals (pseudo-hypoparathyroidism and pseudopseudohypo-parathyroidism), for abnormalities of the nails (hyperthyroidism and hypothyroidism, and hypoparathyroidism), tremor, palmar erythema and sweating of the palms (hyperthyroidism).

Take the pulse (thyroid disease) and the blood pressure (hypertension in Cushing's syndrome, or postural hypotension in Addison's disease). Look for Trousseau's sign (tetany). Test for proximal muscle weakness (thyroid disease, Cushing's syndrome).

Go to the **axillae**. Look for loss of axillary hair (hypopituitarism), or acanthosis nigricans and skin tags (acromegaly).

Examine the **eyes** (hyperthyroidism) and the **fundi** (diabetes, acromegaly). Look at the **face** for hirsutism, or fine-wrinkled hairless skin (panhypopituitarism). Note any skin greasiness, acne or plethora (Cushing's syndrome).

Look at the **mouth** for protrusion of the chin and enlargement of the tongue (acromegaly) or buccal pigmentation (Addison's disease).

Examine the **neck** for thyroid enlargement. Note any neck webbing (Turner's syndrome). Palpate for supraclavicular fat pads (Cushing's syndrome).

Inspect the **chest** wall for hirsutism or loss of body hair, reduction in breast size in women (panhypopituitarism) or gynaecomastia in men. Look for nipple pigmentation (Addison's disease).

Examine the **abdomen** for hirsutism, central fat deposition, purple striae (Cushing's syndrome) and the **external genitalia** for virilisation or atrophy Look at the **legs** for diabetic changes.

Measure the body **weight** and **height**, and examine the **urine**.

References

1. Alvi A, Johnson JT. The neck mass. A challenging differential diagnosis. *Postgrad Med* 1995; 97:87–90, 93–94. Reviews how the history and examination narrow the differential diagnosis.
2. Siminoski K. Does this patient have a goiter? *JAMA* 1995; 273:813–817. A guide to examining the thyroid.
3. Wallace C, Siminoski K. The Pemberton sign. *Ann Intern Med* 1996; 125:568–569. Describes the sign, due to a retrosternal goitre compressing cephalic venous inflow (and in some tracheal airflow).
4. McGee S, *Evidence-based physical diagnosis*, 2nd edn. St Louis: Saunders, 2007.
5. Braunstein GD. Gynecomastia. *N Engl J Med* 1993; 328:490–495. A good review.
6. Edelson GW, Armstrong DG, Lavery LA, Ciacco G. The acutely infected diabetic foot is not adequately evaluated in an inpatient setting. *Arch Intern Med* 1996; 156:2372–2378. All patients evaluated had undergone a less than adequate foot examination. Of admitted patients, 31% did not have their pedal pulses documented; 60% of the admitted patients were not evaluated for the presence or absence of protective sensation.

Suggested reading

Greenspan FS, Gardner DG, eds. *Basic and clinical endocrinology*, 8th edn. New York: Lange Medical/ McGraw Hill, 2007.

Hegedus L. Clinical practice. The thyroid nodule. *N Engl J Med* 2004; 351:1764–1771.

Kronenberg HM, Melmed S, Polonsky KS, Larsen PR. *Williams textbook of endocrinology*, 11th edn. Philadelphia: Saunders, 2007.

Chapter 11

The nervous system

Who could have foretold, from the structure of the brain, that wine could derange its functions?

Hippocrates (460–375 BC)

The neurological history

The neurological history begins in detail with the presenting problem or problems (Table 11.1). The patient should be allowed to describe the symptoms in his or her own words to begin with,

and then the clinician needs to ask questions to clarify information and obtain more detail. It is particularly important to ascertain the *temporal course of the illness*, as this may give important information about the underlying aetiology.

An acute onset of symptoms (within minutes to an hour) is suggestive of a vascular or convulsive problem (e.g. the explosive severe headache of subarachnoid haemorrhage or the rapid onset of a seizure).

For these episodes of sudden onset, a precipitating event (e.g. exercise) or warning (*aura*) may be present. The aura that precedes a seizure may be localising (e.g. auditory hallucinations, an unusual smell or taste, loss of speech, or motor changes) or non-localising (e.g. a feeling of apprehension). The occurrence of an aura followed by sudden unconsciousness is very suggestive of the diagnosis of a major seizure or complex partial seizure.

A *stroke* or *cerebrovascular accident* usually causes symptoms which appear over minutes or are present when the patient wakes from sleep. There is a focal problem with function of the brain. Patients may be unable to move one side of the body (hemiplegia) or have difficulty with speech or swallowing, There may have been previous episodes. When there is resolution of the symptoms within 24 hours the episode is called a *transient ischaemic attack*—TIA). The rapid onset of focal symptoms almost always has a vascular cause— embolism, infarction or haemorrhage. If the patient can answer questions it is important to ask about the onset of the symptoms and about risk factors for stroke (*Questions box 11.1*).

The sudden onset of weakness on one side of the body followed by resolution and a severe headache is characteristic of hemiplegic migraine. Sudden resolution without headache suggests a transient

TABLE 11.1 Neurological history

Presenting symptoms*
Headache, facial pain
Neck or back pain
Fits, faints or funny turns
Dizziness or vertigo
Disturbances of vision, hearing or smell
Disturbances of gait
Loss of or disturbed sensation, or weakness in limb(s)
Disturbances of sphincter control (bladder, bowels)
Involuntary movements or tremor
Speech and swallowing disturbance
Altered cognition

Risk factors for cerebrovascular disease
Hypertension
Smoking
Diabetes mellitus
Hyperlipidaemia
Atrial fibrillation, bacterial endocarditis, myocardial
    infarction (emboli)
Haematological disease
Family history of stroke

* Note particularly the temporal course of the illness, whether symptoms suggest focal or diffuse disease, and the likely level of involvement of the nervous system.

Questions box 11.1

Questions to ask the (non-aphasic) patient with a possible stroke or transient ischaemic attack

1 What have you noticed has been wrong?
2 How quickly did it come on? How long ago?
3 Has it improved or gone away now?
4 Have you ever had a stroke before? How did that affect you?
5 Have you had high blood pressure or cholesterol (risk factors)?
6 Are you a diabetic (risk factor)?
7 Do you smoke (risk factor)?
8 Is there a history of strokes in the family?
9 Have you had palpitations or been told you have atrial fibrillation?
10 Have you been treated with blood-thinning drugs such as aspirin or warfarin?

Questions box 11.2

Questions to ask the patient with a possible neurological problem

1 Can you tell me what has been happening to you?
2 Are you right- or left-handed?
3 Have you had problems with headaches?
4 Have you been dizzy or had problems with your balance?
5 Have you noticed trouble with your speech?
6 Have you had problems with your vision?
7 Have you had weakness in an arm or leg?
8 Have you ever had a seizure or a blackout?
9 Have you ever had a head injury?
10 Have you had any back problems?
11 Have you had any scans of your brain or spinal cord?
12 What medications have you been taking?
13 Have you had high blood pressure?
14 Is there a history of neurological or muscle problems in the family?
15 Do you drink alcohol?

ischaemic episode. The very gradual onset of muscle weakness suggests a muscle abnormality such as myopathy rather than a vascular event.

A subacute onset (hours to days) occurs with inflammatory disorders (e.g. meningitis, cerebral abscess or the Guillain-Barré[a] syndrome—acute inflammatory polyradiculoneuropathy).

A more chronic symptom course suggests that the underlying disorder may be related to either a tumour (weeks to months) or a degenerative process (months to years). Metabolic or toxic disorders may present with any of these time courses.

Based on the history (and physical examination), a judgment is made as to whether the disease process is *localised or diffuse*, and which *levels of the nervous system* are involved (the nervous system may be thought of as having four different levels: the peripheral nervous system, the spinal cord, the posterior fossa, and the cerebral hemispheres). Consideration of the time course and the levels of involvement will usually lead to a logical differential diagnosis of the patient's symptoms. After detailed questions about the presenting problem, ask about previous neurological symptoms and about previous neurological diagnoses or investigations. The patient may know the results of CT or magnetic resonance imaging brain scans performed in the past. A thorough neurological history will include routine questions about possible neurological symptoms (*Questions box 11.2*). If the patient answers 'yes' to any of these, more-detailed questions about the nature of the problem and its time course are indicated.

Headache and facial pain

Headache is a very common symptom (*Questions box 11.3*). It is important, as with any type of pain, to determine the character, severity, site, duration, frequency, radiation, aggravating and relieving factors and associated symptoms.[1,2] Unilateral headache that is preceded by flashing lights or zigzag lines and is associated with light hurting the eyes (photophobia) is likely to be a *migraine with an aura* ('classical migraine'); common migraine has no aura. Pain over one eye (or over the temple) lasting for minutes to hours, associated with lacrimation, rhinorrhoea and flushing of the forehead, and occurring in bouts that last several weeks a few times a year or less, is suggestive of *cluster headache*. This occurs predominantly in males and patients can't stay still. Headache over the occiput and associated with neck stiffness may be from *cervical spondylosis*. *Coital headache*

---

a Georges Guillain (1876–1961), Jean Alexandre Barré (1880–1967) and A Strohl described the syndrome in 1916; Strohl's name was dropped because of anti-German feeling during World War I.

TABLE 11.2 Symptoms and signs of temporal arteritis

Symptoms	Frequency (%)	Positive LR	Negative LR
Headache often present for 2 or 3 months	77	1.5	0.82
Jaw claudication (pain in proximal jaw near TMJ after brief chewing of tough food)	51	4.2	0.72
Malaise	48	1.2	0.94
Polymyalgia rheumatica (shoulder girdle pain and stiffness)	34	0.97	0.99
Visual disturbance (often sudden monocular blindness)	29	0.85	1.2
Examination findings			
Fever	26	–	–
Tender temporal artery (palpated just anterior and superior to the tragus of the ear).	53	2.6	0.82
Enlarged temporal artery	–	4.3	0.67
There can be ischaemic changes of the tongue or scalp.			

TMJ = temporomandibular joint.
Likelihood ratios from McGee S, *Evidence-based physical diagnosis*, 2nd edn. St Louis: Saunders, 2007.

Questions box 11.3

Questions to ask the patient with headache

1 What is it like, e.g. dull, sharp, throbbing or tight?

2 Where do you feel it—at the front or back, on one side or in the face?

3 How severe is it and how long does it last?

4 Has it begun very suddenly and severely?—Subarachnoid haemorrhage

5 Do you get any warning that it is about to start, e.g. flashing lights or zigzag lines in your vision?—Migraine

6 Is it associated with sensitivity to light (photophobia)?—Migraine

7 Do you feel drowsy or nauseated?—Raised intracranial pressure

8 Is the pain on one side over the temple and have you had any blurred vision?—Temporal arteritis

9 Is the pain worst over your cheek bones?—Sinusitis

10 Are the attacks likely to occur in clusters and associated with watering of one eye?—Cluster headache

11 Is there a prolonged feeling of tightness over the head but no other symptoms?—Tension headache

12 Did you drink large amounts of alcohol last night?—Hangover

occurs during intercourse close to orgasm.

A generalised headache that is worse in the morning and is associated with drowsiness or vomiting may reflect *raised intracranial pressure*, while generalised headache associated with photophobia and fever as well as with a stiff neck of more gradual onset may be due to *meningitis*. A persistent unilateral headache over the temporal area associated with tenderness over the temporal artery and blurring of vision suggests *temporal arteritis*.[3,4] This condition (Table 11.2) is often associated with jaw claudication, or jaw pain during eating, which can lead to considerable loss of weight. Headache with pain or fullness behind the eyes or over the cheeks or forehead occurs in *acute sinusitis*. The dramatic and usually instantaneous onset of severe headache that is initially localised but becomes generalised and is associated with neck stiffness may be due to a *subarachnoid haemorrhage*. Morning headaches worse with coughing, especially in an obese patient, may be due to *idiopathic intracranial hypertension*; visual loss may occur.

Finally, the most frequent type of headache is episodic or chronic *tension-type headache*; this is commonly bilateral, occurs over the frontal, occipital or temporal areas, and may be described as a sensation of tightness that lasts for hours and recurs often. There are usually no associated symptoms such as nausea, vomiting, weakness or paraesthesiae (tingling in the limbs), and the headache does not usually wake the patient at night from sleep.

Pain in the face can result from trigeminal neuralgia, temporomandibular arthritis, glaucoma, cluster headache, temporal arteritis, psychiatric disease, aneurysm of the internal carotid or posterior communicating artery, or the superior orbital fissure syndrome.

Faints and fits (see also page 41)

It is important to try to differentiate syncope (transient loss of consciousness) from *epilepsy* (*Questions box 11.4*). However, primary syncopal events can cause a few clonic jerks in a significant number of cases. Generalised tonic-clonic seizures (grand mal epilepsy) cause abrupt loss of consciousness, which may be preceded by an aura. Often the patient is incontinent of urine and faeces,

and the tongue may be bitten. A witness may be able to describe the type of attack that occurred. It is important to try to determine whether any seizure is generalised or localised to one side of the body: a seizure affecting part of the body may indicate a focal lesion in the central nervous system, such as a tumour or abscess. If consciousness is impaired, these partial seizures are described as 'complex'; if consciousness is unimpaired they are termed 'simple'. Idiopathic absence seizures ('petit mal') occur in children. These are frequent brief episodes of loss of awareness often associated with staring. Major motor movements do not occur with this type of epilepsy.

Transient ischaemic attacks (TIAs) affecting the brainstem can occasionally cause blackouts. Use of the term 'drop attacks' means the patient falls but there is no loss of consciousness. In either case the patient falls to the ground without premonition and the attacks are of brief duration. *Hypoglycaemia* can lead to episodes of loss of consciousness. Patients with hypoglycaemia may also report sweating, weakness and confusion before losing consciousness. Bizarre attacks of loss of consciousness occur with *hysteria*.[b] During such attacks the patient may slump to the ground without sustaining any injury and there may be apparent fluctuations in the level of consciousness for a prolonged period.

Dizziness

If a patient complains of dizziness, it is important to determine what is meant by this term. In true *vertigo*, there is actually a sense of motion, usually of the surroundings but also of the head itself (page 41).[5] When vertigo is severe it may not be possible for the patient to stand or walk, and associated symptoms of nausea, vomiting, pallor, sweating and headache may be present. Causes of vertigo include the 'peripheral vestibular lesions':

- benign positioning (positional) vertigo—recurrent brief episodes of vertigo precipitated by a change of head position, due to crystals in the saccule and utricle
- vestibular neuronitis—non-positional vertigo due to inflammation of the acoustic nerve with normal hearing, and
- acute labyrinthitis—associated with hearing loss.

Other causes of vertigo include:

- ototoxic drugs (e.g. aminoglycosides), associated with deafness or tinnitus;

Questions box 11.4

Questions to ask the patient with syncope or dizziness

1 Have you lost consciousness completely? How long for?

2 Do you black out or feel dizzy when you stand up quickly?—Postural hypotension

3 How often have episodes occurred?

4 Was the sensation more one of spinning?—Vertigo

5 Did the episode occur during heavy exercise or when you got up to pass urine at night? Exercise—suggests a left ventricular outflow tract obstruction such as aortic stenosis. Pass urine at night—micturition syncope

6 Have you injured yourself?

7 Do you get any warning?—A feeling of nausea and being in a stuffy room suggests a vasovagal episode; a strange smell or feeling of deja-vu suggests an aura and therefore a seizure

8 Have you passed urine during the episode?—Seizure

9 Have you bitten your tongue?—Seizure

10 Has anyone seen an episode and noticed jerking movements (tonic-clonic movements)?—Makes a seizure more likely but can also occur with cardiac syncope

11 Do you wake up feeling normal or drowsy? Normal—cardiac syncope. Drowsy—seizure

12 What medications are you taking—any antihypertensive medications, cardiac anti-arrhythmic drugs or anti-epileptic drugs?

---

b   Hysteria is an old but still popular term that refers to a presumed psychogenic condition.

- Ménière's disease,[c] which occurs in those over 50 years of age and presents with the triad of episodic vertigo and tinnitus (ringing in the ears) with progressive deafness;
- acoustic neuroma (where patients may also have deafness and tinnitus);
- central causes such as vertebrobasilar TIAs—these may be associated with diplopia (double vision; page 427), visual loss and ataxia; and
- rarely, internal auditory artery occlusion.

Visual disturbances and deafness

Problems with vision can include double vision (diplopia), blurred vision (amblyopia), light intolerance (photophobia) and visual loss. The causes of deafness are summarised on page 348.

Disturbances of gait

Many neurological conditions can make walking difficult. These are described on page 376. Walking may also be abnormal when orthopaedic disease affects the lower limbs or spine. A bizarrely abnormal gait can sometimes be a sign of a hysterical reaction.

Disturbed sensation or weakness in the limbs

Pins and needles in the hands or feet may indicate nerve entrapment or a peripheral neuropathy (page 386) but can result from sensory pathway involvement at any level. The carpal tunnel syndrome is common; here there is median nerve entrapment, and patients experience pain and paraesthesiae in the hand and wrist. Sometimes pain may extend to the arm and even to the shoulder, but paraesthesiae are felt only in the fingers. These symptoms are usually worse at night and may be relieved by dangling the arm over the side of the bed or shaking the hand.

Nerve root, spinal cord and cerebral abnormalities can all cause disturbance of sensation and weakness.

Limb weakness can be caused by lesions at different levels in the motor system. There are a number of patterns of limb and muscle weakness:
- Upper motor neurone (UMN) weakness (page 383) is due to interruption of a neural pathway at a level above the anterior horn cell. The result is an increase in tone and peripheral reflexes. Interruption of this pathway has the greatest effect on the antigravity muscles and is called *pyramidal weakness*. There is little or no muscle wasting.
- Lower motor neurone (LMN) weakness (page 385) is due to a lesion that interrupts the reflex arc between the anterior horn cell and the muscle. There is a reduction in tone and reflexes, fasciculation (irregular contractions of small areas of muscle) may be seen and muscle wasting is prominent.
- Muscle disease causes weakness in a particular muscle or group of muscles. There is wasting, decreased tone, and the reflexes are reduced or absent.
- Disease at the neuromuscular junction (e.g. myasthenia gravis, page 394) causes generalised weakness, which worsens with repetition. The reflexes and tone are often normal.
- Non-organic weakness (e.g. due to hysteria) causes a non-anatomical pattern of weakness in association with normal tone and power and, unless there has been prolonged disuse, normal muscle bulk.

Tremor and involuntary movements

Tremor is a rhythmical movement (Table 11.3). A slow tremor has, by definition, a rate between 3 Hz and 5 Hz. Rapid tremors are faster than 10 Hz. *Resting* tremors are present mostly during relaxation of the muscles, while *intention* tremors occur with deliberate movement and become more pronounced towards the end of the action. Tremors become worse with fatigue or anxiety. Shivering is a type of tremor brought on by cold. It is normal for there to be a fine tremor associated with holding a posture or performing a movement slowly. This is called a *physiological* tremor. It becomes more obvious with fright and fatigue. It is often increased by the beta-agonist drugs used to treat asthma or by caffeine. Thyrotoxicosis is a cause of exaggeration of physiological tremor. These movements are very fine and may be difficult to see unless looked for specifically. *Benign essential (familial)* tremor is an inherited disorder which causes tremor, but no other signs. The tremor is most easily seen when the patient's arms are stretched out; it can become worse during voluntary movements. It usually disappears when the muscles are at complete rest. Parkinson's disease[d] may present with a resting tremor (page 397). Intention (or target-seeking)

---

c   Prosper Ménière (1799–1862), director of the Paris Institution for Deaf-Mutes, characterised this condition just before he died of post-influenzal pneumonia. He was an expert on orchids and a friend of Victor Hugo and Honoré de Balzac. He added the grave accent on the second 'e' in his name himself; the acute accent on the first 'e' was added by his son.

d   James Parkinson (1755–1824), English general practitioner, published an essay on 'The Shaking Palsy' in 1817. He was nearly transported to Australia for reformist activities.

tremor is due to cerebellar disease (page 398). *Chorea* involves involuntary jerky movements (page 399). Definitions of the terms used to describe movement disorders are shown in Table 11.4.

Speech and mental status

Speech may be disturbed by many different neurological diseases and is discussed on page 377. A number of different diseases can also result in delirium or dementia, as described on page 377 and in Chapter 12.

Past health

Inquire about a past history of meningitis or encephalitis, head or spinal injuries, a history of epilepsy or convulsions and any previous operations. Any past history of sexually transmitted disease (e.g. risk factors for HIV infection or syphilis) should be obtained. Ask about risk factors that may predispose to the development of cerebrovascular disease (Table 11.1). A previous diagnosis of peripheral vascular disease or of coronary artery disease indicates an increased risk of cerebrovascular disease. Chronic or paroxysmal atrial fibrillation is associated with a greatly increased risk of embolic stroke, especially for people over the age of 70.

Medication history

Previous and current medications may be the cause of certain neurological or apparently neurological syndromes (Table 11.5).

TABLE 11.5 Drugs and neurology

1 **Anti-hypertensives**
   Therapeutic use: reduction of risk of stroke
   Side-effects: postural dizziness, syncope, depression (methyldopa)

2 **Anti-platelet drugs and anti-coagulants**
   Therapeutic use: reduction of risk of stroke
   Side-effect: cerebral haemorrhage

3 **Statins**
   Therapeutic use: reduction in stroke risk
   Side-effect: myopathy

4 **Major tranquillisers**
   Therapeutic use: treatment of psychoses
   Side-effects: ataxia, sedation, Parkinsonian tremor

5 **Other neurological symptoms associated with drugs**
   Headache: nitrates, sildenafil
   Deafness: aminoglycoside antibiotics, aspirin, frusemide
   Peripheral neuropathy: amiodarone, isoniazid, metronidazole
   Non-Parkinsonian tremor: bronchodilators, amphetamines
   Dysphagia: bisphosphonates
   Confusion and loss of memory: minor tranquillisers
   Seizures: lignocaine

TABLE 11.3 Rates of tremors

Parkinson's disease	3 to 5 Hz
Essential/familial	4 to 7 Hz
Physiological	8 to 13 Hz

TABLE 11.4 Definitions of terms used to describe movement disorders

Akithesia	Motor restlessness; constant semi-purposeful movements of the arms and legs
Asterixis	Sudden loss of muscle tone during sustained contraction of an outstretched limb
Athetosis	Writhing, slow sinuous movements, especially of the hands and wrists
Chorea	Jerky small rapid movements, often disguised by the patient with a purposeful final movement: e.g. the jerky upward arm movement is transformed into a voluntary movement to scratch the head
Dyskinesia	Purposeless and continuous movements, often of the face and mouth; often a result of treatment with major tranquillisers for psychotic illness
Dystonia	Sustained contractions of groups of agonist and antagonist muscles, usually in flexion or extremes of extension; it results in bizarre postures
Hemiballismus	An exaggerated form of chorea involving one side of the body: there are wild flinging movements which can injure the patient (or bystanders)
Myoclonic jerk	A brief muscle contraction which causes a sudden purposeless jerking of a limb
Myokymia	A repeated contraction of a small muscle group; often involves the orbicularis oculi muscles
Tic	A repetitive irresistible movement which is purposeful or semi-purposeful
Tremor	A rhythmical alternating movement

Ask about treatment for neurological disorders with anticonvulsants, anti-Parkinsonian drugs, steroids, immunosuppressants, biological agents, anticoagulants, antiplatelet agents and for other drug treatment that may be associated with neurological problems; use of the contraceptive pill, antihypertensive agents or drugs for other disorders needs to be documented.

Social history

As smoking predisposes to cerebrovascular disease, the smoking history is relevant. It is useful to ask about occupation and exposure to toxins (e.g. heavy metals). Alcohol can also result in a number of neurological diseases (see Table 1.3, page 7).

Family history

Any history of neurological or mental disease should be documented. A number of important neurological conditions are inherited (Table 11.6).

TABLE 11.6 Inherited neurological conditions

X-linked	Colour blindness, Duchenne's and Becker's muscular dystrophy, Leber's* optic atrophy
Autosomal dominant	Huntington's chorea, tuberose sclerosis, dystrophia myotonica
Autosomal recessive	Wilson's disease, Refsum's† disease, Freiderich's ataxia, Tay-Sachs'‡ disease
Increased incidence in families	Alzheimer's§ disease

* Theodor Karl von Leber (1840–1917). German ophthalmologist, professor of ophthalmology at Heidelberg. He began studying chemistry but was advised by Bunsen that there were too many chemists and so changed to studying medicine.
† Siguald Refsum (1907–91), Norwegian neurologist. He described this in 1945, calling it heredotaxia hemerlopica polyneuritiformis. This may be an argument for the use of eponymous names.
‡ Warren Tay (1843–1927), English ophthalmologist, described the ophthalmological abnormalities of the condition. Bernard Sachs (1858–1944), American neurologist and psychiatrist, described the neurological features in 1187. He studied in Germany and was a pupil of von Recklinghausen. The condition was originally called amaurotic family idiocy. This may be another reason to use eponymous names.
§ Alois Alzheimer (1864–1915), Bavarian neuropathologist, described the condition in 1906. His doctoral thesis was on the wax-producing glands of the ear.

The neurological examination
Examination anatomy

More than for any other system of the body, neurological diagnosis depends on localising the anatomical site of the lesion—in the brain, spinal cord or peripheral nerve. Figure 11.1 shows the gross anatomy of the brain and the major functional areas.

As a preliminary to the neurological assessment, the clinician should obtain some biographical information from the patient, including the age, place of birth, handedness, occupation and level of education.

The examination of the nervous system and the interpretation of findings require a lot of practice. In a viva voce examination, this system more than any other system requires a polished technique. The signs need to be elicited carefully because the precise anatomical localisation of any lesions can often be determined this way. It is important, therefore, to remember some elementary neuroanatomy.

Examination can be long and difficult and it is said to take much of a day if absolutely everything that can be done (including psychometric assessment) is done. This is obviously impractical, but a screening examination that will uncover most signs takes only a relatively short time.

In brief, the following aspects of the examination must be attended to:
1 General, including examination for neck stiffness, assessment of the higher centres, speech, and abnormal movements.
2 The cranial nerves II to XII.
3 The upper limbs. Motor system: inspection, tone, power, reflexes, coordination. Sensory system: pinprick sensation, proprioception, vibration sense, light touch.
4 The lower limbs: as for the upper limbs, but including assessment of walking (gait).
5 The skull and spine for local disease.
6 The carotid arteries for bruits.

General signs
Consciousness

Note the level of consciousness. If the patient is unconscious look for responses to various stimuli (page 401).

Neck stiffness

Any patient with an acute neurological illness, or who is febrile or has altered mental status **must** be assessed for signs of meningism.[6]

With the patient lying flat in bed, the examiner slips a hand under the occiput and gently flexes

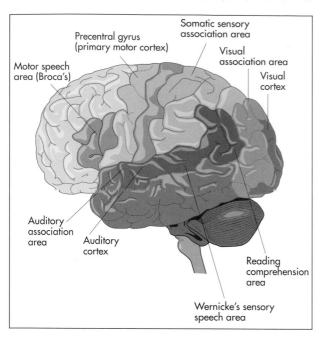

Motor speech area (Broca's)

Motor speech area (Broca's)

Precentral gyrus (primary motor cortex)

Somatic sensory association area

Visual association area

Visual cortex

Auditory association area

Auditory cortex

Reading comprehension area

Wernicke's sensory speech area

Figure 11.1 The functional areas of the brain

the neck passively (i.e. without assistance from the patient). The chin is brought up to approach the chest wall. Meningism may be caused by pyogenic or other infection of the meninges, or by blood in the subarachnoid space secondary to subarachnoid haemorrhage. There is resistance to neck flexion due to painful spasm of the extensor muscles of the neck. Other causes of resistance to neck flexion are characterised by an equal resistance to head rotation. They include: (i) cervical spondylosis; (ii) after cervical fusion; (iii) Parkinson's disease; and (iv) raised intracranial pressure, especially if there is impending tonsillar herniation. The *Brudzinski sign*[e] is spontaneous flexion of the hips during flexion of the neck by the examiner and indicates meningism.

Kernig's sign[f] should also be elicited if meningitis is suspected. Flex each hip in turn, then attempt to straighten the knee while keeping the hip flexed. This is greatly limited by spasm of the hamstrings (which in turn causes pain) when there is meningism due to an inflammatory exudate around the lumbar spinal roots.

Although the diagnostic value has been questioned (combined meningeal signs had a positive LR of 0.92 and a negative LR of 0.88),[6] we have found these signs useful clinically (and they have excellent specificity).

Handedness

Shake the patient's hand and ask if he or she is right- or left-handed. This is polite and allows the examiner to assess the likely dominant hemisphere. Ninety-four per cent of right-handed people and about 50% of left-handed people have a dominant left hemisphere. There is division of function between the two hemispheres, the most obvious distinction being that the dominant hemisphere controls language and mathematical functions.

Orientation

Test orientation in *person*, *place* and *time* by asking the patient his or her name, present location and the date (normal patients who have been in hospital for long periods often get the day wrong as one day seems very much like another in hospital). Disorientation is not a specific localising sign and may be acute and reversible (delirium) or chronic and irreversible (dementia). The mini-mental state examination (Table 12.7, page 420) is a useful way to document the progress of a confusional state or dementia over time.

The cranial nerves[g]
Examination anatomy

The cranial nerves (Figure 11.2) arise as direct extensions of the brain (I and II) or from the brainstem (midbrain, pons and medulla)—Figures 11.10 (page 337), 11.13 (page 340) and 11.14 (page 341).

If possible, position the patient so that he or she is sitting over the edge of the bed. Look at the head, face and neck. If hydrocephalus has occurred in infancy—before closure of the cranial sutures—the head and face may resemble an inverted triangle. Acromegaly (page 307), Paget's disease (page 320) or basilar invagination (page 321) may be obvious. A careful *general inspection* may reveal signs easily missed when each cranial nerve is examined separately. This is particularly true of ptosis (page 337), proptosis (page 303), pupillary inequality (page 336), skew deviation of the eyes

---

e   Josef Brudzinski (1874–1917), Polish paediatrician , described this in 1909.
f   Vladimir Kernig (1840–1917), St Petersburg neurologist, described this in 1882.

g   The anatomy and function of the cranial nerves was well established by the late 19th century. Galen identified at least seven of the cranial nerves in the 2nd century. These were probably the optic, oculomotor, the sensory part of the trigeminal, the motor part of the trigeminal, facial, vestibular, the glossopharyngeal (including the vagus and accessory) and the hypoglossal.

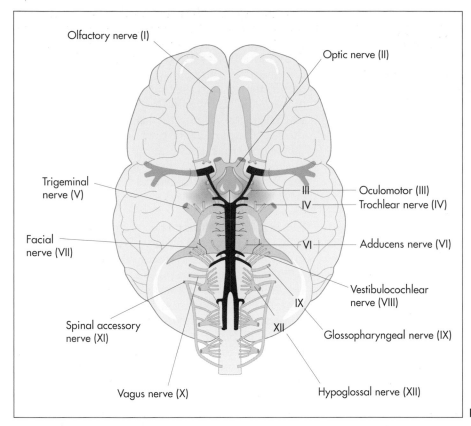

Olfactory nerve (I)

Optic nerve (II)

Trigeminal nerve (V)

III — Oculomotor (III)

IV — Trochlear nerve (IV)

Facial nerve (VII)

VI — Adducens nerve (VI)

Vestibulocochlear nerve (VIII)

IX

Spinal accessory nerve (XI)

XII

Glossopharyngeal nerve (IX)

Vagus nerve (X)

Hypoglossal nerve (XII)

Figure 11.2 Cranial nerves

and facial asymmetry. Inspect the whole scalp for craniotomy scars and the skin for neurofibromas (Figure 11.3). Look for skin lesions: for example, a capillary or cavernous haemangioma is seen on the face in the distribution of the trigeminal (V) nerve in the Sturge-Weber syndrome.[h] It is associated with an intracranial venous haemangioma of the leptomeninges and with seizures.

The cranial nerves are usually tested in approximately the order of their number.[7]

The first (olfactory) nerve[i]

Examination anatomy. This is a purely sensory nerve, whose fibres arise in the mucous membrane of the nose and pass through the cribriform plate of the ethmoid bone to synapse in the olfactory bulb. From here the olfactory tract runs under the frontal lobe and terminates in the medial temporal lobe on the same side.

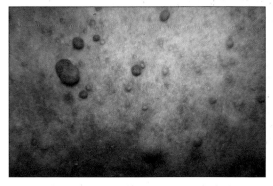

Figure 11.3 Subcutaneous neurofibromas in neurofibromatosis type I, associated with optic nerve and pontine gliomas (acoustic neuromas occur in type II)

Examination of the nose and sense of smell. Note the external appearance of the nose. Look for rash or deformity. Then examine the nasal vestibule by elevating the tip of the nose (in adults a speculum is usually needed to give an adequate view).

The first nerve is not tested routinely. If the patient complains of loss of smell (anosmia) or there are other signs suggesting a frontal or temporal lobe lesion, then it should be examined. Anosmic patients sometimes complain of loss of taste rather

h   William Allen Sturge (1850–1919), British physician, described this in 1879, and Frederick Parkes Weber (1863–1962), London physician, described it in 1922.
i   Samuel von Sommerring (1755–1830) is responsible for the modern classification of 12 cranial nerves. He separated the vestibular from the facial, and the glossopharyngeal from the vagus and accessory.

than of smell because the sense of smell plays a large part in the appreciation of taste. Test each nostril separately with a series of bottles containing essences of familiar smells, such as coffee, vanilla and peppermint (this is traditional, but not very reliable). Pungent substances such as ammonia should not be used, first because they upset the patient and second because noxious stimuli of this sort are detected by sensory fibres of the fifth (trigeminal) nerve. An easy way to test smell is to use the isopropyl alcohol wipes present in most hospital clinics. These have a distinctive and non-pungent smell.

Examination of the nasal passages must be performed if anosmia is present. Polyps and mucosal thickening may be seen and may explain the findings.

Causes of anosmia. Most cases of anosmia are bilateral. Causes include: (i) upper respiratory tract infection (commonest); (ii) smoking and increasing age; (iii) ethmoid tumours; (iv) basal skull fracture or frontal fracture, or after pituitary surgery; (v) congenital—for example, Kallmann's syndrome (hypogonadotrophic hypogonadism); (vi) meningioma of the olfactory groove; and (vii) following meningitis. The main unilateral causes are head trauma without a fracture, or an early meningioma of the olfactory groove.[j]

The second (optic) nerve

Examination anatomy. The optic nerve is not really a nerve but an extension of fibres of the central nervous system that unites the retinas with the brain. It is purely sensory, contains about a million fibres and extends for about 5 cm (Figure 11.4), passing through the optic foramen close to the ophthalmic artery and joining the nerve from the other side at the base of the brain to form the optic chiasm. The spatial orientation of fibres from different parts of the fundus is preserved so that fibres from the lower part of the retina are found in the inferior part of the chiasm, and vice versa. Fibres from the temporal visual fields (the nasal halves of the retinas) cross in the chiasm, whereas those from the nasal visual fields do not. Fibres for the light reflex from the optic chiasm finish in the superior colliculus, whence connections occur with both third nerve nuclei. The remainder of the fibres leaving the chiasm are concerned with vision, and travel in the optic tract to the lateral geniculate body. From here the fibres form the optic radiation and pass through the posterior part of the internal capsule, finishing in the visual cortex of the occipital lobe. In their course they splay out so that fibres serving the lower quadrants course through the parietal lobe, while those for the upper quadrants traverse the temporal lobe. The result of the decussation of fibres in the optic chiasm is that fibres from the left visual field terminate in the right occipital lobe, and vice versa.

History. The majority of visual symptoms involve reduction in visual acuity. These are discussed in detail with the physical examination findings. Some patients notice a more specific change, which will help direct the examination. Ask about the time course of the visual disturbance and whether it seems to involve the vision of one eye or one visual field. Sudden loss of vision in one eye (often described as the awareness of a curtain being drawn across the eye) may be due to an embolus to the retina. These are called *negative* visual symptoms. There is usually, but not always, spontaneous return of vision. This is called *amaurosis fugax*. Migraine attacks may be preceded by subjective visual changes, including scintillating scotomas, photophobia, blurred vision or hemianopia. Visual hallucinations such as flashing lights and distortions of vision are called *positive* visual symptoms. They can occur in psychotic states or as the aura of an epileptic seizure.

More gradual loss of vision has many possible causes.

Examination. Assess visual acuity, visual fields and the fundi.

Visual acuity is tested with the patient wearing his or her spectacles, if used for reading or driving, as refractive errors are *not* considered to be cranial nerve abnormalities. Use a hand-held eye chart or a Snellen's chart[k] on the wall. Each eye is tested separately, while the other is covered by a small card.

Formal testing with a standard Snellen's chart requires the patient to be 6 metres from the chart. Unless a very large room is available, this is done using a mirror. Normal visual acuity is present when the line marked 6 can be read correctly with

---

j   Other abnormalities of smell are hyperosmia and parosmia. *Hyperosmia* is an increase in the sensitivity of the sense of smell. It is often a sign of psychosis or hysteria but may occur with migraine, during menstruation and in cases of encephalitis. *Parosomia* is a perversion of the sense of smell. It can occur following trauma to the head and in some psychoses. Olfactory hallucinations are more often than not a result of an organic lesion and suggest an irritating lesion in the olfactory cortex.

k   Hermann Snellen (1834–1908), Dutch ophthalmologist, invented this chart in 1862.

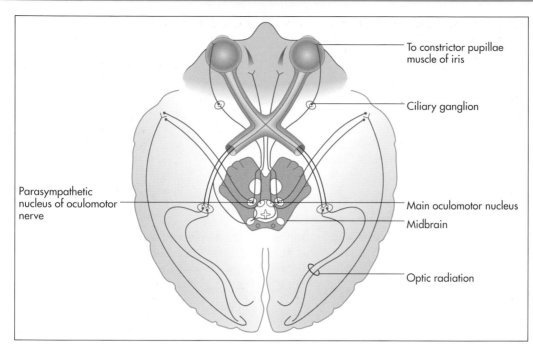

Figure 11.4 The optic pathways and visual reflexes (Adapted from Snell RS, Westmoreland BF, *Clinical neuroanatomy for medical students*, 4th edn. Boston: Little Brown, 1997.)

each eye (6/6 acuity). If poor visual acuity improves when the patient is asked to read the chart through a pin-hole, refractive error is likely to be the cause. A patient who is unable to read even the largest letter of the chart should be asked to count fingers held up in front of each eye in turn, and if this is not possible, then perception of hand movement is tested. Failing this, light perception only may be present.

Any abnormality of the lens, cornea, fundus or optic nerve pathway can cause reduction in visual acuity:

- *Causes of bilateral blindness of rapid onset* include bilateral occipital lobe infarction; bilateral occipital lobe trauma; bilateral optic nerve damage, as with methyl alcohol poisoning; and hysteria.
- *Sudden blindness in one eye* can be due to retinal artery or vein occlusion, temporal arteritis, non-arteritic ischaemic optic neuropathy and occasionally optic neuritis or migraine.
- *Bilateral blindness of gradual onset* may be caused by cataracts; acute glaucoma; macular degeneration; diabetic retinopathy (vitreous haemorrhages); bilateral optic nerve or chiasmal compression; and bilateral optic nerve damage—for example, tobacco *amblyopia* (blindness due to retinal disease).

Visual fields are examined by *confrontation* (Figure 11.5). Always remove a patient's spectacles

first. The examiner's head should be level with the patient's head. Use a white- or red-tipped hat pin or pen. Test each eye separately. The examiner holds the pin at arm's length with the coloured head upwards. It should be positioned halfway between the patient and the examiner, and brought in from just outside the examiner's peripheral vision until the patient can see it. Make sure the patient is staring directly at the examiner's eye and explain that he or she is looking for the first sight of the pin out of the corner of the eye. When the right eye is being tested the patient should look straight into the examiner's left eye. The patient's head should be at arm's length and the eye not being tested should be covered. The pin should be brought into the visual field from the four main directions, diagonally towards the centre of the field of vision.

Next the blind spot can be mapped out by asking about disappearance of the pin around the centre of the field of vision of each eye. The pin is moved slowly across the field of vision. A large central scotoma will lead to its apparent temporary disappearance and then reappearance. Only a gross enlargement may be detectable.

If a patient has such poor acuity that a pin is difficult to see, the fields should be mapped with the fingers. The examiner's fingers can also be used to perform a quick screening test of the visual fields. Usually two fingers are held up and brought into the centre of vision in the four quadrants. The examiner wriggles the fingers and asks the patient to say 'yes' when movement of the fingers is first

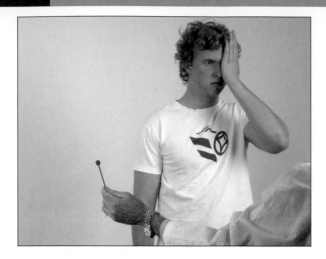
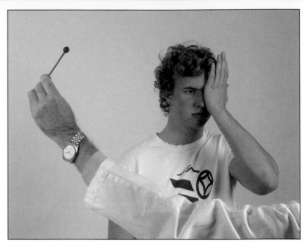

Figure 11.5 Visual field testing: 'Tell me when you first see the red pin come into view'

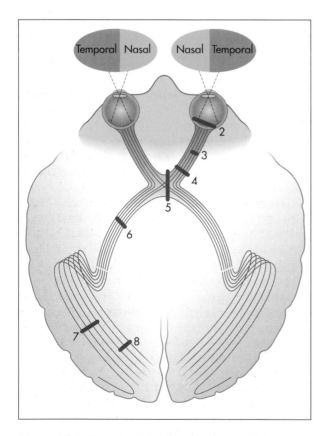

Figure 11.6 The visual fields and optic pathways
Numbers indicate sites of lesions producing field defects shown in Figure 11.7.
(Adapted from Snell RS, Westmoreland BF, *Clinical neuroanatomy for medical students*, 4th edn. Boston: Little Brown, 1997.)

1. TUNNEL VISION
   Concentric diminution, e.g. glaucoma, papilloedema, syphilis

2. ENLARGED BLIND SPOT
   Optic nerve head enlargement

3. CENTRAL SCOTOMATA
   Optic nerve head to chiasmal lesion, e.g. demyelination, toxic, vascular, nutritional

4. UNILATERAL FIELD LOSS
   Optic nerve lesion, e.g. vascular tumour

5. BITEMPORAL HEMIANOPIA
   Optic chiasm lesion, e.g. pituitary tumour, sella meningioma

6. HOMONYMOUS HEMIANOPIA
   Optic tract to occipital cortex, e.g. vascular, tumour (NB: incomplete lesion results in macular (central) vision sparing)

7. UPPER QUADRANT HOMONYMOUS HEMIANOPIA
   Temporal lobe lesion, e.g. vascular, tumour

8. LOWER QUADRANT HOMONYMOUS HEMIANOPIA
   Parietal lobe lesion

Figure 11.7 Visual field defects with lesions at various levels along the optic pathway, at sites indicated in Figure 11.6
(Adapted from Bickerstaff ER, Spillane JA. *Neurological examination in clinical practice*, 5th edn. Oxford: Blackwell, 1989.)

seen. The following patterns of visual field loss may be detected (Figures 11.6 and 11.7):

- *Concentric diminution of the field (tunnel vision)* may be caused by glaucoma; retinal abnormalities such as chorioretinitis or retinitis pigmentosa; papilloedema; or acute ischaemia, as with migraine. Normally even a reduced field of vision widens as objects are moved further away. Tubular diminution of the visual fields suggests hysteria. There is always a small area close to the centre of the visual fields where there is no vision (the blind spot). This is the area where the optic disc is seen on fundoscopy and is the point where the optic nerve joins the retina. The blind spot enlarges with papilloedema.
- *Central scotomata, or loss of central (macular) vision,* may be due to demyelination of the optic nerve (multiple sclerosis causes unilateral or asymmetrical bilateral scotomata); toxic causes, such as methyl alcohol (symmetrical bilateral scotomata); nutritional causes, such as tobacco or alcohol amblyopia (symmetrical central or centrocecal scotomata); vascular lesions (unilateral); and gliomas of the optic nerve (unilateral).
- *Total unilateral visual loss* is due to a lesion of the optic nerve or to unilateral eye disease.
- *Bitemporal hemianopia* is due to a lesion that affects the centre of the optic chiasm, damaging fibres from the nasal halves of the retinas as they decussate. This will result in loss of both temporal halves of the visual fields. Causes include a pituitary tumour, a craniopharyngioma and a suprasellar meningioma.
- *Binasal hemianopia* is very rare and is due to bilateral lesions affecting the uncrossed optic fibres, such as atheroma of the internal carotid siphon.
- *Homonymous hemianopia* is due to a lesion that damages the optic tract or radiation, affecting the visual field on the right or left side. For example, left temporal and right nasal field loss will occur with a right-sided lesion. The exact nature of the defect depends on the site of interruption of the fibres. In the optic tract the defect is usually complete—there is no macular sparing. In the more posterior optic radiation the macular vision is usually spared if the cause is ischaemia, but not if a destructive process such as tumour or haemorrhage is responsible. The macular cortical area is thought to have some additional blood supply from the anterior and middle cerebral arteries.
- *Homonymous quadrantanopia* is loss of the upper or lower homonymous quadrants of the visual fields. This may be due to temporal lobe lesions (e.g. vascular lesions or tumours), which cause upper quadrantanopia, or parietal lobe lesions (e.g. vascular lesions or tumours), which cause lower quadrantanopia.

The presence of an abnormality has diagnostic value (positive LRs 4.2 to 6.8),[8] but absence is largely unhelpful.

Fundoscopy does not begin with the examination of the fundus, but rather with visualisation of the cornea with the ophthalmoscope. Use the right eye to look in the patient's right eye, and vice versa. This prevents contact between the noses of the patient and the examiner in the midline. Keep your head vertical so that the patient can fix with the other eye.

Begin with the ophthalmoscope on the +20 lens setting, with the patient gazing into the distance. This prevents reflex pupil contraction, which occurs if the patient attempts to accommodate. Look first at the cornea and iris, and then at the lens. Large corneal ulcers may be visible, as may undulation of the rim of the iris, which is due to previous lens extraction and is called iridodonesis.

By racking the ophthalmoscope down towards 0, the focus can be shifted towards the fundus. Opacities in the lens (cataracts) may prevent inspection of the fundus. When the retina is in focus, search first for the optic disc. This is done by following a large retinal vein back towards the disc. All these veins radiate from the optic disc.

The margins of the disc must be examined with care. The disc itself is usually a shallow cup with a clearly outlined rim. Loss of the normal depression of the optic disc will cause blurring at the margins and is called papilloedema (Figure 11.8a). It indicates raised intracranial pressure. If papilloedema is suspected, the retinal veins should be examined for spontaneous pulsations. When these are present raised intracranial pressure is excluded, but their absence does not prove the pressure is raised.[9] If the appearance of papilloedema is associated with demyelination in the anterior part of the optic nerve, it is called papillitis (Table 13.3, page 428). These two can be distinguished because papillitis causes visual loss but papilloedema does not.

Next note the colour of the optic disc. Normally it is a rich yellow colour in contrast to the rest of the fundus which is a rich red colour. The fundus may be pigmented in some diseases and in patients with pigmented skin. When the optic disc has a

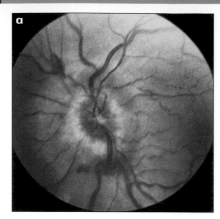

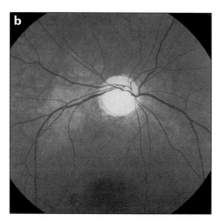

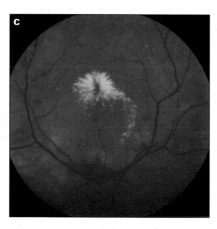

Figure 11.8 Fundoscopy in the neurological patient
(a) Papilloedema. (b) Optic atrophy. (c) Grade 4 hypertensive retinopathy, with papilloedema, a 'macular star' of hard exudates collecting around the fovea, and retinal oedema.

pale insipid white colour, optic atrophy is usually present (Figure 11.8b).

Each of the four quadrants of the retina should be examined systematically for abnormalities. Look especially for diabetic and hypertensive changes (Figure 11.8c). Note haemorrhages or exudates.

The third (oculomotor), fourth (trochlear) and sixth (abducens) nerves—the ocular nerves

Examination anatomy. The size of the pupils depends on a balance of parasympathetic and sympathetic innervation. The parasympathetic innervation to the eyes is supplied by the Edinger-Westphal nucleus[l] of the third nerve (stimulation of these fibres causes pupillary constriction: *miosis*). The sympathetic innervation to the eye (stimulation causes pupillary dilatation: *mydriasis*) is as follows: fibres from the hypothalamus go to the ciliospinal centre in the spinal cord at C8, T1 and T2, synapse, and second-order neurones exit via the anterior ramus in the thoracic trunk and synapse in the superior cervical ganglion in the neck. Third-order neurones travel from here with the internal carotid artery to the eye. In addition, the pupillary reflexes (Figure 11.9) depend for their afferent limb on the optic nerve (Figure 11.4). Constriction of the pupil in response to light is relayed by the optic nerve and tract to the superior colliculus and then to the Edinger-Westphal nucleus of the third nerve in the midbrain. Efferent motor fibres from the oculomotor nucleus (Figure 11.10) travel in the wall of the cavernous sinus, where they are in association with the fourth, ophthalmic division of the fifth, and the sixth cranial nerves (see Figure 10.10, page 308). These nerves leave the skull together through the superior orbital fissure. The iridoconstrictor fibres terminate in the ciliary ganglion, whence postganglionic fibres arise to innervate the iris. The rest of the third nerve supplies all the ocular muscles except the superior oblique (fourth nerve) and the lateral rectus (sixth nerve) muscles. The third nerve also supplies the levator palpebrae superioris, which elevates the eyelid (Figure 11.11).

Examination. Assess the pupils and movements of the eye.

The pupils. With the patient looking at an object at an intermediate distance, examine the pupils for size, shape, equality and regularity. Slight differences in pupil size (up to 20%) may be normal.[m]

---

l   Ludwig Edinger (1855–1918), Frankfurt neurologist, and Carl Friedrich Otto Westphal (1833–90), Berlin neurologist.
m   Gross differences are abnormal and called *anisocoria*. A small amount of fluctuation in the size of the pupils is normal and called *pupillary unrest*. More pronounced rhythmical contraction and dilatation of the pupils is called *hippus*; this may follow recovery from a third nerve palsy or occur during sleepiness. This is not often of any significance and is not a localising sign.

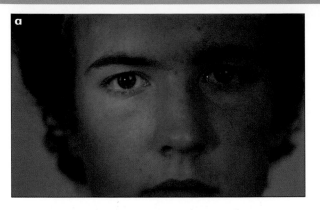 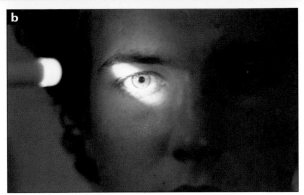

Figure 11.9 Cranial nerves II and III
(a) The pupils: inspect for size and symmetry. (b) Testing the pupillary reflex.

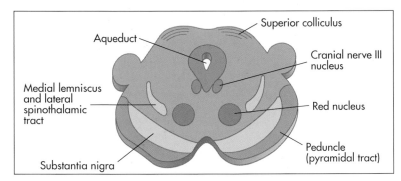

Figure 11.10 (left) Anatomy of the midbrain

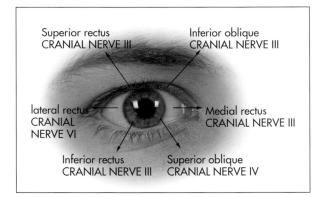

Figure 11.11 The eye muscles and nerve innervation

Look for *ptosis* (drooping) of one or both eyelids. Remember that *ectropion* or drooping of the lower lid is a common degenerative problem in old age but can also be caused by a seventh nerve palsy or facial scarring. There is often eye irritation and watering associated with it because of defective tear drainage.

Test the *light reflex*. Using a pocket torch, shine the light from the side (so the patient does not focus on the light and accommodate) into one of the pupils to assess its reaction to light. Inspect both

pupils and repeat this procedure on the other side. Normally the pupil into which the light is shone constricts briskly—this is the *direct* response to light. Simultaneously, the other pupil constricts in the same way. This is called the *consensual* response to light.

Move the torch in an arc from pupil to pupil. If an eye has optic atrophy or severely reduced visual acuity from another cause, the affected pupil will dilate paradoxically after a short time when the torch is moved from the normal eye to the abnormal eye. This is called an *afferent pupillary defect* (or the Marcus Gunn pupillary sign[n]). It occurs because an eye with severely reduced acuity has reduced afferent impulses so that the light reflex is markedly decreased. When the light is shone from the normal eye to the abnormal one the pupil dilates, as reflex pupillary constriction in the abnormal eye is so reduced that relaxation after the consensual response dominates.

Now test *accommodation*. Ask the patient to look into the distance and then to focus his or her

n   Robert Marcus Gunn (1850–1909), London ophthalmologist, described the defect in 1883.

eyes on an object such as a finger or a white-tipped hat pin brought to a point about 30 cm in front of the nose. There is normally constriction of both pupils—the accommodation response. It depends on a pathway from the visual association cortex descending to the third nerve nucleus. Causes of an absent light reflex with an intact accommodation reflex include a midbrain lesion (e.g. the Argyll Robertson pupil of syphilis), a ciliary ganglion lesion (e.g. Adie's pupil[o]) or Parinaud's syndrome[p] (page 340). Failure of accommodation alone may occur occasionally with a midbrain lesion or with cortical blindness.

Eye movements. Here failure of eye movement, double vision (diplopia) and nystagmus are assessed.

Normally the eyes move in parallel except during convergence. When they move out of alignment the patient is said to have *strabismus* or a *squint*. This abnormality may be due to a cranial nerve palsy (III, IV or VI), and in these cases the angle of alignment changes depending on the direction of gaze (an *incomitant* squint). When the malalignment of the eye movement remains constant for any direction of gaze the squint is said to be *concomitant*. Concomitant squints are common in children and may be idiopathic or occasionally caused by an intracranial mass. Strabismus is associated with diplopia unless one of the images has been suppressed by the brain. This can happen quite quickly in children and may lead to severe visual loss in that eye—*amblyopia*.

Ask the patient to look at the invaluable hat pin. (The presence of these pins in the lapel of a well-cut white coat or expensive suit often indicates that the wearer is a neurologist.) Assess voluntary eye movements in both eyes first. Ask the patient to look laterally right and left, then up and down (Figure 11.12). Remember the lateral rectus (sixth nerve) only moves the eyes horizontally outwards, while the medial rectus (third nerve) only moves the eyes horizontally inwards. The remainder of the muscle movements are a little more complicated. When the eye is abducted, the elevator is the superior rectus (third nerve), while the depressor is the inferior rectus (third nerve). When the eye is adducted, the elevator is the inferior oblique (third nerve) while the depressor is the superior oblique (fourth nerve) (Figure 11.11). The practical upshot of all this is that the testing of pure movement (that

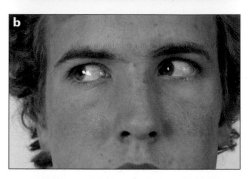

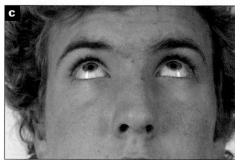

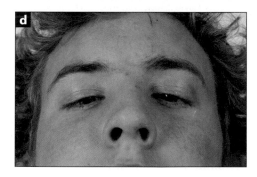

Figure 11.12 The cranial nerves III, IV and VI: voluntary eye movements
(a) 'Look to the left.' (b) 'Look to the right.' (c) 'Look up.' (d) 'Look down.'

is, one muscle only) for elevation and depression is performed first with the eye adducted and then with it abducted. Therefore, ask the patient to follow the moving hat pin, held by the examiner 30–40 cm from the patient and moved in an H pattern, with

---

o William Adie (1886–1935), Australian neurologist working in Britain, described this in 1931.
p Henri Parinaud (1844–1905), French ophthalmologist, described this in 1889.

both eyes and to say if double images are seen in any direction.

Diplopia can be an early sign of ocular muscle weakness because the light falls on different parts of the corresponding retinas due to slight movement differences. If diplopia is present, further testing is necessary. The false image is usually paler, less distinct and always more peripheral than the real one. Ask the patient whether the two images lie side by side or one above the other. If they are side by side, only the lateral or medial recti can be responsible. If they lie one above the other, then either of the obliques or the superior or inferior recti may be involved. To decide which pair of muscles is responsible, ask in which direction there is maximum image separation. Separation is greatest in the direction in which the weak muscle has its purest action. At the point of maximum separation, cover one eye and find out which image disappears. Loss of the lateral image indicates that the covered eye is responsible. Diplopia that persists when one eye is covered can be due to astigmatism, a dislocated lens or hysteria.

Note failure of movement of either eye in any direction. This indicates ocular muscle involvement. If any abnormality is detected, then each eye must be tested separately. The other eye is covered with a card or with the examiner's hand. Abnormal eye movement may be due to III, IV or VI nerve palsy, or to an abnormality of conjugate gaze.

Features of a third nerve lesion. These are complete ptosis (partial ptosis may occur with an incomplete lesion); divergent strabismus (eye 'down and out'); and dilated pupil which is unreactive to direct light (the consensual reaction in the opposite normal eye is intact) and unreactive to accommodation. Always try to exclude a fourth (trochlear) nerve lesion when a third nerve lesion is present. One way to do this is by tilting the head to the same side as the lesion. The affected eye will intort if the fourth nerve is intact (remember SIN—the *Superior* oblique **IN**torts the eye).

Aetiology of a third nerve palsy. Third nerve lesions are most commonly related to trauma or are idiopathic. Central causes include vascular lesions in the brainstem, tumours and rarely demyelination.

Peripheral causes include: (i) compressive lesions, such as an aneurysm (usually on the posterior communicating artery), tumour, basal meningitis, nasopharyngeal carcinoma or orbital lesions—for example, Tolosa-Hunt syndrome (superior orbital fissure syndrome—painful lesions of III, IV, VI

and the first division of V); and (ii) ischaemia or infarction, as in arteritis, diabetes mellitus and migraine.

Features of a fourth nerve lesion. Test this nerve by asking the patient to turn the eye in and then try to look down: a lesion results in paralysis of the superior oblique with weakness of downward (and outward) movement. The patient may walk around with his or her head tilted away from the lesion—that is, to the opposite shoulder (this allows the patient to maintain binocular vision).

An isolated fourth nerve palsy is rare and is usually idiopathic or related to trauma. It may occasionally occur with lesions of the cerebral peduncle.

Features of a sixth nerve lesion. These are failure of lateral movement, convergent strabismus and diplopia. These signs are maximal on looking to the affected side, and the images are horizontal and parallel to each other. The outermost image from the affected eye disappears on covering this eye (this image is usually also more blurred).

Aetiology of a sixth nerve palsy. Bilateral lesions may be due to trauma or Wernicke's encephalopathy (a syndrome of ophthalmoplegia, confusion and ataxia which is often associated with Korsakoff's psychosis due to thiamine deficiency). Mononeuritis multiplex and raised intracranial pressure are also causes of sixth nerve palsy.

Unilateral sixth nerve lesions are most commonly idiopathic or related to trauma. They may have a central (e.g. vascular lesion or tumour) or peripheral (e.g. raised intracranial pressure or diabetes mellitus) origin.

Abnormalities of conjugate gaze. Normal eye movements occur in an organised fashion so that the visual axes remain in the same plane throughout. There are centres for conjugate gaze in the frontal lobe for saccadic movements and in the occipital lobe for pursuit movements. Conjugate movement to the right is controlled from the left side of the brain. From these centres fibres travel to the region of the sixth nerve nucleus, from which area the medial longitudinal fasciculus coordinates movement with the contralateral third nerve (medial rectus) nucleus (Figure 11.13). A brainstem lesion causes ipsilateral paralysis of horizontal conjugate gaze, and a frontal lobe lesion causes contralateral paralysis of horizontal conjugate gaze.

There are a number of possible causes for deviation of the eyes to one side. For example,

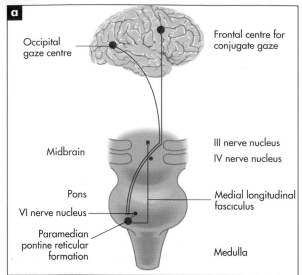

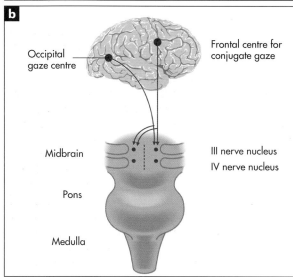

Figure 11.13 Horizontal (a) and vertical (b) eye movements

(Adapted from Lance JW, McLeod JG. *A physiological approach to clinical neurology*, 3rd edn. London: Butterworths, 1981.)

deviation of the eyes to the left can result from: (i) a destructive lesion (usually vascular or neoplastic), which involves the pathways between the *left* frontal lobes and the oculomotor nuclei; (ii) a destructive lesion of the *right* side of the brainstem; or (iii) an irritative lesion, such as an epileptic focus, of the *right* frontal lobe, which stimulates deviation of the eyes to the left.

Supranuclear palsy is loss of vertical or horizontal gaze or both (Figure 11.13). The clinical features that distinguish this from third, fourth and sixth nerve palsies include: (i) both eyes are affected; (ii) pupils may be fixed and are often unequal; (iii) there is usually no diplopia; and (iv) the reflex eye movements—for example, on flexing and extending the neck—are usually intact.

- *Progressive supranuclear palsy* (or Steele Richardson Olszewski syndrome[q]): here there is loss of vertical and later of horizontal gaze, which is associated with extrapyramidal signs, neck rigidity and dementia. Reflex eye movements on neck flexion and extension are preserved until late in the course of the disease.
- *Parinaud's syndrome* is loss of vertical gaze often associated with nystagmus on attempted convergence (see below). There are pseudo-Argyll Robertson pupils. The causes of Parinaud's syndrome include a pinealoma, multiple sclerosis and vascular lesions.
- Involuntary upward deviation of the eyes (*oculogyric crises*) occurs with post-encephalitic Parkinson's disease and may be seen in patients sensitive to phenothiazine derivatives or in patients on levodopa therapy.

One-and-a-half syndrome is rare but important to recognise. These patients have a horizontal gaze palsy when looking to one side (the 'one') plus impaired adduction on looking to the other side (the 'and-a-half'). Other features often include turning out (exotropia) of the eye opposite the side of the lesion (paralytic pontine exotropia). One-and-a-half syndrome can be caused by a stroke (infarct), plaque of multiple sclerosis or tumour in the dorsal pons.

Nystagmus. The eyes are normally maintained at rest in the midline by the balance of tone between opposing ocular muscles. Disturbance of this tone, which depends on impulses from the retina, the muscles of the eyes themselves and various vestibular and central connections, allows the eyes to drift in one direction. This drift is corrected by a quick movement (saccadic) back to the original position. When these movements occur repeatedly nystagmus is said to be present. The direction of the nystagmus is defined as that of the fast (correcting) movement, although it is the slow drift that is abnormal. Nystagmus from any cause tends to be accentuated by gaze in a direction away from the midline. In many instances nystagmus is not present when the eyes are at rest, and is only detected when the eyes are deviated (gaze-evoked nystagmus). At the extremes of gaze, fine nystagmus is normal

q   J Steele and J Richardson, Canadian neurologists, described this in 1964.

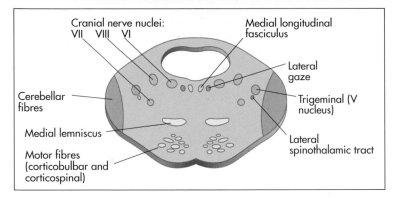

Figure 11.14 Anatomy of the pons

(physiological). Therefore test for nystagmus by asking the patient to follow your pin out to 30 degrees from the central gaze position.

Nystagmus may be jerky or pendular.

Jerky horizontal nystagmus may be due to (i) a vestibular lesion (acute lesions cause nystagmus away from the side of the lesion while chronic lesions cause nystagmus to the side of the lesion); (ii) a cerebellar lesion (unilateral diseases cause nystagmus to the side of the lesion); (iii) toxic causes, such as phenytoin and alcohol (may also cause vertical nystagmus but less often); and (iv) *internuclear ophthalmoplegia*. Internuclear ophthalmoplegia is present when there is nystagmus in the abducting eye and failure of adduction of the other (affected) side. This is due to a lesion of the medial longitudinal fasciculus. The most common cause in young adults with bilateral involvement is multiple sclerosis; in the elderly, vascular disease is an important cause.

Jerky vertical nystagmus may be due to a brainstem lesion. (Vertical nystagmus means nystagmus where the oscillations are in a vertical direction.) Upbeat nystagmus suggests a lesion in the midbrain or floor of the fourth ventricle, while downbeat nystagmus suggests a foramen magnum lesion. Phenytoin or alcohol can also cause this abnormality.

With **pendular nystagmus** the nystagmus phases are equal in duration. Its cause may be retinal (decreased macular vision, e.g. albinism) or congenital. This condition is thought to occur as a result of poor vision or increased sensitivity to light. It develops in childhood and occurs as the patient performs searching movements in an attempt to fixate or improve the visual impulses.

A summary of how to approach the medical eye examination is provided on in Chapter 13.

The fifth (trigeminal) nerve

Examination anatomy. This nerve contains both sensory and motor fibres. Its motor nucleus and its sensory nucleus for touch lie in the pons (Figure 11.14), its proprioceptive nucleus lies in the midbrain, while its nucleus serving pain and temperature sensation descends through the medulla to reach the upper cervical cord. It is the largest of the cranial nerves.

The nerve itself leaves the pons from the cerebellopontine angle and runs over the temporal lobe in the middle cranial fossa. At the petrous temporal bone the nerve forms the trigeminal (Gasserian[r]) ganglion and from here the three sensory divisions arise. The first (ophthalmic) division runs in the cavernous sinus with the third nerve and emerges from the superior orbital fissure to supply the skin of the forehead, the cornea and conjunctiva. The second (maxillary) division emerges from the infraorbital foramen and supplies skin in the middle of the face and the mucous membranes of the upper part of the mouth, palate and nasopharynx. The third and largest (mandibular) division runs with the motor part of the nerve, leaving the skull through the foramen ovale to supply the skin of the lower jaw and mucous membranes of the lower part of the mouth (Figures 11.15 and 11.16).

Pain and temperature fibres from the face run from the pons through the medulla as low as the upper cervical cord, terminating in the spinal tract nucleus as they descend. The second-order neurones arise in this nucleus and ascend again as the ventral trigeminothalamic tract. Touch and proprioceptive fibres terminate in the pontine or main sensory and mesencephalic nuclei, respectively, to form the dorsal and ventral mesencephalic tracts. Because of this segregation in the brainstem, lesions of the medulla or upper spinal cord can cause a *dissociated sensory loss of the face*—loss of pain and temperature sensation, but retention of touch and proprioception.

r   Johann Laurenz Gasser (1723–65), professor of anatomy, Vienna.

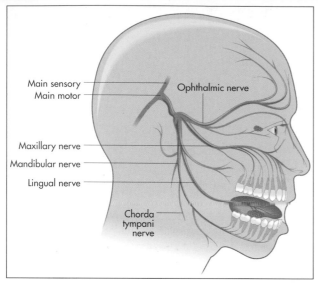

Figure 11.15 The trigeminal nerve (cranial nerve V)

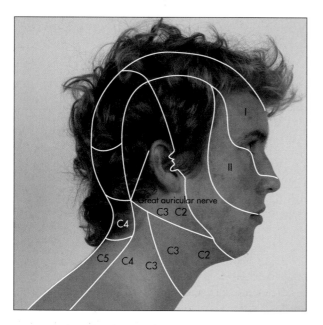

Figure 11.16 Dermatomes of the head and neck

The motor part of the nerve supplies the muscles of mastication.

History. Pain in the distribution of part of the trigeminal nerve is common. *Tic douloureux* (*trigeminal neuralgia*) is a sudden severe shooting pain in one of the divisions of the nerve. It is more common in elderly people. The occurrence in a young woman suggests multiple sclerosis. The pain is brief but very distressing. It may be precipitated by an activity such as eating or brushing the teeth. The pain is caused by a pontine lesion or by compression of the trigeminal nerve by a vascular abnormality. Pain due to sinusitis, dental abscess, malignant disease of the sinuses and herpes zoster may be felt in a trigeminal nerve distribution. Muscle weakness of the trigeminal nerve may lead the patient to complain of difficulty eating or talking.

Examination. Test the *corneal reflex*. Lightly touch the cornea (*not* the conjunctiva) with a wisp of cottonwool brought to the eye from the side. Reflex blinking of *both* eyes is a normal response. Ask the patient whether he or she feels the touch of the cottonwool. The sensory component of the reflex is mediated by the ophthalmic division of the fifth nerve, while the reflex blink (motor) results from facial nerve innervation of the orbicularis oculi muscles. Absence of corneal sensation is associated with corneal ulceration.

Note: If blinking occurs only with the contralateral eye this indicates an ipsilateral seventh nerve palsy. The patient will then still feel the touch of the cottonwool on the cornea.

Test *facial sensation* in the three divisions of the nerve, comparing each side with the other (Figure 11.17). Test first with the sharp end of a new neurological pin for pain sensation (never use an old pin in these days of hepatitis B, HIV etc).[10] The pin is applied lightly to the skin and the patient is asked whether it feels sharp or dull. Some examiners ask patients to shut their eyes. Loss of pain sensation will result in the pinprick feeling dull. An area of dull sensation should be mapped by testing pinprick sensation progressively: testing should go *from the dull to the sharp area*. Test also

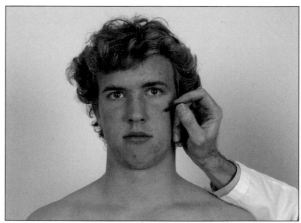

Figure 11.17 Facial sensation V, maxillary division: 'Does this feel sharp or blunt?'—test all three divisions on each side

above the forehead progressively back over the top of the head. If the ophthalmic division is affected sensation will return when the C2 dermatome is reached (Figure 11.16). It is important to exercise caution: too sharp a pin will leave a little trail of bloody spots, which is embarrassing. Temperature is not tested routinely unless syringobulbia is suspected, as temperature loss usually accompanies loss of pain sensation.

The patient keeps the eyes closed and a new piece of cottonwool is used to test light touch in the same way. The patient should be instructed to say 'yes' each time the touch of the cottonwool is felt (do *not* stroke the skin). Proprioception loss is not routinely tested on the face (and indeed it would be rather a difficult thing to do!).

Now examine the *motor division* of the nerve. Begin by inspecting for wasting of the temporal and masseter muscles. Ask the patient then to clench the teeth and palpate for contraction of the masseter above the mandible (Figure 11.18). The strength of these muscles can be tested by asking the patient to bite forcefully onto a wooden tongue depressor with the molar teeth. The depth of the teeth marks on each side give an indication of the relative strengths of the muscles. The examiner can attempt to withdraw the tongue depressor as the patient bites it. A bite of normal strength will prevent this. Then get the patient to open the mouth (pterygoid muscles) and hold it open while the examiner attempts to force it shut. A unilateral lesion of the motor division causes the jaw to deviate towards the weak (affected) side.

Test the *jaw jerk* or *masseter reflex*. The patient lets the mouth fall open slightly and the examiner's finger is placed on the tip of the jaw and tapped lightly with a tendon hammer (Figure 11.19). Normally there is a slight closure of the mouth or no reaction at all. In an upper motor neurone lesion above the pons the jaw jerk is greatly exaggerated. This is commonly seen in pseudobulbar palsy).[s]

Causes of a fifth nerve palsy. Central (pons, medulla and upper cervical cord) causes include a vascular lesion, tumour or syringobulbia.

Peripheral (middle fossa) causes include an aneurysm, tumour (secondary or primary) or chronic meningitis.

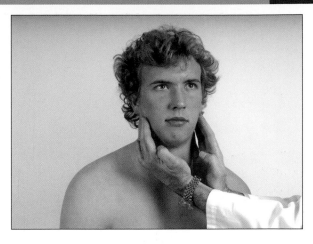

Figure 11.18 Cranial nerve V (motor): 'Clench your jaw'—feel the masseter muscles

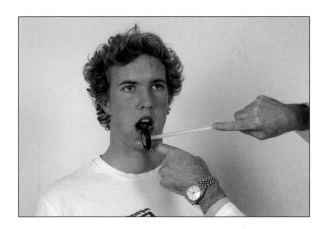

Figure 11.19 Cranial nerve V: the jaw jerk

Trigeminal ganglion (petrous temporal bone) causes include a trigeminal neuroma, meningioma, or fracture of the middle fossa.

Cavernous sinus causes involve the ophthalmic division only and are usually associated with third, fourth and sixth nerve palsies. They include aneurysm, tumour or thrombosis.

Remember, if there is total loss of sensation in all three divisions of the nerve, this suggests that the level of the lesion is at the ganglion or the sensory root—for example, an acoustic neuroma (Figure 11.20). If there is total sensory loss in one division only, this suggests a postganglionic lesion. The ophthalmic division is most commonly affected because it runs in the cavernous sinus and through the orbital fissure, where it is vulnerable to a number of different insults.

If there is dissociated sensory loss (loss of pain, but preservation of touch sensation) this

---

s   Testing of the sneeze reflex is not routine. Here stimulation or irritation of the nasal mucosa with a hair or small piece of string is followed by contraction of the muscles of the nasopharynx and thorax. The afferent limb of this arc is through the trigeminal nerve and the efferent limb through the facial, glossopharyngeal, vagus and trigeminal nerves, and the motor nerves of the cervical spine. The reflex centre is in the brainstem and upper spinal cord.

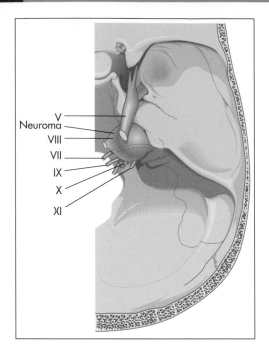

V
Neuroma
VIII
VII
IX
X
XI

Figure 11.20 Cerebellopontine angle tumour
A neuroma arising from the acoustic (VIII) nerve compresses adjacent structures, including the trigeminal (V) and facial (VII) nerves and the brainstem and cerebellum (removed to permit the cranial nerves to be seen).
(Adapted from Simon RP, Aminoff MJ, Greenberg DA, *Clinical neurology 1989*. Appleton & Lange, 1989.)

suggests a brainstem or upper cord lesion, such as syringobulbia, foramen magnum tumour, or infarction in the territory of the posterior inferior cerebellar artery. If touch sensation is lost but pain sensation is preserved, this is usually due to an abnormality of the pontine nuclei, such as a vascular lesion or tumour. Motor loss can also be central or peripheral.

Irritative motor changes. Convulsive seizures that involve the precentral gyrus can include clenching of the jaw and biting of the tongue. Parkinson's disease and essential tremor can cause a rhythmic tremor of the lips or jaw. *Trismus* is a forceful clenching of the jaw that can occur in tetanus and encephalitis. The patient may be unable to open the mouth. Repetitive chewing and yawning movements can occur as an effect of antipsychotic drugs (*tardive orofacial dyskinesias*).

The seventh (facial) nerve

Examination anatomy. The seventh nerve nucleus lies in the pons next to the sixth cranial nerve nucleus (Figure 11.14). The nerve (Figure 11.21) leaves the pons with the eighth nerve through the cerebellopontine angle. After entering the facial canal it enlarges to become the geniculate ganglion. The branch that supplies the stapedius muscle is given off from within the facial canal. The chorda

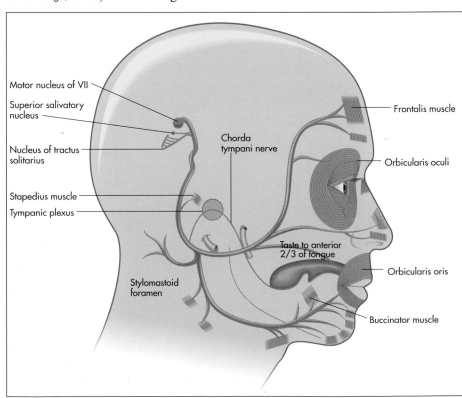

Motor nucleus of VII
Superior salivatory nucleus
Nucleus of tractus solitarius
Stapedius muscle
Tympanic plexus
Chorda tympani nerve
Stylomastoid foramen
Taste to anterior 2/3 of tongue
Frontalis muscle
Orbicularis oculi
Orbicularis oris
Buccinator muscle

Figure 11.21 The facial nerve (cranial nerve VII)
Note: The branches of the facial nerve: 'Two zebras bit my car'—**t**emporal, **z**ygotic, **b**uccal, **m**andibular, **c**ervical.

tympani (containing taste fibres from the anterior two-thirds of the tongue) joins the nerve in the facial canal. The seventh nerve leaves the skull via the stylomastoid foramen. It then passes through the middle of the parotid gland and supplies the muscles of facial expression. The frontalis muscle receives upper motor innervation bilaterally, the other muscles receive innervation from the contralateral cortex.

History. The patient may have noticed the onset of difficulty with speaking and keeping liquids in the mouth or may have noticed facial asymmetry in the mirror. He or she may be aware of dryness of the eyes (decreased lacrimation) or the mouth (decreased salivary production). Paralysis of the stapedius muscle can cause *hyperacusis* or intolerance of loud or high-pitched sounds. Normal contraction of the stapedius muscle occurs in response to loud noises such as popular music and dampens movement of the ossicles.

Examination. Inspect for *facial asymmetry*, as a seventh nerve palsy can cause unilateral drooping of the corner of the mouth, and smoothing of the wrinkled forehead and the nasolabial fold (Figure 11.22). However, with bilateral facial nerve palsies symmetry can be maintained.

Test the *muscle power*. Ask the patient to look up so as to wrinkle the forehead (Figure 11.23). Look for loss of wrinkling and feel the muscle

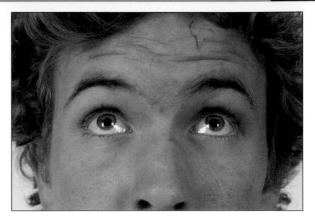

Figure 11.23 Cranial nerve VII: 'Look up to wrinkle your forehead'

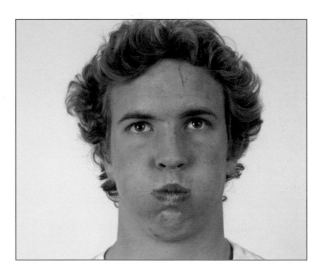

Figure 11.24 Cranial nerve VII: 'Puff out your cheeks'

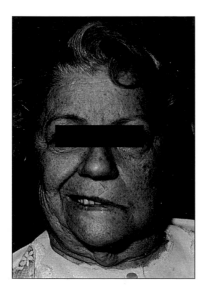

Figure 11.22 Left upper motor neurone facial weakness, showing drooping of the corner of the mouth, flattened nasolabial fold, and sparing of the forehead; the lesion is in the right side of the brain

strength by pushing down against the corrugation on each side. This movement is relatively preserved on the side of an upper motor neurone lesion (a lesion that occurs above the level of the brainstem nucleus) because of bilateral cortical representation of these muscles. The remaining muscles of facial expression are usually affected on the side of an upper motor neurone lesion, although occasionally the orbicularis oculi muscles are preserved. Ask the patient to puff out the cheeks (Figure 11.24). Look for asymmetry.

In a lower motor neurone lesion (at the level of the nucleus or nerve root), all muscles of facial expression are affected on the side of the lesion.

Next ask the patient to shut the eyes tightly (Figure 11.25). Compare how deeply the eyelashes are buried on the two sides and then try to force

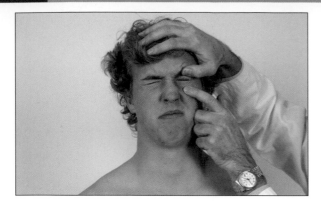

Figure 11.25 Cranial nerve VII: 'Shut your eyes tight and stop me opening them'

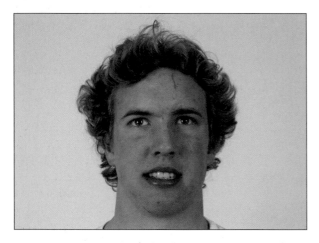

Figure 11.26 Cranial nerve VII: 'Show me your teeth'
(Before asking this question, make sure the patient's teeth are not in a container beside the bed.)

open each eye. Check whether Bell's phenomenon[t] is evident. Bell's phenomenon is present in everyone, although not usually visible unless a person has a VII nerve palsy. In this case, when the patient attempts to shut the eye on the side of a lower motor neurone VII nerve palsy, there is upward movement of the eyeball and incomplete closure of the eyelid. Next ask the patient to grin (Figure 11.26) and compare the nasolabial grooves, which are smooth on the weak side.

If a lower motor neurone lesion is detected, check quickly for the ear and palatal vesicles of herpes zoster of the geniculate ganglion—the Ramsay Hunt[u] syndrome.

A facial paralysis due to a cortical lesion may spare facial movements due to emotion such as crying or smiling, and indeed these movements may be exaggerated. The opposite abnormality (preservation of voluntary but loss of emotional movements) can also occur as a result of lesions in a number of areas, including the frontal lobes.

Examining for taste on the anterior two-thirds of the tongue is not usually required. If necessary, it can be tested by asking the patient to protrude the tongue to one side: sugar, vinegar, salt and quinine (sweet, sour, saline and bitter) are placed one at a time on each side of the tongue. The patient indicates the taste by pointing to a card with the various tastes listed on it. The mouth is rinsed with water between each sample.

Causes of a seventh (facial) nerve palsy. Vascular lesions or tumours are the common causes of **upper motor neurone lesions (supranuclear)**. Note that lesions of the frontal lobes may cause weakness of the emotional movements of the face alone; voluntary movements are preserved.

In **lower motor neurone lesions**, *pontine* causes (often associated with V and VI lesions) include vascular lesions, tumours, syringobulbia or multiple sclerosis. *Posterior fossa* lesions include an acoustic neuroma, a meningioma or chronic meningitis. At the level of the *petrous temporal bone*, Bell's palsy (an idiopathic acute paralysis of the nerve; Figure 11.27), a fracture, the Ramsay Hunt syndrome or otitis media may occur, while the parotid gland may be affected by a tumour or sarcoidosis. Remember, Bell's palsy is the most common cause (up to 80%) of a facial nerve palsy.[v]

Regrowth of the nerve fibres that occurs as the patient recovers from Bell's palsy can lead to aberrant connections. The most striking is the regrowth of fibres meant for the salivary gland to the lacrimal gland in up to 5% of patients. This leads to tear formation when a patient eats—crocodile tears.

Bilateral facial weakness may be due to the Guillain-Barré syndrome, sarcoidosis, bilateral parotid disease, Lyme disease or rarely mononeuritis multiplex. Myopathy and myasthenia gravis can also cause bilateral facial weakness, but in these cases it is not due to facial nerve involvement.

Unilateral **loss of taste**, without other abnormalities, can occur with middle-ear lesions

---

t   Sir Charles Bell (1774–1842), professor of anatomy at London's Royal College of Surgeons, later professor of surgery at Edinburgh, described facial nerve palsy in 1821.
u   James Ramsay Hunt (1874–1937), American neurologist.

v   A patient with an old Bell's palsy may exhibit *synkinesis*. When the patient blinks the corner of the mouth twitches; when the lips are protruded the affected eye closes.

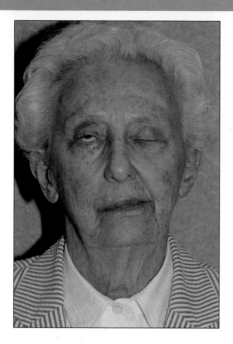

Figure 11.27 Bell's palsy
(From Mayo Clinic Images, with permission. © Mayo Clinic Scientific Press and CRC Press.)

involving the chorda tympani or lingual nerve, but these are very rare.

Irritative changes. Tonic and clonic movements of the facial muscles can occur in seizures. Various abnormal movements of the facial muscles can occur as a result of basal ganglia or extrapyramidal abnormalities (page 396). These include athetoid and dystonic (page 399) movements. Irritative lesions in the brainstem can cause increased secretion of saliva (*sialorrhoea*). This can also occur in Parkinson's disease or accompany attacks of nausea.

The eighth (acoustic) nerve

Examination anatomy. The eighth (acoustic) nerve has two components: the cochlear, with afferent fibres subserving hearing; and the vestibular, containing afferent fibres subserving balance. Fibres for hearing originate in the organ of Corti[w] and run to the cochlear nuclei in the pons. From here there is bilateral transmission to the medial geniculate bodies and thence to the superior gyrus of the temporal lobes. Fibres for balance begin in the utricle and semicircular canals, and join auditory fibres in the facial canal. They then enter the brainstem at the cerebellopontine angle. After entering the pons, vestibular fibres run widely throughout the brainstem and cerebellum.

History. Loss of hearing may have been noticed by the patient or complained of by his or her relatives or friends. Unilateral hearing loss is much more likely to be due to a nerve lesion and must be identified. One should also find out if this has been of gradual or sudden onset, whether there is a family history of deafness, and whether there has been an occupational or recreational exposure to loud noise (e.g. boilermaker, retired rock musician) without hearing protection. There may be a history of trauma or recurrent ear infections.

Examination of the ear and hearing. Look to see if the patient is wearing a hearing aid; remove it. Examine the pinna and look for scars behind the ears. Pull on the pinna gently (it is tender if the patient has external ear disease or temporomandibular joint disease). Feel for nodes (pre- and post-auricular) that may indicate disease of the external auditory meatus.

Inspect the patient's external auditory meatus. The adult canal angulates, so in order to see the eardrum it is necessary to pull up and backwards on the auricle before inserting the otoscope. The normal eardrum (tympanic membrane) is pearly grey and concave. Look for wax or other obstructions, and inspect the eardrum for inflammation or perforation (see Chapter 13).

Next test hearing. A simple test involves covering the opposite auditory meatus with a finger, moving it about as a distraction while whispering a number in the other ear. This should be standardised by the use of set numbers for different tones. For example, the number 68 is used to test high tone and 100 to test low tone. Whispering should be performed towards the end of expiration in an attempt to standardise the volume and at about 60 cm from the ear. The examiner's larynx should not vibrate if the whispering is soft enough. If partial deafness is suspected, perform Rinné's and Weber's tests:

- **Rinné's test**[x]—a 256 Hz vibrating tuning fork is placed on the mastoid process, behind the ear, and when the sound is no longer heard it is placed in line with the external meatus (Figure 11.28). Normally the note is audible at the external meatus. If a patient has nerve deafness the note is audible at the external meatus, as air and bone conduction are reduced equally,

---

w Alfonso Corti (1822–1888), Italian anatomist, described this in 1851.

x Heinrich Adolf Rinné (1819–1968), German ear specialist, described his test in 1855.

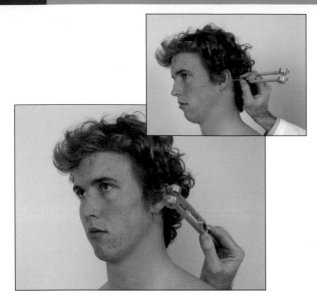

Figure 11.28 Cranial nerve VIII, Rinné's test: 'Where does it sound louder?'

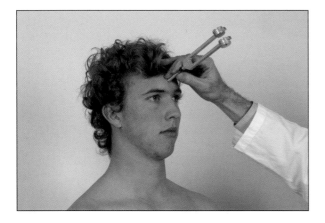

Figure 11.29 Cranial nerve VIII, Weber's test: 'Is the buzzing louder on one side?'

so that air conduction is better (as is normal). This is termed Rinné-positive. If there is a conduction (middle ear) deafness, no note is audible at the external meatus. This is termed Rinné-negative.

- **Weber's[y] test**—a vibrating 256 Hz tuning fork is positioned on the centre of the forehead (Figure 11.29). Normally the sound is heard in the centre of the forehead. Nerve deafness causes the sound to be heard better in the normal ear. A patient with a conduction deafness finds the sound louder in the abnormal ear.

Causes of deafness. Unilateral nerve deafness may be due to (i) tumours, such as an acoustic neuroma; (ii) trauma, such as fracture of the petrous temporal bone; or (iii) vascular disease of the internal auditory artery (rare).

Bilateral nerve deafness may be due to (i) environmental exposure to noise; (ii) degeneration, such as presbyacusis; (iii) toxicity, such as aspirin, streptomycin or alcohol; (iv) infection, such as congenital rubella syndrome, congenital syphilis; or (vi) Ménière's disease.

Brainstem disease is a rare cause of bilateral deafness.

Conduction deafness may be due to (i) wax; (ii) otitis media; (iii) otosclerosis; or (iv) Paget's disease of bone.

Examination of vestibular function. If a patient complains of vertigo, the *Hallpike[z] manoeuvre* should be performed. The patient sits up; having warned him or her what is about to occur, the examiner grasps the patient's head between the hands and gets him or her to lie back quickly so that the head lies 30 degrees below the horizontal. At the same time, the head is rotated 30 degrees towards the examiner. Ask the patient to keep the eyes open. If the test is positive, after a short latent period vertigo and nystagmus (rotatory) towards the affected (lowermost) ear occur for several seconds and then abate and are not reproducible for 10 to 15 minutes. This result is seen in the condition called *benign paroxysmal positioning vertigo* (BPPV). It occurs with repositioning of the head and then abates so that the old name, *benign positional vertigo*, is not really appropriate. It is due to a disorder in the utricle and occurs, for example, following infection, trauma or vascular disease. It is caused by the presence of concretions in the semicircular canals. Inertia of these concretions following movement of the head causes the illusion of movement and nystagmus. If there is no latent period, no fatiguability or the nystagmus persists or is variable, this suggests that there is a lesion of the brainstem (e.g. multiple sclerosis) or cerebellum (e.g. metastatic carcinoma).

Causes of vestibular abnormalities. Labyrinthine causes include acute labyrinthitis, motion sickness, streptomycin toxicity or, rarely, Ménière's disease.

Vestibular causes include vestibular neuronitis as well as many of the causes of nerve deafness.

In the brainstem, vascular lesions, tumours of

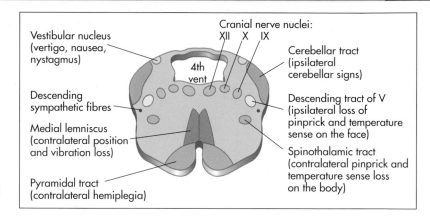

Figure 11.30 Anatomy of the medulla
Shows correlation between lesions and clinical features.

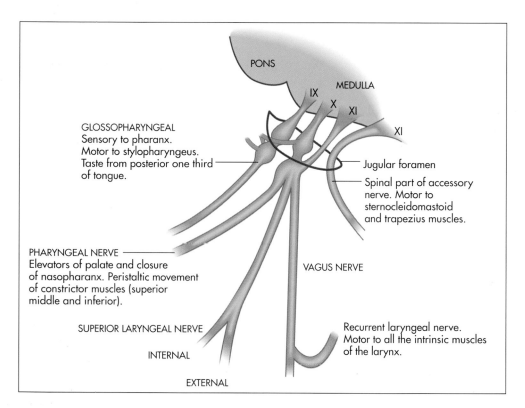

Figure 11.31 The lower cranial nerves—glossopharyngeal (IX), vagus (X) and accessory (XI)
(Adapted from Walton JN, *Brain's diseases of the nervous system*, 10th edn. Oxford: Oxford University Press, 1993.)

the cerebellum or fourth ventricle, demyelination or vasospastic conditions such as migraine may involve the central connections of the vestibular system.

Vertigo may be associated with temporal lobe dysfunction (e.g. ischaemia or complex partial seizures).

The ninth (glossopharyngeal) and tenth (vagus) nerves

Examination anatomy. These nerves have motor, sensory and autonomic functions. Nerve fibres from nuclei in the medulla (Figure 11.30) form multiple nerve rootlets as they exit the medulla. These join to form the ninth and tenth nerves, and also contribute to the eleventh nerve. The nerves emerge from the skull through the jugular foramen (Figure 11.31). The ninth nerve receives sensory fibres from the nasopharynx, pharynx, middle and inner ear and from the posterior third of the tongue (including taste fibres). It also carries secretory fibres to the parotid gland. The tenth nerve receives sensory fibres from the pharynx

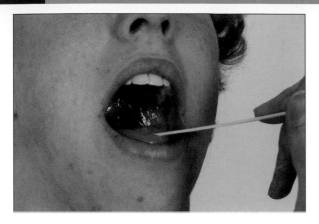

Figure 11.32 Cranial nerve X: 'Say "Ah"'—look for asymmetrical movement of the uvula

and larynx, and innervates muscles of the pharynx, larynx and palate.

History. A lesion of the glossopharyngeal nerve may cause the patient no definite symptoms, but difficulty in swallowing dry foods may have been noticed. *Glossopharyngeal neuralgia* is a tic douloureux of the ninth nerve. The patient experiences sudden shooting pains which radiate from one side of the throat to the ear. There may be trigger areas in the throat and attacks can be brought on by chewing or swallowing.

Unilateral vagus nerve paralysis may cause difficulty in initiating the swallowing of solids and liquids and hoarseness.

Examination. Ask the patient to open the mouth and inspect the palate with a torch. Note any displacement of the uvula. Then ask the patient to say 'Ah!' (Figure 11.32). Normally the posterior edge of the soft palate—the *velum*[aa]—rises symmetrically. If the uvula is drawn to one side this indicates a unilateral tenth nerve palsy. Note that the uvula is drawn towards the normal side.

Testing for the *gag reflex* (ninth is the sensory component and tenth the motor component) is traditional but not necessary.[11] A better alternative is to touch the back of the pharynx on each side with a spatula (rather than the soft palate). The patient is asked if the touch of the spatula (ninth) is felt each time. Normally, there is reflex contraction of the soft palate. If contraction is absent and sensation is intact this suggests a tenth nerve palsy. The most common cause of a reduced gag reflex is old age. Of more concern to the examiner is the patient with an

exaggerated but still normal reflex. This can lead to vomiting onto the examining clinician.

Ask the patient to speak in order to assess hoarseness (which may occur with a unilateral recurrent laryngeal nerve lesion), and then to cough. Listen for the characteristic bovine cough that occurs with recurrent laryngeal nerve lesions. It is not necessary routinely to test taste on the posterior third of the tongue (ninth nerve).

Test the patient's ability to swallow a small amount of water and watch for regurgitation into the nose, or coughing.

Causes of a ninth (glossopharyngeal) and tenth (vagus) nerve palsy. Central causes are vascular lesions (e.g. lateral medullary infarction, due to vertebral or posterior inferior cerebellar artery disease), tumours, syringobulbia and motor neurone disease. **Peripheral (posterior fossa) lesions** comprise aneurysms at the base of the skull, tumours, chronic meningitis or the Guillain-Barré syndrome.

The eleventh (accessory) nerve

Examination anatomy. The central portion of this nerve arises in the medulla close to the nuclei of the ninth, tenth and twelfth nerves and its spinal portion arises from the upper five cervical segments. It leaves the skull with the ninth and tenth nerves through the jugular foramen (Figure 11.31). Its central division provides motor fibres to the vagus and the spinal division innervates the trapezius and sternocleidomastoid muscles. The motor fibres that supply the sternocleidomastoid muscle are thought to cross twice so that cortical control of the muscle is ipsilateral. This makes sense when one remembers that the muscle turns the head to the opposite side. This means that the hemisphere which receives information from and controls one side of the body also turns the head to face that side.

Examination. Ask the patient to shrug the shoulders (Figure 11.33). Feel the bulk of the trapezius muscles and attempt to push the shoulders down. Then instruct the patient to turn the head to the side against resistance (the examiner's hand) (Figure 11.34). Remember that the right sternocleidomastoid turns the head to the left. Feel the muscle bulk of the sternocleidomastoids.

Weakness of these muscles is less common than *torticollis*, which is due to overactivity of multiple neck muscles. It is a complex movement disorder. The head appears turned to one side either permanently or in spasms. Ask the patient to turn

---

aa   Velum means 'curtain' in Latin.

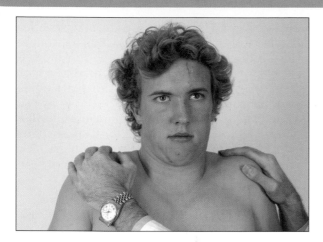

Figure 11.33 Cranial nerve XI: 'Shrug your shoulders—push up hard'

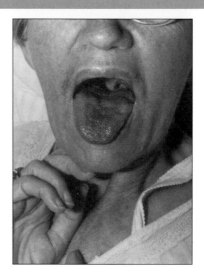

Figure 11.35 Fasciculations of the tongue in motor neurone disease

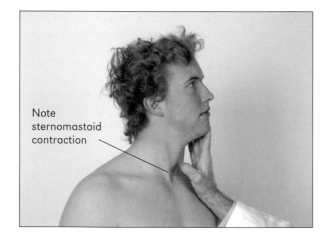

Note sternomastoid contraction

Figure 11.34 Cranial nerve XI: 'Turn your head against my hand'

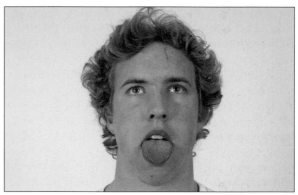

Figure 11.36 Cranial nerve XII: 'Stick out your tongue'

the head to face forwards. This is usually possible at least briefly, but look to see whether he or she needs to use the hands to push the head straight.

Causes of eleventh nerve palsy. Unilateral causes are trauma involving the neck or the base of the skull, poliomyelitis, basilar invagination (platy-basia), syringomyelia and tumours near the jugular foramen. **Bilateral** causes comprise motor neurone disease, poliomyelitis and the Guillain-Barré syndrome. *Note:* Bilateral sternocleidomastoid and trapezius weakness also occurs in muscular dystrophy (especially dystrophia myotonica).

The twelfth (hypoglossal) nerve
Examination anatomy. This nerve also arises from the medulla. It leaves the skull via the hypoglossal foramen. It is the motor nerve for the tongue.

History. The patient with bilateral hypoglossal nerve paresis may have noticed difficulty in swallowing and a sensation of choking if the tongue slips back into the throat. There are no sensory changes caused by hypoglossal nerve abnormalities, and unilateral disease rarely causes symptoms.

Examination. Inspect the tongue at rest on the floor of the mouth. The normal tongue may move a little, especially when protruded, but is not wasted. Look for wasting and fasciculations (fine, irregular, non-rhythmical muscle fibre contractions). These signs indicate a lower motor neurone lesion. Fasciculations may be unilateral or bilateral (Figure 11.35).

Ask the patient to poke out the tongue (Figure 11.36), which may deviate towards the weaker (affected) side if there is a unilateral lower motor

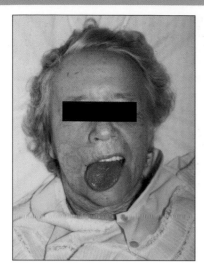

Figure 11.37 Right hypoglossal (XII) nerve palsy—lower motor neurone lesion

neurone lesion (Figure 11.37). The tongue, like the face and palate, has a bilateral upper motor neurone innervation in most people, so a unilateral upper motor neurone lesion often causes no deviation.

A clinically obvious upper motor neurone lesion of the twelfth nerve is usually bilateral and results in a small immobile tongue. The combination of bilateral upper motor neurone lesions of the ninth, tenth and twelfth nerves is called pseudobulbar palsy.

A lower motor neurone lesion of the twelfth nerve causes fasciculation, wasting and weakness. If the lesion is bilateral it causes dysarthria.

Movement disorders may affect the tongue. In Parkinson's disease there may be a coarse tremor of the tongue, made worse by speaking or protruding the tongue. Athetoid, choreiform and tardive dyskinesia can all involve the tongue (page 399).

Causes of twelfth nerve palsy. Bilateral upper motor neurone lesions may be due to vascular lesions, motor neurone disease or tumours, such as metastases to the base of the skull.

Unilateral lower motor neurone lesions with a *central* cause include vascular lesions, such as thrombosis of the vertebral artery; motor neurone disease; and syringobulbia. *Peripheral* causes include: in the posterior fossa, aneurysms or tumours, chronic meningitis and trauma; in the upper neck, tumours or lymphadenopathy; and the Arnold-Chiari malformation.[bb] The Arnold-

Chiari malformation is a congenital malformation of the base of the skull with herniation of a tongue of cerebellum and medulla into the spinal canal, causing lower cranial nerve palsies, cerebellar limb signs (due to tonsillar compression) and upper motor neurone signs in the legs.

Causes of **bilateral lower motor neurone lesions** include motor neurone disease, the Guillain-Barré syndrome, poliomyelitis and the Arnold-Chiari malformation.

Multiple cranial nerve lesions

The anatomical courses of the cranial nerves means they can be affected in groups by single lesions that damage them when they run close to each other. Certain disease processes may also interfere with a number of the cranial nerves. There are a number of syndromes that result from abnormalities of groups of cranial nerves:

1　Unilateral III, IV, V and VI involvement suggests a lesion in the cavernous sinus.
2　Unilateral V, VII and VIII involvement suggests a cerebellopontine angle lesion (usually a tumour).
3　Unilateral IX, X and XI involvement suggests a jugular foramen lesion.
4　Combined bilateral X, XI and XII suggests bulbar palsy if lower motor neurone changes are present and pseudobulbar palsy if there are upper motor neurone signs. The clinical features of pseudobulbar and bulbar palsies are shown in Table 11.7, and the causes of multiple cranial nerve palsies are listed in Table 11.8.
5　Weakness of the eye and facial muscles that worsens with repeated contraction suggests myasthenia.

The head and neck

Inspect and palpate the skull for lumps, such as a meningioma or a sarcoma. Auscultate the skull by placing the diaphragm of the stethoscope on the frontal bone, and then on the lateral occipital bones, and then the bell over each eye (with the opposite eye open). Ask the patient to hold his or her breath each time. Bruits heard over the skull may be due to an arterio-venous malformation, advanced Paget's disease or a vascular meningioma, or they may be conducted from the carotids. Then auscultate over the carotid arteries for a carotid bruit.

The limbs and trunk
History

A variety of symptoms suggest that a patient may have a neurological problem involving the limbs and trunk and that these need to be examined. The exact nature of the symptoms will often suggest

---

bb　Julies Arnold (1835–1915) and Hans Chiari (1851–1916), German pathologists, described this in 1894.

TABLE 11.7 Clinical features of pseudobulbar and bulbar palsies

Feature	Pseudobulbar (bilateral UMN lesions of IX, X and XII)	Bulbar (bilateral LMN lesions of IX, X and XII)
Gag reflex	Increased or normal	Absent
Tongue	Spastic	Wasted, fasciculations
Jaw jerk	Increased	Absent or normal
Speech	Spastic dysarthria	Nasal
Other	Bilateral limb UMN (long tract) signs	Signs of the underlying cause—e.g. limb fasciculations
	Labile emotions	Normal emotions
Causes	Bilateral cerebrovascular disease (e.g. both internal capsules)	Motor neurone disease
		Guillain-Barré syndrome
	Multiple sclerosis	Poliomyelitis
	Motor neurone disease	Brainstem infarction

UMN = upper motor neurone; LMN = lower motor neurone.

TABLE 11.8 Causes of multiple cranial nerve palsies

Nasopharyngeal carcinoma

Chronic meningitis—e.g. carcinoma, haematological malignancy, tuberculosis, sarcoidosis

Guillain-Barré syndrome (spares sensory nerves)

Brainstem lesions. These are usually due to vascular disease causing crossed sensory or motor paralysis (i.e. cranial nerve signs on one side and contralateral long tract signs). Patients with a brainstem tumour (e.g. in the cerebellopontine angle) may also have similar signs

Arnold-Chiari malformation

Trauma

Paget's disease

Mononeuritis multiplex (rarely), e.g. diabetes mellitus

the correct diagnosis and where the examination should be directed. A thorough examination is still essential, however, if unexpected findings are not to be missed.

The patient may present with symptoms that are purely or predominately sensory or motor (*Questions box 11.5*), or related to disorders of movement such as tremor. Sensory symptoms include pain, numbness and paraesthesiae (tingling or pins and needles). It is important to find out if there is involvement of more than one modality, something the patient may not have noticed. The distribution, time of onset and duration may give clues to the aetiology of the symptoms or at least

as to where the sensory examination should be concentrated.

A family history of a similar problem may help provide the diagnosis in conditions such as muscular dystrophy. A previous injury may be responsible, for example, for a peripheral nerve problem but not remembered until asked about specifically.

Examination anatomy

Muscle weakness has four major causes:

1 Pyramidal or upper motor neurone weakness, which is caused by a lesion in the brain proximal to the 'pyramids' in the brainstem. This is where the nerve fibres decussate or cross to the other side before travelling down the spinal cord (Figure 11.38).
2 Lower motor neurone weakness, which is caused by a nerve lesion within the spinal cord or peripheral nerve.
3 Abnormalities of the neuromuscular junction (myasthenia gravis).
4 Muscle disease.

General examination approach

It is most important to have a set order of examination of the limbs for neurological signs so that nothing important is omitted. The following scheme is a standard approach.

1 **Motor system**
   General inspection
   - Posture
   - Muscle bulk
   - Abnormal movements

Questions box 11.5

Questions to ask the patient with muscle weakness

1   Have you felt weakness on both sides of the body?—Suggests spinal cord disease, myopathy or myasthenia gravis (transverse myelitis)

2   Is the weakness just on one side of the body or face?—Transient ischaemic attack or stroke

3   Has the weakness affected just an arm or leg or part of a limb?—Peripheral neuropathy or radiculopathy, stroke or multiple sclerosis

4   Have you had trouble getting up from a chair or brushing your hair or lifting your head?—Proximal muscle weakness (myasthenia gravis, diabetic amyotrophy [involves lower limbs], polymyositis)

5   Have you had trouble swallowing or difficulty speaking?—Myasthenia gravis, polymyositis

6   Have you noticed double vision?—Myasthenia gravis, cranial nerve mononeuritis multiplex

7   Are you taking any medications?—Steroid-induced proximal myopathy

8   Have you had problems with your neck or back or with severe arthritis?—Radiculopathy

9   Have you had a cancer diagnosed at any stage?—Paraneoplastic, Eaton Lambert syndrome

10 Is there any problem like this in the family?—Familial myopathy, Charcot-Marie-Tooth disease

11 Have you had HIV infection?—Various neurological lesions and drug reactions

12 Have you ever had multiple sclerosis diagnosed?

13 Are you a diabetic?—Mononeuritis multiplex, amyotrophy

Fasciculations
Tone
Power
Reflexes
Coordination.
2   **Sensory system**
Pain and temperature
Vibration and proprioception
Light touch.

General inspection

1   Stand back and look at the patient for an *abnormal posture*—for example, one due to hemiplegia caused by a stroke. In this case the upper limb is flexed and there is adduction and pronation of the arm, while the lower limb is extended.

2   Look for *muscle wasting,* which indicates a denervated muscle, a primary muscle disease or disuse atrophy. Compare one side with the other for wasting and try to work out which muscle groups are involved (proximal, distal or generalised, symmetrical or asymmetrical).

3   Inspect for *abnormal movements*, such as tremor of the wrist or arm.

4   Inspect the *skin*—for example, for evidence of neurofibromatosis, cutaneous angiomata in a segmental distribution (associated with syringomyelia) or herpes zoster. Look for scars from old injuries or surgical treatment. Note the presence of a urinary catheter.

The upper limbs

The motor system[cc]

General. Shake hands with the patient and introduce yourself. A patient who cannot relax his or her hand grip has myotonia (an inability to relax the muscles after voluntary contraction). The commonest cause of this is the muscle disease dystrophia myotonica (page 392). Once your hand has been extracted from the patient's, and after pausing briefly for the vitally important general inspection, ask the patient to undress so that the arms and shoulder girdles are completely exposed.

Sit the patient over the edge of the bed if this is possible. Next ask the patient to hold out both hands, palms upward, with the arms extended and the eyes closed (Figure 11.39). Watch the arms for evidence of drifting (movement of one or both arms from the initial neutral position). There are only three causes for drift of the arms:

1   Upper motor neurone (pyramidal) weakness. The drift of the affected limb(s) here is due to muscle weakness and tends to be in a downward direction. The drifting typically starts distally with the fingers and spreads proximally. There may be slow pronation of the wrist and flexion of the fingers and elbow.

2   Cerebellar disease. The drift here is usually upwards. It also includes slow pronation of the wrist and elbow.

3   Loss of proprioception. The drift here (pseudo-athetosis) is really a searching movement and usually affects only the fingers. It is due to loss of joint position sense and can be in any direction.

---

cc   Aretaeus of Cappadocia reasoned, in 150 AD, that the nerves cross (decussate) between the brain and the periphery and that injury to the right side of the head causes abnormalities of the left side of the body.

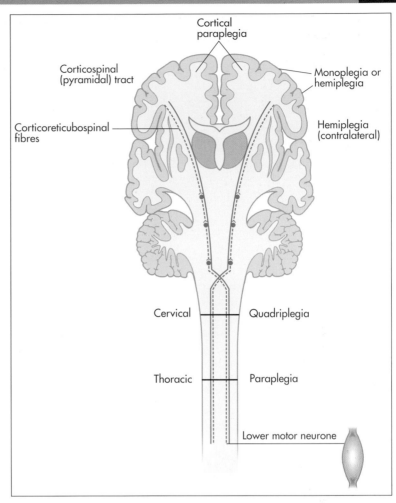

Figure 11.38 Upper and lower motor neurone lesions
(Adapted from Lance JG, McLeod JW, *A physiological approach to clinical neurology*, 3rd edn. London: Butterworths, 1981.)

Ask the patient to relax the arms and rest them on his or her lap. Inspect the large muscle groups for *fasciculations* (Table 11.9). These are irregular contractions of small areas of muscle which have no rhythmical pattern. Fasciculation may be coarse or fine and is present at rest, but not during voluntary movement.[dd] If present with weakness and wasting, fasciculation indicates degeneration of the lower motor neurone. It is usually benign if unassociated with other signs of a motor lesion.

Tone. Tone is tested at both the wrists and elbows. Rotation of the wrists with supination and pronation of the elbow joints (supporting the patient's elbow with one hand and holding the hand with the other)

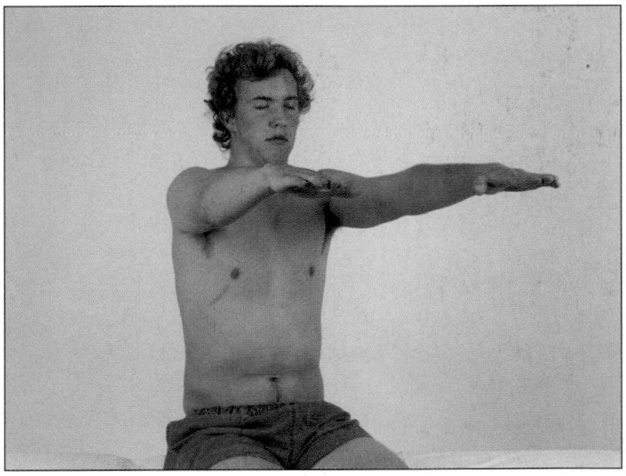

Figure 11.39 Testing for arm drift: 'Shut your eyes and hold your arms out straight. Now turn your palms upwards.'

---

dd If no fasciculation is seen, tapping over the bulk of the brachioradialis and biceps muscles with the finger or with a tendon hammer, and watching again has been recommended, but this is controversial. Most neurologists do not do this. The reason is that fasciculations are spontaneous. Any muscle movement from a local stimulus is not spontaneous. Even if they occur they may have nothing to do with fasciculations.

TABLE 11.9 Causes (differential diagnosis) of fasciculations
Motor neurone disease
Motor root compression
Peripheral neuropathy—e.g. diabetic
Primary myopathy
Thyrotoxicosis
Note: Myokymia resembles coarse fasciculation of the same muscle group, and is particularly common in the orbicularis oculi muscles, where it is usually benign. Focal myokymia, however, often represents brainstem disease, e.g. multiple sclerosis or glioma. Fibrillation is seen only on the electromyogram.

briefly), according to the following modified Medical Research Council scheme (although this lacks sensitivity at the higher grades because work against gravity may only make up a small component of a muscle's function, e.g. the finger flexors):

0   Complete paralysis (no movement).
1   Flicker of contraction possible.
2   Movement is possible when gravity is excluded.
3   Movement is possible against gravity but not if any further resistance is added.
4–   Slight movement against resistance.
4   Moderate movement against resistance.
4+   Submaximal movement against resistance.
5   Normal power.[ee]

is performed passively, and the patient should be told to relax to allow the examiner to move the joints freely.

If the patient resists these movements the joints should be moved unpredictably and at different rates. When the arm is raised by the examiner and dropped, it will fall suddenly if tone is reduced. With experience it is possible to decide if tone is normal or increased (hypertonic, as in an upper motor neurone or extrapyramidal lesion). Hypotonia is a difficult clinical sign to elicit and probably not helpful in the assessment of a lower motor neurone lesion.

The cogwheel rigidity of Parkinson's disease is an important abnormality of tone in the upper limbs and should be recognised. It is best assessed by having the patient move the other arm up and down as the examiner moves the hand and forearm, testing tone at the wrist and elbow.

Myotonia as described above is also an abnormality of tone that is worse after active movement. In these patients, tone is usually normal at rest but after sudden movements there may be a great increase in tone and the patient is unable to relax the muscle. Tapping over the body of a myotonic muscle causes a dimple of contraction, which only slowly disappears (*percussion myotonia*). This is best tested by tapping the thenar eminence or by asking the patient to make a tight fist and then open the hand quickly. The opening of the fist is very slow when the muscles are myotonic.

Power. Muscle strength is assessed by gauging the examiner's ability to overcome the patient's full voluntary muscle resistance. To decide whether the power is normal, the patient's age, gender and build should be taken into account. Power is graded based on the maximum observed (no matter how

If power is reduced, decide whether this is symmetrical or asymmetrical, whether it involves only particular muscle groups, or whether it is proximal, distal or general. It is also important to consider whether any painful joint or muscle disease is interfering with the assessment (see Chapter 9). Asymmetrical muscle weakness is most often the result of a peripheral nerve, brachial plexus or root lesion, or an upper motor neurone lesion. As each movement is tested the important muscles involved should be observed or palpated.

Shoulder
- *Abduction*—mostly deltoid and supraspinatus—(C5, C6): the patient should abduct the arms with the elbows flexed and resist the examiner's attempt to push them down (Figure 11.40).
- *Adduction*—mostly pectoralis major and latissimus dorsi—(C6, C7, C8): the patient should adduct the arms with the elbows flexed and not allow the examiner to separate them.

Elbow
- *Flexion*—biceps and brachialis—(C5, C6): the patient should bend the elbow and pull so as not to let the examiner straighten it out (Figure 11.41).
- *Extension*—triceps brachii—(C7, C8): the patient should bend the elbow and push so as not to let the examiner bend it (Figure 11.42).

Wrist
- *Flexion*—flexor carpi ulnaris and radialis—(C6,

---

ee You should not be able to overcome a normal adult patient's power, at least in the legs.

C7): the patient should bend the wrist and not allow the examiner to straighten it.

- *Extension*—extensor carpi group—(C7, C8): the patient should extend the wrist and not allow the examiner to bend it (Figure 11.43).

Fingers

- *Extension*—extensor digitorum communis, extensor indicis and extensor digiti minimi—(C7, C8): the patient should straighten the fingers and not allow the examiner to push

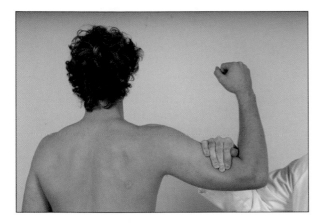

Figure 11.40 Testing power—shoulder abduction: 'Stop me pushing your arm down'

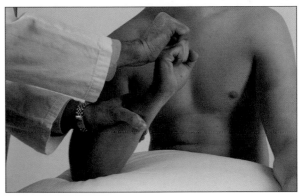

Figure 11.43 Testing power—wrist extension: 'Stop me bending your wrist'

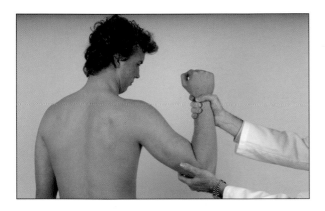

Figure 11.41 Testing power—elbow flexion: 'Stop me straightening your elbow'

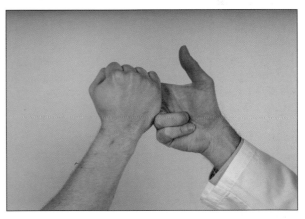

Figure 11.44 Testing power—finger flexion: 'Squeeze my fingers hard' (don't offer more than two fingers)

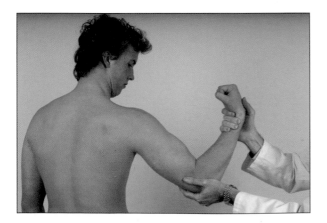

Figure 11.42 Testing power—elbow extension: 'Stop me bending your elbow

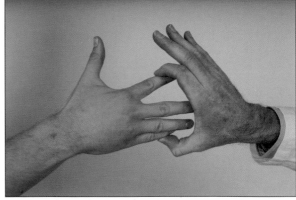

Figure 11.45 Testing power—finger abduction: 'Stop me pushing your fingers together'

them down (push with the side of your hand across the patient's metacarpophalangeal joints).

- *Flexion*—flexor digitorum profundus and sublimis—(C7, C8): the patient squeezes two of the examiner's fingers (Figure 11.44).
- *Abduction*—dorsal interossei—(C8, T1): the patient should spread out the fingers and not allow the examiner to push them together (Figure 11.45).
- *Adduction*—volar interossei—(C8, T1): the patient holds the fingers together and tries to prevent the examiner from separating them further.

Reflexes. The sudden stretching of a muscle usually evokes brisk contraction of that muscle or muscle group. This reflex is usually mediated via a neural pathway synapsing in the spinal cord. It is subject to regulation via pathways from the brain. As the reflex is a response to stretching of a muscle, it is correctly called a muscle stretch reflex rather than a tendon reflex. The tendon merely transmits stretch to the muscle.

Tendon hammers are available in a number of designs. Sir William Gowers[ff] used the ulnar side of his hand or part of his stethoscope. In Australia and Britain, the Queen Square hammer[gg] is in common use (Figure 11.46). The Taylor hammer is popular in America; it is shaped like a tomahawk and has a broad rubber edge for most tendons and a more pointed side for the cutaneous reflexes.

Reflexes are graded from absent to greatly increased (Table 11.10).

Make sure the patient is resting comfortably with the elbows flexed and hands lying pronated on the lap and not overlapping one another.

To test the **biceps jerk (C5, C6)**, place one forefinger on the biceps tendon and tap this with the tendon hammer (Figure 11.47). The hammer should be held near its end and the head allowed to fall with gravity onto the positioned forefinger. The examiner soon learns not to hit too hard. Normally, if the reflex arc is intact, there is a brisk contraction of the biceps muscle with flexion of the forearm at the elbow, followed by prompt relaxation. Practice will help the examiner decide whether the response

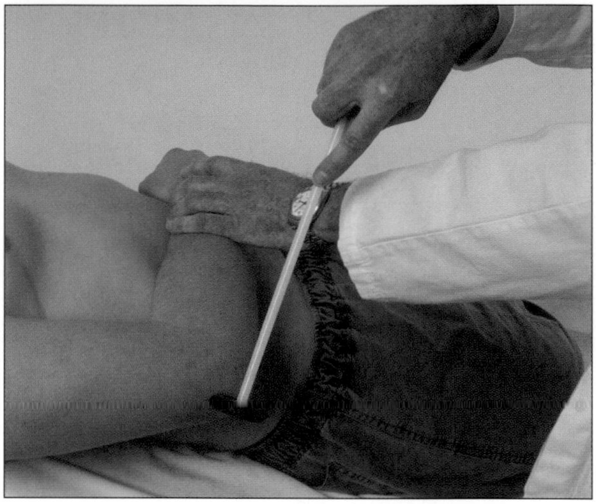

Figure 11.46 A Queen Square patellar hammer

TABLE 11.10 Classification of muscle stretch reflexes	
0	= absent
+	= present but reduced
++	= normal
+++	= increased, possibly normal
++++	= greatly increased, often associated with clonus (page 368)

is within the normal range. When a reflex is greatly exaggerated, it can be elicited away from the usual zone.

If a reflex appears to be absent, always test following a *reinforcement manoeuvre*. For example, ask the patient to clench the teeth tightly just before you let the hammer fall. Supraspinal and fusiform mechanisms have been identified to explain reinforcement, but it works partly as a distraction, especially if the reflex is absent because an anxious patient has contracted opposing muscle groups. Merely talking to the patient may provide enough distraction for the reflex to be elicited. Sometimes normal reflexes can be elicited only after reinforcement, but they should still be symmetrical.

An increased jerk occurs with an upper motor neurone lesion (page 354). A decreased or absent reflex occurs with a breach in any part of the reflex motor arc—the muscle itself (e.g. myopathy), the motor nerve (e.g. neuropathy), the anterior spinal cord root (e.g. spondylosis), the anterior horn cell (e.g. poliomyelitis) or the sensory arc (sensory root or sensory nerve).

---

ff Sir William Gowers (1845–1915), professor of clinical medicine at University College Hospital, London, and neurologist to the National Hospital for Nervous Diseases, Queen Square, London. He was also an artist who illustrated his own books and had paintings exhibited at the Royal Academy.

gg The Queen Square hammer was invented by Miss Wintle, staff nurse at Queen Square. She made hammers from brass wheels covered by a ring pessary and mounted on a bamboo handle; she sold these to medical students and resident medical officers.

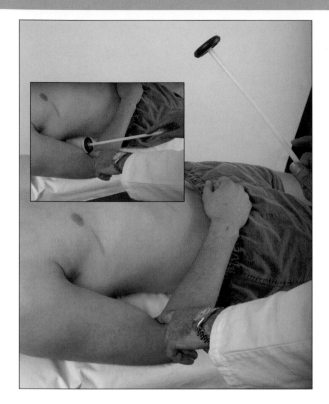

Figure 11.47 The biceps jerk examination

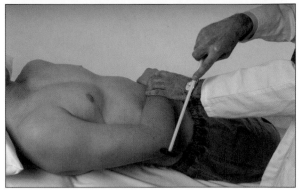

Figure 11.48 The triceps jerk examination

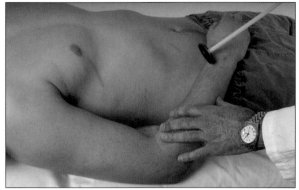

Figure 11.49 The supinator jerk strike zone

To test the **triceps jerk (C7, C8)**, support the elbow with one hand and tap over the triceps tendon (Figure 11.48). Normally, triceps contraction results in forearm extension.

To test the **brachioradialis (supinator) jerk (C5, C6)**, strike the lower end of the radius just above the wrist (Figure 11.49). To avoid hurting the patient by striking the radial nerve directly, place your own first two fingers over this spot and then strike the fingers, as with the biceps jerk. Normally, contraction of the brachioradialis causes flexion of the elbow.

If elbow extension and finger flexion is the only response when the patient's wrist is tapped, the response is said to be inverted, known as the *inverted brachioradialis (supinator) jerk*. The triceps contraction causes elbow extension instead of the usual elbow flexion. This is associated with an absent biceps jerk and an exaggerated triceps jerk. It indicates a spinal cord lesion at the C5 or C6 level due, for example, to compression (e.g. disc prolapse), trauma or syringomyelia. It occurs because a lower motor neurone lesion at C5 or C6 is combined with an upper motor neurone lesion affecting the reflexes below this level.

To test **finger jerks (C8)**, the patient rests the hand palm upward, with the fingers slightly flexed.

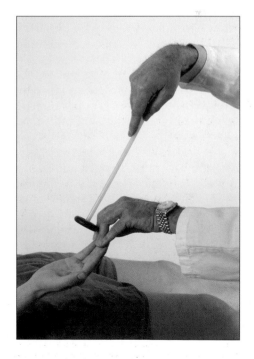

Figure 11.50 The finger jerk examination

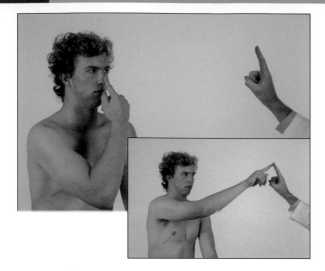

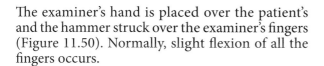

Figure 11.51 Finger–nose test: 'Touch your nose with your forefinger and then reach out and touch my finger'

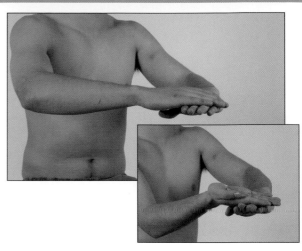

Figure 11.52 Testing for dysdiadochokinesis in the upper limbs: 'Turn your hand over, backwards and forwards on the other one, as quickly and smoothly as you can'

The examiner's hand is placed over the patient's and the hammer struck over the examiner's fingers (Figure 11.50). Normally, slight flexion of all the fingers occurs.

Coordination. The cerebellum has multiple connections (afferent and efferent) to sensory pathways, brainstem nuclei, the thalamus and the cerebral cortex. Via these connections the cerebellum plays an integral role in coordinating voluntary movement. A standard series of simple tests is used to test coordination. Always demonstrate these movements for the patient's benefit.

Finger–nose test. Ask the patient to touch his or her nose with the index finger and then turn the finger around and touch the examiner's outstretched forefinger at nearly full extension of the shoulder and elbow (Figure 11.51). The test should be done both briskly and slowly, and repeated a number of times with the patient's eyes open and later closed. Slight resistance to the patient's movements by the examiner pushing on his or her forearm during the test may unmask less-severe abnormalities.

Look for the following abnormalities: (i) intention tremor, which is tremor increasing as the target is approached (there is no tremor at rest); and (ii) past-pointing, where the patient's finger overshoots the target towards the side of cerebellar abnormality. These abnormalities occur with cerebellar disease.

Rapidly alternating movements. Ask the patient to pronate and supinate his or her hand on the dorsum of the other hand as rapidly as possible (Figure 11.52). This movement is slow and clumsy in cerebellar disease and is called dysdiadochokinesis.[hh]

Rapidly alternating movements may also be affected in extrapyramidal disorders (e.g. Parkinson's disease) and in pyramidal disorders (e.g. internal capsule infarction).

Rebound. Ask the patient to lift the arms rapidly from the sides and then stop. Hypotonia due to cerebellar disease causes delay in stopping the arms. This method of demonstrating rebound is preferable to the more often used one where the patient flexes the arm at the elbow against the examiner's resistance. When the examiner suddenly lets go, violent flexion of the arm may occur and, unless prevented, the patient can strike himself or herself in the face. Therefore, only medical students trained in self-defence should use this method.[ii]

Muscle weakness may also cause clumsiness, but motor testing should have revealed any impairment of this sort.

The sensory system

To test sensation, which can be a difficult assessment and frustratingly time-consuming, use the following routine.[12]

---

hh Actually, dysdiadochokinesis is the inability to perform alternating movements of both wrists with the arms and forefingers extended. *Diadochi* is a Greek word meaning succession. The problem here is with successive movements. The Diadochi were the successors of Alexander the Great. They divided his empire.

ii Nick Talley has a black belt in Tae Kwon Do and Tang Soo Do.

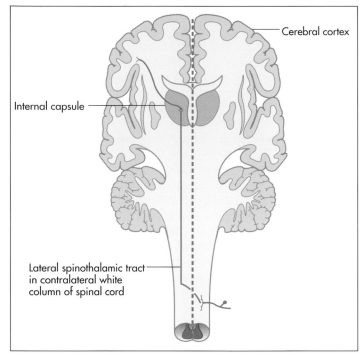

Figure 11.53 Pain and temperature pathways
(Adapted from Snell RS, Westmoreland BF, *Clinical neuroanatomy for medical students*, 4th edn. Boston: Little Brown, 1997.)

Spinothalamic pathway (pain and temperature). Pain and temperature fibres enter the spinal cord and cross, a few segments higher, to the opposite spinothalamic tract (Figure 11.53). This tract ascends to the brainstem.

Pain (pinprick) testing. Using a new pin,[10] demonstrate to the patient that this induces a relatively sharp sensation by touching lightly a normal area, such as the anterior chest wall. Then ask the patient to say whether the pinprick feels sharp or dull. Begin proximally on the upper arm and test in each dermatome—the area of skin supplied by a vertebral spinal segment (Figure 11.54). Also compare right with left in the same dermatome. Map out the extent of any area of dullness. Always do this by going from the area of dullness to the area of normal sensation.

Temperature testing. This can be done in a similar fashion, using test tubes filled with hot (40–45 degrees) and cold (5–10 degrees) water. Cold sensation can also be tested with a metal object, such as a tuning fork. Absence of ability to feel heat is almost always associated with inability to feel cold. Temperature differences of 2–5 degrees can usually be distinguished. These tests are performed only in special circumstances—for example, for suspected syringomyelia.

Posterior columns (vibration and proprioception[jj]). These fibres enter and ascend ipsilaterally in the posterior columns of the spinal cord to the nucleus gracilis and nucleus cuneatus in the medulla, where they decussate (Figure 11.55).

Vibration testing. Use a 128 Hz tuning fork (not a 256 Hz fork). Ask the patient to close the eyes, and then place the vibrating tuning fork on one of the distal interphalangeal joints. The patient should be able to describe a feeling of vibration. The examiner then deadens the tuning fork with

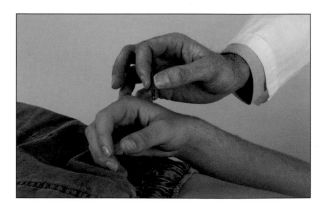

Figure 11.54 Testing for pinprick (pain) sensation with a disposable neurology pin: 'Does this feel sharp or blunt?'

jj In 1826 Sir Charles Bell recognised that there was a 'sixth sense', which was later called proprioception. Vibration sense had been recognised in the 16th century and tests for it developed in the 19th century by Rinné and others. Rydel and Seiffer found that vibration sense and proprioception were carried in the posterior columns of the spinal cord.

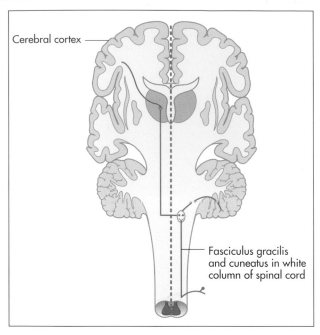

Cerebral cortex

Fasciculus gracilis and cuneatus in white column of spinal cord

Figure 11.55 Vibration and joint position sense pathways
(Adapted from Snell RS, Westmoreland BF, *Clinical neuroanatomy for medical students*, 4th edn. Boston: Little Brown, 1997.)

the hand, and the patient should be able to say exactly when this occurs. Compare one side with the other. If vibration sense is reduced or absent, test over the ulnar head at the wrist, then the elbows (over the olecranon) and then the shoulders to determine the level of abnormality. Although the tuning fork is traditionally placed only over bony prominences, vibration sense is just as good over soft tissues.

Proprioception testing. Use the distal interphalangeal joint of the patient's little finger. When the patient has his or her eyes open, grasp the distal phalanx from the sides and move it up and down to demonstrate these positions. Then ask the patient to close the eyes while these manoeuvres are repeated randomly. Normally, movement through even a few degrees is detectable, and should be reported correctly. If there is an abnormality, proceed to test the wrists and elbows similarly. As a rule, sense of position is lost before sense of movement, and the little finger is affected before the thumb.

Light-touch testing. Some fibres travel in the posterior columns (i.e. ipsilaterally) and the rest cross the middle line to travel in the anterior spinothalamic tract (i.e. contralaterally). For this reason light touch is of the least discriminating value. Irritation of light-touch receptors is probably

responsible for paraesthesiae—for example following ischaemia of a limb.

Test light touch by touching the skin with a wisp of cottonwool. Ask the patient to shut the eyes and say 'yes' when the touch is felt. Do not stroke the skin because this moves hair fibres. Test each dermatome,[kk] comparing left and right sides.

Interpretation of sensory abnormalities. Try to fit the distribution of any sensory loss into a dermatome (due to a spinal cord or nerve root lesion), a single peripheral nerve territory, a peripheral neuropathy pattern (glove distribution, page 386), or a hemisensory loss (due to spinal cord or upper brainstem or thalamic lesion).

Sensory dermatomes of the upper limb (Figure 11.56) can be recognised by memorising the following rough guides: C5 supplies the shoulder tip and outer part of the upper arm; C6 supplies the lateral aspect of the forearm and thumb; C7 supplies the middle finger; C8 supplies the little finger; T1 supplies the medial aspect of the upper arm and elbow.

Examination of the peripheral nerves of the upper limb

A lesion of a peripheral nerve causes a characteristic motor and sensory loss.[13] Peripheral nerve lesions may have local causes, such as trauma or compression, or may be part of a mononeuritis multiplex, where more than one nerve is affected by systemic disease.

The radial nerve (C5–C8). This is the *motor nerve* supplying the triceps and brachioradialis and the extensor muscles of the hand. The characteristic deformity that results from radial nerve injury is *wrist drop*. To demonstrate this, if it is not already obvious, get the patient to flex the elbow, pronate the forearm and extend the wrist and fingers. If a lesion occurs above the upper third of the upper arm, the triceps muscle is also affected. Therefore test elbow extension, which will be absent if the lesion is high.

Test *sensation* using a pin over the area of the anatomical snuff box. Sensation here is lost with a radial nerve lesion before the bifurcation into posterior interosseous and superficial radial nerves at the elbow (Figure 11.57).

---

kk The human dermatomes (which he called *pain spots*) were first mapped by Sir Henry Head (1861–1940). He was most famous for his experimental cutting of his own radial nerve. This enabled him to chart the order of return of the sensory modalities.

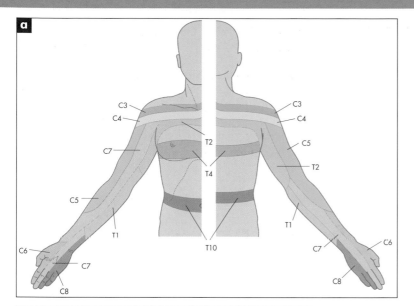

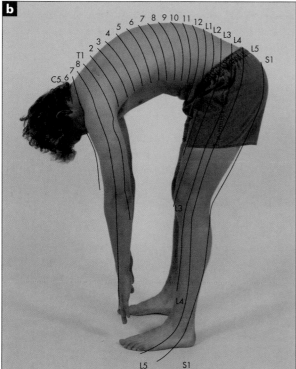

Figure 11.56 Dermatomes of the upper limb and trunk
(a) The dermatomes explained. (b) The distribution of the dermatomes makes more sense if we are thought of as quadrupedal.

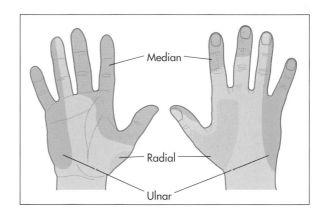

Figure 11.57 Average loss of pain sensation (pinprick) with lesions of the major nerves of the upper limbs

The median nerve (C6–T1). This nerve contains the *motor* supply to all the muscles on the front of the forearm except the flexor carpi ulnaris and the ulnar half of the flexor digitorum profundus. It also supplies the following short muscles of the hand (LOAF)—the *Lateral* two lumbricals, *Opponens* pollicis, *Abductor* pollicis brevis, and in many people the *Flexor* pollicis brevis.

Lesion at the wrist (carpal tunnel).[14,15] Use the pen-touching test to assess for weakness of

the abductor pollicis brevis. Ask the patient to lay the hand flat, palm upwards on the table, and attempt to abduct the thumb vertically to touch the examiner's pen held above it (Figure 11.58). This may be impossible if there is a median nerve palsy at the wrist or above. Remember, however, that most patients with the carpal tunnel syndrome have normal power and may indeed have symptoms but no signs at all.

Lesion in the cubital fossa. Ochsner's clasping

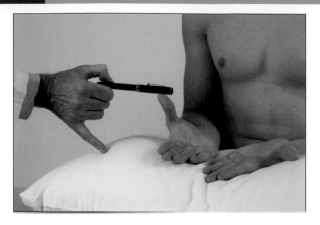

Figure 11.58 Pen-touching test for loss of abductor pollicis brevis: 'Lift your thumb straight up to touch my pen'

test[ll] (for loss of flexor digitorum sublimis). Ask the patient to clasp the hands firmly together (Figure 11.59a)—the index finger on the affected side fails to flex with a lesion in the cubital fossa or higher (Figure 11.59b).

For the *sensory* component of the median nerve, test pinprick sensation over the hand. The constant area of loss includes the palmar aspect of the thumb, index, middle and lateral half of the ring fingers (Figure 11.57). The palm is spared in median nerve lesions in the carpal tunnel.

The ulnar nerve (C8–T1). This nerve contains the *motor* supply to all the small muscles of the hand (except the LOAF muscles), flexor carpi ulnaris and the ulnar half of flexor digitorum profundus. Look for wasting of the small muscles of the hand and for partial clawing of the little and ring fingers (a claw-like hand). Clawing is hyperextension at the metacarpophalangeal joints and flexion of the interphalangeal joints. Note that clawing is more pronounced with an ulnar nerve lesion at the wrist, as a lesion at or above the elbow also causes loss of the flexor digitorum profundus, and therefore less flexion of the interphalangeal joints. This is the 'ulnar nerve paradox', in that a more distal lesion causes greater deformity.

Froment's sign.[mm] Ask the patient to grasp a piece of paper between the thumb and lateral aspect of the forefinger with each hand. The affected thumb will flex because of loss of the adductor of the thumb.

Causes of a true claw hand are shown in Table 11.11, while causes of wasting of the small muscles of the hand are shown in Table 11.12; see also Figure 11.60.

For the *sensory* component of the ulnar nerve, test for pinprick loss over the palmar and dorsal aspects of the little finger and the medial half of the ring finger (Figure 11.57).

The brachial plexus. Brachial plexus lesions vary from mild to complete; motor and/or sensory fibres may be involved. Nerve roots form trunks, which divide into cords and then form peripheral nerves (see Tables 11.13 and 11.14). The anatomy is shown in Figure 11.61.

[ll] Albert Ochsner (1858–1925), American surgeon of Swiss extraction, who claimed descent from Andreas Vesalius, the great anatomist.

[mm] Jules Froment (1878–1946), Professor of Medicine, Lyons, France, described the sign in 1915.

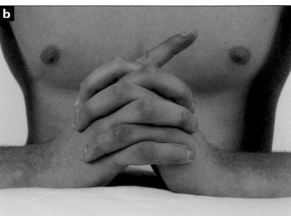

Figure 11.59 Ochsner's clasping test
(a) Normal. (b) Abnormal due to loss of function of the flexor digitorum (simulated demonstration).

TABLE 11.11 Causes (differential diagnosis) of a true claw hand (all fingers clawed)

Ulnar and median nerve lesion (ulnar nerve palsy alone causes a claw-like hand)

Brachial plexus lesion (C8–T1)

Other neurological disease—e.g. syringomyelia, polio

Ischaemic contracture (late and severe)

Rheumatoid arthritis (advanced, untreated disease)

TABLE 11.12 Causes (differential diagnosis) of wasting of the small muscles of the hand

Spinal cord lesions
Syringomyelia
Cervical spondylosis with compression of the C8 segment
Tumour
Trauma

Anterior horn cell disease
Motor neurone disease, poliomyelitis
Spinal muscular atrophies, e.g. Kugelberg-Welander* disease

Root lesion
C8 compression

Lower trunk brachial plexus lesion
Thoracic outlet syndromes
Trauma, radiation, infiltration, inflammation

Peripheral nerve lesions
Median and ulnar nerve lesions
Peripheral motor neuropathy

Myopathy
Dystrophia myotonica—forearms are more affected than the hands
Distal myopathy

Trophic disorders
Arthropathies (disuse)
Ischaemia, including vasculitis
Shoulder hand syndrome

Note: Distinguishing an ulnar nerve lesion from a C8 root/lower trunk brachial plexus lesion depends on remembering that sensory loss with a C8 lesion extends proximal to the wrist, and the thenar muscles are involved with a C8 root or lower trunk brachial plexus lesion. Distinguishing a C8 root from a lower trunk brachial plexus lesion is difficult clinically, but the presence of a Horner's syndrome or an axillary mass suggests the brachial plexus is affected.
* Eric Klas Kugelberg (1913–83), professor of clinical neurophysiology at the Karolinska Institute in Stockholm, and Lisa Welander (1909–2001) described this in 1956. Lisa Welander was Sweden's first woman professor of neurology.

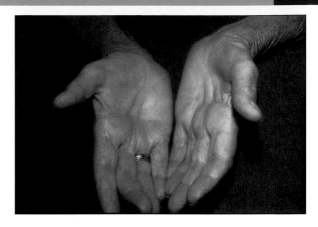

Figure 11.60 Motor neurone disease
Shows wasting of the small muscles of the hand.

Patients with brachial plexus lesions may complain of pain or weakness in the shoulders or arms. Pain is often prominent, especially when there has been nerve root avulsion. A neurological cause is more likely if there is dull pain that is difficult to localise, if the pain is not related to limb movement and is worse at night, and if there is no associated tenderness. The patient may be unable to get comfortable. An orthopaedic or traumatic cause is more likely if the pain is much worse with movement, or there are signs of inflammation, joint deformity or local tenderness. Most plexus lesions are supraclavicular (i.e. proximal), especially when they occur after trauma. When infraclavicular (i.e. distal) lesions occur they are usually less severe.

Examine the arms and shoulder girdle (Table 11.15). Remember that the dorsal scapular nerve (which supplies the rhomboid muscles) comes from the C5 nerve root proximal to the upper trunk, and so rhomboid function is usually spared in upper trunk lesions. Typical lesions of the brachial plexus are described in Table 11.16. The cervical rib syndrome may cause a lower brachial plexus lesion (Table 11.17). Table 11.18 suggests a scheme for distinguishing plexus and nerve root lesions.

Ask the patient to stand facing away from you with the arms and hands stretched out to touch and push against the wall. Winging of the scapulae is seen typically in fascio-scapular-humeral dystrophy (Figure 11.62).

Causes of brachial plexus lesions include:
1 Inflammation, autoimmune disorders (more often upper plexus).
2 Radiotherapy (more often upper plexus).
3 Cancer (more often lower plexus). *Cancer* causes a brachial plexus lesion by local invasion. The

TABLE 11.13 Nerve roots and brachial plexus trunks

Nerve roots	Trunks	Muscles supplied
C5 and 6	Upper	Shoulder (especially biceps and deltoid)
C7	Middle	Triceps and some forearm muscles
C8 and T1	Lower	Hand and some forearm muscles

TABLE 11.14 Brachial plexus cords, nerves and their supplied muscles

Cords	Nerves formed	Muscles supplied
Lateral	Musculocutaneous, median	Biceps, pronator teres, flexor carpi radialis
Medial	Median and ulnar	Hand muscles
Posterior	Axillary and radial	Deltoid, triceps and forearm extensors

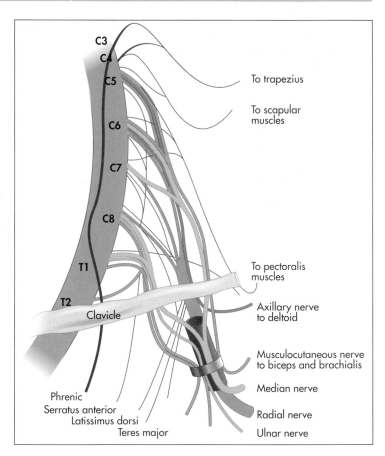

Figure 11.61 The brachial plexus
(Adapted from Chusid JG, *Correlative neuroanatomy and functional neurology*, 19th edn. Los Altos: Lange Medical, 1985.)

lower trunk is usually affected first. These plexus lesions are usually painful and progress rapidly. Weakness and sensory loss are both present.

4 Trauma: direct (motor vehicle accident, surgery including sternotomy, lacerations and gunshots), traction (birth injuries, motor vehicle accidents, sporting injuries such as rugby tackles—more often upper plexus), chronic compression (thoracic outlet, 'backpack palsy', fractures with bone displacement).

The lower limbs

Begin by testing *gait*, if this is possible (see page 376).

Inspect the legs with the patient lying in bed with the legs and thighs entirely exposed (place a towel over the groin). Note whether there is a urinary catheter present, which may indicate that there is spinal cord compression or other spinal cord disease, particularly multiple sclerosis.

TABLE 11.15 Shoulder girdle examination

Method

Abnormalities are likely to be due to a muscular dystrophy, single nerve or a root lesion. Inspect each muscle, palpate its bulk and test function as follows:

1 *Trapezius (XI, C3, C4):* ask the patient to elevate the shoulders against resistance and look for winging of the upper scapula.

2 *Serratus anterior (C5–C7):* ask the patient to push the hands against the wall and look for winging of the lower scapula.

3 *Rhomboids (C4, C5):* ask the patient to pull both shoulder blades together with the hands on the hips.

4 *Supraspinatus (C5, C6):* ask the patient to abduct the arms from the sides against resistance.

5 *Infraspinatus (C5, C6):* ask the patient to rotate the upper arms externally against resistance with the elbows flexed at the sides.

6 *Teres major (C5–C7):* ask the patient to rotate the upper arms internally against resistance.

7 *Latissimus dorsi (C7, C8):* ask the patient to pull the elbows into the sides against resistance.

8 *Pectoralis major, clavicular head (C5–C8):* ask the patient to lift the upper arms above the horizontal and push them forward against resistance.

9 *Pectoralis major, sternocostal part (C6–T1) and pectoralis minor (C7):* ask the patient to adduct the upper arms against resistance.

10 *Deltoid (C5, C6) (and axillary nerve):* ask the patient to abduct the arms against resistance.

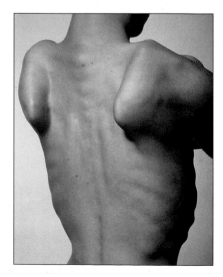

Figure 11.62 Winging of the scapulae, often a result of muscular dystrophy
(From Mir MA, *Atlas of Clinical Diagnosis*, 2nd edn. Edinburgh: Saunders, 2003, with permission.)

TABLE 11.16 Brachial plexus lesions

Complete lesion (rare)

1 Lower motor neurone signs affect the whole arm

2 Sensory loss (whole limb)

3 Horner's syndrome (an important clue)

Note: This is often painful.

Upper lesion (Erb Duchenne*) (C5, C6)

1 Loss of shoulder movement and elbow flexion—the hand is held in the waiter's tip position

2 Sensory loss over the lateral aspect of the arm and forearm

Lower lesion (Klumpke†) (C8, T1)

1 True claw hand with paralysis of all the intrinsic muscles

2 Sensory loss along the ulnar side of the hand and forearm

3 Horner's syndrome

* Wilhelm Heinrich Erb (1840–1921), Germany's greatest neurologist.

† Auguste Déjérine-Klumpke (1859–1927), French neurologist, described this lesion as a student. She was an American, but was educated in Switzerland. As a final-year student she married the great French neurologist Jules Déjérine.

TABLE 11.17 Cervical rib syndrome

Clinical features

1 Weakness and wasting of the small muscles of the hand (claw hand)

2 C8 and T1 sensory loss

3 Unequal radial pulses and blood pressure

4 Subclavian bruits on arm manoeuvring (may be present in normal people)

5 Palpable cervical rib in the neck (uncommon)

The motor system

Fasciculations and muscle wasting. Inspect for fasciculations. Look for muscle wasting. Feel the muscle bulk of the quadriceps and calves. Then run a hand along each shin, feeling for wasting of the anterior tibial muscles.

Tone. Test tone at the knees and ankles. Place one hand under a chosen knee and then abruptly pull the knee upwards, causing flexion. When the patient is relaxed this should occur without resistance. Then, supporting the thigh, flex and extend the knee at increasing velocity, feeling for resistance to muscle stretch (tone). Tone in the legs may also be tested by sitting the patient with legs hanging freely over the edge of the bed. A leg (of the patient) is raised

TABLE 11.18 Distinguishing brachial plexus lesions and nerve root compression

	Root	Plexus
Previous trauma	Occasionally	Some types
Insidious onset	Usually	Some types
Neck pain	Yes	No
Unilateral interscapular pain	Yes	No
Weakness	Mild–moderate	Often severe
Pattern of weakness	Most commonly triceps (C7 lesions, the most commonly affected root)	Usually shoulder and biceps or hand

by the examiner to the horizontal and suddenly let go. The leg will oscillate up to half a dozen times in a normal person who is completely relaxed. If hypotonia is present, as occurs in cerebellar disease, the oscillations will be wider and more prolonged. If increased tone or spasticity is present, the movements will be irregular and jerky.

Next test for *clonus* of the ankle and knee. This is a sustained rhythmical contraction of the muscles when put under sudden stretch. It is due to hypertonia from an upper motor neurone lesion. It represents an increase in reflex excitability (from increased alpha motor neurone activity).

Sharply dorsiflex the foot with the knee bent and the thigh externally rotated. When ankle clonus is present, recurrent ankle plantar flexion movement occurs. This may persist for as long as the examiner sustains dorsiflexion of the ankle. Test for patellar clonus (which is not so common) by resting the hand on the lower part of the quadriceps with the knee extended and moving the patella down sharply. Sustained rhythmical contraction of the quadriceps occurs as long as the downward stretch is maintained.

Power. Test power next.
Hip
- *Flexion*—psoas and iliacus muscles—(L2, L3): ask the patient to lift up the straight leg and not let you push it down (having placed your hand above the knee) (Figure 11.63).
- *Extension*—gluteus maximus—(L5, S1, S2): ask the patient to keep the leg down and not let you pull it up from underneath the calf or ankle (Figure 11.64).
- *Abduction*—gluteus medius and minimus, sartorius and tensor fasciae latae—(L4, L5, S1): ask the patient to abduct the leg and not let you push it in (Figure 11.65).
- *Adduction*—adductors longus, brevis and magnus—(L2, L3, L4): ask the patient to keep

the leg adducted and not let you push it out (Figure 11.66).

Knee
- *Flexion*—hamstrings (biceps femoris, semimembranosus, semitendinosus)—(L5, S1): ask the patient to bend the knee and not let you straighten it (Figure 11.67). If there is doubt about the real strength of knee flexion, it should be tested with the patient in the prone position. Here possible help from hip flexion is prevented and the muscles can be palpated during contraction.
- *Extension*—quadriceps femoris (this muscle is three times as strong as its antagonists, the hamstrings)—(L3, L4): with the knee slightly bent, ask the patient to straighten the knee and not let you bend it (Figure 11.68).

Ankle
- *Plantar flexion*—gastrocnemius, plantaris, soleus—(S1, S2): ask the patient to push the foot down and not let you push it up (Figure 11.69).
- *Dorsiflexion*—tibialis anterior, extensor digitorum longus and extensor hallucis longus—(L4, L5): ask the patient to bring the foot up and not let you push it down (Figure 11.70). The power of the ankle joint can also be tested by having the patient stand up on the toes (plantar flexion) or on the heels (dorsiflexion); these movements may also be limited if coordination is impaired.

Tarsal joint
- *Eversion*—peroneus longus and brevis, and extensor digitorum longus—(L5, S1): ask the patient to evert the foot against resistance (Figure 11.71).
- *Inversion*—tibialis posterior, gastrocnemius and hallucis longus—(L5, S1): with the foot

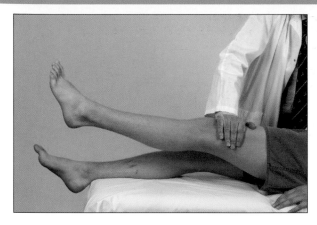

Figure 11.63 Testing power—hip flexion: 'Lift your leg up and don't let me push it down'

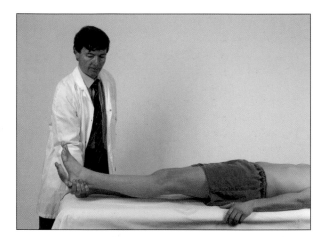

Figure 11.64 Testing power—hip extension: 'Push your heel down and don't let me pull it up'

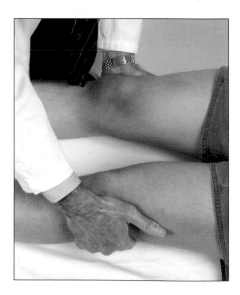

Figure 11.65 Testing power—hip abduction: 'Don't let me push your knees together'

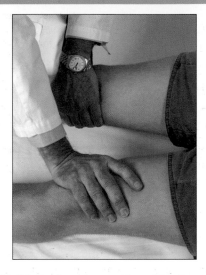

Figure 11.66 Testing power—hip adduction: 'Don't let me push your knees apart'

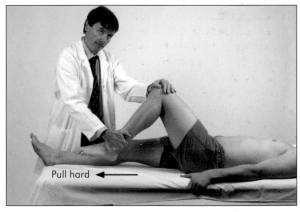

Pull hard

Figure 11.67 Testing power—knee flexion: 'Bend your knee and don't let me straighten it'; pull hard

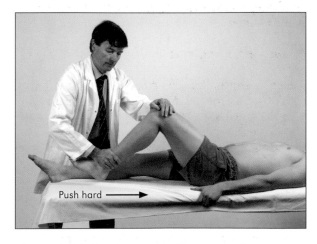

Push hard

Figure 11.68 Testing power—knee extension: 'Straighten your knee and don't let me bend it'; push hard

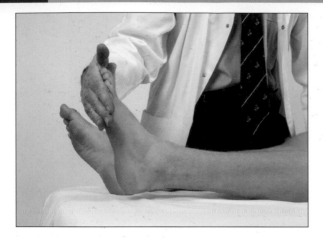

Figure 11.69 Testing power—ankle, plantar flexion: 'Don't let me push your foot up'

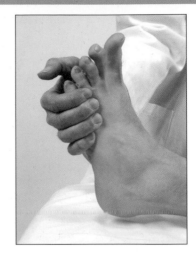

Figure 11.71 Testing power—ankle (tarsal joint) eversion: 'Stop me turning your foot inwards'

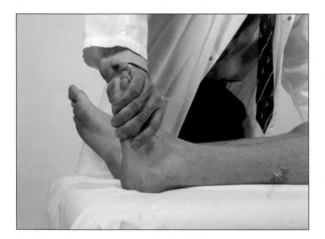

Figure 11.70 Testing power—ankle, dorsiflexion: 'Don't let me push your foot down'

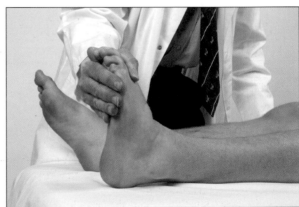

Figure 11.72 Testing power—ankle (tarsal joint) inversion: 'Stop me turning your foot outwards'

in complete plantar flexion, ask the patient to invert the foot against resistance (Figure 11.72).

Non-organic or hysterical unilateral limb weakness may be detected by Hoover's test. Normally when a patient attempts to resist movement, the contralateral limb works to support the effort. For example when a patient attempts to extend the leg against resistance, the other leg pushes down into the bed. If this movement is absent Hoover's[nn] sign is positive.

Quick test of lower limb power. The clinician in a hurry can test lower limb power quickly by asking the patient to:

1. stand up on his or her toes (S1) (Figure 11.73a);
2. stand up on the heels (L4, L5) (Figure 11.73b);
3. squat and stand again (L3, L4) (Figure 11.73c).

This tests ankle, knee and hip power. Inability to perform any of the tests suggests a need to test more formally.

Reflexes. Test the following reflexes.

Knee jerk (L3, L4). Slide one arm under the knees so that they are slightly bent and supported. The tendon hammer is allowed to fall onto the infrapatellar tendon (Figure 11.74). Normally, contraction of the quadriceps causes extension of the knee. Compare the two sides. If the knee jerk appears to be absent on one or both sides, it should be tested again following a reinforcement manoeuvre. Ask the patient to interlock the fingers and then pull apart hard at the moment before the hammer

---

[nn] Charles Hoover also described an important sign of chronic obstructive pulmonary disease (page 122).

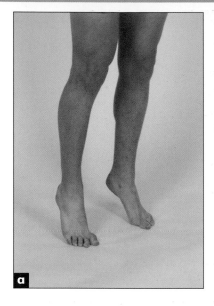
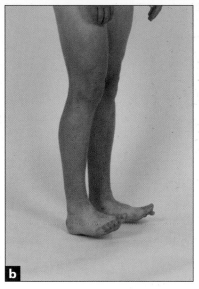
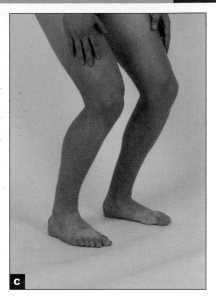

Figure 11.73 Quick test of lower limbs power
(a) 'Stand up on your toes.' (b) 'Now lift up on your heels.' (c) 'Now squat and stand up again.'

strikes the tendon (Jendrassik's manoeuvre[oo]) (Figure 11.75). This manoeuvre has been shown to restore an apparently absent ankle jerk in 70% of elderly people. A reinforcement manoeuvre such as this, or teeth-clenching or grasping an object, should be used if there is difficulty eliciting any of the muscle stretch reflexes.

Ankle jerk (S1, S2). Have the foot in the mid-position at the ankle with the knee bent, the thigh externally rotated on the bed, and the foot held in dorsiflexion by the examiner. The hammer is allowed to fall on the Achilles tendon (Figure 11.76). The normal response is plantar flexion of the foot with contraction of the gastrocnemius muscle. Again, test with reinforcement if appropriate. This reflex can also be tested with the patient kneeling (page 308) or by tapping the sole of the foot.[16]

Plantar reflex (L5, S1, S2). After telling the patient what is going to happen, use a blunt object (such as the key to an expensive car) to stroke up the lateral aspect of the sole, and curve inwards before it reaches the toes, moving towards the middle metatarsophalangeal (MTP) joint (Figure 11.77). The patient's foot should be in the same position as for testing the ankle jerk. The normal response is flexion of the big toe at the MTP joint in patients over one year of age. The extensor

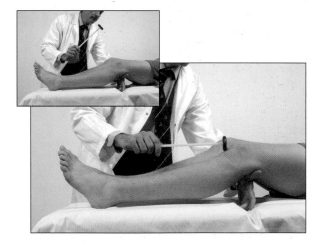

Figure 11.74 The knee jerk examination

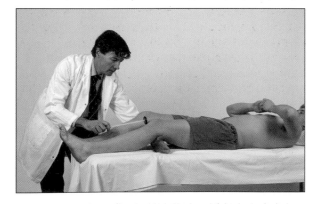

Figure 11.75 The knee jerk with reinforcement: 'Grip your fingers and pull your hands apart'

---

oo Ernst Jendrassik (1858–1921), Budapest physician.

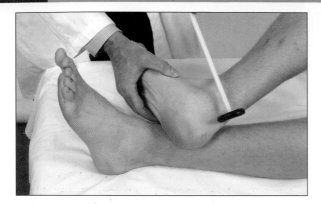

Figure 11.76 The ankle jerk (first method, see also page 308): the examiner dorsiflexes the foot slightly to stretch the tendon

(Babinski[pp])[17] response is abnormal and is characterised by extension of the big toe at the MTP joint (the upgoing toe) and fanning of the other toes. This indicates an upper motor neurone (pyramidal) lesion, although the test's reliability can be relatively poor. Bilateral upgoing toes may also be found after a generalised seizure, or in a patient in coma.

Coordination. Test for cerebellar disease with three manoeuvres.

Heel–shin test. Ask the patient to run the heel of one foot up and down the opposite shin at a moderate pace and as accurately as possible (Figure 11.78). In cerebellar disease the heel wobbles all over the place, with oscillations from side to side and overshooting. Closing the eyes makes little difference to this in cerebellar disease, but if there is posterior column loss the movements are made worse when the eyes are shut—that is, there is 'sensory ataxia'.

Toe–finger test. Unfortunately, a toe–nose test is not a practical way of assessing the lower limbs, so a toe–finger test is used. Ask the patient to lift the foot (with the knee bent) and touch the examiner's finger with the big toe. Look for intention tremor.

Foot-tapping test. Rapidly alternating movements are tested by getting the patient to tap the sole of the foot quickly on the examiner's hand or tap the heel on the opposite shin. Look for loss of rhythmicity.

The sensory system

As for the upper limb, test for pain sensation first

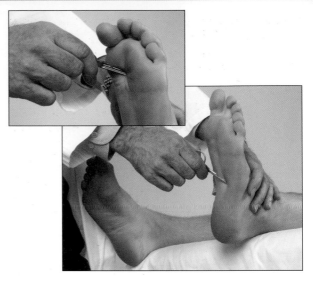

Figure 11.77 The plantar reflex examination

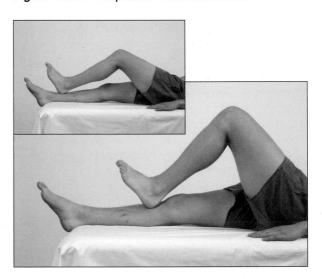

Figure 11.78 The heel–shin test: 'Run your heel down your shin smoothly and quickly'

in each dermatome, comparing the right with the left side (Figure 11.79). Map out any abnormality and decide on the pattern of loss.

Then test vibration sense over the ankles and, if necessary, on the knees and the anterior superior iliac spines (Figure 11.80). Next test proprioception, using the big toes (Figure 11.81) and, if necessary, the knees and hips.

Finally, test light touch (Figure 11.82).

Dermatomes. Memorise the following rough guide (Figure 11.83): L2 supplies the upper anterior thigh; L3 supplies the area around the front of the knee; L4 supplies the medial aspect of the leg; L5 supplies

---

pp   Josef Babinski (1857–1932), Parisian neurologist of Polish extraction, described this sign in 1896. (It was probably first described by Remak in 1893.) Babinski was a famous gourmet and assistant to Charcot.

the lateral aspect of the leg and the medial side of the dorsum of the foot; S1 supplies the heel and most of the sole; S2 supplies the posterior aspect of the thigh; S3, S4 and S5 supply concentric rings around the anus.

Sensory levels. If there is peripheral sensory loss in the leg, attempt to map out the upper level

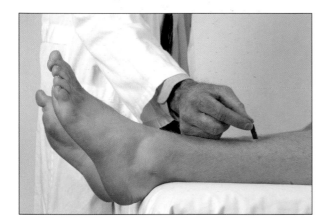

Figure 11.79 Testing pinprick (pain) sensation in the lower limbs (do not draw blood with the pin)

with a pin, moving up at 5 cm intervals initially, from the leg to the abdomen, until the patient reports it is sharp. This may involve testing over the abdominal or even the chest dermatomes. Establishing a sensory level on the trunk indicates the spinal cord level that is affected. Remember, a level of hyperaesthesia (increased sensitivity) often occurs above the sensory level and it is the upper level of this that should be determined, as it usually indicates the highest affected spinal segment. Also remember that the level of a vertebral body only corresponds to the spinal cord level in the upper cervical cord because the spinal cord is shorter than the spinal canal. The C8 spinal segment lies opposite the C7 vertebra. In the upper thoracic cord there is a difference of about two segments and in the mid-thoracic cord three segments. All the lumbosacral segments are opposite the T11 to L1 vertebrae.

The superficial or cutaneous reflexes

These reflexes occur in response to light touch or scratching of the skin or mucous membranes. The stimulus is more superficial than the tendon (muscle stretch) reflexes. As a rule these reflexes

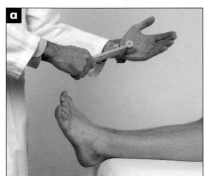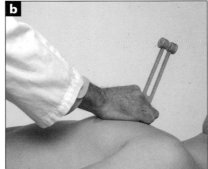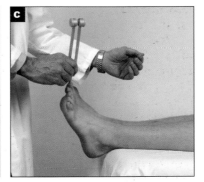
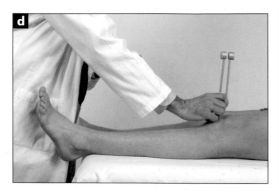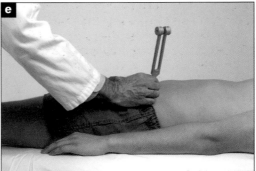

Figure 11.80 Testing vibration sense in the lower limbs
(a) Strike a 128 Hz tuning fork confidently on your thenar eminence. (b) Demonstrate the vibration of the tuning fork on the patient's sternum: 'Can you feel this vibration?' (c) Place the tuning fork on the great toe: 'Can you feel the vibration there? Tell me when it stops.' (d) If vibration sense is absent on the great toe, try testing on the patella. (e) If vibration sense is absent at the knee, try testing on the anterior superior iliac spine.

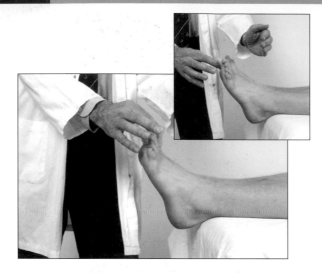

Figure 11.81 Position sense: 'Shut your eyes and tell me whether I have moved your toe up or down'

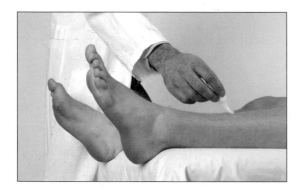

Figure 11.82 Testing light-touch sensation (do not stroke the skin with the cottonwool)

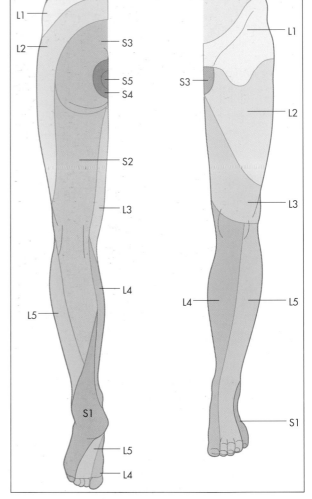

Figure 11.83 Dermatomes of the lower limbs

occur more slowly after the stimulus, are less constantly present and fatigue more easily.

Examples include the palmar or grasp reflex, the cremasteric reflex and the abdominal reflexes and the plantar responses.

The abdominal reflexes (epigastric T6–T9, mid-abdominal T9–T11, lower abdominal T11–L1). Test these by lightly stroking the abdominal wall diagonally towards the umbilicus in each of the four quadrants of the abdomen (Figure 11.84). Reflex contractions of the abdominal wall are *absent* in upper motor neurone lesions above the segmental level and also in patients who have had surgical operations interrupting the nerves. They disappear in coma and deep sleep, and during anaesthesia. They are usually difficult to elicit in obese patients

and can also be absent in some normal people (20%). Their absence in the presence of increased tendon reflexes is suggestive of corticospinal tract abnormality.

The cremasteric reflexes (L1–L2). Stroke the inner part of the thigh in a downward direction; normally contraction of the cremasteric muscle pulls up the scrotum and testis on the side stroked. It may be absent in elderly men and in those with a hydrocele or varicocele, or after an episode of orchitis.

Saddle sensation and anal reflex. Test now for saddle sensation if a cauda equina lesion is suspected (e.g. because of urinary or faecal incontinence). The only sensory loss may be on the buttocks or around the anus (S3–S5). In this case also test the anal reflex (S2, S3, S4): normal contraction

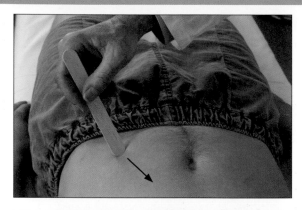

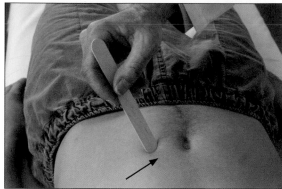

Figure 11.84 Abdominal reflex: stroke towards the umbilicus from each quadrant and watch for abdominal muscle contraction

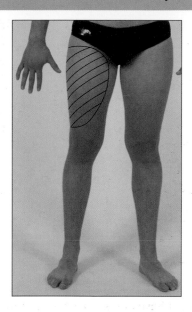

Figure 11.85 Distribution of the lateral cutaneous nerve of the thigh

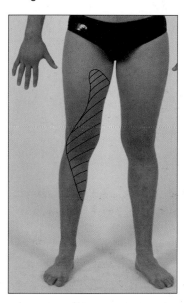

Figure 11.86 Sensory distribution of the femoral nerve

of the external sphincter in response to pinprick of the perianal skin is abolished in patients with a lesion of the sacral segments of the cauda equina. If, however, the lowest sacral segments are spared but the higher ones are involved, this suggests that there is an intrinsic cord lesion.

Spine. Examine the spine and perform the straight-leg raising test.

Examination of the peripheral nerves of the lower limb

Lateral cutaneous nerve of the thigh. Test for sensory loss (Figure 11.85). A lesion of this nerve usually occurs because of entrapment between the inguinal ligament and the anterior superior iliac spine. It causes a sensory loss over the lateral aspect of the thigh with no motor loss detectable. If painful, it is called *meralgia paraesthetica*.

Femoral nerve (L2, L3, L4). Test for weakness of knee extension (quadriceps paralysis). Hip flexion weakness is only slight, and adductor strength is preserved. The knee jerk is absent. The sensory loss involves the inner aspect of the thigh and leg (Figure 11.86).

Sciatic nerve (L4, L5, S1, S2). This nerve supplies all the muscles below the knee and the hamstrings. Test for loss of power below the knee resulting in a footdrop (plantar flexed foot) and for weakness of knee flexion. Test the reflexes: with a sciatic nerve lesion the knee jerk is intact but the ankle jerk and plantar response are absent. Test sensation on the posterior thigh, lateral and posterior calf, and on the foot (lost with a proximal nerve lesion)(Figure 11.87).

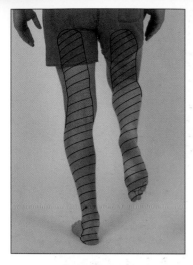

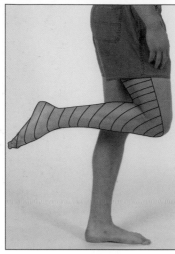

Figure 11.87 Sensory distribution of the sciatic nerve

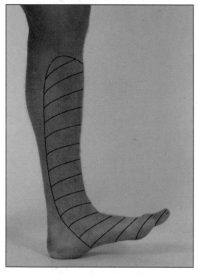

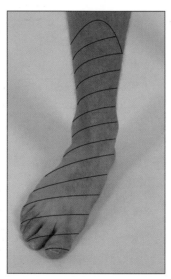

Figure 11.88 Sensory distribution of the common peroneal nerve (compression at the fibular neck)

Common peroneal nerve (L4, L5, S1). This is a major terminal branch of the sciatic nerve. It supplies the anterior and lateral compartment muscles of the leg (Figure 11.88). On inspection one may notice a footdrop (Table 11.19). Test for weakness of dorsiflexion and eversion. Test the reflexes, which will all be intact. Test for sensory loss. There may be only minimal sensory loss over the lateral aspect of the dorsum of the foot. Note that these findings can be confused with an L5 root lesion, but the latter includes weakness of knee flexion and loss of foot inversion as well as sensory loss in the L5 distribution.

Gait
Method
Make sure the patient's legs are clearly visible. Now ask the patient to walk normally for a few metres and then turn around quickly and walk back. Then ask the patient to walk heel-to-toe to exclude a midline cerebellar lesion (Figure 11.89). Ask the patient to then walk on the toes (an S1 lesion will

TABLE 11.19 Causes (differential diagnosis) of footdrop

Common peroneal nerve palsy
Sciatic nerve palsy
Lumbosacral plexus lesion
L4, L5 root lesion
Peripheral motor neuropathy
Distal myopathy
Motor neurone disease
Stroke—anterior cerebral artery or lacunar syndrome ('ataxic hemiparesis')

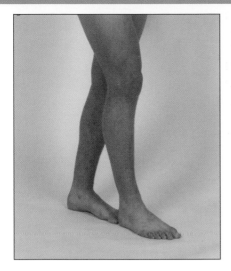

Figure 11.89 Cerebellar testing—heel–toe walking

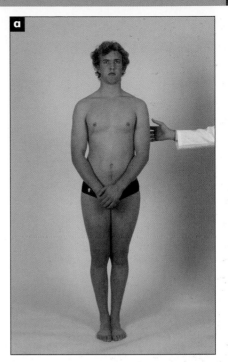

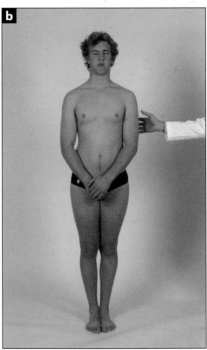

make this difficult or impossible) and then on the heels (an L4 or L5 lesion causing footdrop will make this difficult or impossible).

Test for proximal myopathy by asking the patient to squat and then stand up, or sit in a low chair and then stand.

To test *station* (Romberg[qq] test), ask the patient to stand erect with the feet together and the eyes open (Figure 11.90a). Once the patient is stable ask him or her to close the eyes (Figure 11.90b). Compare the steadiness shown with the eyes open, then closed for up to 1 minute. Even in the absence of neurological disease a person may be slightly unsteady with the eyes closed, but the sign is positive if marked unsteadiness occurs to the point where the patient looks likely to fall. Normal people can maintain this position easily for 60 seconds. The Romberg test is positive when unsteadiness increases with eye closure. This is usually seen with the loss of proprioceptive sensation.

Marked unsteadiness with the eyes open is seen with cerebellar or vestibular dysfunction.

Gait disorders are summarised in Table 11.20.

Speech and higher centres

At this stage of the examination dysarthria (difficulty with articulation), dysphonia (altered quality of the voice with reduction in volume as a result of vocal cord disease) or dysphasia (dominant higher centre disorder in the use of symbols for

Figure 11.90 Romberg test
(a) 'Stand with your feet together.'
(b) 'Now shut your eyes. I won't let you fall.'

communication—language) may be obvious. If not, before going on to compartmentalised tests, the clinician should get the patient to talk freely— *propositional* or *free* speech. In a normal clinical encounter this comes from history taking. In viva

---

qq Moritz Heinrich von Romberg (1795–1873), Berlin professor, wrote the first modern neurology textbook. His original description of the sign was of patients with tabes dorsalis (dorsal column disease caused by syphilis).

TABLE 11.20 Gait disorders

Hemiplegia: the foot is plantar flexed and the leg is swung in a lateral arc

Spastic paraparesis: scissors gait

Parkinson's disease:
- hesitation in starting
- shuffling
- freezing
- festination
- propulsion
- retropulsion

Cerebellar: a drunken gait which is wide-based or reeling on a narrow base; the patient staggers towards the affected side if there is a unilateral cerebellar hemisphere lesion

Posterior column lesion: clumsy slapping down of the feet on a broad base

Footdrop: high-stepping gait

Proximal myopathy: waddling gait

Prefrontal lobe (apraxic): feet appear glued to floor when erect, but move more easily when the patient is supine

Hysterical: characterised by a bizarre, inconsistent gait

voce or observed standardised clinical examinations (OSCEs), ask the patient to describe the room, his or her clothes, or job or daily activities, in order to promote flowing speech. Then test *comprehension*. This is done first without eliciting language—for example, 'Touch your chin, then your nose and then your ear'; and then with yes and no questions—for example, 'Do you put your shoes on before your socks?' Then test *repetition*—for example, 'Repeat the phrase "no ifs, ands or buts"'.

To complete the screening, ask the patient to *name two objects* pointed at, and to *say a phrase* such as 'British Constitution' or 'West Register St' (page 396).

There is no need to examine further if no abnormality of speech is detected in this way.

If there is an abnormality, proceed as outlined in Table 11.21.

Dysphasia

There are four main types of dysphasia:[18] receptive, expressive, nominal and conductive. The expressive aphasias are forms of motor *apraxia*. This means the inability to perform deliberate actions in the absence of paralysis.

1 **Receptive (posterior) dysphasia.** This is where the patient cannot understand the spoken (*auditory dysphasia*) or written word (*alexia*).

This condition is suggested when the patient is unable to understand any commands or questions or to recognise written words in the absence of deafness or blindness. Speech is fluent but disorganised. It occurs with a lesion (infarction, haemorrhage or space-occupying tumour) in the dominant hemisphere in the posterior part of the first temporal gyrus (Wernicke's area[rr]).

2 **Expressive (anterior) dysphasia.** This is present when the patient understands, but cannot answer appropriately. Speech is non-fluent. This occurs with a lesion in the posterior part of the dominant third frontal gyrus (Broca's area[ss]). Certain types of speech may be retained by these patients. These include *automatic speech*. The patient may be able to recite word series such as the days of the week or letters of the alphabet. Sometimes *emotional speech* may be preserved so that when frustrated or upset the patient may be able to swear fluently. In the same way the patient may be able to sing familiar songs while unable to speak the words. It is important to remember that unless the lesion responsible for these defects is very large there may be no reduction in the patient's higher intellectual functions, memory or judgment. Some of these patients may incorrectly be considered psychotic, because of their disorganised speech.

3 **Nominal dysphasia.** All types of dysphasia cause difficulty naming objects. There is also a specific type of nominal dysphasia. Here objects cannot be named (e.g. the nib of a pen) but other aspects of speech are normal. The patient may use long sentences to overcome failure to find the correct word (circumlocution). It occurs with a lesion of the dominant posterior temporoparietal area. Other causes include encephalopathy or the intracranial pressure effects of a distinct space-occupying lesion; it may also occur in the recovery phase from any dysphasia. Its localising value is therefore doubtful.

4 **Conductive dysphasia.** Here patients repeat statements and name objects poorly, but can follow commands. This is thought to be caused by a lesion of the arcuate fasciculus and/or other fibres linking Wernicke's and Broca's areas.

To examine for dysphasia in more detail refer to Table 11.21. If the speech is fluent, but conveys

rr   Karl Wernicke (1848–1904), professor of neurology at Breslau, described receptive aphasia in 1874. He was killed while riding his bicycle.
ss   Pierre Broca (1824–1880), professor of surgery at Paris, described this area in 1861. He described muscular dystrophy before Duchenne.

TABLE 11.21 Examination of a patient with dysphasia

Fluent speech (receptive, conductive or nominal aphasia, usually)

1 Name objects. Patients with nominal, conductive or receptive aphasia will name objects poorly.
2 Repetition. Conductive and receptive aphasic patients cannot repeat 'no ifs, ands or buts'.
3 Comprehension. Only receptive aphasic patients cannot follow commands (verbal or written): 'Touch your nose, then your chin and then your ear'.
4 Reading. Conductive and receptive aphasic patients may have difficulty (dyslexia).
5 Writing. Conductive aphasic patients have impaired writing (dysgraphia) while receptive aphasic patients have abnormal content of writing. Patients with dominant frontal lobe lesions may also have dysgraphia.

Non-fluent speech (expressive aphasia, usually)

1 Naming of objects. This is poor but may be better than spontaneous speech.
2 Repetition. May be possible with great effort. Phrase repetition (e.g. 'No ifs, ands or buts') is poor.
3 Comprehension. Often mildly impaired despite popular belief, but written and verbal commands are followed.
4 Reading. Patients may have dyslexia.
5 Writing. Dysgraphia may be present.
6 Look for hemiparesis. The arm is more affected than the leg.
7 As patients are usually aware of their deficit they are often frustrated and depressed.

information with paraphasic errors, such as 'treen' for 'train' (i.e. a word of similar sound or spelling to the one intended is used),[tt] the main possibilities are nominal, receptive and conductive dysphasia. Test for these by asking the patient to name an object, repeat a statement after you, and then follow commands. Then, if the above are abnormal, ask the patient to read and write, but remember that the occasional patient may be illiterate.

If the speech is slow, hesitant and non-fluent, expressive dysphasia is more likely and exactly the same procedure is followed. It is important to note that many dysphasias will have mixed elements. Large lesions in the dominant hemisphere may cause global dysphasia.

Dysarthria

Here there is no disorder of the content of speech but a difficulty with articulation. It can occur because of abnormalities at a number of levels. Upper motor neurone lesions of the cranial nerves, extrapyramidal conditions (e.g. Parkinson's disease) and cerebellar lesions cause disturbances to the rhythm of speech.

Ask the patient to say a phrase such as 'British Constitution' or 'Peter Piper picked a peck of pickled peppers'.

Pseudobulbar palsy is an upper motor neurone weakness that causes a spastic dysarthria (it sounds as if the patient is trying to squeeze out words from tight lips), paralysis of the facial muscles and difficulty chewing and swallowing. The cause is infarction in both internal capsules. This causes interruption of the descending pyramidal tracts to the brainstem motor nuclei. The jaw jerk is usually increased. These patients tend to be very emotional and laugh and cry inappropriately. Their facial expressions become very animated at these times in contrast to their inability to control their facial expressions voluntarily.[uu] This phenomenon occurs because the nuclei that control motor responses to emotion do not reside in the motor cortex.

Patients who have bilateral lesions of the ninth and tenth cranial nerves are at risk of aspirating fluids or solids into their lungs if they try to eat or drink. Certain bedside tests can be performed to see if it is safe for them to eat or drink. These traditionally include the level of consciousness, gag reflex, pharyngeal sensation and testing swallowing water. *Good signs guide 11.1* shows the likelihood ratios for these and other tests. The water swallowing test involves asking patient to sip repeatedly 5–10 mL of water. Coughing, choking or a fall in blood arterial oxygen saturation makes the test positive.

Bulbar palsies cause a nasal speech, while *facial muscle* weakness causes slurred speech. *Extrapyramidal disease* can be responsible for monotonous speech, as it causes bradykinesia and muscular rigidity. Other causes of dysarthria include alcohol intoxication and *cerebellar disease*. These result in loss of coordination and slow, slurred and often explosive speech, or speech broken up into syllables, called scanning speech.

Mouth ulceration or disease may occasionally mimic dysarthria. Each of these causes must be considered and examined for as appropriate.

Dysphonia

This is alteration of the sound of the voice, such

[tt]   Sometimes a word of similar meaning is used (e.g. 'go' for 'start'): this is called *semantic paraphrasia*.

[uu]   This syndrome should probably be called *'pseudo-pontine-bulbar palsy'* since the motor nuclei of the fifth and seventh nerves are in the pons, not the medulla (bulbs).

GOOD SIGNS GUIDE 11.1 Risk of aspiration after stroke

	Likelihood ratio if:	
	Present	Absent
Voice and cough		
Abnormal voluntary cough	1.9	0.6
Dysphonia	1.3	0.4
Examination		
Drowsiness	3.4	0.5
Abnormal sensation—face and tongue	NS	NS
Absent pharyngeal sensation	2.4	0.03
Abnormal gag reflex	1.5	0.6
Tests		
Water swallow test	3.2	0.4
Oxygen desaturation 2 min after swallowing	3.1	0.3

Adapted with permission from McGee S, *Evidence-based physical diagnosis*, 2nd edn. St Louis: Saunders, 2007.

TABLE 11.22 Symptoms and signs in higher centre dysfunction

Parietal lobe
Dysphasia (dominant)
Acalculia,* agraphia,* left–right disorientation,* finger agnosia*
Sensory and visual inattention,[†] construction and dressing apraxia,[†] spatial neglect and inattention,[†] lower quadrantic hemianopia,[‡] astereognosis[‡]
Seizures

Temporal lobe
Memory loss
Upper quadrantic hemianopia
Dysphasia (receptive if dominant lobe)
Seizures

Frontal lobe
Personality change
Primitive reflexes, e.g. grasp, pout
Anosmia
Optic nerve compression (optic atrophy)
Gait apraxia
Leg weakness (parasagittal)
Loss of micturition control
Dysphasia (expressive), dysgraphia
Seizures

Occipital lobe
Homonymous hemianopia
Alexia (inability to read; word blindness)
Seizures (flashing light aura)

* Gerstmann's syndrome: dominant hemisphere parietal lobe only.
[†] Non-dominant parietal lobe signs.
[‡] Non-localising parietal lobe signs.

as huskiness of the voice with decreased volume. It may be due to laryngeal disease (e.g. following a viral infection or a tumour of the vocal cord), or to recurrent laryngeal nerve palsy.

The cerebral hemispheres

Parietal, temporal and frontal lobe functions are tested if the patient is disoriented or has dysphasia, or if dementia is suspected. If the patient has a receptive aphasia, however, these tests cannot be performed. Their examination is otherwise not routine (Table 11.22). Students should already be familiar with the method of examining the cranial nerves and limbs.

Parietal lobe function

The parietal lobe is concerned with the reception and analysis of sensory information.

Dominant lobe signs. A lesion of the dominant parietal lobe in the angular gyrus causes a distinct clinical syndrome called Gerstmann's syndrome. Test for this in the following manner.

1 Ask the patient to perform simple arithmetical calculations, e.g. serial 7s (take 7 from 100, then 7 from the answer, and so on). The inability to do this at least with partial accuracy is called *Acalculia*.

2 Ask the patient to write—inability is called *Agraphia*.

3 Test for left–right disorientation by asking the patient to show you his or her right and then left hand. If this is correctly performed, ask the patient to touch his or her left ear with the right hand and vice versa. Inability to do this is called *Left–right disorientation*.

4 Ask the patient to name his or her fingers—inability to do this is called *Finger agnosia*. This inability may extend to identification of the examiner's fingers. The *agnosias* are receptive defects involving the inability to understand the meaning of stimulations of different types.

A mnemonic for these four dominant parietal lobe signs is **AALF**. Remember that Gerstmann's syndrome[vv] can be diagnosed only if the higher centres are intact. A demented patient would not be able to perform many of these tests.

Non-dominant and non-localising parietal lobe signs (*cortical sensation*). Cortical sensations are those that require processing at a higher level than simple sensation. They rely on an intact simple sensation, especially touch and pinprick.

- *Graphesthesia* is the ability to recognise numbers or letters drawn on the skin. Use a pointed object or pencil to draw numbers on the skin (Figure 11.91).
- *Tactile extinction* is the ability to feel a stimulus when it is applied to each side separately, but not on one side when both sides are stimulated. The patient (with eyes shut) is touched first on one hand and then on the other, and then on both together. Ask on which side the touch is felt. The normal response is 'both' when stimulation is applied to each side. It is important that the hands be touched simultaneously.

Now test for general signs of parietal lobe dysfunction.

- Look for *sensory* and *visual inattention*. When one arm or leg is tested at a time, sensation is normal, but when both sides are tested

vv Josef Gerstmann (1887–1969), Austrian-born neuropsychiatrist who worked in the United States.

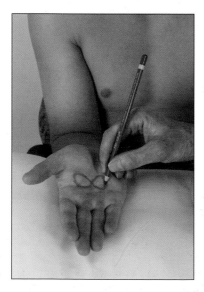

Figure 11.91 Agraphesthesia: 'What number have I drawn?' Patient's reply: 'One'
Avoid the use of an indelible pencil.

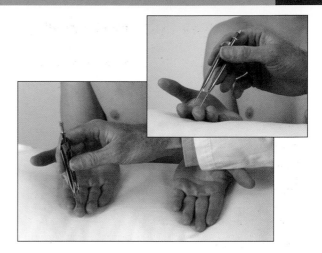

Figure 11.92 Two-point discrimination: 'Can you feel one point or two?'

simultaneously the sensation is appreciated only on the normal side. A right-sided parietal lesion will lead to inattention on the left side and vice versa.

- Formal *visual field testing* is also important, as parietal, temporal and occipital lesions can give distinctive defects.
- Examine now for *astereognosis (tactile agnosia)*, which is the inability, with eyes closed, to recognise an object placed in the hand when the ordinary sensory modalities are intact. A parietal lobe lesion results in astereognosis on the opposite side.
- *Agraphesthesia* may also be present; this is the inability to appreciate a number drawn on the hand on the opposite side to a parietal lesion (Figure 11.91).
- *Two-point discrimination* testing involves the ability to distinguish a single point from two points close together (Figure 11.92). The minimal separation that can be distinguished is about 3 cm on the hand or foot and 0.6 cm on the fingertips. A compass can be used for this test. Ask the patient to shut the eyes and then say whether one or two points can be felt. Bring the compass points closer together and test intermittently with just one point.
- Examine for *dressing* and *constructional apraxia*. Dressing apraxia is tested by taking the patient's pyjama top or cardigan, turning it inside out and asking him or her to put it back on. Patients with a non-dominant parietal lobe lesion may find this impossible to do. Constructional apraxia is tested by asking the patient to copy an object that you have drawn (e.g. a tree or a house—Figure 11.93a & b).

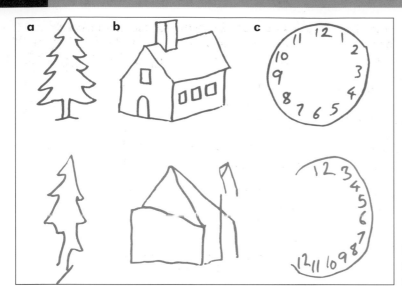

Figure 11.93 Lower figures show constructional apraxia (a & b) and spatial neglect (c)

- Next test *spatial neglect* by asking the patient to fill in the numbers on an empty clock face (Figure 11.93c). Patients with a right parietal lesion may fill in numbers only on the left side (the other side of the clock face is ignored). Spatial neglect also occurs with dominant parietal lobe lesions but is less common.

Temporal lobe function

This lobe is concerned with short-term and long-term memory. Test short-term memory by the name, address, flower test—ask the patient to remember a name, address and the names of three flowers, and repeat them immediately. Then ask the patient five minutes later to repeat the names again. Test long-term memory by asking, for example, what year World War II ended. Memory may be impaired in dementia from any cause.

An alert patient with a severe memory disturbance may make up stories to fill any gaps in his or her memory. This is called *confabulation*, and is typical of the syndrome of Korsakoff's psychosis[ww] (amnesic dementia). Confabulation can be tested by asking the patient whether he or she has met you before. However, be prepared for the very long, detailed and completely false story that may follow.

Korsakoff's psychosis occurs most commonly in alcoholics (where there is loss of nerve cells in the thalamic nuclei and mammillary bodies), and rarely with head injury, tumour, anoxic encephalopathy or encephalitis. It is characterised by retrograde amnesia (memory loss for events before the onset of the illness) and an inability to memorise new information, in a patient who is alert, responsive and capable of problem-solving.

Frontal lobe function

Frontal lobe damage as a result of tumours or surgery (or both), or diffuse disease such as dementia or HIV infection, may cause changes in emotion, memory, judgment, carelessness about personal habits, and disinhibition. There may be persistent or alternating irritability and euphoria.[xx] These features may be clear when the history is taken but may need to be reinforced by interviewing relatives or friends. Changes of this sort in a previously reserved personality may be obvious and very distressing to relatives.

Assess first the *primitive reflexes*. There is controversy concerning their significance; they are not normally present in adults but may reappear in normal old age.[19] The presence of an isolated primitive reflex may not be abnormal, but multiple primitive reflexes are usually associated with diffuse cerebral disease involving the frontal lobes and frontal association areas more than other parts of the brain. Dementia, encephalopathy and neoplasms are all possible causes.

1 Grasp reflex: the examiner runs his or her fingers across the palm of the patient's hand, which will grasp the examining fingers involuntarily on the side contralateral to the lesion.
2 Palmomental reflex: ipsilateral contraction of

---

ww Sergei Sergeyevich Korsakoff (1853–1900), Russian psychiatrist and great humanitarian, described the syndrome in 1887.

xx Euphoria may cause a lack of seriousness, and the repetition of bad jokes and puns (*witzelsucht*).

the ipsilateral mentalis muscle occurs when the examiner strokes the thenar eminence firmly with a key or thumb nail. Contraction of the mentalis causes protrusion and lifting of the lower lip. This is best considered as the beginning of a wince in response to pain. The response can also be elicited by painful stimulus to other parts of the body. The response is bilateral in about 50% of cases. A unilateral lesion does not necessarily correspond to the side of the lesion in the brain.

3 Pout and snout reflexes: stroking or tapping with the tendon hammer over or above the upper lip induces pouting movements of the lips. This can occur with many intracranial lesions. The sucking reflex is an extension of this. The stimulation may produce sucking, chewing and swallowing movements. It is not a localising sign.

Next ask the patient to *interpret a proverb*, such as 'A rolling stone gathers no moss'. Patients with frontal lobe disease give concrete explanations of proverbs. Test for loss of smell (*anosmia*) and for *gait apraxia*, where there is marked unsteadiness in walking, which can be bizarre—the feet typically behave as if glued to the floor, causing a strange shuffling gait. Look in the *fundi*; you may rarely see optic atrophy on the side of a frontal lobe space-occupying lesion caused by compression of the optic nerve, and papilloedema on the opposite side due to secondarily raised intracranial pressure (Foster Kennedy[yy] syndrome).

Correlation of physical signs and neurological disease
Upper motor neurone lesions
In neurology a clinical diagnosis is made by defining the deficit that is present, deciding on its anatomical level and then considering the likely causes. It is important to be able to distinguish *upper motor neurone* signs (*Good signs guide 11.2*) from *lower motor neurone* signs (Figure 11.38, page 355; see also Table 11.26, page 386). The former occur when a lesion has interrupted a neural pathway at a level above the anterior horn cell: for example, motor pathways in the cerebral cortex, internal capsule, cerebral peduncles, brainstem or spinal cord. When this occurs there is greater weakness of abductors and extensors in the upper limb, and flexors and abductors in the lower limb, as the normal function of this pathway is to mediate voluntary contraction

yy Robert Foster Kennedy (1884–1952), a New York neurologist.

GOOD SIGNS GUIDE 11.2 Unilateral hemisphere lesion

Sign	Positive LR	Negative LR
Upper limb drift	33.0	0.2
Facial weakness	32.3	0.2
Hemiparesis	31.7	0.3
Wrist extensor weakness	29.0	0.3
Babinski response	19.0	0.6
Hemianopia	NS	0.7
Hemisensory disturbance	NS	0.7

NS = not significant.
From McGee S, *Evidence-based physical diagnosis.* 2nd edn. St Louis: Saunders, 2007.

TABLE 11.23 Level of upper motor neurone lesion

1	Leg affected: L1 or above
2	Arm affected: C3 or above
3	Face affected: pons or above
4	Diplopia: midbrain or above

of the antigravity muscles. All muscles, however, are usually weaker than normal. Muscle wasting is slight or absent, probably because there is no loss of trophic factors normally released from the lower motor neurone. The disuse that results from severe weakness may, however, cause some atrophy.

Upper motor neurone signs occur when the lesion is in the brain or spinal cord above the level of the lower motor neurone (Table 11.23).

Spasticity occurs because of destruction of the corticoreticulospinal tract, resulting in stretch reflex hyperactivity.

Monoplegia is paralysis affecting only one limb, when there is a motor cortex or partial internal capsule lesion. *Hemiplegia* affects one side of the body due to a lesion affecting projection of pathways from the contralateral motor cortex.

Paraplegia affects both legs, while *quadriplegia* affects all four limbs, and is the result of spinal cord trauma or, less often, a brainstem lesion (e.g. basilar artery thrombosis).

Causes of hemiplegia (upper motor neurone lesion)
Vascular disease (stroke or TIA). Thrombosis, embolism or haemorrhage occur in specific vascular territories (Figure 11.94).[20] Thrombus induces

TABLE 11.24 Intracerebral thrombosis or embolism: clinical features

Middle cerebral artery	Posterior cerebral artery	Anterior cerebral artery	Vertebral/basilar (brainstem)
Main branch Infarction middle third of hemisphere: UMN face, arm>leg; homonymous hemianopia; aphasia or non-dominant hemisphere signs (depends on side); cortical sensory loss	**Main branch*** Infarction of thalamus and occipital cortex: hemianaesthesia (loss of all modalities); homonymous hemianopia (complete); colour blindness	UMN leg>arm; cortical sensory loss leg only; (if corpus callosum affected) urinary incontinence	'Crossed' motor/sensory (e.g. left face, right arm); bilateral extremity motor/sensory; Horner's syndrome (Chapter 13); cerebellar signs; lower cranial nerve signs
Perforating artery Internal capsule infarction: UMN face, UMN arm>leg			

UMN = upper motor neurone lesion.
* Effects variable because of anastomoses with distal middle cerebral artery branches and supply from posterior communicating artery, but one would examine particularly for occipital and temporal lobe dysfunction.

symptoms and signs in a slow stepwise progression. Embolic strokes are worse at the onset. Symptoms lasting less than 24 hours are called transient ischaemic attacks (TIAs). Lesions in the territory of the *internal carotid artery* result in hemiplegia on the opposite side of the body if a large area of the internal capsule or hemisphere is involved. Homonymous hemianopia, hemianaesthesia and dysphasia may occur (Table 11.24). Stenosis of the internal carotid artery in the neck may be associated with a bruit.[21]

Haemorrhagic strokes often involve the internal capsule and putamen (causing a contralateral hemiparesis and often sensory loss), or the thalamus (causing a contralateral hemianaesthesia).

Lesions in the territory of the *vertebrobasilar artery* may produce cranial nerve palsies, cerebellar signs, Horner's syndrome (Chapter 13) and sensory loss, as well as upper motor neurone signs (often bilateral because of the close proximity of structures in the brainstem). For example, a lesion in the midbrain may be associated with a third nerve paralysis and upper motor neurone signs on the opposite side. Hemianaesthesia and homonymous hemianopia may occur if the posterior cerebral arteries are affected. An important syndrome to recognise is the *lateral medullary syndrome* (Table 11.25). Atheroma in the ascending aorta is increasingly recognised as a source of cerebral emboli.

Compressive and infiltrative lesions. Tumours tend to occur in the lobes of the brain, and focal signs will depend on the tumour site. Signs localised

TABLE 11.25 Lateral medullary syndrome ('Wallenberg's* syndrome')

Occlusion of the vertebral, or posterior inferior cerebellar or lateral medullary arteries causes ipsilateral and 'crossed' neurological signs

- Cerebellar signs (ipsilateral)
- Horner's syndrome (ipsilateral)
- Lower cranial nerves (IX, X)—palate and vocal cord weakness (ipsilateral)
- Facial sensory loss of pain (ipsilateral)
- Arm and leg sensory loss of pain (contralateral)
- No upper motor neuron weakness

* Adolf Wallenberg (1862–1942), professor of medicine, Danzig.

to the parietal, temporal, occipital or frontal lobe suggest this disease process (see Table 11.22).

There may, however, be false localising signs in the presence of raised intracranial pressure: for example, a unilateral or bilateral sixth nerve palsy (because of the nerve's long intracranial path). Papilloedema is usually associated if there is raised intracranial pressure.

Demyelinating disease. Multiple sclerosis results in lesions in different areas usually with a relapsing and remitting course.

Infection. Human immunodeficiency virus (HIV) infection.

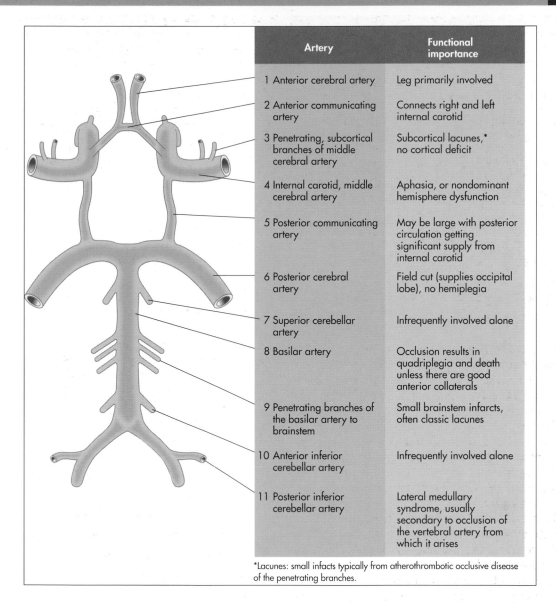

Artery	Functional importance
1 Anterior cerebral artery	Leg primarily involved
2 Anterior communicating artery	Connects right and left internal carotid
3 Penetrating, subcortical branches of middle cerebral artery	Subcortical lacunes,* no cortical deficit
4 Internal carotid, middle cerebral artery	Aphasia, or nondominant hemisphere dysfunction
5 Posterior communicating artery	May be large with posterior circulation getting significant supply from internal carotid
6 Posterior cerebral artery	Field cut (supplies occipital lobe), no hemiplegia
7 Superior cerebellar artery	Infrequently involved alone
8 Basilar artery	Occlusion results in quadriplegia and death unless there are good anterior collaterals
9 Penetrating branches of the basilar artery to brainstem	Small brainstem infarcts, often classic lacunes
10 Anterior inferior cerebellar artery	Infrequently involved alone
11 Posterior inferior cerebellar artery	Lateral medullary syndrome, usually secondary to occlusion of the vertebral artery from which it arises

*Lacunes: small infacts typically from atherothrombotic occlusive disease of the penetrating branches.

Figure 11.94 Anatomy of the circle of Willis, showing the functional importance of the arterial blood supply
(Adapted from Weiner HL, Levitt LP, *Neurology for the house officer*, 6th edn. Baltimore: Williams & Wilkins, 2000.)

Lower motor neurone lesions

Lower motor neurone lesions interrupt the spinal reflex arc and therefore cause muscle wasting, reduced or absent reflexes and sometimes fasciculations. This results from a lesion of the spinal motor neurones, motor root or peripheral nerve (Table 11.26).

Motor neurone disease

This disease of unknown aetiology results in pathological changes in the anterior horn cells, the motor nuclei of the medulla and the descending tracts. It therefore causes a combination of upper motor neurone and lower motor neurone signs, although one type may predominate.

Importantly, fasciculations are almost always present. The muscle stretch reflexes are usually present (often increased) until late in the course of the disease, and there are rarely any objective sensory changes (15%–20% of patients report sensory symptoms).

Peripheral neuropathy

Distal parts of the nerves are usually involved first because of their distance from the cell bodies, causing a distal loss of sensation or motor function,

TABLE 11.26 Upper and lower motor neurone lesions (see also Figure 11.38, page 355)

Signs of upper motor neurone (pyramidal) lesions

1 Weakness is present in all muscle groups, but in the lower limb may be more marked in the flexor and abductor muscles. In the upper limb, weakness may be most marked in the abductors and extensors. There is very little muscle wasting.
2 Spasticity: increased tone is present (may be clasp-knife) and often associated with clonus.
3 The reflexes are increased except for the superficial reflexes (e.g. abdominal), which are absent.
4 There is an extensor (Babinski) plantar response (upgoing toe).

Signs of lower motor neurone lesions

1 Weakness may be more obvious distally than proximally, and the flexor and extensor muscles are equally involved. Wasting is a prominent feature.
2 Tone is reduced.
3 The reflexes are reduced and the plantar response is normal or absent.
4 Fasciculation may be present.

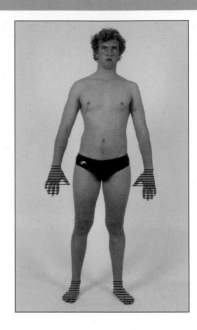

Figure 11.95 Peripheral neuropathy: glove and stocking sensory loss

or both, in the limbs. A typical sensory change is a symmetrical glove and stocking loss to all modalities (see Figure 11.95). This is unlike the pattern found with individual nerve or nerve root disease, which should be suspected if sensory loss is asymmetrical or confined to one limb. Peripheral muscle weakness may be present due to motor nerve involvement. Occasionally motor neuropathy may occur without sensory change. In the latter case, reflexes are reduced but may not be absent in the distal parts of the limbs (Table 11.27).

Guillain-Barré syndrome (acute inflammatory polyradiculoneuropathy)

This disease, thought to have an immune basis, may begin 7 to 10 days after an infective illness. It results in flaccid proximal and distal muscle paralysis, which typically ascends from the lower to the upper limbs. Wasting is rare. The reflexes are reduced or absent. The cranial nerves can be affected; occasionally disease is confined to these. Sensory loss is minimal or absent. Unlike transverse myelitis, the sphincters are little affected. Weakness of the respiratory muscles can be fatal but the disease is usually self-limiting. HIV infection can cause a similar syndrome.

Multiple sclerosis

This disease with unknown cause is characterised by scattered areas of inflammation in the central nervous system (CNS). A careful history is necessary as the diagnosis depends on the occurrence of at least two neurological episodes separated in time and place within the CNS; see Table 11.28.

The examination

The signs can be very variable. Look particularly for signs of spastic paraparesis and posterior column sensory loss as well as cerebellar signs.

Examine the cranial nerves. Look carefully for loss of visual acuity, optic atrophy, papillitis and scotomata (usually central). *Internuclear ophthalmoplegia* is an important sign and is almost diagnostic in a young adult. Internuclear ophthalmoplegia is weakness of adduction in one eye as a result of damage to the ipsilateral medial longitudinal fasciculus; there may be nystagmus in the abducting eye. Bilateral internuclear ophthalmoplegia is almost always caused by MS.

Other cranial nerves may rarely be affected (III, IV, V, VI, VII, pseudobulbar palsy) by lesions within the brainstem. Charcot's triad for multiple sclerosis consists of nystagmus, intention tremor and scanning speech, but occurs in only 10% of patients.

Look for Lhermitte's[zz] sign (an electric-shock-like sensation in the limbs or trunk following neck flexion). This can also be caused by other disorders of the cervical spine, such as subacute combined

---

zz Jacques Jean Lhermitte (1877-01939), French neurologist and neuropsychiatrist.

TABLE 11.27 Peripheral neuropathy (Figure 11.95)

Causes (differential diagnosis) of peripheral neuropathy

1 Drugs—e.g. isoniazid, vincristine, phenytoin, nitrofurantoin, cisplatinum, heavy metals, amiodarone
2 Alcohol abuse (with or without vitamin B_1 deficiency)
3 Metabolic—e.g. diabetes mellitus, chronic kidney disease (renal failure)
4 Guillain-Barré syndrome
5 Malignancy—e.g. carcinoma of the lung (paraneoplastic neuropathy), leukaemia, lymphoma
6 Vitamin deficiency (e.g. B_{12}) or excess (e.g. B_6)
7 Connective tissue disease or vasculitis—e.g. PAN, SLE
8 Hereditary—e.g. hereditary motor and sensory neuropathy
9 Others, e.g. amyloidosis, HIV infection
10 Idiopathic

Causes of a predominant motor neuropathy

1 Guillain-Barré syndrome, chronic inflammatory polyradiculoneuropathy
2 Hereditary motor and sensory neuropathy
3 Diabetes mellitus
4 Others—e.g. acute intermittent porphyria, lead poisoning, diphtheria, multifocal conduction block neuropathy

Causes of a painful peripheral neuropathy

1 Diabetes mellitus
2 Alcohol
3 Vitamin B_1 or B_{12} deficiency
4 Carcinoma
5 Porphyria
6 Arsenic or thallium poisoning

PAN = polyarteritis nodosa; SLE = systemic lupus erythematosus; HIV = human immunodeficiency virus.

TABLE 11.28 Clinical manifestations suggestive of multiple sclerosis

• Internuclear ophthalmoplegia (affected eye—weak adduction; other eye on abduction horizontal nystagmus)

• Optic neuritis (central visual loss, eye pain, pale optic disc)

• Marcus Gunn pupil

• Upper motor neurone weakness

• Cerebellar signs

• Posterior columns sensory loss

• Faecal/urinary incontinence

degeneration of the cord, cervical spondylosis, cervical cord tumour, foramen magnum tumours, nitrous oxide abuse, and from mantle irradiation.

Thickened peripheral nerves

If there is evidence of a peripheral nerve lesion, peripheral neuropathy or a mononeuritis multiplex (Table 11.29), palpate for thickened nerves. The median nerve at the wrist, the ulnar nerve at the elbow, the greater auricular nerve in the neck and the common peroneal nerve at the head of the fibula are the most easily accessible. If nerves are thickened consider the following diagnoses:

• Acromegaly
• Amyloidosis
• Chronic inflammatory demyelinating polyradiculoneuropathy
• Leprosy
• Hereditary motor and sensory neuropathy (autosomal dominant) (Table 11.35, page 394)
• Other—e.g. sarcoidosis, diabetes mellitus, neurofibromatosis.

Spinal cord compression (Figures 11.96 to 11.100)

It is important to remember that a spinal cord lesion causes lower motor neurone signs at the level of the lesion and upper motor neurone signs below that level (Table 11.30). Don't forget the spinal cord's anatomy and vascular supply (Figure 11.96). Examine any suspected case as follows.

After carefully examining the lower limbs (see above) determine the level of any sensory impairment (Table 11.31). Then examine the back for signs of a local lesion. Look for deformity, scars

TABLE 11.29 Mononeuritis multiplex

Definition: mononeuritis multiplex refers to the separate involvement of more than one peripheral (or less often cranial) nerve by a single disease

Acute causes (usually vascular)
Polyarteritis nodosa
Diabetes mellitus
Connective tissue disease—e.g. rheumatoid arthritis, systemic lupus erythematosus

Chronic causes
Multiple compressive neuropathies
Sarcoidosis
Acromegaly
HIV infection
Leprosy
Lyme disease
Others—e.g. carcinoma (rare)

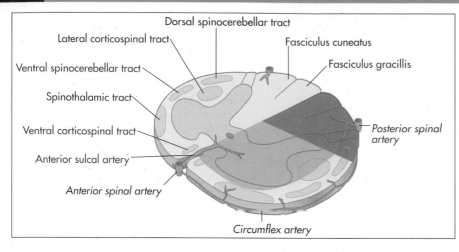

Figure 11.96 Anatomy and vascular supply of the spinal cord
Note: Anterior spinal artery occlusion spares posterior column function.

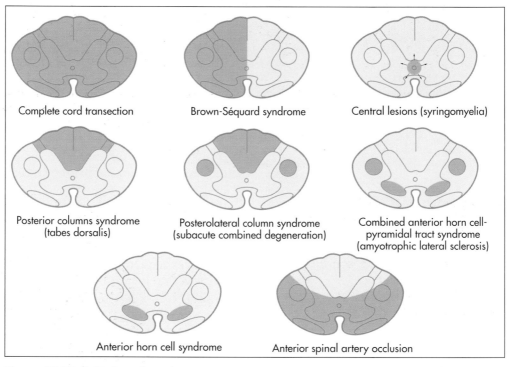

Figure 11.97 Spinal cord syndromes
(Adapted from Brazis PW, *Localisation in clinical neurology*, Philadelphia: Lippincott, Williams & Wilkins, 2001.)

and neurofibromas. Palpate for vertebral tenderness and auscultate down the spine for bruits. Next examine the upper limbs and cranial nerves to determine the upper level if this is not already obvious.

Important spinal cord syndromes
Brown-Séquard syndrome[aaa]

Clinical features are shown in Figure 11.101. These signs result from hemisection of the cord.

- **Motor changes:** (i) upper motor neurone signs below the hemisection on the same side as the lesion; (ii) lower motor neurone signs at the level of the hemisection on the same side.
- **Sensory changes:** (i) pain and temperature

[aaa] Charles Edouard Brown-Séquard (1817–1894) succeeded Claude Bernard at the College de France. He was the son of an American sea captain (pirate) and a French woman. He was born in Mauritius at a time when it was under British rule. With this background he roved around the world, working in Paris, Mauritius, London and New York. His syndrome usually arose from failed murder attempts. Traditionally Mauritian cane cutters, when trying to murder someone, used a very long thin knife which was slipped between the ribs from behind, to cut the aorta or penetrate the heart. Only such a knife could have caused a cord hemitransection.

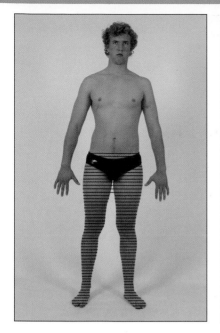

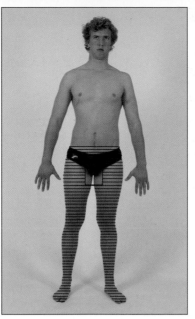

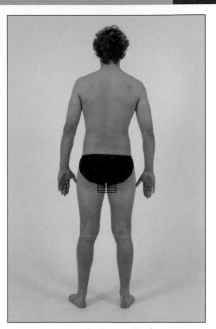

Figure 11.98 Sensory loss with transverse section of the spinal cord

Figure 11.99 Pattern of sensory loss with intrinsic spinal cord disease
For example, central tumour or less commonly with extrinsic compression of the spinal cord—sacrum is spared.

Figure 11.100 Conus medullaris or cauda equina lesion—saddle anaesthesia

loss on the opposite side to the lesion—note that the upper level of sensory loss is usually a few segments below the level of the lesion; (ii) vibration and proprioception loss occur on the same side; (iii) detection of light touch is often normal.

- **Causes:** (i) multiple sclerosis; (ii) angioma; (iii) trauma; (iv) myelitis; (v) post-radiation myelopathy.

Subacute combined degeneration of the cord (vitamin B₁₂ deficiency)

Clinical features are (i) posterior column loss symmetrically (vibration and joint position sense), causing an ataxic gait; (ii) upper motor neurone signs in the lower limbs symmetrically with absent ankle reflexes; knee reflexes may be absent or, more often, exaggerated. There may also be (iii) peripheral sensory neuropathy (less common and mild); (iv) optic atrophy; (v) dementia.

Dissociated sensory loss

This usually indicates spinal cord disease but may occur with a peripheral neuropathy.

- **Causes of spinothalamic loss only:** (i) syringomyelia; (ii) Brown-Séquard syndrome (contralateral leg); (iii) anterior spinal artery

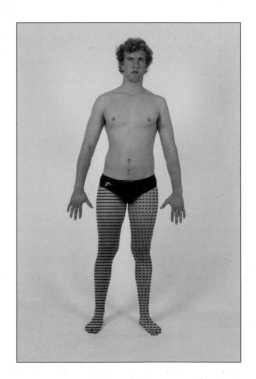

Figure 11.101 Brown-Séquard syndrome
Loss of pain and temperature on the opposite side to the lesion, with loss of vibration and proprioception on the same side as the lesion.

TABLE 11.30 Important motor and reflex changes of spinal cord compression

See Figures 11.98 to 11.100 for sensory changes.

Upper cervical

Upper motor neurone signs in the upper and lower limbs.

C5
- Lower motor neurone weakness and wasting of rhomboids, deltoids, biceps and brachioradialis.
- Upper motor neurone signs affect the rest of the upper and all the lower limbs. The biceps jerk is lost. The brachioradialis jerk is inverted.

C8
- Lower motor neurone weakness and wasting of the intrinsic muscles of the hand.
- Upper motor neurone signs in the lower limbs.

Midthoracic

Intercostal paralysis.
Upper motor neurone signs in the lower limbs.
Loss of upper abdominal reflexes at T7 and T8.

T10–T11
- Loss of the lower abdominal reflexes and upward displacement of the umbilicus.
- Upper motor neurone signs in the lower limbs.

L1
- Cremasteric reflex is lost (normal abdominal reflexes).
- Upper motor neurone signs in the lower limbs.

L4
- Lower motor neurone weakness and wasting of the quadriceps.
- Knee jerks lost.
- Ankle jerks may be hyperreflexic with extensor plantar response (upgoing toes), but more often the whole conus is involved, causing a lower motor neurone lesion.

L5–S1
- Lower motor neurone weakness of knee flexion and hip extension (S1) and abduction (L5) plus calf and foot muscles.
- Knee jerks present.
- No ankle jerks or plantar responses.
- Anal reflex present.

S3–S4
- No anal reflex.
- Saddle sensory loss.
- Normal lower limbs.

Causes of spinal cord compression

1 Vertebral
- Spondylosis
- Trauma
- Prolapse of a disc
- Tumour
- Infection

2 Outside the dura
- Lymphoma, metastases
- Infection—e.g. abscess

3 Within the dura but extramedullary
- Tumour—e.g. meningioma, neurofibroma

4 Intramedullary*
- Tumour—e.g. glioma, ependymoma
- Syringomyelia
- Haematomyelia

* Lower motor neurone signs may extend for several segments, and spastic paralysis occurs late, unlike the situation with extramedullary lesions.

TABLE 11.31 Important patterns of abnormal sensation

Sign	Location of lesion
Total unilateral loss of all forms of sensation	Thalamus or upper brainstem (extensive lesion)
Pain and temperature loss on one side of face and opposite side of body	Medulla involving descending nucleus of spinal tract of the fifth nerve and ascending spinothalamic tract (lateral medullary lesion) (Figure 11.102)
Bilateral loss of all forms of sensation below a definite level	Spinal cord lesion (if only pain and temperature affected: anterior cord lesion)
Unilateral loss of pain and temperature below a definite level	Partial unilateral spinal cord lesion on opposite side (Brown-Séquard syndrome) (Figure 11.101)
Loss of pain and temperature over several segments but normal sensation above and below	Intrinsic spinal cord lesion near its centre anteriorly (involves the crossing fibres), e.g. syringomyelia, intrinsic cord tumour (Note: more posterior lesions cause proprioceptive loss)
Loss of sensation over many segments with sacral sparing	Intrinsic cord compression more likely
Saddle sensory loss (lowest sacral segments)	Cauda equina lesion (touch preserved in conus medullaris lesions)
Loss of position and vibration sense only	Posterior column lesion
Glove and stocking loss (hands and feet)	Peripheral neuropathy
Loss of all forms of sensation over a well-defined body part only	Posterior root lesion (purely sensory) or peripheral nerve (often motor abnormality associated)

thrombosis; (iv) lateral medullary syndrome (contralateral to the other signs) (Figure 11.102); (v) small fibre peripheral neuropathy (e.g. diabetes mellitus, amyloid).

- **Causes of dorsal column loss only:** (i) subacute combined degeneration; (ii) Brown-Séquard syndrome (ipsilateral leg); (iii) spinocerebellar degeneration (e.g. Friedreich's[bbb] ataxia); (iv) multiple sclerosis; (v) tabes dorsalis; (vi) peripheral neuropathy (e.g. diabetes mellitus, hypothyroidism); (vii) sensory neuronopathy (a dorsal root ganglionopathy which may be caused by carcinoma, diabetes mellitus or Sjögren's syndrome).

Syringomyelia (a central cavity in the spinal cord)

- **Clinical triad:** (i) loss of pain and temperature over the neck, shoulders and arms (a 'cape' distribution); (ii) amyotrophy (atrophy and areflexia) of the arms; (iii) upper motor neurone signs in the lower limbs.

There may also be thoracic scoliosis due to asymmetrical weakness of the paravertebral muscles.

[bbb] Nicholaus Friedreich (1825–1882), German physician, described this in 1863. He was professor of pathology at Heidelberg. *Pes cavus* is also called Friedreich's foot.

An extensor plantar response plus absent knee and ankle jerks

- **Causes:** (i) subacute combined degeneration of the cord (B$_{12}$ deficiency); (ii) conus medullaris lesion; (iii) combination of an upper motor neurone lesion with cauda equina compression or peripheral neuropathy, such as a stroke in a diabetic; (iv) syphilis (taboparesis); (v) Friedreich's ataxia; (vi) motor neurone disease; (vii) human T-cell lymphotropic virus (HTLV-I) infection.

A summary of the features that differentiate intramedullary from extramedullary cord lesions is presented in Table 11.32.

Myopathy

Muscle weakness can be due to individual peripheral nerve lesions, mononeuritis multiplex, peripheral neuropathy or spinal cord disease. Each of these has a characteristic pattern. Primary disease of muscle (myopathy) also causes weakness. There is no sensory loss with myopathy, which is an important clue. The motor weakness is similar to that of the lower motor neurone type. There are two major patterns: proximal myopathy and distal myopathy.

Proximal myopathy is the more common form. On examination there is proximal muscle wasting and weakness (Tables 11.33 and 11.34;

TABLE 11.32 Differentiating intramedullary from extramedullary cord lesions

Intramedullary	Extramedullary
Root pains rare	Root pains common
Late onset of corticospinal signs	Early onset of corticospinal signs
Lower motor neurone signs extend for several segments	Lower motor neurone signs localised
Dissociated sensory loss (pain and temperature) may be present	Brown-Séquard syndrome if lateral cord compression
Normal or minimally altered cerebrospinal fluid findings	Early, marked cerebrospinal fluid abnormalities
May have sacral sparing	

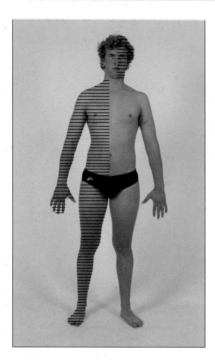

Figure 11.102 Pattern of sensory loss in the lateral medullary syndrome

TABLE 11.33 Causes (differential diagnosis) of proximal weakness and myopathy

Causes of proximal weakness
Myopathy (q.v.)
Neuromuscular junction disease, e.g. myasthenia gravis
Neurogenic, e.g. motor neurone disease, polyradiculopathy, Kugelberg-Welander disease (proximal muscle wasting and fasciculation due to anterior horn cell disease—autosomal recessive)

Causes of myopathy
Hereditary muscular dystrophy (Table 11.34)
Congenital myopathies (rare)
Acquired myopathy (mnemonic, PACE, PODS):
   Polymyositis or dermatomyositis (Figure 11.104)
   Alcohol, AIDS (HIV infection)
   Carcinoma
   Endocrine—e.g. hyperthyroidism, hypothyroidism, Cushing's syndrome, acromegaly, hypopituitarism

   Periodic paralysis (hyperkalaemic, hypokalaemic or normokalaemic)
   Osteomalacia
   Drugs—e.g. clofibrate, chloroquine, steroids, zidovudine
   Sarcoidosis

Note: Causes of *proximal myopathy with a peripheral neuropathy* include:
Paraneoplastic syndrome
Alcohol
Hypothyroidism
Connective tissue diseases

Figures 11.103 and 11.104). Reflexes involving these muscles may be reduced. This can be caused by genetic (e.g. muscular dystrophy) or acquired disease. *Distal myopathy* also occurs and is always genetic, although peripheral neuropathy is a much more common cause of distal muscle weakness. If the distal limbs are affected, consider hereditary motor and sensory neuropathy (Table 11.35). Motor neurone disease also causes weakness without any sensory loss.

Dystrophia myotonica

If this disease (which is inherited as an autosomal-dominant condition) is suspected because of an inability on the part of the patient to let go when shaking hands (myotonia), or because general inspection reveals the characteristic appearance (Figure 11.105), examine as follows.

Observe the face for frontal baldness (the patient may be wearing a wig), the expressionless triangular facies, atrophy of the temporalis muscle and partial ptosis. Thick spectacles, a traditional sign of this disease, are not often seen now because of lens replacement surgery. The eyes should still be examined, as these patients can develop characteristic iridescent cataracts and subcapsular fine deposits.

TABLE 11.34 Muscular dystrophies

1 Duchenne's* (pseudohypertrophic)
- Affects only males (sex-linked recessive)
- Calves and deltoids: hypertrophied early, weak later
- Proximal weakness: early
- Dilated cardiomyopathy

2 Becker[†]
- Affects only males (sex-linked recessive)
- Similar clinical features to Duchenne's except for less heart disease, a later onset and less-rapid progression

3 Limb girdle
- Males or females (autosomal recessive), onset in the third decade
- Shoulder or pelvic girdle affected
- Face and heart usually spared

4 Facioscapulohumeral
- Males or females (autosomal dominant)
- Facial and pectoral weakness with hypertrophy of deltoids

5 Dystrophia myotonica (autosomal dominant)

* Guillaume Duchenne (1806–75), brilliant eccentric who founded French neurology. He died of a stroke.
[†] Peter Becker (b. 1908), German professor of genetics.

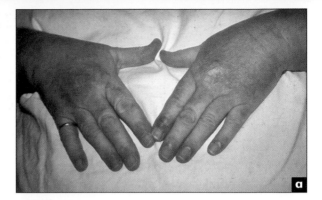
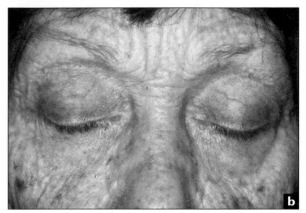

Figure 11.104 Dermatomyositis
(a) Gottren's sign in dermatomyositis—heliotrope (lilac-coloured) flat topped papules, which occur over the knuckles, but may also be seen over the elbows or knees and may ulcerate. (b) Dermatomyositis may also cause a heliotrope rash on the face (especially on the eyelids, upper cheeks and forehead), periorbital oedema, erythema, maculopapular eruptions and scaling dermatitis. Dermatomyositis and the closely related condition polymyositis are idiopathic myopathies. Up to 10% of adult patients with dermatomyositis may have an underlying malignancy.
(From McDonald FS, ed., *Mayo Clinic images in internal medicine*, with permission. © Mayo Clinic Scientific Press and CRC Press.)

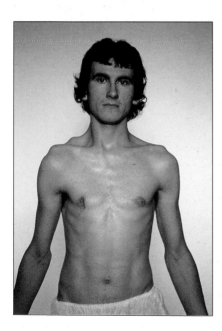

Figure 11.103 Fascioscapular muscular dystrophy
(From Mir MA, *Atlas of Clinical Diagnosis*, 2nd edn. Edinburgh: Saunders, 2003.)

Look at the neck for atrophy of the sternocleido-mastoid muscles and then test neck flexion (neck flexion is weak while extension is normal).

Go to the upper limbs. Shake hands and test for percussion myotonia. Tapping over the thenar eminence causes contraction and then slow relaxation of abductor pollicis brevis. Examine the arm now for signs of wasting and weakness distally (forearms are usually affected first) and proximally. There are no sensory changes.

Go to the chest and look for gynaecomastia (uncommon). Examine the cardiovascular system for cardiomyopathy. Next palpate the testes for atrophy. Examine the lower limbs. The tibial nerves are affected first. Always ask to test the urine for sugar (diabetes mellitus is associated with this disease).

Note: Muscle myotonia can also occur in the hereditary diseases myotonia congenita (autosomal dominant or recessive) and hereditary paramyotonia (autosomal dominant cold-induced myotonia).

Myasthenia gravis

Myasthenia gravis is an autoimmune disease of the neuromuscular junction. There are circulating antibodies against acetylcholine receptors. It differs from the proximal myopathies in that muscle power decreases with use. There is little muscle wasting and no sensory change.

It is necessary to test for muscle fatigue. Test the oculomotor muscles by asking the patient to sustain an upward gaze by looking up at the ceiling for 1 minute, and watch for progressive ptosis (Figure 11.106). Test the Peek sign for orbicularis oculi weakness. Ask the patient to close the eyes; if positive, within 30 seconds the lid margin will begin to separate, showing the sclera. This test strongly increases the likelihood of myasthenia (positive LR = 30.0).[22] Then test the proximal limb girdle muscles—ask the patient to hold the arms above the head. The examiner can repeatedly press the abducted arms down until they weaken. Power will decrease with repeated muscle contraction.

Look for a thymectomy scar (over the sternum)—thymectomy is often undertaken as treatment for generalised myasthenia.

The cerebellum (Figure 11.107)

If the patient complains of clumsiness or problems with coordination of movement, a cerebellar examination is indicated. Signs of cerebellar disease occur on the same side as the lesion in the brain. This is because most cerebellar fibres cross twice in the brainstem, both on entry to and exit from the cerebellum. Proceed as follows with the examination.

TABLE 11.35 Features of hereditary motor and sensory neuropathy (Charcot-Marie-Tooth* disease)
1 Pes cavus (short-arched feet)
2 Distal muscle atrophy due to peripheral nerve degeneration. This does not usually extend above the elbows or above the middle third of the thighs. Peroneal muscle atrophy gives the legs the shape of an inverted champagne bottle
3 Absent reflexes
4 Slight or no sensory loss in the limbs
5 Thickened nerves
6 Optic atrophy, Argyll Robertson pupils (rare)
* Jean Martin Charcot (1825–93), Parisian physician and neurologist; Pierre Marie (1853–1940), Parisian neurologist and Charcot's greatest pupil; and Howard Henry Tooth (1856–1926), London physician, who described the condition independently in 1886. Type I is usually autosomal dominant.

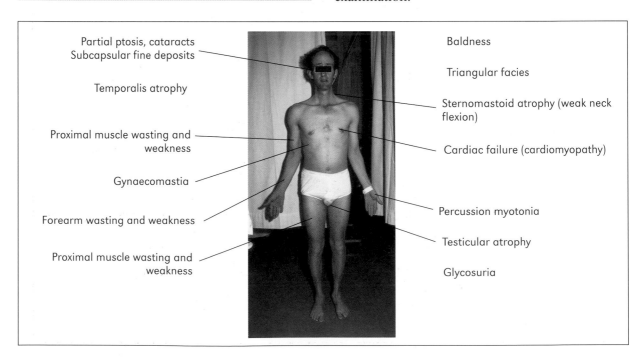

Partial ptosis, cataracts
Subcapsular fine deposits

Temporalis atrophy

Proximal muscle wasting and weakness

Gynaecomastia

Forearm wasting and weakness

Proximal muscle wasting and weakness

Baldness

Triangular facies

Sternomastoid atrophy (weak neck flexion)

Cardiac failure (cardiomyopathy)

Percussion myotonia

Testicular atrophy

Glycosuria

Figure 11.105 Dystrophia myotonica

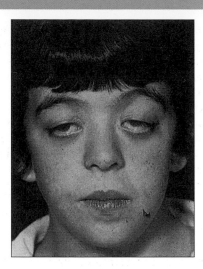

Figure 11.106 Bilateral ptosis after upward gaze in myasthenia gravis

Look first for nystagmus—usually jerky horizontal nystagmus with an increased amplitude on looking towards the side of the lesion. The direction of fast movement is the side of the lesion. Assess speech next. Ask the patient to say 'British Constitution' or 'West Register Street' (Figure 11.108). Cerebellar speech is jerky, explosive and loud, with an irregular separation of syllables.

Go to the upper limbs. Ask the patient to extend the arms and look for upward arm drift due to hypotonia of the agonist muscles. Test tone. Hypotonia[ccc] is due to loss of a facilitatory influence on the spinal motor neurones.

Next perform the finger–nose test. The patient touches the nose, then rotates the finger and touches the examiner's finger. Note any intention tremor (tremor which increases as the target is approached—this is due to loss of cerebellar connections in the brainstem) and past-pointing

(the patient overshoots the target). Test rapidly alternating movements: the patient taps alternately the palm and back of one hand on the other hand or thigh. Inability to perform this movement smoothly

[ccc] The concepts of hypotonia, rebound and pendular jerks in cerebellar disease stem from Gordon Holmes' 1917 description of signs in acute unilateral cerebellar disease. They may well not exist in other cerebellar problems. Students will, however, still be expected to know how to test for these signs.

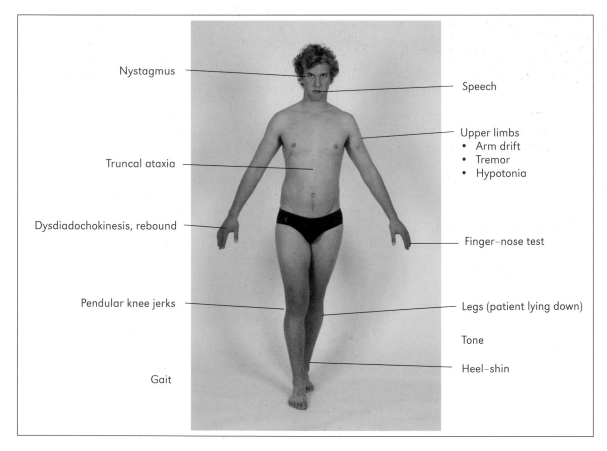

Figure 11.107 The cerebellar examination

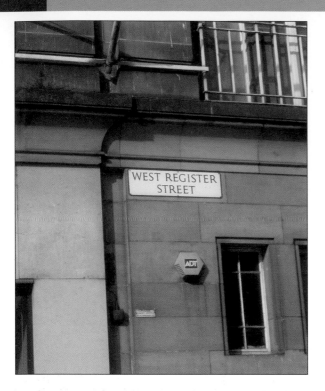

Figure 11.108 West Register Street, Edinburgh

is called dysdiadochokinesis. Now test rebound—ask the patient to lift the arms quickly from the sides, then stop (incoordination of antagonist and agonist action causes the patient to be unable to stop the arms). Before testing, always demonstrate these movements for the patient's benefit.

Go on to examine the legs. Again, test tone here. Then perform the heel–shin test looking for accuracy of fine movement when the patient slides the heel down the shin slowly on each side for several cycles. Then ask the patient to lift the big toe up to touch the examiner's finger, and look for intention tremor and past-pointing. Ask the patient then to tap each heel on the other shin.

Look for truncal ataxia by asking the patient to fold the arms and sit up. While the patient is sitting, ask him or her to put the legs over the side of the bed and test for pendular knee jerks (the lower leg continues to swing a number of times before coming to rest—this is evidence of hypotonia).

Test gait (the patient will stagger towards the affected side if there is a unilateral cerebellar hemisphere lesion).

If there is an obvious unilateral cerebellar problem examine the cranial nerves for evidence of a cerebellopontine angle tumour (fifth, seventh and eighth nerves affected) or the lateral medullary syndrome, and auscultate over the cerebellum.

Always look in the fundi for papilloedema. Next examine for peripheral signs of malignant disease and for vascular disease (carotid or vertebral bruits). Examine the base of the skull for scars from previous neurosurgery.

If there is evidence of a midline lesion, such as truncal ataxia, abnormal heel–toe walking or abnormal speech, consider either a midline tumour or a paraneoplastic syndrome (Table 11.36). If there is bilateral disease, look for signs of multiple sclerosis, Friedreich's ataxia (pes cavus is the most helpful initial clue) (Table 11.37) and hypothyroidism (rare). Alcoholic cerebellar degeneration (which affects the anterior lobe of the cerebellar vermis) classically spares the arms. If there are, in addition, upper motor neurone signs, consider the causes in Table 11.38.

Remember that there are important reciprocal connections between the cerebellum and the parietal and frontal lobes. These explain the problems cerebellar abnormalities can cause with functions other than coordination. Loss of verbal fluency, grammatical problems with speech, difficulty with memory and planning can all sometimes be features of cerebellar disease.

Parkinson's disease

This is a common extrapyramidal disease of middle to old age (1% of people older than 65) where there is degeneration of the substantia nigra and its pathways. This results in dopamine deficiency and a relative excess of cholinergic transmission in the caudate nucleus and putamen, which causes excessive supraspinal excitatory drive. There may be a history of insidious and asymmetrical onset. Non-specific symptoms (sleep abnormalities, constipation, depression and dementia) may precede or accompany the classic tremor.

Examine as follows.[23]

Inspection

Note the lack of facial expression, which leads to a mask-like facies. The posture is characteristically flexed and there are few spontaneous movements.

Gait and movements

Ask the patient to rise from a chair, walk, turn quickly, stop and start.

The characteristic gait is described as *shuffling*—there are small steps, and the patient hardly raises the feet from the ground. There is often difficulty in initiating walking, but once it begins the patient hurries (festination) and has difficulty stopping. The Parkinsonian patient seems always to be trying to catch up with the centre of gravity. There is a lack of the normal arm swing. Walking heel-to-toe will be difficult.

Testing for *propulsion* or *retropulsion* (propulsion involves pushing the patient from behind and retropulsion pushing from in front) is of uncertain value and must be done with some caution because the patient may be unable to stop and may fall over. The examiner can stand behind the patient and pull him or her backwards, but should stand braced to catch the patient.

Bradykinesia (a decrease in the speed and amplitude of complex movements) may be the result of a lesion in the nigrostriatal pathway (a dopaminergic pathway), which affects connections between the caudate nucleus, putamen and motor cortex, causing abnormal movement programming and abnormal recruitment of single motor units. Two simple tests (Figure 11.109) for this are *finger tapping* and *twiddling*. Ask the patient to tap the fingers in turn onto a surface repeatedly, quickly and with both hands at once. Twiddling is rotating the hands around each other in front of the body. These movements are slow and clumsy in Parkinsonian patients but obviously depend on motor and cerebellar function as well. Difficulty getting out of a chair can be another sign of bradykinesia and patients often have difficulty turning over in bed.

Kinesia paradoxica is the striking ability of a patient to perform rapid movements (especially if startled) but not slow ones; for example, the patient may be able to run down the stairs in response to a fire alarm but be unable to stop at the bottom—this is *not* a recommended test.

Tremor

Have the patient return to bed. Look for a resting tremor, which is often asymmetrical. The characteristic movement is described as pill-rolling. Movement of the fingers at the metacarpophalangeal joints is combined with the movements of the

---

TABLE 11.36 Causes of cerebellar disease

Rostral vermis lesion (only lower limbs affected)
Usually due to alcohol

Unilateral
1 Space-occupying lesion (tumour, abscess, granuloma)
2 Ischaemia (vertebrobasilar disease)
3 Multiple sclerosis
4 Trauma

Bilateral
1 Drugs—e.g. phenytoin
2 Alcohol (both acutely and chronically, possibly due to thiamine deficiency)
3 Friedreich's ataxia
4 Hypothyroidism
5 Paraneoplastic syndrome
6 Multiple sclerosis
7 Trauma ('punch drunk')
8 Arnold-Chiari malformation
9 Large space-occupying lesion, cerebrovascular disease

Midline
1 Paraneoplastic syndrome
2 Midline tumour

TABLE 11.37 Clinical features of Friedreich's ataxia (autosomal recessive)

This is usually a young person with:

1 Cerebellar signs (bilateral) including nystagmus
2 Pes cavus.* Cocking of the toes. Kyphoscoliosis
3 Upper motor neurone signs in the limbs (although reflexes are absent)
4 Peripheral neuropathy
5 Posterior column loss in the limbs
6 Cardiomyopathy (ECG abnormalities occur in more than 50% of cases)
7 Diabetes mellitus (common)
8 Optic atrophy (uncommon)
9 Normal mentation

* Other causes of pes cavus include hereditary motor and sensory neuropathy, spinocerebellar degeneration or neuropathies in childhood.

TABLE 11.38 Causes of spastic and ataxic paraparesis (upper motor neurone and cerebellar signs combined)

In adolescence
Spinocerebellar degeneration—e.g. Marie's spastic ataxia

In young adults
Multiple sclerosis
Spinocerebellar degeneration
Syphilitic meningomyelitis
Arnold-Chiari malformation or other lesion at the craniospinal junction

In later life
Multiple sclerosis
Syringomyelia
Infarction (in upper pons or internal capsule on one side—'ataxic hemiparesis')
Lesion at the craniospinal junction—e.g. meningioma

Note: Unrelated diseases that are relatively common (e.g. cervical spondylosis and cerebellar degeneration from alcohol) may cause a similar clinical picture.

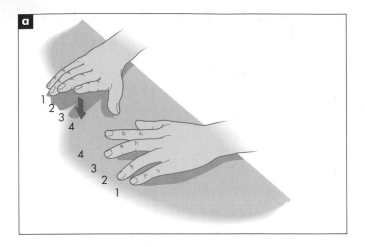

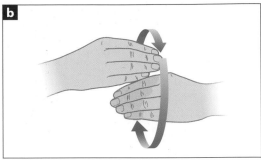

Figure 11.109 Detecting bradykinesia
(a) Tapping the fingers. (b) Twiddling.

thumb. Various attending movements may also occur at the wrist. On finger–nose testing the resting tremor decreases, but a faster action tremor may supervene.

Tremor can be facilitated by getting the patient to perform 'serial 7s'—take 7 from 100, then 7 from the answer and so forth (mental stimulation)—or to move the contralateral limb (e.g. by rapidly opposing the contralateral thumb and fingers). Other types of tremor are summarised in Table 11.39.

Tone

Test tone at both wrists. The characteristic increase in tone is called cogwheel or plastic (lead pipe) rigidity. Tone is increased with an interrupted nature, the muscles giving way with a series of jerks. If hypertonia is not obvious, obtain reinforcement by asking the patient to turn the head from side to side or to wave the contralateral arm. Cogwheel rigidity occurs because the exaggerated stretch reflex is interrupted by tremor.

Remember, the signs are often asymmetrical early in the course of Parkinson's disease.

Face

There may be *titubation* (tremor) of the head, absence of blinking, dribbling of saliva and lack of facial expression. Test the *glabellar tap* (reflex)—keeping your finger out of the patient's line of vision, tap the middle of the forehead (glabella) with your middle finger (Figure 11.110). This sign is positive when the patient continues to blink as long as the examiner taps. Normal people blink only a couple of times and then stop. The glabellar reflex is a primitive reflex which is also frequently present in frontal lobe disease.

Assess *speech*, which is typically monotonous,

TABLE 11.39 A classification of non-physiological tremor*
1 Parkinsonian—resting tremor
2 Postural/action tremor; present throughout movement; the following most often cause a static or postural tremor of the outstretched arms: (a) idiopathic (most common) (b) anxiety (c) drugs (d) familial (e) thyrotoxicosis
3 Essential/familial
4 Intention tremor (cerebellar disease); increases towards the target
5 Midbrain ('red nucleus') tremor—abduction-adduction movements of upper limbs with flexion-extension of wrists (usually associated with intention tremor)
* Tremor is a rhythmic oscillation of a part of the body around a fixed point. NB: Flapping (asterixis) is not strictly a tremor but a sudden brief loss of tone in hepatic failure, cardiac failure, respiratory failure or renal failure (metabolic encephalopathies).

soft and faint, lacking intonation. Sometimes palilalia is present; this is repetition of the end of a word (the opposite of stuttering).

Now test the ocular movements, particularly for *weakness of upward gaze*. Isolated failure of upward gaze is a feature of Parkinson's disease. There is a separate group of patients with marked rigidity and paralysis of gaze who should be diagnosed as having progressive supranuclear palsy rather than Parkinson's disease. These people develop loss first of downward gaze, then of upward gaze and finally of horizontal gaze.

Feel the brow for greasiness (seborrhoea)

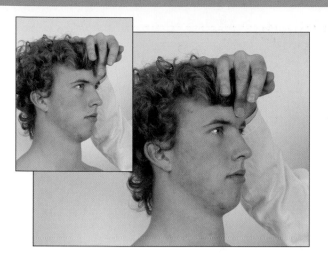

Figure 11.110 The glabellar tap (Wilson's sign)

GOOD SIGNS GUIDE 11.3 Parkinson's disease

Sign	Positive LR	Negative LR
Rigidity, tremor and bradykinesia all present	2.2	0.5
Difficulty walking (heel–toe)	2.9	0.32
Asymmetrical onset, no atypical features and no alternative diagnosis	4.1	0.4
Glabellar tap	4.5	0.13

From McGee S, *Evidence-based physical diagnosis*, 2nd edn. St Louis: Saunders, 2007.

TABLE 11.40 Causes of Parkinson's syndrome

Idiopathic: Parkinson's disease

Drugs: e.g. phenothiazines, methyldopa

Post-encephalitis (now very rare)

Other: toxins (carbon monoxide, manganese), Wilson's disease, progressive supranuclear palsy, Steele-Richardson syndrome, Shy-Drager syndrome, syphilis, tumour (e.g. giant frontal meningioma)

Atherosclerosis is a controversial cause

or sweatiness, due to associated autonomic dysfunction. Orthostatic hypotension may also be present for the same reason.

The palmomental reflex is commonly present in these patients and tends to be more prominent in those with severe akinesia. Dementia develops in 30% of patients.

Writing

Ask the patient to write his or her name and address. *Micrographia* (small writing) is characteristic. The patient may also be unable to do this because of the development of dementia, a late manifestation. Test the higher centres if appropriate. See *Good signs guide 11.3*.

Causes of Parkinson's syndrome

These are shown in Table 11.40.

Other extrapyramidal movement disorders (dyskinesia)

Chorea

Here there is a lesion of the corpus striatum, which causes non-repetitive, abrupt, involuntary jerky movements. These may be unilateral or generalised. Often the patient attempts to disguise this by completing the involuntary movements with a voluntary one. In this disease, dopaminergic pathways dominate over cholinergic transmissions.

Chorea can usefully be distinguished from hemiballismus, athetosis and pseudoathetosis. *Hemiballismus* is due to a subthalamic lesion on the side opposite the movement disorder. It causes unilateral wild throwing movements of the proximal joints. There may be skin excoriation due to limb trauma. These movements may persist during sleep. *Athetosis* or *dystonia* is due to a lesion of the outer segment of the putamen and causes slow sinuous writhing distal movements that are present at rest. *Pseudoathetosis* is a description given to athetoid movements in the fingers in patients with severe proprioceptive loss (these are especially prominent when the eyes are shut).

If the patient has chorea, proceed as follows. First shake hands. There may be tremor and dystonia superimposed on lack of sustained hand grip ('milkmaid's grip'). Ask the patient to hold out the hands, then look for a choreic (dystonic) posture. This typically involves finger and thumb hyperextension and wrist flexion.

Go to the face and look at the eyes for exophthalmos (thyrotoxicosis), Kayser-Fleischer rings (Wilson's disease) and conjunctival injection (polycythaemia). Ask the patient to poke out the tongue and note frequent retraction of the tongue (serpentine movements). Look for skin rashes (e.g. systemic lupus erythematosus, vasculitis). If the patient is young, examine the heart for signs of rheumatic fever (Sydenham's[ddd] chorea).

Test the reflexes. The abdominal reflexes are usually brisk, but tendon reflexes are reduced and may be pendular (due to hypotonia).

Assess the higher centres for dementia (Huntington's chorea[eee]).

Causes of chorea are shown in Table 11.41.

Dystonia

The patient manifests an involuntary abnormal posture with excessive co-contraction of antagonist muscles. Dystonia may be focal (e.g. spasmodic torticollis), segmental or generalised. Other forms of movement disorder may be present (e.g. myoclonic dystonia). The acute onset of dystonia is seen most commonly as a side-effect of various drugs (e.g. levodopa, phenothiazines, metoclopramide).

The unconscious patient

The rapid and efficient examination of the unconscious patient is important. The word COMA provides a mnemonic for four major groups of causes of unconsciousness.

C—CO_2 narcosis (respiratory failure: uncommon).
O—Overdose: for example, tranquillisers, alcohol, salicylates, carbon monoxide, antidepressants.
M—Metabolic: for example, hypoglycaemia, diabetic ketoacidosis, uraemia, hypothyroidism, hepatic coma, hypercalcaemia, adrenal failure.
A—Apoplexy: for example, head injury, cerebrovascular accident (infarction or haemorrhage), subdural or extradural haematoma, meningitis, encephalitis, epilepsy.

Coma occurs when the reticular formation is damaged by a lesion or metabolic abnormality, or when the cortex is diffusely damaged.

General inspection

Remember A–B–C: *Airway*, *Breathing* and *Circulation*.

Airway and breathing

Look to see if the patient is breathing, as indicated by chest wall movement. If not, urgent attention is required, including clearing the airway and providing ventilation. Note particularly the pattern of breathing (see Table 5.11, page 112). Cheyne-Stokes respiration (which may indicate diencephalic injury, but is not specific), irregular ataxic breathing (Biot's breathing, from an advanced brainstem lesion), and deep rapid respiration (e.g. Kussmaul breathing, secondary to a metabolic acidosis, as in diabetes mellitus) are important signs to look for.

Circulation

Look for signs of shock, dehydration and cyanosis. A typical cherry-red colour occurs rarely in cases of carbon monoxide poisoning. Take the pulse rate and blood pressure.

Posture

Look for signs of trauma. Note any neck hyperextension (from meningism in children or cerebellar tonsillar herniation).

Look for:

1 A *decerebrate* or extensor posture, which may be held spontaneously or occur in response to stimuli, and which suggests severe midbrain disease. The arms are held extended and internally rotated and the legs are extended.
2 A *decorticate* or flexor posture, which suggests a lesion above the brainstem. It can be unilateral or bilateral. There is flexion and internal rotation of the arms and extension of the legs.

Involuntary movements

Recurrent or continuous convulsions, which may be focal or generalised, suggest status epilepticus.

TABLE 11.41 Causes of chorea
Drugs: e.g. excess levodopa, phenothiazines, the contraceptive pill, phenytoin
Huntington's disease (autosomal dominant)
Sydenham's chorea (rheumatic fever) and other postinfectious states (both rare)
Senility
Wilson's disease
Kernicterus (rare)
Vasculitis or connective tissue disease—e.g. systemic lupus erythematosus (very rare)
Thyrotoxicosis (very rare)
Polycythaemia or other hyperviscosity syndromes (very rare)
Viral encephalitis (very rare)

[ddd] Thomas Sydenham (1624–89). He was a captain in Cromwell's army and became the most famous English physician of his time, providing clinical descriptions of gout (from which he suffered), fevers, hysteria and venereal disease. He was called the Father of English Clinical Medicine.

[eee] George Huntington (1850–1916), American general practitioner. He described this disease in his only clinical paper in 1872, when he was 22.

TABLE 11.42 Glasgow coma scale

Add up the score for 1, 2 and 3. Score of 4 or less = very poor prognosis, score >11 = good prognosis for recovery.

1 Eyes	Open	Spontaneously	4
		To loud verbal command	3
		To pain	2
	No response		1
2 Best motor response	To verbal command	Obeys	6
	To painful stimuli	Localises pain	5
		Flexion—withdrawal	4
		Abnormal flexion posturing	3
		Extension posturing	2
		No response	1
3 Best verbal response		Oriented	5
		Confused, disoriented	4
		Inappropriate words	3
		Incomprehensible sounds	2
		None	1

Myoclonic jerks can occur after hypoxic injury and as a result of metabolic encephalopathy. Remember that complex partial seizure status epilepticus can cause a reduced level of consciousness without convulsive movements.

Level of consciousness

Tickle the patient's nose with cottonwool and watch for facial movements. This is less likely to harm the patient than the traditional method of firm pressing of knuckles over the sternum to cause pain.

Determine the level of consciousness. *Coma* is unconsciousness with a reduced response to external stimuli. Coma in which the patient responds semi-purposefully is considered light. In deep coma there is no response to any stimuli and no reflexes are present (it is usually due to a brainstem or pontine lesion, though drug overdosage, such as with barbiturates, can be responsible).

Stupor is unconsciousness, but the patient can be aroused. Purposeful movements occur in response to painful stimuli.

Drowsiness resembles normal sleepiness. The patient can be fairly easily roused to normal wakefulness, but when left alone falls asleep again. The Glasgow coma scale (Table 11.42) is used to assess the depth of coma more accurately: record the subscores and total scores.

The neck

If there is no evidence of neck trauma, assess for neck stiffness and Kernig's sign (for meningitis or subarachnoid haemorrhage).

The head and face

Inspect and palpate for head injuries, including Battle's sign,[fff] bruising behind the ear indicating a fracture of the base of the skull. Look for facial asymmetry (i.e. facial weakness). The paralysed side of the face will be sucked in and out with respiration. A painful stimulus (e.g. pressing the supraorbital notch) may produce grimacing and make facial asymmetry more obvious. Note jaundice (e.g. hepatic coma) or manifestations of myxoedema.

The eyes

Inspect the pupils. Very small pupils (but reactive to light) occur in pontine lesions and with narcotic overdoses. One small pupil occurs in Horner's syndrome (e.g. as part of the lateral medullary syndrome or in hypothalamus injury; see Chapter 13). Two midpoint non-reactive pupils suggest midbrain disease, anoxia or drugs (anticholinergics). One dilated pupil suggests a subdural haematoma, raised intracranial pressure (unilateral tentorial herniation) or a subarachnoid haemorrhage from a posterior communicating artery aneurysm. Widely dilated pupils may occur

---

fff   William Battle (1855–1936), surgeon, St Thomas's Hospital, London.

when increased intracranial pressure and coning cause secondary brainstem haemorrhage, or with anticholinergic drugs.

Conjunctival haemorrhage suggests skull fracture. Look in the fundi for papilloedema, diabetic or hypertensive retinopathy, or subhyaloid haemorrhage. The locked-in syndrome is rare; in a lower brainstem lesion patients are awake but can only control their eye movements.

Look at the position of the eyes. Particular cranial nerve palsies may cause deviation of an eye in various directions. The sixth nerve is particularly vulnerable to damage because of its long intracranial course. Deviation of both eyes to one side in the unconscious patient may be due to a destructive lesion in a cerebral hemisphere, which causes fixed deviation towards the side of the lesion. An irritative (epileptic) focus causes the direction of gaze to be away from the lesion. Upward or downward eye deviation suggests a brainstem problem. Trapping of the globe or extraocular muscles by fracture may also lead to an abnormal eye position or to an abnormal eye movement.

Perform *doll's eye testing* by lifting the patient's eyelids and rolling the head from side to side. When vestibular reflexes are intact (i.e. an intact brainstem), the eyes maintain their fixation as if looking at an object in the distance, but change their position relative to the head. This is the normal 'doll's eye phenomenon'. Brainstem lesions or drugs affecting the brainstem cause the eyes to move with the head, so that fixation is not maintained.

Ears and nostrils

Look for any bleeding or drainage of cerebrospinal fluid (the latter indicating a skull fracture). A watery discharge can be simply tested for glucose. The presence of glucose confirms that it is cerebrospinal fluid.

The tongue and mouth

Trauma may indicate a previous seizure, and corrosion around the mouth may indicate ingestion of a corrosive poison. Gum hyperplasia suggests that the patient may be taking phenytoin for epilepsy. Smell the breath for evidence of alcohol poisoning, diabetic ketosis, hepatic coma or uraemia. Remember that alcohol ingestion may be associated with head injury. Test the gag reflex; its absence may indicate brainstem disease or deep coma, but is not a specific sign. Bite marks on the tongue suggest that an epileptic seizure may have been the cause of unconsciousness.

The upper and lower limbs

Look for injection marks (drug addiction, diabetes mellitus). Test tone in the normal way and by picking up the arm and letting it fall. Compare each side, assessing for evidence of hemiplegia. In coma and acute cerebral hemiplegia, the muscle stretch reflexes may be normal or reduced at first on the paralysed side. Later the muscle stretch reflexes become increased and the cutaneous reflexes are absent.

Test for pain sensation by placing a pen over a distal finger or toe just below the nail bed. Press firmly and note if there is arm or leg withdrawal. Test all limbs. There will be no response to pain if sensation is absent or if the coma is deep. If sensation is intact but the limb is paralysed, there may be grimacing with movement of the other limbs.

The presence of grimacing or purposeful movements is important. Segmental reflexes alone can cause the limb to move in response to pain.

The body

Look for signs of trauma. Examine the heart, lungs and abdomen.

The urine

Note whether there is incontinence. Test the urine for glucose and ketones (diabetic ketoacidosis), protein (uraemia) and blood (trauma).

The blood glucose

Always prick the finger, place a drop of blood on an impregnated test strip, and test for hypoglycaemia or hyperglycaemia. If this cannot be done immediately, give the patient a bolus of intravenous glucose anyway (which will not usually harm the patient in diabetic ketoacidosis, but will save the life of a patient with hypoglycaemia). If there is any suspicion of Wernicke's encephalopathy, thiamine must be given as well.

The temperature

Hypothermia (e.g. exposure or hypothyroidism) or fever (e.g. meningitis) must be looked for.

Stomach contents

While protecting the airway, examine stomach contents by inserting a nasogastric tube and washing out the stomach if a drug overdose is suspected, or if no other diagnosis is obvious.

Coma scale

It is most useful to score the depth of coma, as changes in the level of consciousness can then be judged more objectively (Table 11.42).

Summary

Examining the nervous system: a suggested method (Figure 11.111)

Handedness, orientation and speech

Ask the patient if he or she is right- or left-handed. As a screening assessment, ask for the patient's name, present location and the date. Next ask the patient to name an object pointed at and have him or her point to a named object in the room, to test for dysphasia. Ask the patient to say 'British Constitution' to test for dysarthria.

Neck stiffness and Kernig's sign

Ask the patient to lie flat and attempt gently to flex the head by placing a hand under the occiput. Flex the patient's hip with the knee bent and then attempt to straighten the leg.

Cranial nerves

The patient should sit over the edge of the bed if possible. Begin by general inspection of the head and neck looking for craniotomy scars, neurofibromas, facial asymmetry, ptosis, proptosis, skew deviation of the eyes or inequality of the pupils.

The second nerve. Test visual acuity with the patient wearing his or her spectacles. Each eye is tested separately, while the other is covered with a small card.

Examine the visual fields by confrontation using a hat pin or fingers. The examiner's head should be level with the patient's head. Each eye is tested separately. If visual acuity is very poor, the fields are mapped using the fingers.

Look into the fundi.

The third, fourth and sixth nerves. Look at the pupils, noting the shape, relative sizes and any associated ptosis. Use a pocket torch and shine the light from the side to gauge the reaction of the pupils to light. Assess quickly both the direct and consensual responses. Look for an afferent pupillary defect by moving the torch in an arc from pupil to pupil. Test accommodation by asking the patient to look into the distance and then at the hat pin or finger held about 30 cm from the nose.

Assess eye movements with both eyes first, getting the patient to follow the pin in each direction. Look for failure of movement and for nystagmus. Ask about diplopia in each direction.

The fifth nerve. Test the corneal reflexes gently and ask the patient if the touch of the cottonwool on the cornea can be felt. The sensory component of this reflex is V and the motor component VII.

Test facial sensation in the three divisions: ophthalmic, maxillary and mandibular. Test pain sensation with the pin first and map any area of sensory loss from dull to sharp. Test light touch as well so that sensory dissociation can be detected if present.

Examine the motor division of the fifth nerve by asking the patient to clench the teeth while you feel the masseter muscles. Then get the patient to open the mouth while you attempt to force it closed; this is not possible if the pterygoid muscles are working. A unilateral lesion causes the jaw to deviate towards the weak (affected) side.

Test the jaw jerk. This is increased in cases of pseudobulbar palsy.

The seventh nerve. Test the muscles of facial expression. Ask the patient to look up and wrinkle the forehead. Look for loss of wrinkling and feel the muscle strength by pushing down on each side. This is preserved in upper motor neurone lesions because of bilateral cortical representation of these muscles.

Next ask the patient to shut the eyes tightly and compare the two sides. Tell the patient to grin and compare the nasolabial grooves.

The eighth nerve. Softly whisper a number 60 cm away from each ear. Examine the external auditory canals and the eardrums if this is indicated.

The ninth and tenth nerves. Look at the palate and note any uvular displacement. Ask the patient to say 'Ah' and look for symmetrical movement of the soft palate. With a unilateral lesion the uvula is drawn towards the unaffected (normal) side. Test gently for sensation on the palate (the ninth nerve). Ask the patient to speak to assess hoarseness, and to cough. A bovine cough suggests bilateral recurrent laryngeal nerve lesions.

The twelfth nerve. While examining the mouth, inspect the tongue for wasting and fasciculation. Next ask the patient to protrude the tongue. With a unilateral lesion the tongue deviates towards the weaker (affected) side.

The eleventh nerve. Look for torticollis. Ask the patient to shrug the shoulders and feel the trapezius as you push the shoulders down. Then ask the patient to turn the head against resistance and also feel the bulk of the sternomastoid. Then examine the skull and auscultate for carotid bruits.

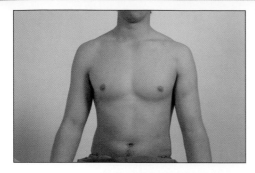

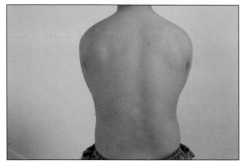

Figure 11.111 The nervous system examination

1 HIGHER CENTRES EXAMINATION GUIDE

Lying or sitting

1 **General inspection**
Obvious cranial nerve or limb lesions
Ask patient about handedness, level of education
Shake hands

2 **Orientation**
Time
Place
Person

3 **Speech**
Name objects (nominal dysphasia)

4 **Parietal lobes**
Dominant (Gerstmann's syndrome)
- Acalculia—(mental arithmetic)
- Agraphia (write)
- Left–right disorientation
- Finger agnosia (name fingers)
Non-dominant
- Dressing apraxia
Both
- Sensory inattention
- Visual inattention
- Cortical sensory loss (loss of graphaesthesia, two-point discrimination, joint position sense and stereognosis)
- Constructional apraxia

5 **Memory (temporal lobe)**
Short-term (e.g. names of flowers)
Long-term

6 **Frontal lobe**
Reflexes—grasp—pout—palmar mental
Proverb interpretation
Smell
Fundi
Gait

7 **Other**
Visual fields
Bruits
Blood pressure, etc.

2 NECK STIFFNESS AND KERNIG'S SIGN

3 CRANIAL NERVES
- II Visual acuity and fields; fundoscopy
- III IV VI Pupils and eye movements
- V Corneal reflexes
- VII Facial muscles
- VIII Hearing
- IX X Palate and gag
- XI Trapezius and sternomastoids
- XII Tongue

4 UPPER LIMBS EXAMINATION GUIDE

1 **General inspection** (patient sitting to begin with)
Scars
Skin (e.g. neurofibromata, café-au-lait)
Abnormal movements

2 **Shake hands**

3 **Motor system**
Inspect arms, shoulder girdle—extend both arms
- Wasting
- Fasciculation
- Tremor
- Drift
Palpate
- Muscle bulk
- Muscle tenderness
Tone
- Wrist
- Elbow
Power
- Shoulder
- Elbow
- Wrist
- Fingers
- Ulnar, median nerve function
Reflexes
- Biceps
- Triceps
- Supinator
- Finger
Coordination
- Finger–nose test—intention tremor, past-pointing
- Dysdiadochokinesis
- Rebound

4 **Sensory system**
Pain (pinprick)
Vibration (128 Hz tuning fork)
Proprioception—distal interphalangeal joint (each hand)
Light touch (cottonwool)

5 **Other**
Thickened nerves (wrist, elbow)
Axillae
Neck
Lower limbs
Cranial nerves
Urine analysis, etc.

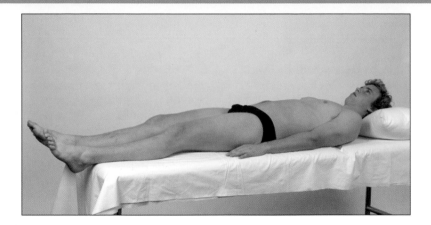

5   LOWER LIMBS EXAMINATION GUIDE

Patient lying
1   **General inspection**
    Scars, skin
    Urinary catheter
2   **Gait**
3   **Motor system**
    Inspect
    • Wasting
    • Fasciculation
    • Tremor
    Palpate
    • Muscle bulk
    • Muscle tenderness
    Tone
    • Knee—and test for clonus
    • Ankle—and test for clonus
    Power
    • Hip
    • Knee
    • Ankle
    • Foot

Reflexes
    • Knee
    • Ankle
    • Plantar
Coordination
    • Heel–shin test
    • Toe–finger test
    • Foot tapping test
4   **Sensory system**
    Pain
    Vibration
    Proprioception
    • Light touch
5   **Saddle region sensation**
6   **Anal reflex**
7   **Back**
    Deformity
    Scars
    Tenderness
    Bruits

Upper limbs

Shake the patient's hand firmly. Ask him or her to sit over the side of the bed facing you, if possible.

Examine the *motor system* systematically every time. Inspect first for wasting (both proximally and distally) and fasciculations. Don't forget to include the shoulder girdle in your inspection.

Ask the patient to hold both hands out (palms up) with the arms extended and close the eyes. Look for drifting of one or both arms (upper motor neurone weakness, cerebellar lesion or posterior column loss). Also note any tremor, or pseudoathetosis due to proprioceptive loss.
• Feel the muscle bulk next, both proximally and distally, and note any muscle tenderness.
• Test tone at the wrists and elbows by passively moving the joints at varying velocities.
• Assess power at the shoulders, elbows, wrists and fingers.

• If indicated, test for an ulnar nerve lesion (Froment's sign) and a median nerve lesion (pen-touching test).
• Examine the reflexes: biceps (C5, C6), triceps (C7, C8) and brachioradialis (C5, C6).
• Assess coordination with finger–nose testing and look for dysdiadochokinesis and rebound.
Motor weakness can be due to an upper motor neurone lesion, a lower motor neurone lesion or a myopathy. If there is evidence of a lower motor neurone lesion, consider anterior horn cell, nerve root or brachial plexus lesions, peripheral nerve lesions or a motor peripheral neuropathy.

Examine the *sensory system* after motor testing, because this can be time-consuming.

First test the spinothalamic pathway (pain and temperature). Demonstrate to the patient the sharpness of a pin on the anterior chest wall or forehead. Then ask him or her to close the eyes and tell you if the sensation is sharp or dull. Start proximally and test each dermatome. Map the abnormal area. As you are assessing, try to fit any sensory loss into dermatomal (cord or nerve root lesion), peripheral nerve, peripheral neuropathy (glove) or hemisensory (cortical or cord) distribution. It is not usually necessary to test temperature.

Next test the posterior column pathway (vibration and proprioception). Use a 128 Hz tuning fork to assess vibration sense. Place the vibrating fork on a distal interphalangeal joint when the patient has the eyes closed and ask whether it can be felt. If so, ask the patient to tell you when the vibration ceases and then, after a short wait, stop the vibrations. If the patient has deficient sensation, test at the wrist, then elbow, then at the shoulder.

Examine proprioception first with the distal interphalangeal joint of the little finger. When the patient has the eyes open grasp the distal phalanx from the sides and move it up and down to demonstrate, then ask the patient to close the eyes; repeat the manoeuvre. Normally, movement through even a few degrees is detectable, and the patient can tell whether it is up or down. If there is an abnormality, test larger movements and then proceed to test the wrist and elbows similarly if necessary.

Test light touch with cottonwool. Touch the skin lightly (do not stroke) in each dermatome.

Feel for thickened nerves—the ulnar at the elbow, the median at the wrist and the radial at the wrist—and feel the axillae if there is evidence of a proximal lesion. Note any scars, and finally examine the neck if relevant.

Lower limbs

Test the stance and gait first if possible. Then put the patient in bed with the legs entirely exposed. Place a towel over the groin—note whether a urinary catheter is present.

Look for muscle wasting and fasciculations. Note any tremor. Feel the muscle bulk of the quadriceps and run your hand up each shin, feeling for wasting of the anterior tibial muscles.

Test tone at the knees and ankles. Test clonus at this time. Push the lower end of the quadriceps sharply down towards the knee. Sustained rhythmical contractions indicate an upper motor neurone lesion. Also test the ankle by sharply dorsiflexing the foot with the knee bent and the thigh externally rotated.

Assess power next at the hips, knees and ankles.

Elicit the reflexes: knee (L3, L4), ankle (S1, S2) and plantar response (L5, S1, S2).

Test coordination with the heel–shin test, toe–finger test and tapping of the feet.

Examine the sensory system as for the upper limbs: pinprick, then vibration and proprioception, and then light touch. If there is a peripheral sensory loss, attempt to establish a sensory level by moving the pin up the leg and onto the abdomen and, if necessary, onto the chest. Examine sensation in the saddle region and test the anal reflex (S2, S3, S4).

Go to the back. Look for deformity, scars and neurofibromas. Palpate for tenderness over the vertebral bodies and auscultate for bruits. Perform the straight leg-raising test.

References

1. Sturm JW, Donnan GA. Diagnosis and investigation of headache. *Aust Fam Phys* 1998; 27:587–589. An accurate clinical history is the key to diagnosing the cause of headache.

2. Marks DR, Rapoport AM. Practical evaluation and diagnosis of headache. *Seminars in Neurology* 1997; 17: 307–312. The history should include information about the onset, intensity, associated autonomic symptoms and trigger factors of headache. Special attention must be paid to the frequency of analgesic use, both prescription and over-the-counter, to identify analgesic rebound headache.

3. Hellmann D. Temporal arteritis: a cough, headache and tongue infarction. *JAMA* 2002; 287:2996–3000.

4. Smetana GW, Shmerling RH. Does this patient have temporal arteritis? *JAMA* 2002; 287:92–101.

5. Froehling DA, Silverstein MD, Mohr DN, Beatty CW. Does this dizzy patient have a serious form of vertigo? *JAMA* 1994; 271:385–388. Helps the clinician distinguish vertigo from other causes of dizziness.

6. Thomas KE, Hasbun R, Jekel J et al. The diagnostic accuracy of Kernig's sign, Brudzinski's sign, and nuchal rigidity in adults with suspected meningitis. *Clin Infect Dis* 2002; 35:46–52.

7. Steinberg D. Scientific neurology and the history of the clinical examination of the cranial nerves. *Semin Neurol* 2002; 22:349–356. An interesting historical review that explains the background to the modern understanding of cranial nerve function and structure.

8. McGee S, *Evidence-based physical diagnosis*, 2nd edn. St Louis: Saunders, 2007.

9. Levin DE. The clinical significance of spontaneous pulsations of the retinal vein. *Arch Neurol* 1978; 35:37–40. Elevated intracranial pressure is excluded if pulsations are observed in the retinal veins. However, the absence of pulsations in the retinal veins does not necessarily mean that intracranial pressure is elevated.

10. Nelson KR. Use new pins for each neurologic examination [Letter]. *New Engl J Med* 1986; 314:581. A cautionary tale.

11. Ruffin et al. Gag reflex in disease [Letter]. *Chest* 1987; 92:1130. This suggests that many normal people may have an absent gag reflex.

12. Freeman C, Okun MS. Origins of the sensory examination in neurology. *Semin Neurol* 2002; 22:399–407

13. Medical Research Council. *Aids to the investigation of peripheral nerve injury*. London: Her Majesty's Stationery Office, 1972. Presents, in a clear and straightforward manner, bedside methods for testing the innervation of all important muscles. An invaluable guide.

14. Katz JN, Larson MG, Sabra A et al. The carpal tunnel syndrome: diagnostic utility of the history and physical examination findings. *Ann Intern Med* 1990; 112:321–327. Unfortunately, individual symptoms and signs have limited diagnostic usefulness. Tinel's sign appears to be of little value.

15. D'Arcy DA, McGee S. The rational clinical examination. Does this patient have carpal tunnel syndrome? *JAMA* 2000; 283:3110–3117. Weak thumb abduction and self-reported sensory symptoms (drawn on a diagram) are useful to predict abnormal median nerve conduction testing.

16. Schwartz RS et al. A comparison of two methods of eliciting the ankle jerk. *Aust NZ J Med* 1990; 20:116–119. The ankle jerk can be tested by tapping the sole of the foot.

17. Lance JW. The Babinski sign. *J Neurol Neurosurg Psychiatry* 2002; 73(4):360–362 A clear explanation of the history and clinical relevance of this most important of neurological signs.

18. Damasio AR. Aphasia. *N Engl J Med* 1992; 326:531–539. A very detailed review.

19. Anonymous. Forgotten symptoms and primitive signs. *Lancet* 1987; 1:841–842. This puts many of the frontal lobe signs into perspective and suggests they are sometimes only of historical interest.

20. Goldstein LB, Matchar DB. Clinical assessment of stroke (the Rational Clinical Examination). *JAMA* 1994; 271:1114–1120. Discusses the limitations of physical examination in identifying the lesion.

21. Sauve JS, Laupacis A, Ostbyte T et al. Does this patient have a clinically important carotid bruit? (The Rational Clinical Examination.) *JAMA* 1993; 270:2843–2846. Describes how to interpret the findings of a carotid bruit. Distinguishing high grade from moderate symptomatic carotid stenosis based on the bruit itself is difficult and the absence of a bruit does not mean the absence of a significant carotid stenosis.

22. Scherer K, Bedlack RS, Simel DL. Does this patient have myasthenia gravis? *JAMA* 2005; 293:1906–1914. Speech failure when speaking over a prolonged period and the Peek test increased the likelihood of myasthenia; their absence was unhelpful.

23. Rao G, Fisch L, Srinivason S et al. Does this patient have Parkinson disease? *JAMA* 2003; 289:347–353. Rigidity, the glabella tap and walking (heel–toe) seem to be useful signs of Parkinsonism.

Suggested reading

Fuller G. *Neurological examination made easy*, 4th edn. Edinburgh: Churchill Livingstone, 2008.

Gates P. The rule of 4 of the brainstem: a simplified method for understanding brainstem anatomy and brainstem vascular syndrome for the non-neurologist. *Intern Med J 2005*; 35:263–266. A simple method is described to localise brainstem vascular syndromes.

Khaw PT, Elkinton AR, eds. *ABC of eyes*, 4th edn. London: BMJ Publishing Group, 2004.

Morris JGL. *The neurological short case*, 2nd edn. London: Edward Arnold, 2005.

Rae-Grant AD. *Weiner and Levitt's Neurology*, 8th edn. Philadelphia: Lippincott, Williams & Wilkins, 2008.

Chapter 12

The psychiatric history and mental state examination

Law number four: the patient is the one with the disease.

House of God: Samuel Shem

This chapter deals with the psychiatric history and the mental state examination. The practising clinician must have an understanding of psychiatric illness and know how to perform a psychiatric interview and a mental state examination. This is because there is considerable overlap between psychiatric and physical illness.

Psychiatric disorders (especially anxiety and depression) are common, and people suffering from these conditions often have medical problems. Appropriate management of these patients will require an understanding of the intercurrent psychiatric disorder and the effect of that disorder on the primary medical problem. A medical illness may, in some instances, present as a psychiatric illness. For example, some endocrine disorders, such as myxoedema, may present with depression. On the other hand, some psychiatric disorders may present medically. Panic disorder (or acute anxiety) may be mistaken for an acute myocardial infarction. Furthermore, a patient's psychological state may interfere with the course of a medical illness; it may lead in some cases to exaggeration of the symptoms and in others to denial of the severity of physical symptoms.

The psychiatric history generally follows the same format as the standard medical history, and the principles described in Chapters 1 and 2 apply just as much here as in any history taking.[1] One should inquire about the history of the present illness, the past psychiatric and medical history, and the social and family history. However, the psychiatric history aims to elicit more detail about the patient's illness from a broad perspective, focusing not only on symptoms but also on the patient's social background, psychological functioning and life circumstances (a biopsychosocial approach). There is, therefore, more attention paid to the developmental, personal and social history than is normal for a standard medical history.

The method of psychiatric history taking is somewhat different from the standard medical interview. The psychiatric interview aims to be therapeutic as well as diagnostic. In the course of the interview it is hoped that the patient will be able to talk about his or her problems and their context. In doing so, patients will gain some relief from their distress by airing their problems. For this to take place, the clinician's attitude needs to be unhurried, patient and understanding. The psychiatric history also aims to gain an understanding of how the patient's problem arose from a biological, interpersonal, social and psychological perspective, so that the best management plan can be worked out.

Obtaining the history

The clinician taking a psychiatric history wants the patient to tell his or her story in his or her own words. In this way the patient will be more likely to report the most important aspects of the illness. This is best achieved using a non-directive approach with open-ended questions. Open-ended questions are those to which the patient will respond with narrative (or a description about what has been happening) rather than a simple factual response. They give the patient an opportunity to talk about his or her problems. Closed questions are more likely to elicit 'yes' or 'no' responses. For example, in the assessment of a patient with depression, a closed question would be: 'Have you been depressed?' An open-ended question would be: 'Tell me about how you have been feeling.' At first glance it might appear that the open-ended question is less efficient, as it could take a longer time to find out about a range of symptoms. However, with a careful and judicious approach, open-ended questioning—by permitting the patient to tell the story—will enable the clinician to get a comprehensive history efficiently. This is not to say that targeted, more-closed questions must not be used—they are necessary to elicit certain symptoms.

While the patient is telling his or her story, the clinician should begin to formulate hypotheses about the problem or diagnosis. These hypotheses are tested by asking more-focused questions later in the interview, at which point a diagnostic hypothesis can be rejected or pursued further. For example, a patient may describe tiredness and lethargy, an inability to concentrate and loss of appetite. These symptoms will suggest a diagnosis of depression. Follow-up questions should focus on this possibility. The clinician should ask questions about other symptoms of depression such as: 'How have you been feeling in yourself?', 'What has your mood been like?' and 'How have you been sleeping?'

Introductory questions

The psychiatric interview should start off with non-threatening questions. After introducing yourself, it can be useful to begin by asking about basic demographic information (age, marital state, occupation, whom the patient lives with) and then making the patient feel at ease by discussing some neutral topic.

History of the presenting illness

In assessing the history of the presenting illness, one needs to cover a number of areas.

1. The problem

Find out the nature of the patient's problem, and the patient's perception of his or her difficulties. This can, of course, be difficult if the patient is psychotic and does not believe a problem exists at all. In these cases a corroborative history must be taken. For example, a manic patient may consider that there is nothing wrong and that his or her behaviour is reasonable, whereas his or her partner is able to recognise that ordering an expensive new sports car when the family is impoverished is a problem.

A range of symptoms commonly found in psychiatric disorders needs to be reviewed in the course of assessing the history of the present illness. These include mood change, anxiety, worry, sleep pattern, appetite, hallucinations and delusions. A set of simple screening questions for each of the major diagnoses is listed within Table 12.1. It is especially useful to ask about symptoms of anxiety and depression (the most common psychiatric disorders). The definitions of other symptoms are given in Table 12.2. It is important to ask about drug usage (legal and illegal) as well as alcohol and caffeine (which may be associated with anxiety disorders).

2. Precipitating events

Psychiatric illness rarely occurs for no reason and there is generally an event that has precipitated the illness. Such events include a range of experiences which may have affected the patient, or a member of the patient's social network. Events such as physical illness, drug treatment or treatment non-compliance may be implicated as precipitants. The last-mentioned is important, as patients with

---

TABLE 12.1 The common psychiatric disorders* and their screening questions

MOOD (AFFECTIVE) DISORDERS

Mood disorders have a pathological disturbance in mood (depression or mania) as the predominant feature. They are distinguished from 'normal' mood changes by their persistence, duration and severity, together with the presence of other symptoms and impairment of functioning.

1. Manic-depressive illness—bipolar disorder

Bipolar disorder is a broad term to describe a recurrent illness characterised by episodes of either mania or depression, with a return to normal functioning between episodes of illness.

a. Mania	Questions box 12.1
A disorder demonstrated by change in mood (*elation*), thought form (*grandiosity*) and behaviour disturbance (*increased energy and disinhibition*).	**Questions to ask the patient with possible mania**
Frequently associated symptoms: increased talkativeness, distractibility, decreased need for sleep, loss of inhibition (e.g. engaging in reckless behaviour such as spending sprees, sexual indiscretion or social overfamiliarity).	1 Have you felt especially good about yourself?
	2 Have you been needing less sleep than usual?
	3 Do you feel that you are special or that you have special powers?
	4 Have you been spending more than usual?

* Based on the WHO International Classification of Disease 10th ed (ICD-10). ICD-II will be published in 2014.

TABLE 12.1 (continued) The common psychiatric disorders* and their screening questions

b. Depression

A disorder characterised by depressed mood (or loss of pleasure) and the presence of somatic (*sleep disturbance, change in appetite, fatigue and weight*), psychological (*low self-esteem, worry- anxiety, guilt, suicidal ideation*), affective (*sadness, irritability, loss of pleasure and interest in activities*) and psychomotor (*retardation or agitation*) symptoms.

Questions box 12.2

Questions to ask the patient with possible depression

1 How have you been feeling in yourself?
2 What has your mood been like?
3 Have you been feeling sad, blue, down or depressed?
4 Have you lost interest in things you usually enjoy?
5 How have you been sleeping?

ANXIETY DISORDERS

Anxiety disorders are those in which the person experiences excessive levels of anxiety. Anxiety may be somatic (*palpitations, difficulty breathing, dry mouth, nausea, frequency of micturition, dizziness, muscular tension, sweating, abdominal churning, tremor, cold skin*) or psychological (*feelings of dread and threat, irritability, panic, anxious anticipation, inner [psychic] tension, worrying over trivia, difficulty concentrating, initial insomnia, inability to relax*).

1. Generalised anxiety disorder (GAD)

A chronic disorder characterised by a tendency to worry excessively about everyday things.
It is accompanied by: symptoms of anxiety or tension; mental tension (*feeling tense or nervous, poor concentration, on edge*); physical tension.

Questions box 12.3

Questions to ask the patient with possible anxiety

1 Have you been feeling nervy or tense?
2 Do you worry a lot about things?
3 Do you worry about things most other people would not worry about?

2. Panic disorder

A disorder characterised by episodes of panic occurring spontaneously in situations where most people would not be afraid.
A panic attack is characterised by the presence of physical symptoms (*palpitations, chest pain, a choking feeling, a churning stomach, dizziness, feelings of unreality*) or fear of some disaster (*losing control or going mad, heart attack, sudden death*). They begin suddenly, build up rapidly, and may last only a few minutes.

Questions box 12.4

Questions to ask the patient with possible panic disorder

1 Have you ever had an attack of acute anxiety or panic?
2 Did this occur in a situation in which most people would not feel afraid?
3 Can these attacks happen at any time?

3. Agoraphobia (phobic anxiety)

A disorder in which an individual avoids places (such as supermarkets or trains) in which they fear they may have a panic attack and cannot escape.

Questions box 12.5

Questions to ask the patient with possible phobic anxiety

1 Do you avoid going out?
2 Do you avoid going to places because you fear you may have an anxiety attack?

4. Obsessive–compulsive disorder

A disorder in which the person has either obsessions or compulsions which interfere with everyday life.

Questions box 12.6

Questions to ask the patient with possible obsessive–compulsive disorder

1 Are there any rituals or habits that you have to carry out every day?
2 Do they cause you problems?
3 Do you ever have a thought going round in your head that you can't get rid of?

STRESS-RELATED DISORDERS

1. Acute stress disorders

Individuals may present shortly after a traumatic event with a range of symptoms, such as *anxiety, depression, disturbed sleep, problems with memory or concentration*. Images, dreams or flashbacks of the traumatic event may also occur.

Questions box 12.7

Questions to ask the patient with possible acute stress disorder

1 Have you been having any problems following ... ?
2 Have you been feeling worried? Or depressed?
3 Have you had trouble sleeping?
4 Do you have bad memories?

* Based on the WHO International Classification of Disease 10th ed (ICD-10). ICD-II will be published in 2014.

TABLE 12.1 (continued) **The common psychiatric disorders* and their screening questions**

2. Post-traumatic stress disorder (PTSD)	**Questions box 12.8**
Onset of persistent problems within 6 months of a traumatic event of exceptional severity. The individual experiences *repetitive and intrusive re-enactments* of the trauma in images, dreams or flashbacks. *Sleep, concentration, memory, mood and attention may be disturbed.* Individuals may feel emotionally detached and avoid things that act as reminders of the traumatic event.	**Questions to ask the patient with possible PTSD** 1 Since ... happened, have you been troubled by bad memories of it? 2 Have you been having nightmares? 3 Have you had trouble with sleep? 4 Have you had trouble with your memory? 5 Are you jumpy?

SCHIZOPHRENIA AND DELUSIONAL DISORDERS

A disorder characterised by disorders of content (*presence of delusions*), thought form (*shown by difficulty understanding the connections between the patient's thoughts*), perception (*hallucinations—predominantly auditory*), behaviour (*erratic or bizarre*) and/or volition (*apathy and withdrawal*).	**Questions box 12.9**
	Questions to ask the patient with possible schizophrenia 1 Have you ever heard people speaking when there is no one around? 2 Do you ever hear voices? 3 Have you heard your thoughts out loud? 4 Do you have any thoughts or beliefs that others might find unusual or strange? 5 Have you felt people may be against you? 6 Have you felt that the TV or radio sends you messages? 7 Do you ever feel as if someone is spying on you or plotting to hurt you? 8 Do you have any ideas that you don't like to talk about because you're afraid other people will think you're mad?

ORGANIC BRAIN DISORDERS

These are disorders in which there is brain dysfunction manifested by cognitive disturbances such as memory loss or disorientation; there may be behavioural disturbance as well.

1. Delirium (acute brain syndrome)	**Questions box 12.10**
A disorder characterised by the acute onset of disturbed consciousness plus changes in cognition that are not due to a pre-existing dementia. It is a direct physiological consequence of a *general medical condition (substance intoxication or withdrawal, use of a medication, exposure to a toxin, or a combination of these factors).* Delirium is characterised by *confusion and clouding of consciousness.* This may be accompanied by *poor memory, disorientation, inattention, agitation, emotional upset, hallucinations, visions or illusions, suspiciousness and disturbed sleep (reversal of sleep pattern).*	**Questions to ask the patient with possible delirium** 1 What day is it today? 2 How long have you been here? 3 What is the name of the place we are in? 4 Do you remember my name? Mental state examination (page 416)
2. Dementia (chronic brain syndrome)	**Questions box 12.11**
A generalised impairment of intellect, memory and personality with no impairment of consciousness. Characterised by *loss of memory* (especially short-term memory), *loss of orientation and deterioration in social functioning and behaviour and emotional control* (may be easily upset—tearful or irritable).	**Questions to ask the patient with possible dementia** 1 What day is it today? 2 How long have you been here? 3 What is the name of the place we are in? 4 Do you remember my name? Mental state examination (page 416)

* Based on the WHO International Classification of Disease 10th ed (ICD-10). ICD-II will be published in 2014.

TABLE 12.1 (continued) The common psychiatric disorders* and their screening questions

OTHER DISORDERS

There are a number of other psychiatric disorders which may present with physical problems, or may be seen in an emergency department with some complication (particularly after attempted suicide).

A. Eating disorders (anorexia nervosa and bulimia nervosa)

Here the sufferer (generally female) has a disturbed body image with an unreasonable fear of being fat, and makes extensive efforts to lose weight (strict dieting, vomiting, use of purgatives, excessive exercise). She may deny that weight or eating habits are problems.

Bulimia nervosa is characterised by binge eating followed by vomiting or purging. *Anorexia nervosa* is characterised by excessive dieting, but there may also be binges followed by vomiting or purging. Anorexic patients will be grossly underweight and may show signs of malnutrition. Amenorrhoea is generally present.

Questions box 12.12

Questions to ask the patient with a possible eating disorder

1 Do you worry about your weight?
2 Do you think that you are fat?
3 Do you diet?
4 Have you ever made yourself sick after a meal?

B. Somataform disorders

1. Somatisation disorder

A disorder characterised by multiple physical complaints that cannot be satisfactorily explained by physical disease. An individual with this disorder will have complaints in several bodily systems (e.g. gastrointestinal, cardiac, respiratory, musculoskeletal, menstrual).

Questions box 12.13

Questions to ask the patient with possible somatoform disorder

1 Do you have any other medical problems?
2 Have you had symptoms that your doctor has not been able to find a cause for?
3 Are you often sick?

2. Hypochondriacal disorder

These patients fear they have a serious illness despite repeated medical reassurance. They often seek repeated medical opinions. In some cases the disorder becomes delusional, e.g. of parasitic skin infection.

Questions box 12.14

Questions to ask the patient with possible hypochondriacal disorder†

1 Have you been very worried about your health?
2 What do you think might be wrong?
3 What have your doctors told you?

3. Conversion disorder (hysteria)

These patients usually present with a neurological abnormality that is not fully explained medically. Common symptoms include: blindness, gait disturbances, sensory loss, limb paralysis and loss of speech.

Questions box 12.15

Questions to ask the patient with possible conversion disorder.

1 What have you noticed has been wrong?
2 What tests have you had?
3 What have you been told about your illness?

SUBSTANCE MISUSE

This category includes the misuse of alcohol, illegal drugs and prescription medications.

PERSONALITY DISORDERS

In these disorders the individual, while not having specific symptoms, has behavioural disturbances and problems with impulse control, interpersonal relationships and mood. Individuals who repeatedly attempt suicide often have a personality disorder. They may also have stormy illnesses, causing frequent problems for staff.

Questions box 12.16

Questions to ask the patient with a possible personality disorder

1 Have you ever tried to harm yourself?
2 Have you ever had problems with relationships?

NEURASTHENIA (CHRONIC FATIGUE SYNDROME)

This is a somewhat controversial inclusion in the current WHO classification of psychiatric disorders.

PUERPERAL MENTAL DISORDERS

This category includes post-partum depression and psychosis.

* Based on the WHO International Classification of Disease 10th ed (ICD-10). ICD-II will be published in 2014.
† Alfons Jakob (1884–1931), professor of neurology in Hamburg from 1924, had over 200 cases of neurosyphilis on his ward at a time; he died of osteomyelitis. Jakob described this cerebral atrophy in 1920 and before Hans Creutzeld (1885–1933).

TABLE 12.2 Symptoms of psychiatric illness

Affect	The observable behaviour by which a person's internal emotional state is judged.
Agitation (psychomotor agitation)	Excessive motor activity associated with a feeling of inner tension. The activity is usually non-productive and repetitive and consists of such behaviour as pacing, fidgeting, wringing the hands, pulling the clothes and inability to sit still.
Anxiety	The apprehensive anticipation of future danger or misfortune. It is associated with feelings of tension and symptoms of autonomic arousal.
Conversion symptom (hysteria)	A loss of, or alteration in, motor or sensory function. Psychological factors are judged to be associated with the development of the symptom, which is not fully explained by anatomical or pathological conditions. The symptom is the result of unconscious conflict and is not feigned.
Delusion	A false unshakable idea or belief that is out of keeping with the patient's educational, cultural and social background.
Depersonalisation	An alteration in the awareness of the self—the individual feels as if he or she is unreal.
Derealisation	An alteration in the perception or experience of the external world so that it seems unreal.
Disorientation	Confusion about the time of day, date or season (time), where one is (place) or who one is (person).
Flight of ideas	A nearly continuous flow of accelerated speech with abrupt changes from topic to topic that are usually based on understandable associations, distracting stimuli, or plays on words. When severe, speech may be disorganised or incoherent.
Grandiosity	An inflated appraisal of one's worth, power, knowledge, importance or identity. When extreme, grandiosity may be of delusional proportions.
Hallucination	A sensory perception that seems real, but occurs without external stimulation of the relevant sensory organ. The term *hallucination* is not ordinarily applied to the false perceptions that occur during dreaming, while falling asleep (*hypnagogic*) or when awakening (*hypnopompic*).
Ideas of reference	The feeling that casual incidents and external events have a particular significance and unusual meaning that is specific to the person.
Illusion	A misperception or misinterpretation of a real external stimulus.
Mood	A pervasive and sustained emotion that colours the perception of the world.
Overvalued idea	An unreasonable belief that is held, but not as strongly as a delusion (i.e. the person is able to acknowledge the possibility that the belief may not be true). The belief is not one that is ordinarily accepted by other members of the person's culture or subculture.
Personality	Enduring patterns of perceiving, relating to, and thinking about the environment and oneself.
Phobia	A persistent irrational fear of a specific object, activity or situation (the phobic stimulus) that results in a compelling desire to avoid it.
Pressured speech	Speech that is increased in amount, accelerated, and difficult or impossible to interrupt. Usually it is also loud and emphatic. Frequently the person talks without any social stimulation and may continue to talk even though no one is listening.
Psychomotor retardation	Visible generalised slowing of movements and speech.
Psychotic	Psychotic can be used to mean a loss of contact with reality, but is generally used to imply the presence of delusions or hallucinations.

Based on DSM-IV, APA 1994.[2]

psychiatric illness are often non-compliant, a major contribution to relapse.

3. Risk

An assessment of the patient's risk of harm, either to others or to him- or herself, is essential: this will indicate whether the patient needs to be treated involuntarily. Patients with psychotic illness may, in some circumstances, need to be treated involuntarily under the *Mental Health Act*. While the exact details for involuntary treatment are different under individual mental health acts, the essential features are generally that: (a) a person has a mental illness; and (b) the person is a danger to self or to others. Assessment of danger to others is difficult, with the best predictor being a history of

TABLE 12.3 Assessment of suicide risk

Suicide may be the unfortunate outcome of psychiatric illness but loss of job, family disruption, alcoholism and self-mutilation can also be the distressing result. Assessing the risk of suicide is an essential part of the psychiatric interview. Asking about this does not increase the risk or put the idea into the patient's head. It may reduce the risk, as the patient may feel relief in talking about his or her fears. The risk of suicide is assessed by asking directly whether the person has ever contemplated it.

Have you thought that life was not worth living?

Or

Have you felt so bad that you have considered ending it all?

If 'yes'...

Have you thought of killing yourself?

Have you thought how you might do this?

Have you made any plans for doing this?

TABLE 12.4 Classes of psychiatric drugs and their major indications

1 Anti-anxiety e.g. benzodiazepines, beta-blockers (control somatic symptoms)	For anxiety disorders, insomnia, alcohol withdrawal
2 Antipsychotic e.g. phenothiazine, major tranquillisers	For schizophrenia, mania, delirium
3 Antidepressants e.g. tricyclics, selective serotonin reuptake inhibitors (SSRIs)	For depression, obsessive-compulsive disorder
4 Mood-stabilising e.g. lithium, carbamazepine	For prevention of manic depression or treatment of mania

TABLE 12.5 Common side effects of the antipsychotic drugs

1 Anti-cholinergic—dry mouth, blurred vision, urinary retention, erectile dysfunction

2 Hypersensitivity reactions—photosensitivity dermatitis, cholestatic jaundice, neutrophilia (clozapine)

3 Effects due to dopamine blockade—Parkinsonism, motor restlessness (akathisia), tardive dyskinesia, dystonia, gynaecomastia, malignant neuroleptic syndrome

past threat or harm to others. It is best to err on the side of caution in such cases. Assessment of suicide risk needs to be made with sensitivity and using a direct approach, as shown in Table 12.3.

The past history and treatment history

Both the past psychiatric and medical history should be assessed. The past medical history should be evaluated in the same way as the general medical history. An assessment should be made of stresses that may have contributed to past episodes of illness, and that may have led to relapse. For the past psychiatric history, it is important to obtain not only the diagnosis but also the treatment the patient has had, and its outcome.

Ask about previous non-drug treatment including counselling, psychotherapy and electroconvulsive therapy (ECT), and whether the patient thought the treatment was effective. Was the patient ever admitted to a psychiatric unit, and for how long?

Find out what drug treatment has been tried—the class (Table 12.4) of psychiatric medication, its effectiveness and any side-effects. The antipsychotic drugs in particular have common long term side-effects (Table 12.5).

The family history

There is a familial component in many psychiatric disorders. Two aspects must be assessed in the family history.

First, the patient should be asked tactfully if anyone in the family has had any psychiatric or mental illness or has committed suicide. He or she should also be asked if anyone in the family has had any treatment for psychological problems, such as anxiety, depression, agoraphobia,[a] eating disorders or drug and alcohol problems (these last few areas are often not considered by patients to be psychiatric or mental illnesses).

Second, one should try to determine what sort of family the patient grew up in. Drawing up a family tree is a useful way of finding this out. Factual details about each family member can be included in this family tree (age, mental state, health). In the psychiatric history we also need to know about what type of person each family member is, and how family members get on with each other. It is worth exploring how much care (or neglect) the patient received from each parent, and how controlling or protective each was. These two factors have been shown to be important in contributing to psychiatric illness. One needs to ask about the quality of the parental relationship and the general family atmosphere.

Childhood abuse (physical or sexual)[3] may be an important predisposing event for many illnesses, and should be inquired about. This can be elicited

---

[a] From the Greek, meaning 'fear of the market place'.

by saying something like 'Sometimes children can have had some unpleasant experiences—I wonder if you had any? Did anyone ever harm you? ... or hit you? ... How about interfering with you sexually? ... Could you tell me more about that and what happened?'

Taking a detailed family history in this way sets the scene for the patient's developmental history, which should be taken next.

The social and personal history

Open-ended questions are again the best way to obtain the personal and social history. Ask the patient something like 'Could you tell me a bit about your background, your development, what sort of childhood you had, what are the important things you remember from your childhood?', and then allow the patient to tell his or her own story. During the course of this narrative, the patient may require some prompting to add information about important issues such as the birth history (schizophrenia is known to be associated with perinatal morbidity) and early development, and whether there were significant problems in early childhood, such as head injuries or serious infections. How did the patient cope with early separations, particularly when starting primary school and going on to secondary school (difficulty in separation may be a risk factor for panic disorder or abnormal illness behaviour). The patient should be asked about peer relationships, friendships, school, academic ability, adolescence and teenage relationships. The adult history should focus predominantly on the quality of intimate relationships and the social support network, especially whether there are people in whom the patient can confide.

The patient's living circumstances should be asked about in the same way as for a medical history. There should also be a focus on the patient's occupation: not only on the type of job but also on how he or she copes with work or, if he or she does not work, how that is coped with.

Premorbid personality

An assessment should be made of the patient's premorbid personality. Ask the patient to describe him- or herself. The personality can be described using the predominant trait, such as obsessional, nervy or highly strung; it is not necessary to use official systems to describe a patient's personality. In the assessment of premorbid personality it is important to evaluate both positive and negative aspects of the person, how he or she copes adaptively and maladaptively to life stress, what type of

interests he or she has, and what other strengths and weaknesses are present.

The mental state examination

While assessing the patient, one should carefully make observations about appearance, behaviour, patterns of speech, attitude to the examiner and ways of interacting. These observations are brought together in a systematic fashion in the mental state examination. This is not something that is 'done' at the conclusion of taking a history; it is an essential part of the total process of assessing the patient.[4]

However, there are a number of tests that need to be conducted in a formalised way as part of the mental state examination. These include assessing the cognitive state (orientation, memory, attention, registration) and inquiring about perceptual disturbances and, in some cases, disorders of thought. The mental state examination provides valuable diagnostic information; with some disorders, it is this examination which gives most of the diagnostic clues.

The headings under which the mental state is recorded are shown in Table 12.6, together with some simple bedside tests for assessing cognitive function. Also shown in Table 12.6 are some abnormal features of the mental state examination that are commonly found in psychiatric disorders.

When cognitive dysfunction is suspected, as in patients with dementia,[5] a more detailed examination of cognitive function should be carried out. A widely used tool for doing this is the minimental state examination,[6] which assesses aspects of orientation, memory and concentration. Details of this examination are shown in Table 12.7. Some of the common causes of delirium and dementia are listed in Tables 12.8 and 12.9.

The diagnosis

At the conclusion of the psychiatric history, which should include a general physical examination, a provisional diagnosis and formulation should be made. Essentially, the diagnostic formulation is a means of pulling together, in a succinct yet comprehensive manner, your understanding of the patient's problem.

Psychiatric disorders generally arise through a combination of biological, psychological and psychosocial factors, and each of these needs to be considered when a patient's problem is being assessed (a biopsychosocial approach). The patient's problem needs to be understood longitudinally, by defining biophysical factors that may have predisposed to the illness and, more immediately, may have precipitated the illness,

TABLE 12.6 The mental state examination

	What is assessed, described or observed	Common findings indicating psychopathology	Types of illness
General description			
Appearance	A general description of the patient's appearance, including body build, posture, clothing (appropriateness), grooming (e.g. make-up) and hygiene. Note any physical stigmata (e.g. tattoos) and facial expression (depression, apprehension, worry, etc).	Bizarre appearance	Psychotic disorders (schizophrenia, mania), personality disorder
		Unkempt, poorly groomed	Schizophrenia, depression
		Apprehensive, anxious	Anxiety disorders
		Over-bright clothing	Mania
		Scarred wrists, tattoos	Personality disorder
Behaviour	All aspects of the patient's behaviour. Note the appropriateness of the patient's behaviour within the interview context..	Uncooperative behaviour	Psychotic disorder, personality disorder
	Abnormal motor behaviour: mcnnerisms, stereotyped movements, tics.	Manneristic behaviour	Psychotic disorder
	Variants of normal motor behaviour: restlessness, psychomotor change (agitation, retardation).	Stereotypic behaviour	Psychotic disorders,developmental disability, organic syndromes
		Bizarre behaviour	Psychotic disorders
		Assaultive, threatening	Personality disorders, intoxication, neuro-logical disorders
		Restlessness	Akathisia from antipsychotic medication
		Psychomotor change	Depression
Attitude towards examiner	The way the patient responds to the interviewer, the level of cooperation, willingness to disclose information. A range of attitudes and deviation from appropriateness may occur, ranging from hostility to seductiveness.	Uncooperative attitude, belligerence	Psychotic disorder, personality disorder
		Seductiveness	Personality disorder
Mood and affect			
Mood	A relatively persistent emotional state: describe the depth, intensity, duration and fluctuations of mood. Mood may be neutral, euphoric, depressed, anxious or irritable.	Depressed	Depression
		Anxious/irritable	Depression/anxiety disorders
Affect	The way a patient conveys his cr her emotional state. Affect may be full, blunted, restricted or inappropriate.	Depressed	Depression
		Blunted, restricted	Schizophrenia
Appropriateness	Are the patient's responses appropriate to the matter being discussed?	Inappropriate	Schizophrenia
Speech	The tempo, modulation and quality of the patient's speech should be described here. Note should be made of dysphasia or dysarthria (see Chapter 11).	Increased tempo	Mania, acute schizophrenia
		Slowed	Depression

TABLE 12.6 The mental state examination

	What is assessed, described or observed	Common findings indicating psychopathology	Types of illness
Mood and affect (continued)			
Perceptual disturbances	The presence of hallucinations (auditory, visual, gustatory or tactile) should be noted. It is important to check whether they occurred with a clear sensorium.	Visual hallucinations	Acute brain syndrome, epilepsy, alcohol withdrawal, drug intoxication
	Hypnagogic or hypnopompic hallucinations are normal experiences. Other perceptual disturbances (e.g. illusions, depersonalisation or derealisation) should be noted.	Auditory	Schizophrenia
		Tactile/gustatory	Epilepsy, schizophrenia
Thought			
Thought form	The process of the patient's thinking. This involves the quantity of ideas (pressured thought, poverty of ideas) and the way in which the ideas (thoughts) are produced.	Disorder of thought form	Schizophrenia
	Are they logical and relevant, or are they fragmented and irrelevant? The link between ideas should be assessed—do they flow logically, or are they disconnected and 'fragmented'? Are ideas connected by spurious concepts (rhyming, the way they sound—'clang' associations)?	Flight of ideas	Mania, schizophrenia
		Poverty of ideas	Schizophrenia, mania, depression
Thought content	The content of the patient's thought. Abnormalities range from preoccupation, obsessions, overvalued ideas to delusions. Themes should also be assessed: suicidal or homicidal thoughts or paranoid ideas. In the medical setting, preoccupation with illness (hypochondriacal thoughts) should be assessed, as well as thoughts of omnipotence—denying illness when it is present.	Delusions	Schizophrenia, mania, depression
Sensorium and cognition Listed below are bedside tests for a basic assessment of cognitive function. If abnormalities are detected, a full mini-mental state examination (Table 12.7) should be carried out.			
Alertness and level of consciousness	The level of consciousness should be assessed. Clouding or fluctuating levels of consciousness should be noted.	Clouding	Delirium
Orientation	Orientation to time, place and person. Ask the day, date, month and year. Ask where he or she is, and if he or she knows who he or she is.	Disorientation	Dementia, delirium
Short-term memory	Short-term memory refers to the ability to retain information over a period of 3–5 minutes. Less than this refers to immediate recall. Ask the patient to recall a list of three objects after 3–5 minutes.	Loss of short-term memory	Dementia, delirium

TABLE 12.6 The mental state examination		
Long-term memory	This refers to memory of remote events. Ask the patient to recall events of the previous few days, as well as events of a year ago.	Loss of long-term memory	Dementia
Concentration	Ask the patient to subtract 7 from 100 and keep subtracting 7, or spell 'world' backwards.	Poor concentration	Delirium, acute psychosis
General knowledge and intelligence	Ask about some recent events. Intelligence can be gauged from the language used. Ask the patient to do some simple arithmetical tasks. Literacy should be assessed.	Poor general knowledge	Dementia, delirium
Judgment and insight			
Judgment	The capacity to behave appropriately. Describe a hypothetical situation, and ask how the patient would behave in it (e.g. 'What would you do if you smelt smoke while sitting in a cinema?').	Impaired judgment	Psychoses, dementia, personality disorders
Insight	Determine whether the patient is aware that he or she has a problem, and the level of understanding of this.	Lack of insight	Psychoses, dementia

and factors that may be contributing to the person remaining ill (perpetuating factors). A simple grid can be used for assessing the patient in this manner (Table 12.10). Here biological, psychological or psychosocial factors that predispose to, precipitate or perpetuate the psychiatric illness are identified. Perpetuating factors are very important, particularly among medically ill patients, as it may be the medical or physical illness that maintains the patient's psychiatric problem. By the same token, psychological factors may perpetuate a patient's medical illness.

An example of such a formulation grid is shown in Table 12.11 for a 53-year-old man who becomes depressed after a myocardial infarction. He has a family history of depression (a genetic predisposing factor) and chronic low self-esteem (a psychological predisposing factor), which he coped with by succeeding in business. He has few friends and his marriage is unsatisfactory (a psychosocial factor). He had his infarct one week after he heard that he would not be promoted at work (a psychological factor) and his job was at risk (a psychosocial precipitant). His insecurity about work and his failing marriage, together with his low self-esteem, is maintaining his illness, as are the biological changes to the neurotransmitter system.

Understanding the patient in this manner helps one to plan an effective management approach that will focus on all the relevant factors, so that, for the patient in this example, a combination of antidepressants, marital counselling and assertiveness training (to build self-esteem) can be organised.

A good psychiatric history will provide a comprehensive understanding of the patient and will permit appropriate management to be planned. This is immensely rewarding for the clinician, and will also be of considerable benefit to the patient.

TABLE 12.7 The mini-mental state examination

	Score	Max
Orientation		
'What is the (year) (season) (date) (day) (month)?' Ask for the date, then specifically inquire about parts omitted (e.g. season). Score 1 point for each correct answer.	☐	5
'Where are we (country) (state) (town) (hospital) (ward)?' Ask in turn for each place. Score 1 point for each correct answer.	☐	5
Registration		
'May I test your memory?' Repeat three objects (e.g. pen, watch, book). Score 1 point for each correct answer.	☐	3
Then repeat until the patient learns all three. Count trials and record (up to six).		
Attention and calculation		
'Count backwards from 100 by sevens' (serial 7s). One point for each answer, up to five (93, 86, 79, 72, 65)		
Or		
Spell 'world' backwards. Score 1 point for each letter in correct order.	☐	5
Recall		
Ask the patient to recall the three objects in 'registration', above. Score 1 point for each correct answer.	☐	3
Language		
Ask the patient to name two objects shown (e.g. pen and watch). Score 0–2 points.	☐	2
'Repeat the following: "No ifs, ands or buts".' Score 1 point.	☐	1
Ask the patient to follow a three-stage command: e.g. 'Take this paper in your right hand, fold it in half and put it on the table.' Score 1 point for each step.	☐	3
Read and obey the following:		
CLOSE YOUR EYES. Score 1 point.	☐	1
WRITE A SENTENCE. Do not dictate—must be sensible, but punctuation and grammar are not essential. Score 1 point.	☐	1
'Copy this design.'		
All ten angles must be present, and the two must intersect. Score 1 point.	☐	1
TOTAL	☐	30

Assess patient's level of consciousness along a continuum:

Alert	**Drowsy**	**Stuporose**	**Coma**

Scores of 21–29 indicate mild cognitive impairment. Scores below 20 indicate more severe cognitive impairment, and are likely to be due to dementia, especially if obtained on repeated examinations.

TABLE 12.8 Common causes of delirium

Drug intoxication	Alcohol Anxiolytics Digoxin L-dopa 'Street drugs'
Withdrawal states	Alcohol (delirium tremens) Anxiolytic sedatives
Metabolic disturbance	Uraemia Liver failure Anoxia Cardiac failure Electrolyte imbalance Postoperative states
Endocrine disturbance	Diabetic ketosis Hypoglycaemia
Systemic infections	Pneumonia Urinary tract infection Septicaemia Viral infections
Intracranial infection	Encephalitis Meningitis
Other intracranial causes	Space-occupying lesions Raised intracranial pressure
Head injury	Subdural haemorrhage Cerebral contusion Concussion
Nutritional and vitamin deficiency	Thiamine (Wernicke's encephalopathy) Vitamin B_{12} Nicotinic acid
Epilepsy	Status epilepticus Post-ictal states

TABLE 12.9 Common causes of dementia

Degenerative type	Senile dementia of Alzheimer's Front temporal dementia* Huntington's chorea Parkinson's disease Normal-pressure hydrocephalus Multiple sclerosis
Hereditable Alzheimer's	Mutation of presenilin-1
Intracranial space-occupying lesions	Tumour Subdural haematomas
Traumatic	Head injuries Boxing encephalopathy
Infections and related conditions	Encephalitis Neurosyphilis HIV (AIDS dementia) Jacob-Creutzfeldt disease
Vascular	Multi-infarct dementia Carotid artery occlusion
Metabolic	Uraemia Hepatic failure
Toxic	Alcoholic dementia Heavy-metal poisoning
Anoxia	Anaemia Carbon monoxide poisoning Cardiac arrest Chronic respiratory failure
Vitamin deficiency	Vitamin B_{12} Folic acid Thiamine (Wernicke–Korsakoff's syndrome)
Endocrine	Myxoedema Addison's disease

* Slowing of thought, relative sensory presentation.

TABLE 12.10 A formulation grid

	Predisposing	Precipitating	Perpetuating
Biological			
Psychological			
Psychosocial			

TABLE 12.11 A completed formulation grid (see text)

	Predisposing	Precipitating	Perpetuating
Biological	Genetic predisposition	Acute myocardial infarct	Neurotransmitter changes
Psychological	Low self-esteem	Not promoted	Low self-esteem and insecurity
Psychosocial	Poor social support Dysfunctional marriage		Dysfunctional marriage

References

1. Kopelman MD. Structured psychiatric interview: psychiatric history and assessment of the mental state. *Br J Hosp Med* 1994; 52:93–98.

2. American Psychiatric Association. *Diagnostic and Statistical Manual of Mental Disorders*, 4th edn. Washington, DC: APA, 1994.

3. Drossman DA, Talley NJ, Lesserman J et al. Sexual and physical abuse and gastrointestinal illness. *Ann Intern Med* 1995; 123:782–794. A good clinical summary of the relevance of abuse to illness.

4. Davies T. The ABC of mental health. Mental health assessment. *BMJ* 1997; 314:1536–1539.

5. Johnson J, Sims R, Gottlieb G. Differential diagnosis of dementia, delirium and depression. Implications for drug therapy. *Drugs and Aging* 1994; 5:431–445. The differential diagnosis hinges on a careful clinical evaluation. Dementia is defined as a chronic loss of intellectual or cognitive function of sufficient severity to interfere with social or occupational function. Delirium is an acute disturbance of consciousness marked by an attention deficit and a change in cognitive ability.

6. Folstein MF, Folstein SE, McHugh PR. Mini Mental State. A practical method for grading the cognitive state of patients for the clinician. *J Psychiatr Res* 1975; 12:189–198.

Suggested reading

Balint M. *The doctor, his patient and the illness*, Millennium edn. New York: Churchill Livingstone, 2000.

Gleason OC. Delirium. *Am Fam Physician* 2003; 67:1027–1034.

Morgan H, Blashki G. Fits, faints and funny turns. Could it be a mental disorder? *Aust Fam Physician* 2003; 32:211–213, 216–219.

Stern TA, Fricchione GL, Cassem NH et al. *Massachusetts General Hospital handbook of general hospital psychiatry*, 5th edn. St Louis: Mosby Year Book, 2004.

Zun LS. Evidence-based evaluation of psychiatric patients. *J Emerg Med* 2005; 28:35–39.

Chapter 13

The eyes, ears, nose and throat

Diagnosis is not the end, but the beginning of practice.

Martin H Fischer

The examination of the eyes and ears, nose and throat is important for any medical patient because these small parts of the body may be involved in local or systemic disease.

The eyes

Examination anatomy (Figure 13.1)
The structure of the eye is shown in Figure 13.1. Many of these structures can be examined as outlined below.

Examination method
Sit the patient at the edge of the bed. Stand well back from the patient at first, and note the following.

1 **Ptosis** (drooping of one or both upper eyelids).

2 The **colour of the sclerae:**
- **yellow** (deposits of bilirubin in jaundice)
- **blue** (which may be due to osteogenesis imperfecta, because the thin sclerae allow the choroidal pigment to show through; blue sclerae can also occur in families without osteogenesis imperfecta); blue-grey scleral discoloration occurs in patients with ochronosis, due to the accumulation of homogentisic acid in connective tissue in this inherited condition; the concha of the ear is often affected (Figure 13.2), as are the joints and heart valves
- **red** (*iritis* or *scleritis* which causes central inflammation; or *conjunctivitis*, which causes more-peripheral inflammation often with pus; or *subconjunctival haemorrhage* (which causes influent blood as a result of trauma) (Tables 13.1 and 13.2)

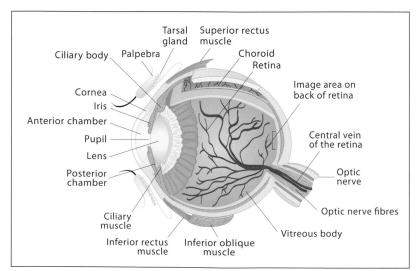

Figure 13.1 The structure of the eye

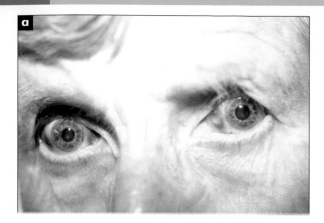

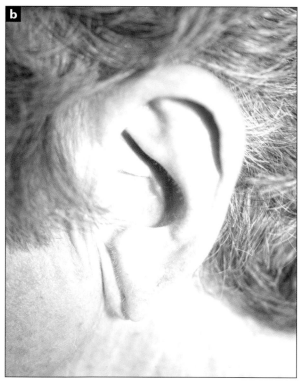

Figure 13.2 Ochronosis
(a) Sclerae. (b) Ears.

- **scleral pallor**, which occurs in anaemia—pull down the lower lid and look for the normal contrast between the pearly white posterior conjunctiva and the red anterior part; loss of this contrast is a reliable sign of anaemia (Figure 13.3).

Look from behind and above the patient for **exophthalmos**, which is prominence of the eyes. If there is actual protrusion of the eyes from the orbits, this is called **proptosis**. It is best detected by looking at the eyes from above the forehead; protrusion beyond the supraorbital ridge is abnormal. If exophthalmos is present, examine specifically for thyroid eye disease: lid lag (the patient follows the examiner's finger as it descends—the upper lid lags behind the pupil), chemosis (oedema of the bulbar conjunctiva), corneal ulceration and ophthalmoplegia (weakness of upward gaze). Look then for any corneal abnormalities, such as band keratopathy or arcus senilis.

3 Look for **corneal ulceration** which may be obvious if severe. A drop of sterile fluorescein will stain corneal ulcers.

4 Proceed then as for the **cranial nerve examination**—that is, testing *visual acuity, visual fields* and *pupillary responses* to light and accommodation. Interruption of the sympathetic innervation of the eye at any point results in *Horner's syndrome (partial ptosis* and a *constricted but reactive pupil)*. Perceptible *anisocoria* (inequality of the diameters of the pupils) has been found in 20% of normal people. Remember also that elderly people quite often have imperceptible pupillary light reactions.

5 Test the **eye movements** (Figure 13.4). Look also for fatiguability of eye muscles by asking the patient to look up at a hat-pin or finger for about half a minute. In myasthenia gravis the muscles tire and the eyelids begin to droop.

6 Test **colour vision** if acuity is not poor. Ishihara test plates (where coloured spots form numbers) can be used. Red desaturation (impaired ability to see red objects) can occur with optic nerve disease. Red-green colour blindness affects 7% of males (X-linked recessive).

7 Test the **corneal reflex**. Consider the possibility that the patient may have a glass eye. This should be suspected if visual acuity is zero in one eye and no pupillary reaction is apparent. Attempts to examine and interpret the fundus of a glass eye will amuse the patient but are always unsuccessful.

8 Perform **fundoscopy**. Successful ophthalmoscopy requires considerable practice. It is important that it be performed in reduced ambient lighting so that the patient's pupils are at least partly dilated and the examiner is not distracted. It can be easier to perform the examination, especially of the fundi, through the patient's spectacles. Otherwise, the patient's refractive error should be corrected by use of the appropriate ophthalmoscope lens. The patient should be asked to stare at a point on the opposite wall or on the ceiling and to ignore the light of the ophthalmoscope. Patients will often attempt to focus on the ophthalmoscope light and should be asked not to do this.

TABLE 13.1 Distinguishing among common causes of a red and painful eye

Disease	Distribution of redness	Corneal surface	Pupil
Bacterial conjunctivitis	Peripheral conjunctiva Bilateral (central sparing)	Normal	Normal
Episcleritis	Segmental, often around cornea Unilateral	Normal	Normal
Acute iritis	Ciliary flush Unilateral	Dull (vision blurred)	Small, irregular shape, may be no light response
Glaucoma	Around cornea Unilateral	Dull	Mid-oval shape, no light response
Corneal ulcer	Around cornea Unilateral	Dull Fluorescein dye stains ulcer	Normal
Subconjunctival haemorrhage	Localised haemorrhage No posterior limit	Normal	Normal
Conjunctival haemorrhage	Localised haemorrhage Posterior limit present	Normal	Normal

TABLE 13.2 Causes of uveitis

Iritis (anterior uveitis)
Idiopathic
Generalised disease
- Seronegative spondyloarthropathies
- Inflammatory bowel disease
- Diabetes mellitus
- Granulomatous disease—e.g. sarcoidosis
- Infections—e.g. gonococcal, syphilis, toxoplasmosis, brucellosis, tuberculosis

Choroiditis (posterior uveitis)
Idiopathic
Generalised disease
- Diabetes mellitus
- Granulomatous disease—e.g. sarcoidosis
- Infections—e.g. toxoplasmosis, syphilis, tuberculosis, toxocaral infection

The uveal tract consists of the anterior uvea (iris) and posterior uvea (ciliary body and choroid).

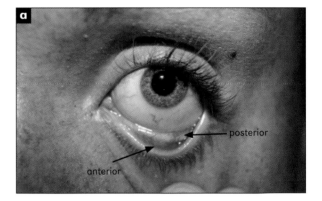
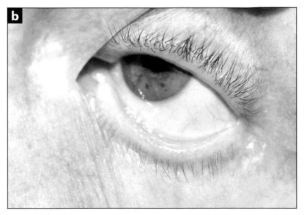

Figure 13.3 (a) Normal sclera (b) Conjunctival pallor in an anaemic patient
Note contrast between anterior and posterior parts in the normal eye.

Begin by examining the **cornea.** Use your right eye to examine the patient's right eye, and vice versa. Turn the ophthalmoscope lens to +20 and examine the cornea from about 20 cm away from the patient. Look particularly for corneal ulceration. Turn the lens gradually down to 0 while moving closer to the patient. Structures, including the *lens, humour* and then the **retina** at increasing distance into the eye, will swim into focus.

Examine the **retinas** (Figure 13.5; see also Figure 11.8, page 336). Focus on one of the

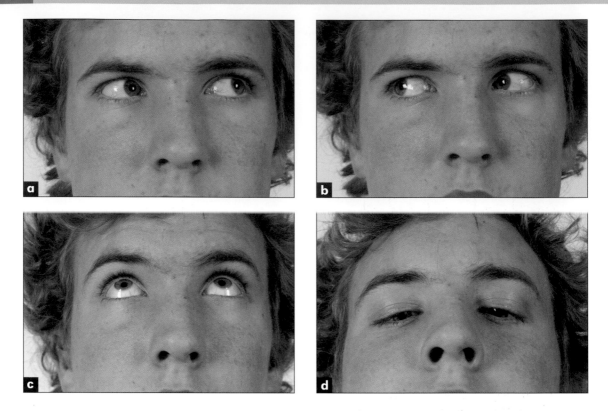

Figure 13.4 The cranial nerves III, IV & VI: voluntary eye movements
(a) 'Look to the left.' (b) 'Look to the right.' (c) 'Look up.' (d) 'Look down.'

retinal arteries and follow it into the optic disc. The normal disc is round and paler than the surrounding retina. The margin of the disc is usually sharply outlined but will appear blurred if there is papilloedema or papillitis, or pale if there is optic atrophy. Look at the rest of the retina, especially for the retinal changes of **diabetes mellitus** or **hypertension**.

There are four types of **haemorrhages**: *streaky haemorrhages* near the vessels (linear or flame-shaped); large *ecchymoses* that obliterate the vessels; *petechiae*, which may be confused with microaneurysms; and *subhyaloid haemorrhages* (large effusions of blood which have a crescentic shape and well-marked borders; a fluid level may be seen). The first two types of haemorrhage occur in hypertensive and diabetic retinopathy. They may also result from any cause of raised intracranial pressure or venous engorgement, or from a bleeding disorder. The third type occurs in diabetes mellitus, and the fourth is characteristic of subarachnoid haemorrhage.

There are two main types of retinal change in **diabetes mellitus**: non-proliferative and

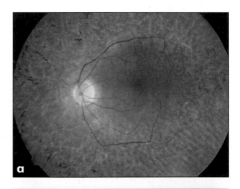

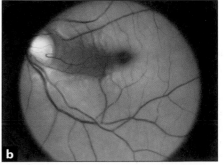

Figure 13.5 Retinal photographs
(a) Retinitis pigmentosa. (b) Central retinal artery occlusion.

proliferative. Non-proliferative changes include: (1) two types of haemorrhages—*dot haemorrhages*, which occur in the inner retinal layers, and *blot haemorrhages*, which are larger and occur more superficially in the nerve fibre layer; (2) *microaneurysms* (tiny bulges in the vessel wall), which are due to vessel wall damage; and (3) two types of exudates—*hard exudates*, which have straight edges and are due to leakage of protein from damaged arteriolar walls, and *soft exudates* (cottonwool spots), which have a fluffy appearance and are due to microinfarcts. Proliferative changes include *new vessel formation*, which can lead to retinal detachment or vitreous haemorrhage.

Hypertensive changes can be classified from grades 1 to 4:

Grade 1—'silver wiring' of the arteries only (sclerosis of the vessel wall reduces its transparency so that the central light streak becomes broader and shinier)

Grade 2—silver wiring of arteries plus arteriovenous nipping or nicking (indentation or deflection of the veins where they are crossed by the arteries)

Grade 3—grade 2 plus haemorrhages (flame-shaped) and exudates (soft—cottonwool spots due to ischaemia, or hard—lipid residues from leaking vessels)

Grade 4—grade 3 changes plus papilloedema.

It is important to describe the changes present rather than just give a grade.

Inspect carefully for **central retinal artery occlusion,** where the whole fundus appears milky-white because of retinal oedema and the arteries become greatly reduced in diameter. This presents with sudden, painless unilateral blindness, and is a medical emergency.

Central retinal vein thrombosis causes tortuous retinal veins and haemorrhages scattered over the whole retina, particularly occurring alongside the veins ('blood and thunder retina'). This presents with sudden painless loss of vision which is not total.

Retinitis pigmentosa causes a scattering of black pigment in a criss-cross pattern. This will be missed if the periphery of the retina is not examined.

In **retinal detachment**, the retina may appear elevated or folded. The patient describes a 'shade coming down', flashes of light or showers of black dots. A diagnosis requires immediate referral to try to prevent total detachment and irrevocable blindness.

White spots occur in **choroiditis** which when active have a fluffy edge (e.g. in toxoplasmosis, sarcoidosis).

Finally, ask the patient to look directly at the light. This allows the examiner to locate and inspect the **macula**. Macular degeneration is the leading cause of blindness; central vision is lost. Drussen formation occurs in macular degeneration—small deposits are seen under the epithelium in the central retina. Macular degeneration may occur secondary to an atrophic or neovascularisation process.

9   **Palpate the orbits** for tenderness. Auscultate the eyes with the bell of the stethoscope—the eye being tested is shut while the other is open and the patient is asked to stop breathing. Listen for a bruit that may be a sign of an arteriovenous malformation or a vascular tumour.

10 **Feel** for the pre-auricular node (adenoviral conjunctivitis).

The causes of common eye abnormalities are summarised in Table 13.3.

Diplopia

Most cases of diplopia (about 60%) are not due to a cranial nerve abnormality. It is important to have an approach to the problem that will help work out the cause.

First find out whether the diplopia is monocular (25%) or binocular. Monocular diplopia persists when one eye is covered. It is usually due to an eye problem such as astigmatism, dislocated lens, uneven contact lens surface or thick spectacles. It disappears if the patient looks through a pin hole. Although it is said to be due to hysteria, this is a very rare cause.

If the diplopia is binocular, consider the common causes:

1   Cranial nerve palsy (III, IV or VI)—look for ptosis, pupil changes (III), abnormal eye movements.

2   Eye muscle disease (myasthenia gravis)—worse later in day, worse after prolonged upward gaze and associated with bilateral ptosis.

3   Thyroid ophthalmopathy—proptosis, lid lag, chemosis.

4   Trauma to the orbit—history or signs of trauma.

5   Internuclear ophthalmoplegia—associated neurological signs.

TABLE 13.3 Causes of eye abnormalities

Cataracts
1 Old age (senile cataract)
2 Endocrine—e.g. diabetes mellitus, steroids
3 Hereditary or congenital—e.g. dystrophia myotonica, Refsum's disease*
4 Ocular disease—e.g. glaucoma
5 Radiation
6 Trauma

Papilloedema vs papillitis

Papilloedema	*Papillitis*
Optic disc swollen without venous pulsation	Optic disc swollen
Acuity normal (early)	Acuity poor
Large blind spot	Large central scotoma
Peripheral constriction of visual fields	Pain on eye movement
Colour vision normal	Onset usually sudden and unilateral
Usually bilateral	Colour vision affected (particularly red desaturation)

Causes of papilloedema
1 Space-occupying lesion (causing raised intracranial pressure) or a retro-orbital mass
2 Hydrocephalus (large cerebral ventricles)
   Obstructive (a block in the ventricle, aqueduct or outlet to the fourth ventricle)—e.g. tumour
   Communicating
   Increased formation of CSF—e.g. choroid plexus papilloma (rare)
   Decreased absorption of CSF—e.g. tumour causing venous compression, subarachnoid space obstruction from meningitis
3 Benign intracranial hypertension (pseudotumour cerebri) (small or normal-sized ventricles)
   (a) Idiopathic
   (b) The contraceptive pill
   (c) Addison's disease
   (d) Drugs—e.g. nitrofurantoin, tetracycline, vitamin A, steroids
   (e) Head trauma
4 Hypertension
5 Central retinal vein thrombosis

Causes of optic atrophy
1 Chronic papilloedema or optic neuritis
2 Optic nerve pressure or division
3 Glaucoma
4 Ischaemia
5 Familial—e.g. retinitis pigmentosa, Leber's disease,[†] Friedreich's ataxia

Causes of optic neuritis
1 Multiple sclerosis
2 Toxic—e.g. ethambutol, chloroquine, nicotine, alcohol
3 Metabolic—e.g. vitamin B12 deficiency
4 Ischaemia—e.g. diabetes mellitus, temporal arteritis, atheroma
5 Familial—e.g. Leber's disease
6 Infective—e.g. infectious mononucleosis

Causes of retinitis pigmentosa
1 Congenital (associated with cataract and deaf-mutism)
2 Laurence-Moon-Biedl syndrome[‡]
3 Hereditary ataxia
4 Familial neuropathy, i.e. Refsum's disease

CSF = cerebrospinal fluid.
* Sigvald Refsum, 20th century Norwegian physician.
[†] Theodor von Leber (1840–1917), Göttingen and Heidelberg ophthalmologist.
[‡] John Laurence (1830–1874), London ophthalmologist; Robert Charles Moon (1844–1914), American ophthalmologist; and Arthur Biedl (1869–1933), professor of physiology, Prague.

TABLE 13.4 Causes of Horner's syndrome

1 Carcinoma of the apex of the lung (usually squamous cell carcinoma)

2 Neck
- Malignancy—e.g. thyroid
- Trauma or surgery

3 Lower trunk brachial plexus lesions
- Trauma
- Tumour

4 Carotid arterial lesion
- Carotid aneurysm or dissection
- Pericarotid tumours (Raeder's syndrome)*
- Cluster headache

5 Brainstem lesions
- Vascular disease (especially the lateral medullary syndrome)
- Tumour
- Syringobulbia

6 Syringomyelia (rare)

* Sweating unaffected, as tumour localised to internal carotid artery.

TABLE 13.5 Important causes of ptosis

Cause	Associated features
Age-related stretching of levator muscle or aponeurosis	Common, often asymmetrical
Orbital tumour or inflammation	Orbital abnormality
Horner's syndrome	Constricted pupil, reduced sweating
Third nerve palsy	Eye 'down and out', dilated pupil
Myasthenia gravis or dystrophical myotonica	Extraocular muscle palsies, muscle weakness
Congenital or idiopathic	

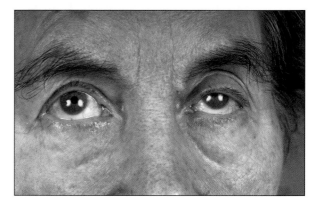

Figure 13.6 Left Horner's syndrome, with partial ptosis and miosis

Horner's syndrome

Examination anatomy

Interruption of the sympathetic innervation of the eye at any point (Figure 13.6) results in Horner's syndrome[a] (Table 13.4).

Clinical approach

The syndrome includes partial *ptosis* (as sympathetic fibres supply the smooth muscle of both eyelids) and a *constricted* pupil (unbalanced parasympathetic action) which reacts normally to light (Figure 13.6). Remember the other causes of ptosis (Table 13.5).

Test for a difference (decrease) in the *sweating* over each eyebrow with the back of the finger (absence of this sign does not exclude the diagnosis).[b]

Horner's syndrome may be part of the *lateral medullary syndrome.*[c]

Next ask the patient to speak and note any hoarseness of the voice, which may be due to recurrent laryngeal nerve palsy from lung carcinoma or from a lower cranial nerve lesion.

Go on now to look at the hands for clubbing and test for weakness of finger abduction. If any of these signs is present, perform a respiratory examination, concentrating on the apices of the lungs for signs of lung carcinoma.

Examine the neck for lymphadenopathy, thyroid carcinoma and a carotid aneurysm or bruit. Syringomyelia may rarely be a cause of this syndrome, so the examination should be completed by testing for dissociated sensory loss. Remember, syringomyelia may cause a bilateral Horner's syndrome.

Iritis

Iritis (anterior uveitis) presents with pain, photophobia and unilateral eye redness (Tables 13.1 and 13.2). On examination of the eye, there is classically a ciliary flush with dilated vessels around the iris. *Hypopyon* refers to pus in the anterior

---

[a] Johann Friedrich Horner (1831–1886), professor of ophthalmology, Zürich, described this in 1869.

[b] Enophthalmos or retraction of the eye, which is often mentioned as a feature of Horner's syndrome, probably does not occur in humans. It may occur in cats. Horner's original paper was very specific about miosis and ptosis, but only casually mentioned that 'the position of the eye seemed very slightly inward'. Apparent enophthalmos results from a combination of ptosis and an elevated lower lid (upside-down ptosis).

[c] Occlusion of any of the following vessels may result in this syndrome: vertebral; posterior inferior cerebellar; superior, middle or inferior lateral medullary arteries.

chamber; a fluid level may be seen. The pupil is usually irregular. There may also be new vessel formation over the iris.

Iritis is associated with inflammatory arthropathies that are linked to HLA-B27 positivity, including ankylosing spondylitis, inflammatory bowel disease, Reiter's syndrome and Behçet's disease with an acute presentation. Chronic iritis can be linked to juvenile rheumatoid arthritis, as well as sarcoidosis and syphilis.

Scleritis presents similarly but with bilateral painful red eyes; it is also associated with the same HLA-B27 arthropathies. Eye movements are painful in scleritis.

Glaucoma

Here prolonged elevation of intraocular pressure induces progressive visual loss. Closed-angle (narrow-angle) glaucoma is due to a rapid pressure increase. Symptoms include severe eye pain, halos around lights and nausea; it is an ocular emergency. The examiner may see a fixed mid-dilated pupil, conjunctival hyperaemia and corneal redness; intraocular pressure on measurement is increased. The condition occurs secondary to iris neovascularisation (e.g. new renal formation in diabetes mellitus) or primarily from an anomalous iris (e.g. genetic).

Shingles

Herpes zoster involving the first (ophthalmic) division of the trigeminal nerve may result in uveitis and keratitis, and threaten vision. The tip of the nose, cornea and iris are all innervated by the nasociliary nerve (a branch of the trigeminal nerve). The appearance of vesicles on the tip of the nose (Hutchinson's[d] vesicles) in patient with herpes zoster indicates an increased risk of ophthalmic complication (LR 3.5).[1]

Eyelid

Two conditions of the eyelid are worth remembering:

1. Stye of the eyelid (*hordeolum*). This is an infection typically caused by *Staphylococcus aureus*; it is tender.
2. A slowly enlarging non-tender nodule of the eyelid is a *chalazion* (sterile inflammation of the meibomian glands if deep, or of the sebaceous glands if superficial). See figure 3.18.

---

d   Sir Jonathon Hutchinson (1828–1913). Among other appointments he was surgeon to Moorfields Eye Hospital. He was president of the Royal College of Surgeons in 1889, elected to the Royal Society in 1882 and knighted in 1908.

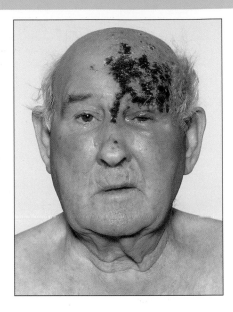

Figure 13.7 Herpes zoster, involving the eye, along the distribution of the ophthalmic branch of the fifth cranial nerve
(From Mir MA, *Atlas of Clinical Diagnosis*, 2nd edn. Edinburgh: Saunders, 2003, with permission.)

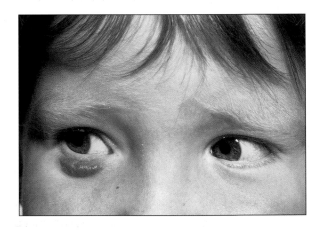

Figure 13.8 A chalazion; unlike styes, chalazions are not usually tender or painful

The ears
Examination anatomy

The pinna, external auditory canal and ear drum are easily assessed with simple equipment (Figure 13.9). Tests of hearing can also provide information about the severity and anatomical site of hearing loss.

Examination method

Ear examination consists of inspection and palpation, auriscopic examination and testing hearing.

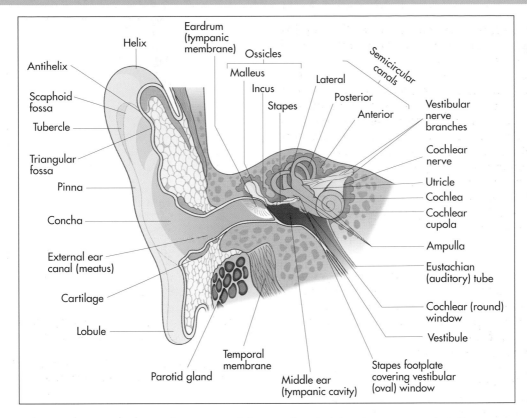

Figure 13.9 Cross-sectional anatomy of the ear showing the pinna, external auditory canal, middle and inner ear

Inspect the position of the **pinna** and note its size and shape. Note any scars or swelling around the ears. Look for an obvious accessory auricle (separate piece of cartilage away from the pinna), cauliflower ears (haematomas from recurrent trauma, which fill in the hollows of the ear) and bat ears (protrusion of the ears from the side of the head).

Look for **inflammation externally** and any obvious ear *discharge.* Otitis externa (swimmer's ear) is redness of the external canal. Necrotising malignant otitis is usually due to *Pseudomonas* infection and damages the deep tissues, sometimes to the bone.

Look for signs of **gouty tophi** (nodular, firm, pale and non-tender chalky depositions of urate in the cartilage of the ear, specific but not sensitive for gout).

Palpate the pinna for swelling or nodules. Pull down the pinna gently; infection of the external canal often causes tenderness of the pinna.

Auriscopic examination of the ears requires use of an earpiece that fits comfortably in the ear canal to allow inspection of the ear canal and tympanic membrane (Figure 13.10). This examination is

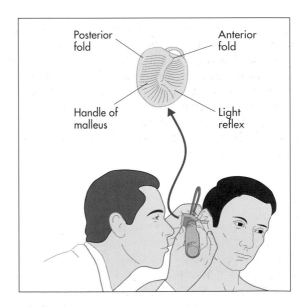

Figure 13.10 Use of the auriscope

essential if there is a history of recent deafness or a painful ear. Examination is also necessary in the patient who has had a head injury. Always examine both ears!

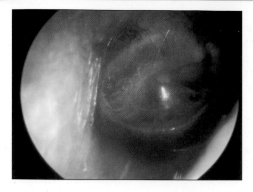

Figure 13.11 The tympanic membrane as viewed through an otoscope
(From Mir MA, *Atlas of Clinical Diagnosis*, 2nd edn. Edinburgh: Saunders, 2003, with permission.)

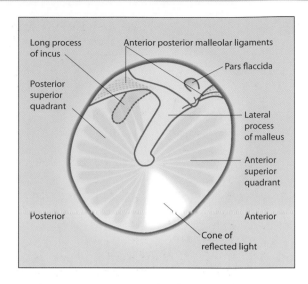

Figure 13.12 The detail of the tympanic membrane
(From Mir MA, *Atlas of Clinical Diagnosis*, 2nd edn. Edinburgh: Saunders, 2003, with permission.)

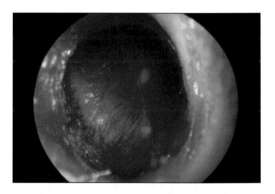

Figure 13.13 Otitis media with hyperaemia of the tympanic membrane
(From Mir MA, *Atlas of Clinical Diagnosis,* 2nd edn. Edinburgh: Saunders, 2003, with permission.)

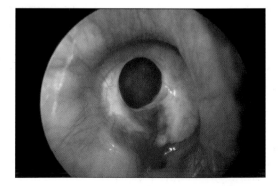

Figure 13.14 Perforated tympanic membrane
(From Mir MA, *Atlas of Clinical Diagnosis*, 2nd edn. Edinburgh: Saunders, 2003, with permission.)

The correct technique is as follows. Ask the patient to turn his or her head slightly to the side, then pull the pinna up, out and back to straighten the ear canal and provide optimal vision. Stretch out the fingers of the hand holding the auriscope to touch the patient's cheek, to steady the instrument and prevent sudden movements of the patient's head. When examining the patient's right ear, the auriscope is preferably held in a *downward position* with the right hand, while using the left hand to pull the pinna. An alternative position involves holding the auriscope upward, but there is a risk that if the patient moves suddenly injury is more likely to occur.

Look at the **external canal** for any evidence of inflammation (e.g. redness or swelling) or discharge. There should be no tenderness unless there is inflammation. *Ear wax* is white or yellowish, and translucent and shiny; it may obscure the view of the tympanic membrane. *Blood* or *cerebrospinal fluid* (watery, clear fluid) may be seen in the canal if there is a fracture at the base of the skull. In patients with herpes zoster, there may be *vesicles* (fluid-filled blisters) on the posterior wall around the external auditory meatus.

Inspect the **tympanic membrane** (ear drum) by introducing the speculum further into the canal in a forward but downward direction. The normal tympanic membrane is greyish and reflects light from the centre at approximately 5 or 7 o'clock (Figures 13.11 and 13.12). Note the colour, transparency and any evidence of *dilated blood vessels* (hyperaemia—a sign of otitis media) (Figure 13.13). Look for *bulging* or *retraction* of the tympanic membrane. Bulging can suggest underlying fluid or pus in the middle ear. Perforation of the tympanic membrane should be noted (Figure 13.14).

If a middle ear infection is suspected, **pneumatic**

auriscopy can be useful. Use a speculum large enough to occlude the external canal snugly. Attach a rubber squeeze bulb to the otoscope. When the bulb is squeezed gently, air pressure in the canal is increased and the tympanic membrane should move promptly inward. Absence of, or a decrease in, movement is a sign of fluid in the middle ear.

To test hearing, whisper numbers 60 cm away from one of the patient's ears while the other ear is distracted by movement of the examiner's finger in the auditory canal. Then repeat the process with the other ear. With practice the normal range of hearing is appreciated. Next perform **Rinne's** and **Weber's** tests (page 347):

1 **Rinne's test**: place a vibrating 256 Hz tuning fork on the mastoid process. When the sound is no longer heard move the fork close to the auditory meatus where, if air conduction is (as is normal) better than bone conduction, it will again be audible.
2 **Weber's test**: place a vibrating 256 Hz fork at the centre of the patient's forehead. Nerve deafness causes the sound to be heard better in the normal ear, but with conduction deafness the sound is heard better in the abnormal ear.

The nose
Examination method
Nose examination consists of **inspection**, **palpation** and **testing the sense of smell**.

Look at the skin. Note any nasal deviation (best seen from behind the patient and looking down). Note any periorbital swelling (e.g. from sinusitis). Inspect the nares by pressing the tip of the nose upwards with the thumb.

Palpate the nasal bones. Then feel for facial swelling or signs of inflammation. Block each nostril to assess any obstruction by asking the patient to inhale. If there is a history of anosmia (loss of smell), test smell as described in Chapter 11 (cranial nerve I).

A saddle-nose deformity (collapse of the nasal septum) can occur in Wegener's granulomatosis and relapsing polychondritis.

Sinusitis
Sinusitis is inflammation of the paranasal sinuses. Pain and tenderness over the sinuses occurs, which in adults is classified as acute if less than 4 weeks in duration, subacute if duration 4–12 weeks and chronic if greater than 12 weeks in duration. Most acute sinusitis is secondary to viral infection.

Acute bacterial sinusitis can occur after viral infection or in the setting of allergic rhinitis, in patients with anatomical abnormalities such as nasal septal deformity or polyps in the nose, or in immunocompromised patients. The commonest bacterial causes of sinusitis are *Streptococcus pneumoniae* and *Haemophilus influenzae*. The four key clinical features suggesting that sinusitis may be bacterial are: (i) worsening symptoms after early improvement (a biphasic illness pattern); (ii) purulent discharge from the nose; (iii) tooth or facial pain over the maxillary sinus (especially if unilateral); and (iv) tenderness over the maxillary sinus (unilaterally). Fever can occur but is rare.

Complications of acute bacterial sinusitis can include orbital cellulitis, meningitis, cavernous sinus thrombosis, brain abscess and osteolitis of the sinus bones. Therefore, if patients present with any of the following warning signs—periorbital oedema, visual changes, or changes in mental status—one should be concerned about complicated bacterial sinusitis. Orbital cellulitis typically presents with erythema of the eyelid, oedema of the eyelid and proptosis.

Potential mimickers of acute bacterial sinusitis include Wegner's granulomatosis, carcinoma or lymphoma, sarcoidosis, and in immuno-compromised or diabetic patients, fungal sinusitis. Chronic sinusitis presents with chronic sinus congestion, postnasal drip, cough, headache and bad breath.

Rhinocerebral mucormycosis is a fungal infection that destroys the sinuses. A black eschar may be seen on the nasal mucosa or palate.

The throat
Examination anatomy
See Figure 13.15.

Examination method
Throat examination consists of **inspection** and **palpation**.

Look in turn at the lips, buccal mucosa, gums, palate and teeth. Note any signs of inflammation (e.g. redness, swelling). Inspect the tongue first in the mouth, then ask the patient to poke it out, and then ask the patient to touch it to the roof of the mouth (so that the examiner may look at the floor of the mouth).

Ask the patient to say 'Ah', then inspect the oropharynx and uvula (there is often a need to press a tongue depressor on the posterior tongue to see properly). Inspect the tonsils (note the size, shape, colour, and note any discharge or membrane—they involute in adults and may not be seen).

Palpate the tongue for lumps (wear gloves). Palpate the salivary glands. Examine the cervical lymph nodes.

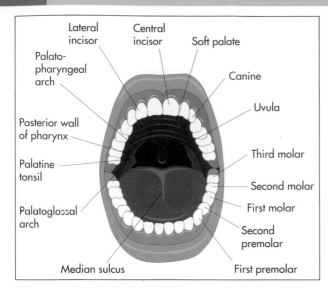

Figure 13.15 The mouth and throat

Pharyngitis

A sore throat due to an exudative pharyngitis in adults is usually secondary to infection. The specific causes of pharyngitis include viruses in about half the cases, while about 10% are due to the group A beta-haemolytic streptococci. *Neisseriae gonorrhea* is a rare cause of pharyngitis in adults; typically there are sexual risk factors present in the history. The two most important viruses are herpes simplex and adenovirus. Many cases are of unknown cause. Clinically, there is redness of the pharynx with or without ulceration.

Clinical criteria are available for determining whether the pharyngitis is likely due to beta-haemolytic streptococcus or not. The *absence* of cough, along with a history of fever, presence of a pharyngeal exudate on examination and anterior cervical adenopathy together strongly predict the presence of this infection, while the absence of the last three strongly suggests that the infection is not due to beta-haemolytic streptococcus. It is important to recognize this because beta-haemolytic streptococcus infection of the pharynx can lead to direct infectious complications (otitis media, sinusitis, peritonsillar abscess [quinsy] and submandibular space infection [Ludwig's^e angina]) and to indirect complications (acute rheumatic fever and glomerulonephritis). Glomerulonephritis is not prevented by antibiotic therapy.

Epiglottitis

A rare cause of sore throat is epiglottitis. This disease classically presents with a triad of sore throat, painful swallowing (odynophagia) and fever. The patient may uncommonly have stridor which may be misdiagnosed as asthma; here there is inspiratory wheeze due to the inflammation of the epiglottis. Pooling of secretions is another clue to the diagnosis. Urgent medical attention is indicated to prevent airway obstruction.

Reference

1. McGee S. *Evidence-based clinical diagnosis*, 2nd edn. St Louis: Saunders, 2007; 694.

---

e Wilhelm Ludwig (1790–1865) was an army surgeon during the Napoleonic wars and a Russian prisoner of war for 2 years. He became court doctor to King Frederick II and was professor of surgery and midwifery at Tübingen. He described submandibular cellulitis in his first paper, published 20 years after he became a professor. The patient described was Queen Catherine of Würtenberg.

Chapter 14

The breasts

Blessed is the physician who takes a good history, looks keenly at his patient and thinks a bit.

Walter C Alvarez (1976)

Breast examination is a vitally important part of the general physical examination. Examinations for breast cancer should be done monthly by the patient and yearly by the doctor in those over the age 40 of years.

History

The history is important. Important questions to ask include the length of time any mass has been present, presence of pain, change in size or texture over time, relationship to menstrual cycle, and any nipple discharge. Ask about previous cyst aspirations.

Find out about risk factors for breast cancer including any family history of breast or ovarian cancer (and age affected), previous personal history of breast cancer, late menopause, late first pregnancy, mantle radiation, heavy alcohol use, and use of oestrogens post-menopausally. A personal history of atypical hyperplasia (ductal or lobular) increases the risk of breast cancer 3 to 5 times. However, three-quarters of patients presenting with a breast cancer have *no* known risk factors.

The breast cancer genes BRCA1 and BRCA2 are associated with a strong risk of breast (and ovarian) cancer, as well as breast cancer in men. For all women from the age of 50 years, screening mammography[1] is generally recommended.

Examination

When it is done properly, the examination takes some time to perform (about 3 minutes per breast).[2] This must obviously be explained to the patient at the start. The patient should be offered a chaperone for the examination.

The examination is only just over 50% sensitive for carcinoma but specificity is as high as 90%. The likelihood ratio of a positive examination is 14.1 and the LR of a negative examination is 0.47.[3]

Inspection

Ask the patient to sit up with her chest fully exposed. There is controversy about the value of inspection of the breasts as part of the examination, but advanced cancers may be obvious at this stage. Look at the *nipples* for retraction (due to cancer or fibrosis; in some patients retraction may be normal) and Paget's disease of the breast (where underlying breast cancer causes a unilateral red, bleeding skin).

Next inspect the rest of the *skin*. Look for visible veins (which if unilateral suggest a cancer), skin dimpling, and for peau d'orange skin (where advanced breast cancer causes oedematous skin pitted by the sweat glands).

A persistent erythematous plaque in the areola area may be contact dermatitis or skin irrigation, but if asymmetric or it has not responded to treatment this may be the malignancy *Paget disease of the breast*.

Ask the patient to *raise her arms above her head* and then lower them slowly. Look for tethering of the nipples or skin, a shift in the relative position of the nipples or a fixed mass distorting the breast (Figure 14.1).

Note whether there are any obvious visible masses in the axillae.

Next ask her to rest her hands on her hips and then press her hands against her hips (the pectoral contraction manoeuvre). This accentuates areas of dimpling or fixation.

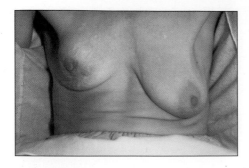

Figure 14.1 Carcinoma of the right breast, showing elevation of the breast, dimpling of skin, and retraction of the nipple

Palpation

Examine both the supraclavicular and axillary regions for lymphadenopathy. It may be difficult, however, to distinguish an axillary fat pad from an enlarged lymph node.

Then ask the patient to lie down. The examination can be performed only if the breast tissue is flattened against the chest wall. If the breasts are large, it can be helpful to have the patient place her hand on her forehead for the palpation of the lateral aspect of the breast and bring her elbow up level with the shoulder for the palpation of the medial side of the breast.

Palpation is performed gently with the pulps of the middle three fingers parallel to the contour of the breast. Feel the four quadrants of each breast systematically (Figure 14.2a). Don't pinch the breast as you may think you then feel a mass. The total examination should involve a rectangular area bordered by the clavicle, sternum, mid-axillary line and the bra line. Start in the axilla and palpate in a line down to the bra line inferiorly. The pattern of palpation is like that of mowing a lawn, a series of vertical strips that cover the whole of the rectangle (Figure 14.2b).

Each area is palpated three times, using small circular movements and slightly increasing pressure. Palpation is more difficult when a breast implant is present. It is probably best to examine such a patient in a supine position and to keep the ipsilateral arm down at her side.

Next feel behind the nipple for lumps and note if any fluid can be expressed: bright blood (from a duct papilloma, fibroadenosis or carcinoma), yellow serous (fibroadenosis) or serous (early pregnancy) fluid, milky (lactation) or green (mammary duct ectasia) fluid.

Don't mistake normal breast structures for a mass![4] You may feel a rib or costochondral junction normally on deep palpation. The inferior ridge

of breast tissue (inframammary fold) may be felt and is symmetrical. You may feel normal rubbery-type plaques (fibroglandular tissue), especially in the upper outer quadrant. It is normal to feel firm breast tissue at the areola border.

Evaluation of a breast lump

The following five points need to be carefully elucidated if a lump is detected.

1 Position—the breast quadrant involved and proximity to the nipple.
2 Size, shape and consistency—a hard, irregular nodule is characteristic of carcinoma.
3 Tenderness—suggests an inflammatory or cystic lesion; breast cancer is usually not tender.
4 Fixation—mobility is determined by taking the breast between the hands and moving it over the

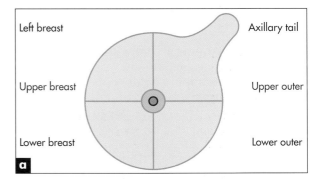

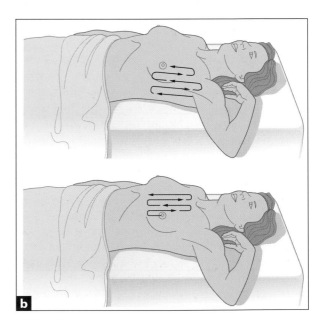

Figure 14.2 Examination of the breast: (a) quadrants; (b) systematic examination

TABLE 14.1 Causes of a breast lump

Non-tender	Tender
Cyst	Cyst
Carcinoma	Breast abscess
Fibroadenosis (chronic mastitis)	Fibroadenosis
Fibroadenoma (benign highly mobile 'breast mouse')	Costal cartilage chondritis
Uncommon causes	Inflammatory breast cancer
• Trauma, fat necrosis	
• Other cysts—e.g. galactocele	
• Other neoplasms—e.g. duct papilloma	
• Chest wall—e.g. lipoma, costal cartilage chondritis (causes tenderness but not a lump) (Tietze's* disease)	

* Alexander Tietze (1864–1927), Chief Surgeon, Allerheiligen Hospital, Breslau, Poland. He described the condition in 1921.

chest wall; in advanced carcinoma the lump may be fixed to the chest wall.

5 Single or multiple lesions present—multiple nodules suggest benign cystic disease or fibroadenosis.

A palpable breast mass is likely to be significant (called a dominant mass) if it is:[4]

1 Clearly 3-dimensional.
2 Distinct from the surrounding tissue.
3 Asymmetrical compared with the other breast.
4 Persistent throughout a menstrual cycle.
5 *Not* smooth, well-demarcated and mobile.

A palpable breast mass is more likely to be malignant if it has the following characteristics:[4]

1 Very firm.
2 Margins seem poorly defined or have an irregular edge.
3 Immobile or fixed.
4 Associated skin dimpling.
5 Associated retraction of the nipple, or nipple scaling.
6 A bloody nipple discharge.
7 Draining lymph nodes are palpable.

Remember that many normal breasts have palpable lumps and that although benign lumps tend to be soft, moveable and regular, they can also have the characteristics of malignant lumps (*Good signs guide 14.1*). Causes of a lump in the breast are listed in Table 14.1.

In men with true gynaecomastia, a disc of breast tissue can be palpated under the areola. This is not present in men who are merely obese. Causes

GOOD SIGNS GUIDE 14.1 Breast lump characteristics and likelihood of cancer in a woman of average risk[3]

Sign	Positive LR
Mass	2.1
Fixed	2.4
Hard	1.6
Irregular	1.8
>2 cm diameter	1.9

From McGee S, *Evidence-based physical diagnosis*, 2nd edn. St Louis: Saunders, 2007.

of breast enlargement in men are presented on page 316.

References

1. Kerlikowske K, Smith-Bindman R, Ljung BM et al. Evaluation of abnormal mammography results and palpable breast abnormalities. *Ann Intern Med* 2003; 139:274–284.
2. Fenton JJ, Rolnick SJ, Harris EL, Barton MB, Barlow WE, Reisch LM, Herrinton LJ, Geiger AM, Fletcher SW, Elmore JG. Specificity of clinical breast examination in community practice. *J Gen Intern Med* 2007 Mar; 22(3):332–327.
3. Barton MB, Harris R, Fletcher SW. Does this patient have breast cancer? *JAMA* 1999; 282:1270–1280. The clinical breast examination may have an overall specificity which is high (94%) but the sensitivity is poor (54%). Unfortunately interobserver variation seems to be high.
4. Pruthi S. Detection and evaluation of a palpable breast mass. *Mayo Clin Proc* 2001; 76:641–647.

Chapter 15

The skin, nails, and lumps

For one mistake made for not knowing, ten mistakes are made for not looking.

JA Lindsay

The dermatological history

With any rash or skin condition, it is important to determine when and where it began, its distribution, whether it has changed over time, its relationship to sun exposure or heat or cold, and any response to treatment[1] (see *Questions box 15.1*). Ask if pruritus is associated; localised pruritus is usually due to dermatological disease. Determine if pain or disturbed sensation has occurred; for example, inflammation and oedema can produce pain in the skin, while disease involving neurovascular bundles or nerves can produce anaesthesia (e.g. leprosy, syphilis). Constitutional symptoms such as fever, headache, fatigue, anorexia and weight loss also need to be documented.

It is important to obtain a past history of rashes or allergic reactions. A past history of asthma, eczema or hay fever suggests atopy. Similarly, evidence of systemic disease in the past may be important in a patient with a rash (e.g. diabetes mellitus, connective tissue disease, inflammatory bowel disease).

A detailed social history needs to be obtained regarding occupation and hobbies, as chemical exposure and contact with animals or plants can all induce dermatitis. All medications that have been taken must be documented. Orally ingested or parenteral medications can cause a whole host of cutaneous lesions and can mimic many skin diseases (Table 15.1). Similarly, a family history of atopic dermatitis, hay fever or skin infestation can be helpful.

Questions box 15.1

Questions to ask the patient with a rash

1 How long have you had the problem?

2 Have you ever had it before?

3 Is it getting worse?

4 What parts of your skin are affected (e.g. sun-exposed areas, areas in contact with clothing or chemicals)?

5 Was the rash flat or raised to begin with, or was it blistered?

6 Is the area itchy?

7 Does anything seem to make it better?

8 Has your diet changed recently?

9 What treatment have you tried for it?

10 Have you had a fever or any joint pains?

11 Have you had problems with allergies?

12 Are you taking any tablets or medicines? Are any of these new (last 2 weeks)?

13 Have you changed your soap, shampoo, deodorant or washing powder recently?

14 What sort of work do you do? Do you come into contact with chemicals at work or with your hobbies?

15 Have you travelled recently? Where to?

16 Has anyone you know got a similar rash?

17 Have you any other problems with your health?

TABLE 15.1 Types of cutaneous drug reactions

1	Acne, e.g. steroids	10	Skin necrosis, e.g. warfarin
2	Hair loss (alopecia), e.g. cancer chemotherapy	11	Drug-precipitated porphyria, e.g. alcohol, barbiturates, sulfonamides, contraceptive pill
3	Pigment alterations: hypomelanosis (e.g. hydroxyquinone, chloroquine, topical steroids), hypermelanosis (page 449)	12	Lichenoid eruptions, e.g. gold, antimalarials, beta-blockers
4	Exfoliative dermatitis or erythroderma (page 448)	13	Fixed drug eruption, e.g. sulfonamides, tetracycline, phenylbutazone
5	Urticaria (hives), e.g. non-steroidal anti-inflammatory drugs, radiographic dyes, penicillin	14	Bullous eruptions, e.g. frusemide, nalidixic acid, penicillamine, clonidine
6	Maculopapular (morbilliform) eruptions, e.g. ampicillin, allopurinol	15	Erythema nodosum or erythema multiforme (page 448)
7	Photosensitive eruptions, e.g. sulfonamides, sulfonylureas, chlorothiazides, phenothiazines, tetracycline, nalidixic acid, anticonvulsants	16	Toxic epidermal necrolysis, e.g. allopurinol, phenytoin, sulfonamides, non-steroidal anti-inflammatory drugs
8	Drug-induced lupus erythematosus, e.g. procainamide, hydralazine	17	Pruritus (page 445)
9	Vasculitis, e.g. propylthiouracil, allopurinol, thiazides, penicillin, phenytoin		

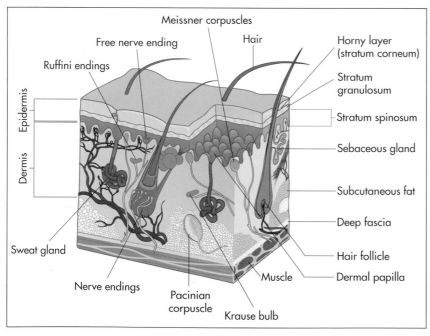

Figure 15.1 The layers of the skin

Examination anatomy

Figure 15.1 shows the three main layers of the skin—epidermis, dermis and subcutaneous fat. These layers can all be involved in skin diseases in varying combinations. For example, most skin tumours arise in the epidermis (Figure 15.2a&b), some bullous eruptions occur at the epidermo-dermal junction, and lipomas are tumours of subcutaneous fat. The skin appendages which include the sweat (eccrine and apocrine) glands, hair follicles (Figure 15.3) and the nails are common sites of infection.

The eccrine glands are present everywhere except in the nail beds and on some mucosal surfaces. They are able to secrete over 5 litres of sweat per day. The apocrine glands are found in association with hair follicles but are confined to certain areas of the body which include the axillae, the pubis, perineum and nipples. They secrete a viscous fluid whose function is unclear in humans.

The nails are formed from heavily keratinised

cells that grow from the nail matrix. The matrix grows in a semilunar shape and appears as the lunules in normal finger and toe nails. Hair is also the product of specialised epithelial cells and grows from the hair matrix within the hair follicle.

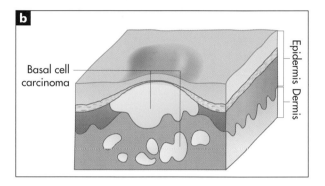

Figure 15.2 (a) Melanoma; (b) Basal cell carcinoma

General principles of physical examination of the skin

The aim of this chapter is to provide an approach to the diagnosis of skin diseases.[2,3] Particular emphasis will be placed on cutaneous signs as indications of systemic disease. Other chapters have included the usual clues that can be used to arrive at a particular diagnosis. This chapter tries to unify the concept of 'inspection' as a valuable starting point in the examination of the patient.

Ask the patient to undress. The whole surface of the skin and its appendages should be carefully inspected (Table 15.2).

When one is examining actual skin lesions, a number of features should be documented. First, each lesion should be *described* precisely, including colour and shape. Use the appropriate dermatological terminology (Table 15.3), even

TABLE 15.2 Considerations when examining the skin

1	Hair
2	Nails
3	Sebaceous glands—oil-producing and present on the head, neck and back
4	Eccrine glands—sweat-producing and present all over the body
5	Apocrine glands—sweat-producing and present in the axillae and groin
6	Mucosa

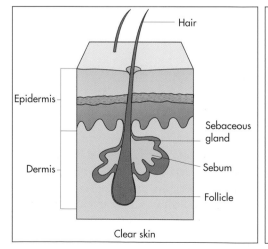
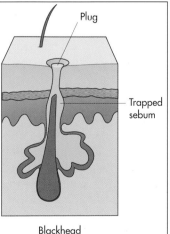
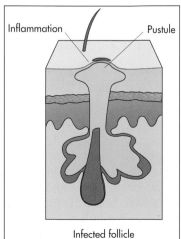

Figure 15.3 Common sites of infection in the skin

TABLE 15.3 Dermatological terms

Term	Definition	Descriptive terms	
Atrophy	Thinning of epidermis with loss of normal skin markings	Annular	Ring-shaped (hollow centre), e.g. tinea infection
Bulla	A large collection of fluid below the epidermis	Arcuate	Curved, e.g. secondary syphilis
Crust	Dried serum and exudate	Circinate	Circular
Ecchymoses	Bruises	Confluent	Lesions that have run together, e.g. measles
Excoriations	Lesions caused by scratching that results in loss of the epidermis	Discoid	Circular without a hollow centre, e.g. lupus
Keloid	Hypertrophic scarring	Eczematous	Inflamed and crusted, e.g. allergic eczema
Macule	A circumscribed alteration of skin colour	Keratotic	Thickened from increased keratin, e.g. psoriasis
Nodule	A circumscribed palpable mass, greater than 1 cm diameter	Lichenified	Thickening and roughening of the epidermis associated with accentuated skin markings
Papule	A circumscribed palpable elevation, less than 1 cm diameter	Linear	In lines, e.g. contact dermatitis
Petechiae	Red, non-blanching spots <5 mm	Nodule	Raised solid lesion >10 mm, e.g. erythema nodosum
Pigment alterations	Increased (hyperpigmentation) or decreased (hypopigmentation)	Papule	Raised solid lesion <10 mm, e.g. wart
Plaque	A palpable disc-shaped lesion	Papulosquamous	Plaques associated with scaling
Purpura	Red, non-blanching spots >5 mm	Reticulated	In a network pattern, e.g. cutaneous parasite
Pustule	A visible collection of pus	Serpiginous	Sinuous
Scales	An accumulation of excess keratin	Zosteriform	Following a nerve distribution
Sclerosis	Induration of subcutaneous tissues, which may involve the dermis		
Ulcer	A circumscribed loss of tissue		
Vesicle	A small collection of fluid below the epidermis		
Wheal	An area of dermal oedema		

though this may seem to make dermatological diseases more, rather than less, mysterious. As many dermatological diagnoses are purely descriptive, a good description will often be of considerable help in making the diagnosis. Second, the *distribution* of the lesions should be noted, as certain distributions suggest specific diagnoses. Third, the *pattern* of the lesions—such as linear, annular (ring-shaped), reticulated (net-like), serpiginous (snake-like) or grouped—also helps establish the diagnosis. Then *palpate* the lesions, noting consistency, tenderness, temperature, depth and mobility. Types of skin lesions are shown in Figure 15.4 and a clinical algorithm for diagnosis is presented in Figure 15.5.

How to approach the clinical diagnosis of a lump

First, determine the lump's site, size, shape, consistency and tenderness. Next, evaluate in what tissue layer the lump is situated. If it is in the *skin* (e.g. sebaceous cyst, epidermoid cyst, papilloma), it should move when the skin is moved, but if it is in the *subcutaneous tissue* (e.g. neurofibroma, lipoma), the skin can be moved over the lump. If it is in the *muscle* or *tendon* (e.g. tumour), then contraction of the muscle or tendon will limit the lump's mobility. If it is in a *nerve*, pressing on the lump may result in pins and needles being felt in the distribution of the nerve, and the lump cannot be moved in the longitudinal axis but can be moved in the transverse axis. If it is in *bone*, the lump will be immobile.

Determine if the lump is *fluctuant* (i.e. contains fluid). Place one forefinger (the 'watch' finger) halfway between the centre and periphery of the lump. The forefinger from the other hand (the 'displacing' finger) is placed diagonally opposite the 'watch' finger at an equal distance from the centre of the lump. Press with the displacing finger and keep the watching finger still. If the lump contains fluid, the watching finger will be displaced in *both* axes of the lump (i.e. fluctuation is present).

Place a small torch behind the lump to determine whether it can be *transilluminated*.

Note any associated signs of *inflammation* (i.e. heat, redness, tenderness and swelling[a]).

Look for similar lumps elsewhere, such as multiple subcutaneous swellings from neurofibromas or lipomas. Neurofibromas are smaller than lipomas. They look hard but are remarkably soft; they occur in neurofibromatosis Type 1 (von Recklinghausen's[b] disease). They continue to increase in number throughout life and are associated with café-au-lait spots and sometimes spinal neurofibromas.

If an inflammatory or neoplastic lump is suspected, remember always to examine the regional lymphatic field and the other lymph node groups.

Correlation of physical signs and skin disease

There are many different skin diseases with varied physical signs. With each major sign the groups of common important diseases that should be considered will be listed.

---

[a] These four cardinal signs were described by Celsus in the 8th volume of his medical book which taught those who were interested surgical techniques. After performing surgery readers were warned to look out for the four cardinal signs of post-surgical inflammation—*calor*, *rubor*, *dolor* and *tumor*. Modern surgeons have added *loss of function* to these signs.

[b] Frederich von Recklinghausen (1833–1910). He was Virchow's assistant in Berlin and then professor of pathology in Strasbourg from 1872. He described this disease in 1882 and haemochromatosis in 1889.

Figure 15.4 Types of skin lesions
(a) Primary skin lesions, palpable with solid mass. (b) Primary skin lesions, palpable and fluid-filled. (c) Special primary skin lesions. (d) Secondary skin lesions, below the skin plane. (e) Secondary skin lesions, above the skin plane. (Adapted from Schwartz M. *Textbook of physical diagnosis*, 4th edn. Philadelphia: Saunders, 2002.)

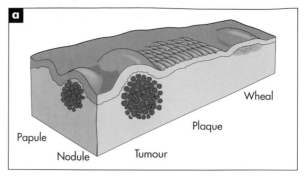
a — Papule, Nodule, Tumour, Plaque, Wheal

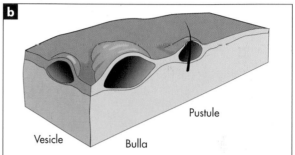
b — Vesicle, Bulla, Pustule

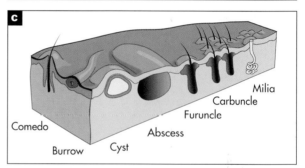
c — Comedo, Burrow, Cyst, Abscess, Furuncle, Carbuncle, Milia

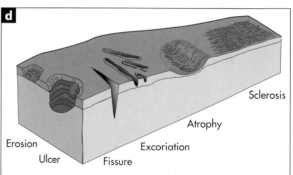
d — Erosion, Ulcer, Fissure, Excoriation, Atrophy, Sclerosis

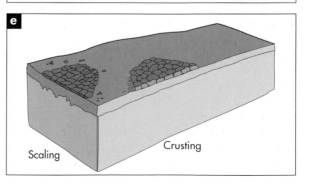
e — Scaling, Crusting

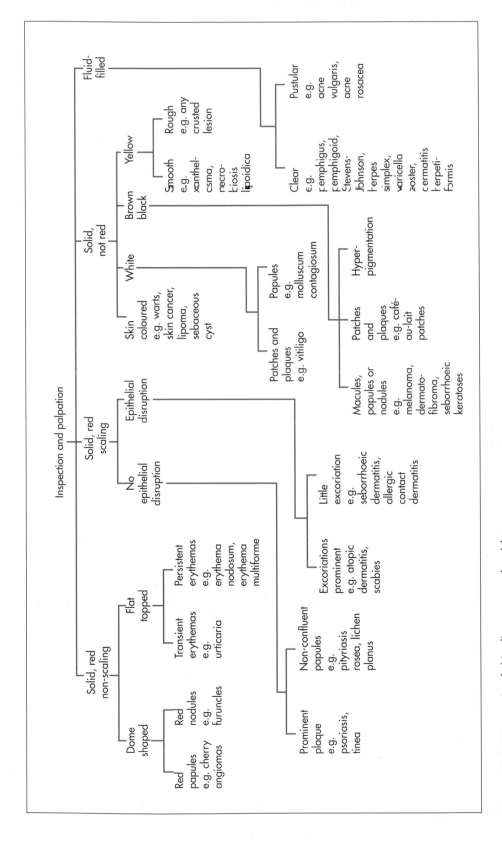

Figure 15.5 Diagnosis of skin disease: an algorithm
(Adapted from Lynch PJ. *Dermatology for the house officer*, 2nd edn. Baltimore: Williams & Wilkins, 1987.)

TABLE 15.4 Primary skin disorders causing pruritus

1 Asteatosis (dry skin)
2 Atopic dermatitis (erythematous, oedematous papular patches on head, neck, flexural surfaces)
3 Urticaria
4 Scabies
5 Dermatitis herpetiformis

TABLE 15.5 Systemic conditions causing pruritus

1 Cholestasis, e.g. primary biliary cirrhosis
2 Chronic renal failure
3 Pregnancy
4 Lymphoma and other internal malignancies
5 Iron deficiency, polycythaemia rubra vera
6 Endocrine diseases, e.g. diabetes mellitus, hypothyroidism, hyperthyroidism, carcinoid syndrome

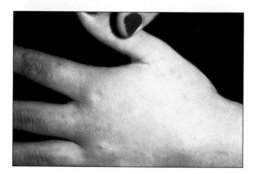

Figure 15.6 Scabies
Scattered fine papules with severe itching. Finger web involvement is common.

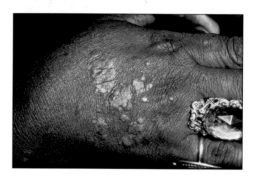

Figure 15.7 Lichen planus
With polygonal flat-topped violaceous lesions.

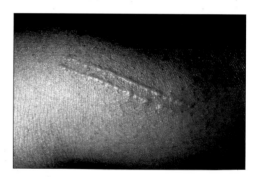

Figure 15.8 Lichen planus
With development of lesions in an area of trauma—the 'Koebner' phenomenon.

Pruritus

Pruritus simply means itching. It may be either generalised or localised. Scratch marks are usually present. Localised pruritus is usually caused by a dermatological condition such as dermatitis or eczema. Generalised pruritus may be caused by primary skin disease, systemic disease or psychogenic factors.

To determine the cause of the pruritus it is essential to examine the skin in detail (Table 15.4). Excoriations are caused by scratching, regardless of the underlying cause. Specific features of cutaneous diseases such as dermatitis, scabies (Figure 15.6) or the blisters of dermatitis herpetiformis should be looked for.

When primary skin diseases have been excluded, a detailed history and examination should be undertaken to consider the various systemic diseases listed in Table 15.5.

Erythrosquamous eruptions

Erythrosquamous eruptions are made up of lesions that are red and scaly. They may be well demarcated or have diffuse borders. They may be itchy or asymptomatic.

When one is attempting to establish a diagnosis of an erythrosquamous eruption, the history is very important. First ask about the time course of the eruption, about a family history of similar skin diseases and whether or not there is a family history of atopy.

The presence or absence of itching and the distribution of the lesions (often on the extensor surfaces of the limbs) also give clues about the diagnosis.

Asymptomatic lesions on the palms and soles are suggestive of secondary syphilis, whereas itchy lesions in the same location would be more suggestive of lichen planus (Figures 15.7 and 15.8). Lichen planus is occasionally associated with

TABLE 15.6 Causes of erythrosquamous eruptions

1 Psoriasis (bright pink plaques with silvery scale)

2 Atopic eczema (diffuse erythema with fine scaling)

3 Pityriasis rosea (paler pink, scaly, macular lesions in a Christmas tree pattern; herald patch; self-limited)

4 Nummular eczema (round patches of subacute dermatitis)

5 Contact dermatitis (irritant or allergic)

6 Dermatophyte infections (ringworm)

7 Lichen planus (violet coloured, small, polygonal papules)

8 Secondary syphilis (flat, red, hyperkeratotic lesions)

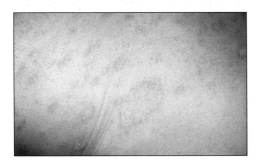

Figure 15.9 Pityriasis rosea
With scattered scaly oval lesions on the trunk and a larger 'herald' patch.

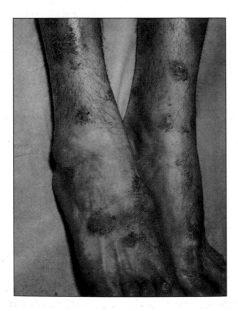

Figure 15.10 Nummular eczema
Typical scattered coin-like lesions of indolent dermatitis.

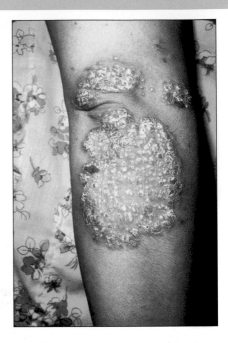

Figure 15.11 Psoriasis
Typical bright red, scaly plaque with silvery scale over a joint.

primary biliary cirrhosis and other liver diseases, chronic graft-versus-host disease and drugs (e.g. gold, penicillamine). Scattered lesions of recent origin on the trunk would be more suggestive of pityriasis rosea (Figure 15.9), whereas more widespread, diffuse and intensely itchy lesions would be more suggestive of nummular eczema (Figure 15.10) (Table 15.6).

Scaly lesions with a well-demarcated edge over the extensor surfaces are usually due to psoriasis (Figures 15.11 and 15.12).

Blistering eruptions

There are a number of different diseases which will present with either vesicles or blisters (Table 15.7). Dermatitis can present as a blistering eruption, particularly acute contact dermatitis (Figure 15.13). See *Questions box 15.2*.

Clinical features of bullous eruptions

Viral blisters such as those of herpes simplex virus infection (Figure 15.14) have a distinctive morphology (grouped vesicles on an erythematous background).

Bullous pemphigoid is a rare disease usually affecting older patients. Blisters are widespread, have a thick roof and tend not to rupture easily.

Pemphigus vulgaris is much more severe. It has thin-roofed blisters that readily rupture and form crusts. The affected superficial skin can be moved

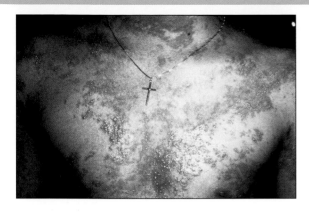

Figure 15.12 Acute widespread pustular psoriasis
Often the eruption is bright red with bizarre patterns and
pustules predominantly at the margins.

TABLE 15.7 Causes of blistering eruptions
1 Traumatic blisters and burns
2 Bullous impetigo
3 Viral blisters (e.g. herpes simplex, varicella)
4 Bullous erythema multiforme
5 Bullous pemphigoid
6 Dermatitis herpetiformis
7 Pemphigus
8 Porphyria
9 Epidermolysis bullosa
10 Dermatophyte infections
11 Acute contact dermatitis

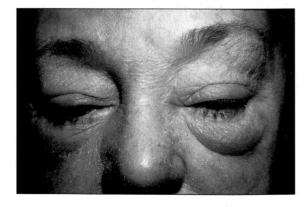

Figure 15.13 Allergic contact dermatitis
From over-the-counter topical medication rubbed over
congested sinuses.

---

[c] Pyotr Vasilyevich Nikolsky (1855–1940), Kiev and Warsaw
dermatologist. Nikolsky's sign also occurs in staphylococcal scalded skin
syndrome and toxic epidermal necrolysis.

Questions box 15.2

**Questions to ask the patient with a blistering
eruption**

! denotes symptoms for the possible diagnosis of an urgent or dangerous problem.

1 Have you had blisters on the backs of your
hands which break easily and are worse if
you have been in the sun?—Porphyria cutanea
tarda

2 Have you had sores or blisters in your mouth
that came on before the skin blisters?—
Pemphigus vulgaris

! 3 Did the inside of your mouth become
ulcerated and painful suddenly?—Stevens-
Johnson syndrome

4 Was the blister on your lip or genitals, and
was it preceded by itching or burning?—
Herpes simplex

! 5 Were the blisters preceded by some days of
severe pain and burning in the areas where
the blisters have broken out?—Herpes zoster

6 Did you notice pink spots on the skin that
were itchy before the blisters appeared?—
Bullous pemphigoid

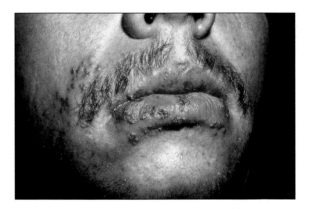

**Figure 15.14 Primary herpes simplex virus infection
in an adult**
Shows typical widespread distribution around the mouth.

over the deeper layer (Nikolsky's[c] sign). Oral ulcers
are common.

Dermatitis herpetiformis is characterised
by a very itchy widespread vesicular or bullous
eruption.

Porphyria cutanea tarda is characterised by
clear or haemorrhagic tense blisters on the hands
and other sun-exposed areas, hyperpigmentation
and increased facial hair; many patients have

TABLE 15.8 Causes of erythroderma

1 Eczema

2 Psoriasis

3 Drugs, e.g. phenytoin, allopurinol

4 Pityriasis rubra pilaris

5 Mycosis fungoides, leukaemia, lymphoma

6 Lichen planus

7 Pemphigus foliaceus

8 Hereditary disorders

9 Dermatophytosis

TABLE 15.9 Causes of pustular and crusted lesions

1 Acne vulgaris (comedones, papules, pustules, cystic lesions, ice pick scars—no telangiectasiae)

2 Acne rosacea (acne-like lesions, erythema and telangiectasia on central face)

3 Impetigo

4 Folliculitis

5 Viral lesions

6 Pustular psoriasis

7 Drug eruptions

8 Dermatophyte infections

Questions box 15.3

Questions to ask the patient with pustular lesions

1 Are you taking cortisone tablets?—Steroid acne

2 Has the skin been painful or have you had a fever?—Pustular psoriasis

3 Have you had psoriasis in the past?

4 Do you find your face becomes flushed easily, for example if you drink hot drinks?—Acne rosacea

5 Are you a diabetic?—Cutaneous candidiasis

6 Do you sweat excessively?—Folliculitis

TABLE 15.10 Causes of dermal plaques

1 Granuloma annulare

2 Necrobiosis lipoidica

3 Sarcoidosis

4 Erythema nodosum

5 Lupus erythematosus

6 Morphoea and scleroderma

7 Tuberculosis

8 Leprosy

hepatitis C and alcohol can induce symptoms (due to decreased uroporphyrinogen decarboxylase).

Erythroderma

Erythroderma is best thought of as the end-stage of numerous skin conditions (Table 15.8). The erythrodermic patient has involvement of nearly all the skin with an erythematous inflammatory process, often with exfoliation. There is usually associated oedema and loss of muscle mass. This represents that most unusual occurrence, a dermatological emergency.

An attempt should be made to determine the underlying cause of the erythroderma, and this is best done based on history and examination. Specific treatment can then be directed at the underlying cause. Some patients with erythroderma will develop profound metabolic changes (including hypoalbuminaemia and extrarenal water loss), and these patients require constant supervision and monitoring until they have recovered from the acute phase of their illness.

The most common cause is eczema, which is usually of the atopic variety. These patients often have an intense pruritus. Some of them will develop a chronic unremitting erythroderma.

Pustular and crusted lesions

The clinical appearance of a *pustular* lesion results from accumulation of neutrophils. Such collections usually indicate an infective process; however, sterile pustules may form as part of a number of skin diseases due to the release of chemotactic factors following an immunological reaction.

A *crust* is a yellowish crystalline material that is found on the skin; it is made up of desiccated serum.

It is essential to determine whether or not a pustular lesion (or a group of pustular lesions) represents a primarily infectious process or an inflammatory dermatological condition. For example, pustular lesions on the hands and feet may either be due to tinea infection or be a primary pustular psoriasis or palmoplantar pustulosis (Table 15.9). See *Questions box 15.3*.

TABLE 15.11 Causes of erythema nodosum

1 Sarcoidosis

2 Streptococcal infections (β-haemolytic)

3 Inflammatory bowel disease

4 Drugs, e.g. sulfonamides, penicillin, sulfonylurea, oestrogen, iodides, bromides

5 Tuberculosis

6 Other infections, e.g. lepromatous leprosy, toxoplasmosis, histoplasmosis, *Yersinia*, *Chlamydia*

7 Systemic lupus erythematosus

8 Behçet's syndrome

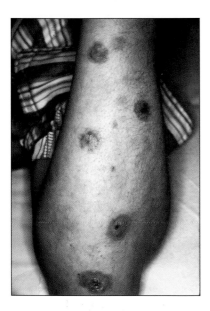

Figure 15.15 Erythema multiforme
Shows classic iris or target lesions, secondary to herpes simplex virus infection of the lips.

Dermal plaques

Plaques are localised thickenings of the skin which are usually caused by changes in the dermis or subcutaneous fat. These may be due to chronic inflammatory processes or scarring sclerotic processes (Table 15.10).

The pattern of involvement of the plaques, the age of the patient and other clinical features should enable a diagnosis to be established.

In *Sweet's syndrome* there are painful red plaques and a high fever (acute febrile neutrophilic dermatosis); 10% have leukaemia.

Erythema nodosum

This is the best known of the group of diseases classified as nodular vasculitis. The lesions of erythema nodosum are usually found below the knee in the pretibial area and are erythematous, palpable and tender (Figure 6.36, page 191). There may be an associated fever (Table 15.11). Sarcoidosis is a common cause, but the skin changes in sarcoid can mimic almost any skin disease (except vesicles).

Erythema multiforme

This is a distinctive inflammatory reaction of skin and mucosa. It is not a systemic disease. Characteristic discrete target lesions occur, particularly on the distal extremities (Figure 15.15). The periphery of these lesions is red, whereas the centre becomes bluish or even purpuric. The lesions can become bullous, and severe cases of this syndrome involve widespread desquamation of the mucosal surfaces (the Stevens-Johnson[d] syndrome). In many cases the condition is precipitated by clinical or subclinical herpes simplex virus infection. Other causes include *Mycoplasma pneumoniae*, histoplasmosis, malignancy, sarcoidosis and drugs (including those that can cause toxic epidermal necrolysis). Sometimes no underlying cause of the erythema multiforme will be established.

Toxic epidermal necrolysis, on the other hand, is a systemic condition and usually secondary to a drug reaction. It results in a peeling of large skin areas. The major causes include penicillin, sulfonamides, phenytoin and non-steroidal anti-inflammatory drugs.

Hyperpigmentation

The presence of hyperpigmentation can be a clue to underlying systemic disease (Table 15.12).

Flushing and sweating

Flushing of the skin may sometimes be observed, especially on the face, by the examiner. Some of the causes of this phenomenon are presented in Table 15.13.

Excessive sweating (hyperhidrosis) can occur with thyrotoxicosis, phaeochromocytoma, acromegaly, hypoglycaemia, autonomic dysfunction, stress, fever and menopause.

Skin tumours

Skin tumours are very common and are usually benign (Table 15.14).[4] Most malignant skin tumours can be cured if they are detected early and treated appropriately (Table 15.15).

---

d   Albert Mason Stevens (1884–1945), New York paediatrician, and Frank C Johnson (1894–1934), American physician.

TABLE 15.12 Causes of diffuse hyperpigmentation

Endocrine disease
Addison's disease (excess ACTH)
Ectopic ACTH secretion (e.g. carcinoma)
The contraceptive pill or pregnancy
Thyrotoxicosis, acromegaly, phaeochromocytoma

Metabolic
Malabsorption or malnutrition
Liver diseases, e.g. haemochromatosis, primary biliary cirrhosis, Wilson's disease
Chronic renal failure
Porphyria
Chronic infection, e.g. bacterial endocarditis
Connective tissue disease, e.g. systemic lupus, scleroderma, dermatomyositis

Racial or genetic

Other
Drugs, e.g. chlorpromazine, busulphan, arsenicals
Radiation

ACTH = adrenocorticotrophic hormone.

TABLE 15.13 Causes of facial flushing

1 Menopause

2 Drugs and foods, e.g. nifedipine, monosodium glutamate (MSG)

3 Alcohol after taking the drug disulfiram (or alcohol alone in some people)

4 Systemic mastocytosis

5 Rosacea

6 Carcinoid syndrome (secretion of serotonin and other mediators by a tumour may produce flushing, diarrhoea and valvular heart disease)

7 Autonomic dysfunction

8 Medullary carcinoma of the thyroid

TABLE 15.14 Benign skin tumours

1 Warts

2 Molluscum contagiosum

3 Seborrhoeic keratoses

4 Dermatofibroma

5 Neurofibroma

6 Angioma

7 Xanthoma

TABLE 15.15 Malignant skin tumours

1 Basal cell carcinoma

2 Squamous cell carcinoma

3 Bowen's* disease (squamous cell carcinoma confined to the epithelial layer of the skin—carcinoma in situ)

4 Malignant melanoma

5 Secondary deposits

* John Templeton Bowen (1857–1941), Boston dermatologist.

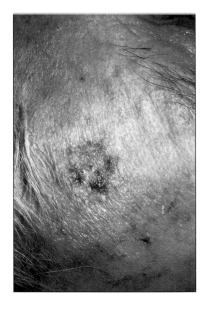

Figure 15.16 Actinic keratosis, slightly eroded and scaly
Higher on the forehead additional granular keratosis could be easily palpated.

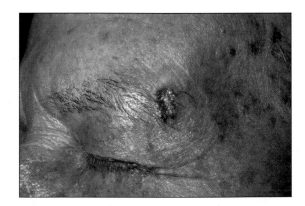

Figure 15.17 Pigmented basal cell carcinoma
With pearly quality and depressed centre, in a patient with sun-damaged skin.

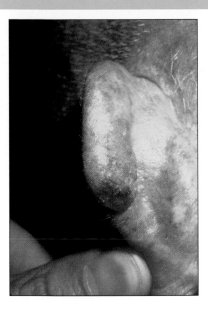

Figure 15.18 Squamous cell carcinoma

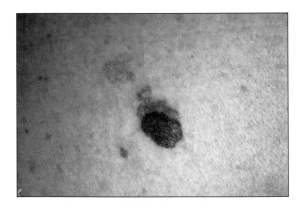

Figure 15.19 Superficial spreading melanoma, still confined to the upper dermis

Skin cancer often occurs in those predisposed individuals (with the fair skin of Celtic or Northern European origin) who undergo chronic exposure to ultraviolet light.

Skin cancers may present as flat scaly lesions or as raised scaly or smooth lesions. They may be large or small and they may eventually ulcerate. All non-healing ulcers should be considered to be skin cancer, until proven otherwise.

The earliest lesions are actinic (solar) keratoses, which are pink macules or papules surmounted by adherent scale (Figure 15.16). Basal cell carcinoma is characteristically a translucent papule with a depressed centre and a rolled border with ectatic capillaries (Figure 15.17). Squamous cell carcinoma is typically an opaque papule or plaque which is often eroded or scaly (Figure 15.18).

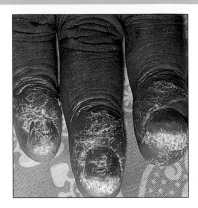

Figure 15.20 Onychomycosis: fungal infection of the nails

Malignant melanomas are usually deeply pigmented lesions that are enlarging and have an irregular notched border (Figure 15.19). There is often variation of pigment within the lesion. Malignant melanoma is likely if the lesion is *Asymmetrical*, has an irregular *Border*, has an irregular *Colour* and is large (*Diameter* >6 mm) and may be *Elevated*, referred to as the ABCDE checklist.[5,6] Patients with numerous large and unusual pigmented naevi (dysplastic naevus syndrome) are at an increased risk of developing malignant melanoma.

The nails

Systemic disease is commonly associated with changes in the patient's finger (and toe) nails and in the nail beds. The slow growth of the nails means that the temporal course of an illness may be seen in nail changes. Many of these findings have been described in other chapters but important features of nail changes are dealt with here.

Fungal infection of the nails (onychomycosis) (Figure 15.20) is their most common abnormality. It makes up 40% of all nail disorders and 30% of all cutaneous fungal infections. The characteristic findings are pitting, thickening, ridging and deformity. The changes can be indistinguishable from those of psoriasis. Candidal nail infections are less common than those due to dermatophytes. Candidal nail infection (diagnosed by microscopy and culture) suggests the possibility of chronic mucocutaneous candidiasis, which is a rare condition associated with polyendocrinopathies.

Nail involvement occurs in about 25% of patients with psoriasis (Figure 15.21). The characteristic abnormality is pitting. This can also occur in fungal infections, chronic paronychia, lichen planus and alopecia areata. Psoriasis is also the most common

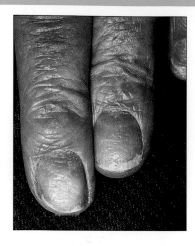

Figure 15.21 Nail involvement occurs in about 25% of patients with psoriasis

cause of onycholysis. Rarer changes in psoriatic nails include longitudinal ridging (onychorrhexis), proximal transverse ridging, subungual hyperkeratosis and yellow-brown discoloration.

Nailfold telangiectasia is an important sign in a number of systemic disorders, including systemic lupus erythematosus, scleroderma and Raynaud's phenomenon. These changes are not very specific and considerable variation in nailfold capillary shape is present in normal people. In patients with dermatomyositis, nailfold telangiectasiae are associated with hypertrophy of the cuticle and small haemorrhagic infarcts.

Raynaud's is also associated with nail changes caused by the inadequate blood supply. These include brittleness, longitudinal ridging, splitting, flattening, onycholysis, koilonychia and a redder than normal nail bed.

Clubbing is an important nail abnormality. It has also been described in patients with HIV infection, and its severity seems proportional to the degree of immunosuppression. HIV infection is also associated with onychomycosis and longitudinal melonychia (dark line in the nail), secondary to treatment with zidovudine.

Summary
The dermatological examination in internal medicine: a suggested method
(Figure 15.22)
Even if the patient shows the examiner only a small single area of abnormality, proceed to examine all the skin.

After obtaining good lighting conditions and asking the patient to disrobe, begin by looking at the **nails and hands**. Paronychia is an infection of the skin surrounding the nails. Other changes to note include pitting (psoriasis, fungal infections) and onycholysis (e.g. thyrotoxicosis, psoriasis). Dark staining under the nail may indicate a subungual melanoma. Linear splinter haemorrhages (e.g. vasculitis) or telangiectasiae (e.g. systemic lupus erythematosus) may be seen in the nail bed.

A purplish discoloration in streaks over the knuckles may indicate dermatomyositis. Also look at the backs of the hands and forearms for the characteristic blisters of porphyria, which occur on the exposed skin. Papules and scratch marks on the backs of the hands, between the fingers and around the wrists may indicate scabies. Viral warts are common on the hands.

Look at the palms for Dupuytren's contracture, pigmented flat junctional moles (which have a high risk of becoming malignant) and xanthomata in the palmar creases.

Next look at the **forearms**, where lichen planus may occur on the flexor surfaces (characterised by small shiny, purple-coloured papules) and psoriasis may be present on the extensor surfaces. Palpable purpura—raised bruising that indicates bleeding into the skin—may be seen on the arms, and indicates vasculitis. Acanthosis nigricans can occur in the axillae.

Inspect the patient's **hair and scalp**. Decide whether or not the hair is dry and whether the distribution is normal. Alopecia may indicate male pattern baldness, recent severe illness, hypothyroidism or thyrotoxicosis. Patches of alopecia occur in the disease alopecia areata. Short broken-off hairs occur typically in systemic lupus erythematosus. In psoriasis there are silvery scales, which may be seen on the skin of the scalp. Metastatic deposits may rarely be felt as firm nodules within the skin of the scalp. Sebaceous cysts are common. The unfortunate examiner may find nits sticking to the head hairs.

Move down now to the **eyebrows** and look for scaling and greasiness, which are found in seborrhoeic dermatitis. A purplish erythema occurs around the eyelids in dermatomyositis. Xanthelasmata are seen near the eyelid.

Look at the **face** for rosacea, which causes bright erythema of the nose, cheeks, forehead and chin, and occasionally pustules and rhinophyma (disfiguring swelling of the nose). Acne causes papules, pustules and scars involving the face, neck and upper trunk. The butterfly rash of systemic lupus erythematosus occurs across the cheeks but is rare. Spider naevi may be present. Ulcerating lesions on the face may include basal cell carcinoma, squamous cell carcinoma or rarely tuberculosis (lupus vulgaris).

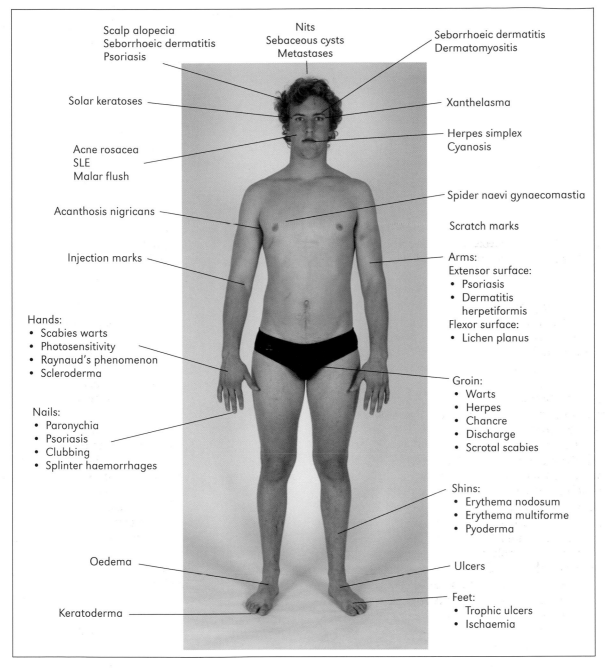

Figure 15.22 Sites of some important skin lesions of the limbs, face and trunk
SLE = systemic lupus erythematosus.

Benign tumours of the face include keratoacanthoma (a volcano-like lesion from a sebaceous gland) and congenital haemangiomas.

Look for the blisters of herpes zoster, which may occur strictly in the distribution of one of the divisions of the trigeminal nerve.

Inspect the **neck**, which is prone to many of the lesions that occur on the face. Rarely, the redundant loose skin of pseudoxanthoma elasticum will be seen around the neck.

Go on to inspect the **trunk**, where any of the childhood exanthems produce their characteristic rashes. Look for spider naevi. Campbell de Morgan spots are commonly found on the abdomen (and chest), as are flat, greasy, yellow-coloured seborrhoeic warts. Erythema marginatum (rheumatic fever) occurs on the chest and abdomen. Herpes zoster may be seen overlying any of the dermatome distributions.

Metastases from internal malignancies may rarely occur anywhere on the skin. Neurofibromas are soft flesh-coloured tumours; when associated with more than five 'café-au-lait' spots (brownish, irregular lesions), they suggest neurofibromatosis (von Recklinghausen's disease). Pigmented moles are seen on the trunk and evidence of malignancy must be looked for with these. The patient's buttocks and sacrum must be examined for bedsores, and the abdomen and thighs may have areas of fat atrophy or hypertrophy from insulin injections.

Go to the **legs**, where erythema nodosum or erythema multiforme may be seen on the shins. Necrobiosis lipoidica diabeticorum affects the skin over the tibia in diabetics. Pretibial myxoedema also occurs over the shins. Look for ulcers on either side of the lower part of the leg. Livedo reticularis is a net-like, red reticular rash that occurs in vasculitis, the anti-phospholipid syndrome and with atheroembolism.

Inspect the **feet** for the characteristic lesion of Reiter's disease called keratoderma blennorrhagica, where crusted lesions spread across the sole because of the fusion of vesicles and pustules. Look at the foot for signs of ischaemia, associated with wasting of the skin and skin appendages. Trophic ulcers may be seen in patients with peripheral neuropathy (e.g. diabetes mellitus). Always separate the toes to look for melanomas.

References

1. Marks R. A diagnostic approach to common dermatology problems. *Aust Fam Phys* 1982; 11:696–702.
2. Ashton RE. Teaching non-dermatologists to examine the skin: a review of the literature and some recommendations. *Brit J Derm* 1995; 132:221–225.
3. Schwarzenberger K. The essentials of the complete skin examination. *Med Clin Nth Am* 1998; 82:981–999.
4. Preston DS, Stern RS. Nonmelanoma cancers of the skin. *N Engl J Med* 1992; 327:649–662. Provides useful information on discriminating between worrying and non-worrying lesions, and includes colour photographs.
5. Whitehead JD, Gichnik JM. Does this patient have a mole or a melanoma? *JAMA* 1998; 279:696–701. The ABCD checklist (asymmetry, border irregularity, irregular colour, diameter >6 mm) has a sensitivity over 90% and a specificity over 95% for identifying malignant melanoma.
6. Abbasi NR, Shaw HM, Rigel DS et al. Early diagnosis of cutaneous melanoma: rewriting the ABC criteria. *JAMA* 2004;292:2771–2776. Changes (evolving) of symptoms or signs (size, shape; pruritus, tenderness, bleeding or colour) are additional evidence for the presence of melanoma.

Suggested reading

Buxton PK. *ABC of dermatology*, 5th edn. London: Wiley & Sons, 2009.

Callen JP, Paller AS, Greer K. eds. *Color atlas of dermatology*, 2nd edn. Philadelphia: WB Saunders, 2000.

Fitzpatrick TB, Johnson RA, Polano MK, Suurmond D, Wolff K. *Color atlas and synopsis of clinical dermatology*, 5th edn. New York: McGraw-Hill, 2005.

Gawkrodger DJ. *Dermatology. An illustrated color text*, 4th edn. New York: Churchill Livingstone, 2008.

Chapter 16

A system for the infectious diseases examination

As it takes two to make a quarrel, so it takes two to make a disease, the microbe and its host.

Charles Chaplain (1856–1941)

We have selected two important presentations to be covered in this chapter to show how infectious diseases can be approached in a systematic manner.

Pyrexia of unknown origin (PUO)

This condition is defined as documented fever (>38°C) of more than 3 weeks' duration, where no cause is found despite basic investigations.[1,2] The most frequent causes to consider are tuberculosis, occult abscess (usually intra-abdominal), osteomyelitis, infective endocarditis, lymphoma or leukaemia, systemic-onset juvenile rheumatoid arthritis, giant cell arteritis and drug fever (drug fever is responsible for 10% of fevers leading to hospital admission[3]). In studies of fever of unknown origin, infection is found to be the cause in 30%, neoplasia in 30%, connective tissue disease in 15% and miscellaneous causes in 15%; in 10% the aetiology remains unknown (Table 16.1). Remember, the longer the duration of the fever, the less likely there is an infectious aetiology. The majority of patients do not have a rare disease but rather a relatively common disease presenting in an unusual way.[4]

History

The history may give a number of clues in these puzzling cases. In some patients a careful history may give the diagnosis where expensive tests have failed. See *Questions box 16.1*.

The time course of the fever and any associated symptoms must be uncovered. Symptoms from the various body systems should be sought methodically.

TABLE 16.1 Common causes of pyrexia of unknown origin

1 Neoplasms
- Hodgkin's and non-Hodgkin's lymphoma, leukaemia, malignant histiocytosis
- Other tumours: hepatic, renal, lung, disseminated carcinoma, atrial myxoma

2 Infections
- Bacterial: e.g. tuberculosis, brucellosis and other bacteraemias, abscess formation (especially pelvic or abdominal), endocarditis, pericarditis, osteomyelitis, cholangitis, pyelonephritis, pelvic inflammatory disease, prostatitis, syphilis, Lyme disease, borreliasis, cat scratch disease, dental abscess
- Viral: e.g. infectious mononucleosis, cytomegalovirus infection, hepatitis B or C, human immunodeficiency virus (HIV) infection, Ross River virus
- Parasitic, rickettsial and others: e.g. malaria, Q fever, toxoplasmosis
- Fungal: e.g. histoplasmosis, cryptococcosis, blastomycosis

3 Connective tissue diseases
- Juvenile rheumatoid arthritis, systemic lupus erythematosus
- Vasculitis, e.g. giant cell arteritis, polyarteritis nodosa

4 Drug fever

5 Miscellaneous
Inflammatory bowel disease, alcoholic liver disease, granulomatous disease (e.g. sarcoid), multiple pulmonary emboli, thyroiditis, adrenal insufficiency, phaeochromocytoma, familial Mediterranean fever and other hereditary periodic fever syndromes, factitious fever

6 Uncertain

Examples include:

1 The gastrointestinal system—diarrhoea, abdominal pain, recent abdominal surgery (inflammatory bowel disease, diverticular disease, cholangitis).
2 The cardiovascular system—heart murmurs, dental procedures (infective endocarditis), chest pain (pericarditis).
3 Rheumatology—joint symptoms, rashes.
4 Neurology—headache (meningitis, cerebral abscess).
5 Genitourinary system—history of renal disease or infection, dysuria
6 Respiratory system—old tuberculosis (TB) or recent TB contact, chest symptoms.

Details of any recent overseas travel are important. Find out also about hobbies and exposure to pets. Occupational exposure may be important. Take a drug history. Find out if the patient is involved in behaviour posing a risk of HIV infection. Patients who are already in hospital may have infected cannulas or old cannula sites.

Fever due to bacteraemia (the presence of organisms in the bloodstream) is associated with a higher risk of mortality. It is present in up to 20% of hospital patients with fever.[5] Certain clinical findings modestly increase the likelihood of the presence of bacteraemia (*Good signs guide 16.1*).

Examination

General

Look at the temperature chart to see whether there is a pattern of fever that is identifiable. Inspect the patient and decide how seriously ill he or she appears. Look for evidence of weight loss (indicating a chronic illness). Note any skin rash (Table 16.2). The details of the examination required will depend on the patient's history.

Hands

Look for the stigmata of infective endocarditis or vasculitic changes. Note whether there is clubbing. The presence of arthropathy or Raynaud's phenomenon may point to a connective tissue disease.

Arms

Inspect for drug injection sites suggesting intravenous drug abuse (see Figure 4.41). Feel for the epitrochlear and axillary nodes (e.g. lymphoma, other malignancy, sarcoidosis, focal infections).

Head and neck

Feel the *temporal arteries* (over the temples). In temporal arteritis these may be tender and thickened.

Questions box 16.1

General questions to ask the patient with a fever

! denotes symptoms for the possible diagnosis of an urgent or dangerous problem.

1 How long have you had high temperatures?
2 Have you taken your own temperature? How high has it been?

! 3 Have you had shivers and shakes (rigors)?
4 Has anyone you know had a similar illness?
5 What medications are you taking?
6 Have you had any recent illnesses?
7 Have you had any recent operations or medical procedures?
8 Have you travelled recently? Where to?
9 Did you take anti-malarial prophylaxis and have the recommended vaccinations for your trip?
10 Have you any pets? Have they been sick lately?

GOOD SIGNS GUIDE 16.1 Clinical findings and bacteraemia

Risk factors	Likelihood ratio if	
	Present	Absent
Age > 50	1.4	0.3
Temperature >38.5	1.2	NS
Rigors	1.8	NS
Tachycardia	1.2	NS
Respiratory rate >20	NS	NS
Hypotension	2.0	NS
Chronic kidney disease	4.6	0.8
Hospitalisation for trauma	3.0	NS
Terminal disease	2.7	NS
Indwelling urinary catheter	2.4	NS
Central venous catheter	2.0	NS
'Toxic appearance'	NS	NS

From McGee S, *Evidence-based physical diagnosis*, 2nd edn. St Louis: Saunders, 2007.

Examine the *eyes* for iritis or conjunctivitis (connective tissue disease—e.g. Reiter's syndrome) or jaundice (e.g. ascending cholangitis, blackwater fever in malaria). Look in the fundi for choroidal tubercles in miliary tuberculosis, Roth's spots in

TABLE 16.2 Differential diagnosis of prolonged fever and rash

1 Viral: e.g. infectious mononucleosis, rubella, dengue fever

2 Bacterial: e.g. syphilis, Lyme disease

3 Non-infective: e.g. drugs, systemic lupus erythematosus, erythema multiforme (which may also be related to an underlying infection)

infective endocarditis, and retinal haemorrhages or the infiltrates of leukaemia or lymphoma.

Inspect the *face* for a butterfly rash (systemic lupus erythematosus, see Figure 9.61, page 284) or seborrhoeic dermatitis, which is common in patients with HIV infection.

Examine the *mouth* for ulcers, gum disease or candidiasis, and the teeth and tonsils for infection (e.g. abscess). Look in the *ears* for otitis media. Feel the *parotid glands* for evidence of infection.

Palpate the cervical lymph nodes. Examine for thyroid enlargement and tenderness (subacute thyroiditis).

Chest

Examine the chest. Palpate for bony tenderness. Carefully examine the respiratory system (e.g. for signs of pneumonia, tuberculosis, empyema, carcinoma) and the heart for murmurs (e.g. infective endocarditis, atrial myxoma) or rubs (e.g. pericarditis).

The abdomen

Examine the abdomen. Inspect for rashes, including rose-coloured spots (in typhoid fever—2- to 4-mm flat red spots, which blanch on pressure and occur on the upper abdomen and lower chest). Examine for evidence of hepatomegaly and ascites (e.g. spontaneous bacterial peritonitis, hepatic carcinoma, metastatic deposits), splenomegaly (e.g. haemopoietic malignancy, infective endocarditis, malaria), renal enlargement (e.g. renal cell carcinoma) or localised tenderness (e.g. collection of pus). Palpate for testicular enlargement (e.g. seminoma, tuberculosis). Feel for inguinal lymphadenopathy.

Perform a rectal examination, feeling for a mass or tenderness in the rectum or pelvis (e.g. abscess, carcinoma, prostatitis). Sigmoidoscopy should also be performed for evidence of inflammatory bowel disease or carcinoma. Perform a vaginal examination to detect collections of pelvic pus or evidence of pelvic inflammatory disease. Look at the penis and scrotum for a discharge or rash.

Central nervous system

Examine the central nervous system for signs of meningism (e.g. chronic tuberculous meningitis, cryptococcal meningitis) or focal neurological signs (e.g. brain abscess, mononeuritis multiplex in polyarteritis nodosa).

HIV infection and the acquired immunodeficiency syndrome (AIDS)

This syndrome, first described in 1981, is caused by the human immunodeficiency virus (HIV).[6,7] This is a T-cell lymphotrophic virus, which results in T4 cell destruction and therefore susceptibility to opportunistic infections and the development of tumours, notably Kaposi's sarcoma[a] and non-Hodgkin's lymphoma.

HIV infection should be suspected particularly if the patient falls into a high-risk group (e.g. male homosexual, intravenous drug abuser, sexual tourist, sexual partner of HIV-infected person, haemophiliac, blood transfusion or blood product recipient, prostitute, or sexual contact with one of these). Examine the patient as follows.

Examination

General inspection

Take the temperature. The patient may appear ill and wasted due to chronic ill-health or chronic opportunistic infection. *Mycobacterium avium* complex (MAC) presents with fever and weight loss.

Look at the skin for rashes:

- The maculopapular rash of acute HIV infection (5- to 10-mm maculopapular lesions on the face and trunk and rarely on the palms and soles).
- Herpes zoster (shingles, which may involve more than one dermatome in this disease and is more commonly seen in early rather than in advanced HIV infection).
- Oral herpes simplex (cold sores) or genital herpes (20%).
- Oral and flexural candidiasis (once the CD4 level is below 200/mm³).
- Molluscum contagiosum (10%), impetigo, seborrhoea (occurs in up to 80% of patients at some time) or other non-specific exanthems.
- Kaposi's sarcoma: red-purple vascular non-tender tumours. These present typically on the skin but can occur anywhere.
- Skin lesions resembling Kaposi's sarcoma may

---

a   Moritz Kohn Kaposi (1837–1902), professor of dermatology, Vienna, described the sarcoma in 1892.

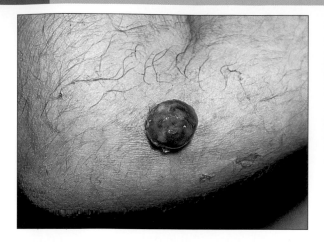

Figure 16.1 Angry red nodule of bacillary angiomatosis

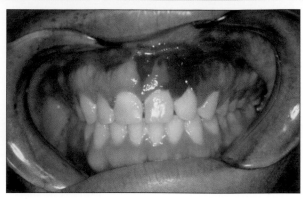

Figure 16.3 Kaposi's sarcoma
(From McDonald FS, ed., *Mayo Clinic images in internal medicine,* with permission. © Mayo Clinic Scientific Press and CRC Press.)

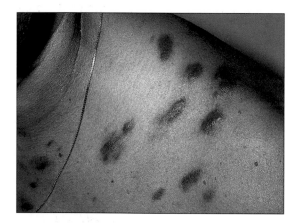

Figure 16.2 Late nodules of Kaposi's sarcoma

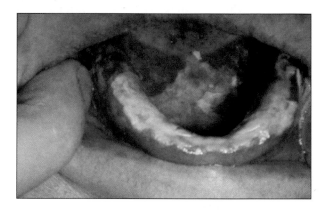

Figure 16.4 Oral candidiasis
(From McDonald FS, ed., *Mayo Clinic images in internal medicine,* with permission. © Mayo Clinic Scientific Press and CRC Press.)

also be seen. These are called bacillary angiomatosis and are caused by *Bartonella henselae* and *Bartonella quintana* (Figures 16.1 and 16.2). Adverse drug reactions are more common in patients with HIV infection and may be the cause of a rash. Look for hyperpigmentation. Patients taking the drug clofamizine for MAC infection usually become deeply pigmented. Areas of peripheral fat atrophy—lipodystrophy— on limbs, cheeks and buttocks may be seen in 20%–30% of patients treated with the protease inhibitor drugs. Some of these patients have fat redistribution with central obesity.

Hands and arms

Look for nail changes including onycholysis. Feel for the epitrochlear nodes; a node 0.5 cm or larger may be characteristic.[8] Note any injection marks.

Face

Inspect the mouth for:
- candidal plaques
- angular stomatitis
- aphthous ulcers
- tongue ulceration (e.g. herpes simplex, cytomegalovirus or candidal infections) or gingivitis.[9]

Periodontal disease is very common. Kaposi's sarcoma (Figures 16.3 and 16.4) may also occur on the hard or soft palate (in which case associated lesions are almost always present elsewhere in the gastrointestinal tract). Oral squamous cell carcinoma and non-Hodgkin's lymphoma are more common in AIDS.

Parotidomegaly is sometimes seen as a result of HIV-associated Sjögren's syndrome. These patients may have dry eyes and mouth for this reason.

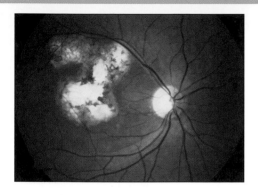

Figure 16.5 Retinal toxoplasmosis—old chorioretinal scar

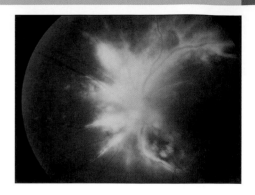

Figure 16.6   Cytomegalovirus retinitis

Hairy leucoplakia is a unique raised or flat, white, painless, and often hairy-looking lesion typically present on the lateral surface of the tongue; it is caused by Epstein-Barr virus infection in HIV-infected persons and is almost diagnostic of HIV infection.

Palpate over the sinuses for tenderness (sinusitis). Examine the cervical and axillary nodes. There may be generalised lymphadenopathy, and all lymph node groups should be examined.

Chest

Note any tachypnoea or dry cough. Chronic cough, either dry or productive of purulent sputum, is common. On auscultation crackles may be present at the bases due to bronchiolitis obliterans. There are often, however, no chest signs despite the presence of pulmonary infiltrates on chest X-ray due to *Pneumocystis jiroveci* (formerly *carinii*) or other opportunistic infections.

Abdomen

Examine for hepatosplenomegaly (e.g. infection, lymphoma). Perform a rectal examination (e.g. perianal ulceration from herpes simplex) and a sigmoidoscopy looking for Kaposi's sarcoma or proctitis (e.g. cytomegalovirus, herpes simplex, amoebic dysentery or pseudomembranous colitis from antibiotic use). Examine the genitals for herpes simplex, warts, discharge or chancre.

Nervous system

Look for signs of meningism (e.g. cryptococcal meningitis). There may be focal signs due to a space-occupying intracranial lesion (e.g. toxoplasmosis, non-Hodgkin's lymphoma).

A syndrome similar to Guillain-Barré and a pure sensory neuropathy can occur. HIV infection itself, opportunistic infection or the drugs used in treatment can be responsible for peripheral sensorimotor neuropathy, polymyositis, radiculopathy, mononeuritis multiplex or a myelopathy.

Look in the fundi for cottonwool spots (common in AIDS patients), scars (e.g. toxoplasmosis—Figure 16.5) or retinitis (e.g. cytomegalovirus-induced retinitis with perivascular haemorrhages and fluffy exudates, which can cause blindness of rapid onset—Figure 16.6).[10] There may be signs of dementia (AIDS encephalopathy).

References

1. Knockaert DC, Vanneste LJ, Vanneste SB, Bobbaers HJ. Fever of unknown origin in the 1980s. An update of the diagnostic spectrum. *Arch Intern Med* 1992; 152: 51–55.

2. Whitby M. The febrile patient. *Aust Fam Phys* 1993; 22:1753–1755, 1758–1761.

3. Arbo M et al. Fever of nosocomial origin: etiology, risk factors and outcomes. *Am J Med* 1993; 95:505–515.

4. Mourad O, Palda V, Detsky AS. A comprehensive evidence based approach to fever of unknown origin. *Arch Intern Med* 2003; 163:545.

5. Bates DW, Cook EF, Goldman L, et al. Predicting bacteremia in hospitalized patients: A prospectively validated model. *Ann Intern Med* 1990; 113:495–500.

6. American College of Physicians and Infectious Diseases Society of America. Human immunodeficiency virus (HIV) infection. *Ann Intern Med* 1994; 120:310–319.

7. Nandwani R. Human immunodeficiency virus medicine for the MRCP short cases. *Br J Hosp Med* 1994; 51:353–356.

8. Malin A, Ternouth I, Sarbah S. Epitrochlear nodes as marker of HIV disease in sub-Saharan Africa. *BMJ* 1994; 309:1550–1551.

9. Weinert ML, Grimes RM, Lynch DP. Oral manifestations of HIV infection. *Ann Intern Med* 1996; 125:485–496. Details the 16 leading oral complications, based on an extensive literature review.

10. De Smet MD, Nessenbatt RB. Ocular manifestations of AIDS. *JAMA* 1991; 266:3019–3022. Provides a very good review of eye changes.

Suggested reading

Edmond RTD, Rowlard HAK. *A color atlas of infectious diseases*, 4th edn. Mosby, 2003.

Appendix I

Writing and presenting the history and physical examination

Experience is never limited, and it is never complete.
Henry James

It is important that the medical record be kept short and simple, yet complete. The following approach is one recommended by the authors. The detail of the history and examination and its record varies of course, depending on whether this is a first visit and on the complexity of the presenting problem. It is not necessary to ask every patient every question.

History

Personal information

Record the name, sex, date of birth and address. Write down the date and time of the examination.

Presenting (principal) symptoms (PS)

A short sentence identifies the *major* symptoms and their duration; it is often useful to quote the patient's own words.

History of present illness (HPI)

Don't record every detail; rather, prepare short prose paragraphs telling the story of the illness in chronological order. Describe the characteristics of each symptom. Note why the patient presents at this time. Also, describe any past medical problems which are related to the current symptoms. Include the relevant positive and negative findings on the system review here. If there are many seemingly unrelated problems, summarise these in an introductory paragraph and present the history of each problem in separate paragraphs.

List **current medications** and doses and the indications for their use, if they are known, and any side-effects or known or measured therapeutic effects. For example, if the patient. takes anti-hypertensive drugs ask whether blood pressure control has been satisfactory as far as the patient knows. Finally, record your impression of the reliability of the information and, if the patient was unable to give the history, describe who was the source.

Past history (PH)

List in chronological order past medical or surgical problems (sometimes called *inactive* problems), past medication use, if relevant, and any history of allergy (particularly drug allergy) or of drug intolerance. Find out exactly what the problem with the drug was. The patient may know the results of certain previous important investigations (e.g. 'the scan showed I had clots in my lung'). A history of blood transfusions should be noted.

Social history (SH)

This may include recording the patient's occupation, schooling, hobbies, marital status, family structure, personal support system, living conditions and recent travel. The number and sex of sexual partners may be relevant. Analgesic use, smoking, alcohol and any recreational drug use should also be described. Ask about ability to perform the activities of daily living (ADL). If a patient has a chronic illness, ask about the effect of this on his or her life.

Family history (FH)

Describe causes of mortality in the first-degree relatives and, if indicated, draw a family tree.

Systems review (SR)

All directly relevant information should be incorporated in the HPI or PH.

Physical examination (PE)

Under each of the major systems, list the relevant

positives and negatives using brief statements. See Appendix II.

Provisional diagnosis

Ask yourself these questions when considering the differential diagnosis of a patient's major symptoms.

1 What is the likely diagnosis based on the patient's age, sex and background?
2 Are there other conditions that resemble the likely diagnosis but can present in the same way?
3 Is there a serious disorder, even if rare, that must not be missed?
4 Could the patient have a specific condition that often masquerades as (or mimics) other conditions (e.g. depression, drugs, diabetes mellitus, thyroid dysfunction, anaemia, malignancy, spinal cord disease, urinary infection, renal failure, alcoholism, syphilis, tuberculosis, HIV, infective endocarditis or connective tissue disease)?
5 Is the patient trying to really tell me that there is an emotional or psychological problem?

Problem list and plans

Using a sentence or two, summarise the most important findings and then give a provisional diagnosis (PD) and differential diagnosis (DD).

Remember Occam's razor: choose the simplest hypothesis to explain observations. Also remember Sutton's law: the famous bank robber said he robbed banks because 'that's where the money is'—i.e. consider a common diagnosis before resorting to a rare one to explain the symptoms and signs.

It is often useful to ask yourself if the patient's problem is a diagnostic or management one (or both). For example, a patient with the new onset of dyspnoea presents a diagnostic problem—What is the cause of the breathlessness?; and a management problem—How should the condition be treated? The patient who presents with a worsening of previously diagnosed angina presents a management problem—How should the symptoms be treated?

List all the active problems that require management. Outline the diagnostic tests and therapy planned for each problem.

Sign your name and then put your name and position underneath.

Continuation notes

Date (and time) each progress note in the record. The SOAP format can be useful (*subjective*, *objective*, *assessment* and *plans*).

Subjective data refer to what the patient tells you;

list relevant current problems and note any new problems. Have the patient's previous symptoms improved on the current treatment?

Objective data are physical or laboratory findings; relevant data for each active problem are summarised.

Assessment refers to the interpretation of any relevant findings for each problem.

Plans describe any interventions that will be started for each problem.

Many patient records are now kept in a computer file. Parts of this can be used to provide referral information for the patient to take to a specialist or if he or she is travelling. It is important that such files be kept up to date and especially that lists of medications that are no longer used are deleted from the current list before it is given to the patient.

Presentation

In their formal examinations and less formally on the wards, students and resident medical officers will often be expected to present the history and physical examination of a patient to an examiner or senior colleague. This is excellent training for clinical practice, as the need to discuss patients with colleagues or specialists arises frequently in both hospital and non-hospital practice.

A successful case presentation is both *succinct* and *relevant*. The examiner is most interested in what the patient's problems are now. One should aim to convey basic biographical information and an assessment of the patient's presenting problem in the first few sentences. It is often helpful to present the case as a diagnostic or management problem, or both.

The information will have been obtained from the patient by taking the history as set out above. The examination of the patient should be performed with particular attention to the areas most likely to be abnormal. This information must then be assembled into a form that can easily be conveyed to others. The following is a suggested method.

1 Begin with a sentence that tells your colleague something about the patient and the clinical problem. For example, one might say 'Mr Jones is a 72-year-old retired cabinet minister who presents with two hours of chest pain which is not typically ischaemic'. This gives an idea about the patient himself and indicates that the problem is likely to be a diagnostic one.
2 One should then go on to explain in what way the pain is atypical of ischaemia and whether it has features suggestive of any other diagnosis.
3 Once the presenting symptom or problem has

been described, relevant past history should be discussed. In a patient with chest pain this would include any previous cardiac history or investigations, and a summary of the patient's risk factors for ischaemic heart disease.

4   Present a list of the patient's current medications.

5   Important previous health problems should be outlined briefly. This retired cabinet minister might also have a history of intermittent claudication and of chronic obstructive pulmonary disease. These facts will affect possible treatment for ischaemic heart disease, e.g. the use of beta-blockers.

6   Present the physical examination in two parts.

(a)   Abnormal and *important* normal examination findings in the presenting system. In this patient's case this would mean giving the pulse rate and blood pressure but not details of normal heart sounds. If there was a history of claudication, the examination of the peripheral pulses should be presented even if it is normal.

(b)   Abnormal findings in the rest of the examination.

7   Offer the most likely diagnosis and the differential diagnosis.

8   Suggest a plan for investigation and treatment.

9   Much more detail will have been obtained in the assessment of the patient than should be presented routinely, but further details may be asked for by your colleague. These may include information about the patient's living conditions and the availability of support from the family. This may determine how soon the patient can be sent home from hospital after treatment.

By the end of your presentation your colleague should know what you think is wrong with the patient and what you intend to do about it.

Suggested reading

Kroenke K. The case presentation: stumbling blocks and stepping stones. *Am J Med* 1985; 79: 605–608.

Appendix II

A suggested method for a rapid screening physical examination

To all students of medicine who listen, look, touch and reflect: may they hear, see, feel and comprehend.

John B Barlow (1986)

Begin by positioning the appropriately undressed patient in bed at 45 degrees. Use this opportunity to make a spot diagnosis if this is possible. Look particularly for any of the diagnostic facies or body habituses. Decide also whether the patient looks ill or well. Note if there is any dyspnoea or other distress. Take the blood pressure. Repeat the measurement a few minutes later if the first reading is high.

Key to Appendix II	
CNS	central (and peripheral) nervous system
CVS	cardiovascular system
ENDO	endocrine system
GIT	gastrointestinal system
HAEM	haematological system
INF	infectious diseases
RENAL	renal system
RESP	respiratory system
RHEUM	rheumatological system

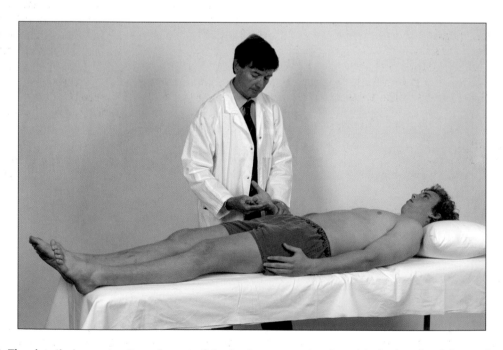

Figure A1 The detailed examination of most of the body systems begins with the hands of the patient

The hands and arms

Begin by picking up the patient's right hand and examine the nails for clubbing (RESP, CVS, GIT) and for the stigmata of infective endocarditis (CVS) or chronic liver disease (GIT) (Figure A1). The nail changes suggesting chronic renal disease or iron deficiency must also be spotted (RENAL, HAEM). Note any evidence of arthropathy (RHEUM). Examine the other hand.

Take the patient's pulse, and note the rate and regularity or irregularity (CVS). While this is being done the arms can be inspected for bruising or scratch marks (GIT, HAEM, RENAL). Determine the state of hydration (GIT, RENAL, CVS). Then examine for axillary lymphadenopathy (HAEM).

The face

Look at the eyes for jaundice (GIT, HAEM) or exophthalmos (ENDO). Look at the face for evidence of a vasculitic rash (RHEUM). Inspect the mouth for mucosal ulcers (RHEUM, GIT, HAEM, INF) and the tongue for glossitis (nutritional deficiencies) or cyanosis (RESP, CVS).

The front of the neck

Feel the carotid pulses and pay careful attention to the state of the jugular venous pressure (CVS). Feel gently for the position of the trachea (RESP). Then palpate the supraclavicular lymph nodes (HAEM, GIT).

The chest

Examine the front of the chest for scars and deformity. Note any spider naevi (GIT) or hair loss (GIT, ENDO). Palpate the chest wall and auscultate the heart (CVS). Then percuss and auscultate the chest (RESP) and examine the breasts.

The back of the chest and neck

Sit the patient up and lean him or her forward. After inspection, test chest expansion of the upper and lower lobes of the lungs. Percuss and auscultate the back of the chest (RESP). Feel for cervical lymphadenopathy (RESP, GIT, HAEM). Then examine formally for a goitre from behind (ENDO). Test for sacral oedema (CVS, RENAL).

The abdomen

Lay the patient flat on one pillow. Inspect the abdomen from the side and then palpate for organomegaly and other abdominal masses. Percuss for shifting dullness if this is appropriate and auscultate over the abdomen. Palpate for inguinal lymphadenopathy and hernias, and in men palpate the testes (GIT, RENAL).

The legs

Look for peripheral oedema (CVS, RENAL) and leg ulcers (HAEM, RHEUM, CVS, CNS). Feel all the peripheral pulses (CVS).

Neurological examination

Find out if the patient is right- or left-handed.

Begin with examination of the higher centres and cranial nerves. Test orientation and note any speech defect. Ask about any noticed problem with the sense of smell (I). Then examine the visual acuity, visual fields, the fundi (II), the pupils and eye movements (III, IV, VI). Screen for the other cranial nerves by testing pain sensation over the face (V), the strength of upper and lower facial muscles (VII), whispered voice hearing (VIII), the palatal movement ('Ah') (IX, X), poking out the tongue (XII), and rotation of the head (XI).

Next look for wasting and fasciculation in the upper limbs. Test tone, power (shoulders, elbows, wrists and fingers), and the biceps, triceps and brachioradialis reflexes. Assess finger–nose movements. Then test pinprick sensation on the tip of the shoulder, outer and inner forearms, and on the median, ulnar and radial areas of the hands.

Go to the lower limbs. Test gait fully: ask the patient to walk away several paces, turn around rapidly and walk back. Then test heel–toe walking (cerebellum), ability to stand on the toes (S1) and heels (L4, L5), and squatting (proximal muscles). Finally look for Romberg's sign (posterior columns). Next, test hip and knee flexion and extension, and dorsiflexion and plantar flexion of the feet in bed. Then do knee, ankle and plantar reflexes, and heel–shin tests. Test pinprick sensation on the middle third of the thighs, both sides of the tibia, the dorsum of the feet, the little toes, on the buttocks, and three levels on the trunk on both sides.

Completing the examination

Thorough physical examination always requires a rectal and pelvic examination, analysis of the patient's urine, a temperature reading, and measurement of height and weight and calculation of the BMI.

Particular details of the examination will be altered depending on what is found. An important guide to the areas where examination should be particularly directed, apart from the history, is the general inspection. A minute or two spent standing back to inspect the patient before the detailed examination begins is never wasted.

Appendix III

The pre-anaesthetic medical evaluation (PAME)

An appropriate medical evaluation of the patient who has been admitted for elective surgery is always required. It includes a history and examination which is sufficient to uncover any likely major problems with anaesthesia or the procedure itself.

The history

The first thing to find out, of course, is the presenting problem, what operation is intended, and whether the surgery is expected to be performed under general or local anaesthesia. Clearly the assessment of a patient having a small lesion removed under local anaesthesia can be briefer than the assessment of a patient undergoing extensive bowel resection under general anaesthesia. As a rule, before any patient undergoes surgery under general anaesthesia or spinal anaesthesia, careful attention must be given to identifying whether he or she is at higher risk.

Cardiovascular history

The most important questions here relate to a history of ischaemic heart disease. Patients who have had a myocardial infarct in the preceding six months should not usually undergo elective surgery; the risks of further infarction or malignant arrhythmia and death are high during this period. A patient who has symptoms of angina which have recently become unstable is also at greater risk. A history of stable angina which has not changed for months or years is not a contraindication to most forms of surgery. The recent placement of a coronary stent may mean that cessation of anti-platelet drugs is not safe for 1 month after insertion of a bare metal stent and 1 year after the insertion of a drug-eluting stent.

Symptoms of cardiac failure should be sought. Any patient with uncontrolled cardiac failure is at considerable risk of severe cardiac failure postoperatively. This is particularly true if large amounts of intravenous fluids are given during and after surgery while the patient's anti-failure drugs (e.g. diuretics) are omitted.

Cardiac drugs should be asked about, particularly anti-anginal and anti-failure drugs. It is important to attempt to ensure that the patient receives these drugs, particularly beta-blockers, on the day of the operation. The surgeon will often require the patient to stop aspirin a week or more before surgery. This is usually a safe thing for the patient to do but may be a problem in the first month at least after a coronary angioplasty because of the risk of thrombosis of the stent in this early period. Previous coronary artery bypass grafting or angioplasty is not a contraindication to surgery.

A history of infective endocarditis or the presence of a prosthetic cardiac valve or complex congenital cardiac condition is an indication for antibiotic prophylaxis for any procedure that may result in bacteraemia – the circulation of bacteria in the blood stream. These procedures include most types of dental work, colonoscopy and surgery on the bowel or bladder, and some gynaecological operations and vaginal delivery.

Patients who take the anticoagulant drug warfarin are a special problem. When the drug is being used to protect the patient from embolic events associated with atrial fibrillation it may be reasonable, on the balance of risks, to have the drug stopped 4 days before surgery and resumed as soon as practical afterwards. If the patient takes the drug to protect a mechanical heart valve from clot, the drug should, in general, be replaced by intravenous unfractionated or subcutaneous fractionated heparin. The last dose of fractionated heparin can be given about 12 hours before surgery and the drug recommenced as soon as the surgeon feels it is safe. Many patients can administer the drug themselves at home. Patients with mechanical valves, especially in the mitral position, are at high risk of embolic events if their warfarin is stopped without replacement with some form of heparin.

The presence of a cardiac pacemaker or implanted defibrillator may be a problem if the surgeon intends to use a diathermy device.

The respiratory history

Inquire about a history of respiratory disease, particularly chronic obstructive pulmonary disease or severe asthma. Patients who have continued to smoke up to the time of their surgery have a much higher risk of postoperative chest infections than those who have not. Even stopping a few weeks before will reduce this risk. Severe respiratory disease is a relative contraindication to surgery. It may be difficult to reverse the anaesthetic and muscle relaxant drugs in such a patient, and he or she may require ventilation postoperatively. Doctors in charge of intensive care units are always happier to be warned that a patient may require ventilation postoperatively than to have it come as a surprise.

Drug therapy for respiratory disease must be asked about. Steroids may impair wound healing, and steroid doses may need to be increased during the operative period because of steroid-induced adrenal suppression.

Other

Inquire about any history of bleeding diathesis, diabetes mellitus, renal disease, hepatitis, jaundice and drug abuse. The control of blood sugar in diabetic patients can be difficult in the perioperative period, especially while normal diet is impossible. The fasting preoperative diabetic on insulin may need to be advised to have half the normal insulin dose on the morning of surgery, possibly with a very early light breakfast. This may be important to avoid ketoacidosis.

Specific inquiries about *previous operations and anaesthetics*, particularly with reference to any complications, should be made. *Allergies* to anaesthetic agents or other drugs must be asked about. Attempt to distinguish a true allergy or anaphylaxis from an adverse effect such as vomiting after a morphine injection. Some operations involve the use of contrast media, and an allergy to iodine may be a contraindication to their use. This risk is now much less with the new non-ionic contrast media. There may occasionally be a *family history of anaesthetic complications* or deaths. This raises the possibility of malignant hyperthermia, which is an inherited disorder leading to fever and muscle destruction after administration of muscle relaxants.

The examination

Examination according to the rapid screening method outlined in Appendix II represents the best approach. Record height, weight and vital signs (pulse rate, blood pressure, respiratory rate). The cardiovascular and respiratory systems must be fully examined. Patients with a short thick neck may be difficult to ventilate and intubate. It is better for the anaesthetist to be aware of this possible problem before the patient is given a muscle relaxant and is unable to breath spontaneously. The presence of loose or fragile teeth must also be noted because of the risk of their dislodgement during attempted intubation.

If a previously undiagnosed symptom or sign of significance is uncovered, some further investigations may be required before surgery, and the operation may have to be deferred. For example, the discovery of a new and significant heart murmur, uncontrolled hypertension, respiratory failure, a bleeding diathesis, uncontrolled diabetes mellitus or renal failure should be brought to the attention of the surgeon and anaesthetist.

Now this is not the end.
It is not even the beginning of the end.
But it is, perhaps, the end of the beginning.
Winston Churchill,
Speech at the Lord Mayor's Day Luncheon,
London, 10 November 1942

Index